Self-Care Deficit Syndrome
  (Specify Feeding, Bathing/Hygiene, Dressing/
  Grooming, Toileting, *Instrumental)
Sudden Infant Death Syndrome, Risk for
Tissue Perfusion, Altered (specify type: Cerebral,
  Cardiopulmonary, Renal, Gastrointestinal,
  Peripheral)

5. **Sleep—Rest**
Disturbed Sleep Pattern
†Sleep, Readiness for Enhanced

6. **Cognitive—Perceptual**
*Comfort, Altered
  Acute Pain
  Chronic Pain
Confusion
  Acute Confusion
  Chronic Confusion
Decisional Conflict
Dysreflexia
Environmental Interpretation Syndrome,
  Impaired
Knowledge Deficit (specify)
†Knowledge, Readiness for Enhanced (specify)
Risk for Aspiration
Sensory—Perceptual Alterations (specify:
  Visual, Auditory, Kinesthetic,
  Gustatory, Tactile, Olfactory)
Thought Processes, Altered
Unilateral Neglect

7. **Self—Perception**
Anxiety
Fatigue
Fear
Hopelessness
Powerlessness
*Disturbed Self-Concept
Disturbed Body Image
Disturbed Personal Identity
Disturbed Self-Esteem
  Chronic Low Self-Esteem
  Situational Low Self-Esteem
†Self-Concept, Readiness for Enhanced

8. **Role—Relationship**
*Communication, Impaired
Communication, Impaired Verbal
†Communication, Readiness for Enhanced
Family Processes, Interrupted: Alcoholism
Family Processes, Readiness for Enhanced
Family Processes, Interrupted

*Grieving
  Grieving, Anticipatory
  Grieving, Dysfunctional
Loneliness, Risk for
Parent–Infant Attachment, Risk for Impaired
Parenting, Impaired
†Parenting, Readiness for Enhanced
Parental Role Conflict
Role Performance, Impaired
Social Interaction, Impaired
Social Isolation

9. **Sexuality—Reproductive**
Sexual Dysfunction
Sexuality Patterns, Ineffective

10. **Coping—Stress Tolerance**
Adjustment, Impaired
Caregiver Role Strain
Coping, Ineffective
  Defensive Coping
  Ineffective Denial
†Coping, Readiness for Enhanced
Coping, Ineffective Family: Disabling
Coping, Ineffective Family: Compromised
Coping, Family: Potential for Growth
Coping, Ineffective Community
Coping, Potential for Enhanced Community
Energy Field Disturbance
Post-Trauma Response
  Rape Trauma Syndrome
Relocation Stress Syndrome
*Self-Harm, Risk for
*Self-Abuse, Risk for
Self-Mutilation, Risk for
*Suicide, Risk for
Violence, Risk for

11. **Value—Belief**
Spiritual Distress
Spiritual Well-Being, Potential for
  Enhanced

†**Collaborative Problems**
Potential Complication (PC): Cardiac/Vascular
PC: Decreased Cardiac Output
PC: Dysrhythmias
PC: Cardiogenic Shock
PC: Thromboembolic/Deep Vein Thrombosis
PC: Hypovolemic Shock
PC: Peripheral Vascular Insufficiency
PC: Hypertension

(continued)

CONDITIONS THAT NECESSITATE NURSING CARE (Continued)

PC: Congenital Heart Disease
PC: Angina
PC: Endocarditis
PC: Pulmonary Embolism
PC: Spinal Shock
PC: Ischemic Ulcers

Potential Complication: Respiratory

PC: Hypoxemia
PC: Atelectasis/Pneumonia
PC: Tracheobronchial Constriction
PC: Pleural Effusion
PC: Tracheal Necrosis
PC: Pneumothorax
PC: Laryngeal Edema

Potential Complication: Renal/Urinary

PC: Acute Urinary Retention
PC: Renal Insufficiency
PC: Bladder Perforation
PC: Renal Calculi

Potential Complication: Gastrointestinal—Hepatic—Biliary

PC: Paralytic Ileus/Small Bowel Obstruction
PC: Hepatic Dysfunction
PC: Hyperbilirubinemia
PC: Evisceration
PC: Hepatosplenomegaly
PC: Curling's Ulcer
PC: Ascites
PC: Gastrointestinal Bleeding

Potential Complication: Metabolic/Immune/Hematopoietic

PC: Hypoglycemia/Hyperglycemia
PC: Negative Nitrogen Balance
PC: Electrolyte Imbalances
PC: Thyroid Dysfunction
PC: Hypothermia (severe)
PC: Hyperthermia (severe)
PC: Sepsis
PC: Acidosis (metabolic, respiratory)
PC: Alkalosis (metabolic, respiratory)
PC: Hypothyroidism/Hyperthyroidism
PC: Allergic Reaction
PC: Donor Tissue Rejection
PC: Adrenal Insufficiency.
PC: Anemia
PC: Thrombocytopenia
PC: Immunodeficiency
PC: Polycythemia

PC: Sickling Crisis
PC: Disseminated Intravascular Coagulation

Potential Complication: Neurologic/Sensory

PC: Increased Intracranial Pressure
PC: Stroke
PC: Seizures
PC: Spinal Cord Compression
PC: Neuroleptic Malignant Syndrome
PC: Meningitis
PC: Cranial Nerve Impairment (specify)
PC: Paralysis
PC: Peripheral Nerve Impairment
PC: Increased Intraocular Pressure
PC: Corneal Ulceration
PC: Neuropathies

Potential Complication: Muscular/Skeletal

PC: Osteoporosis
PC: Joint Dislocation
PC: Compartmental Syndrome
PC: Pathologic Fractures

Potential Complication: Reproductive

PC: Fetal Distress
PC: Postpartum Hemorrhage
PC: Pregnancy-associated Hypertension
PC: Hypermenorrhea
PC: Polymenorrhea
PC: Syphilis
PC: Prenatal Bleeding
PC: Preterm Labor

Potential Complication: Multisystem

PC: Medication Therapy Adverse Effects
PC: Adrenocorticosteroid Therapy Adverse Effects
PC: Antianxiety Therapy Adverse Effects
PC: Antiarrhythmia Therapy Adverse Effects
PC: Anticoagulant Therapy Adverse Effects
PC: Anticonvulsant Therapy Adverse Effects
PC: Antidepressant Therapy Adverse Effects
PC: Antihypertensive Therapy Adverse Effects
PC: Beta-adrenergic Blockers Therapy Adverse Effects
PC: Calcium Channel Blockers Therapy Adverse Effects
PC: Angiotensin-converting Enzyme Therapy Adverse Effects
PC: Antineoplastic Therapy Adverse Effects
PC: Antipsychotic Therapy Adverse Effects

The Functional Health Patterns were identified by M. Gordon in *Nursing diagnosis: Process and application* (New York: McGraw-Hill, 1982) with minor changes by the author.
* These diagnoses are not currently on the NANDA list, but have been included for clarity and usefulness.
† Frequently used collaborative problems are represented on this list. Other situations not listed here could qualify as collaborative problems.

New 21·98

FOURTH EDITION

Nursing Care Plans & Documentation

Nursing Diagnoses and Collaborative Problems

LYNDA JUALL CARPENITO-MOYET, R.N., M.S.N., C.R.N.P.

Family Nurse Practitioner
ChesPenn Health Services
Chester, Pennsylvania

Nursing Consultant
Mickleton, New Jersey

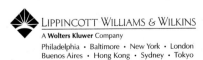

LIPPINCOTT WILLIAMS & WILKINS
A **Wolters Kluwer** Company

Philadelphia · Baltimore · New York · London
Buenos Aires · Hong Kong · Sydney · Tokyo

Senior Acquisitions Editor: Quincy McDonald
Senior Developmental Editor: Renee A. Gagliardi
Editorial Assistant: Marie Rim
Production Editor: Diane Griffith
Senior Production Manager: Helen Ewan
Managing Editor / Production: Erika Kors
Art Director: Carolyn O'Brien
Manufacturing Manager: William Alberti
Indexer: Coughlin Indexing Services, Inc.
Compositor: Circle Graphics
Printer: Courier-Kendallville

4th Edition

9   8   7   6   5   4   3   2   1

Library of Congress Cataloging-in-Publication Data

Carpenito-Moyet, Lynda Juall.
    Nursing care plans & documentation : nursing diagnoses and collaborative problems /
Lynda Juall Carpenito-Moyet.—4th ed.
        p. ; cm.
    Includes bibliographical references and index.
    ISBN 0-7817-3906-3 (alk. paper)
    1. Nursing care plans. 2. Nursing assessment. 3. Nursing diagnosis. I. Title: Nursing
care plans and documentation. II. Title.
    [DNLM: 1. Patient Care Planning. 2. Nursing Process. 3. Nursing Records. WY 100
C294n 2003]
    RT49.C38 2003
    610.73—dc21

                                                                                    2003050142

Care has been taken to confirm the accuracy of the information presented and to describe
generally accepted practices. However, the author, editors, and publisher are not responsible
for errors or omissions or for any consequences from application of the information in this
book and make no warranty, express or implied, with respect to the content of the publication.

The author, editors, and publisher have exerted every effort to ensure that drug selection and
dosage set forth in this text are in accordance with the current recommendations and practice
at the time of publication. However, in view of ongoing research, changes in government
regulations, and the constant flow of information relating to drug therapy and drug reactions,
the reader is urged to check the package insert for each drug for any change in indications
and dosage and for added warnings and precautions This is particularly important when the
recommended agent is a new or infrequently employed drug.

Some drugs and medical devices presented in this publication have Food and Drug Administration (FDA) clearance for limited use in restricted research settings. It is the responsibility
of the health care provider to ascertain the FDA status of each drug or device planned for use
in his or her clinical practice.

LWW.com

DEDICATION

To Pati, my sister
Your lessons to the children you teach
    go beyond the book
You offer strength to those in need
You will not be silenced by power
We have feared together, cried together
    and rejoiced together
Blood has made us sisters, trust has
    made us friends

CONTRIBUTORS

Caroline M. Alterman, M.S.N., C.N.S.
Director, Spinal Cord Injury Program, Lakeshore Rehabilitation Hospital,
Birmingham, Alabama
  (Spinal Cord Injury, 2nd ed.)

Elizabeth Brady-Avis, R.N., M.S.N., C.C.R.N.
Clinical Nurse Specialist, Thomas Jefferson University Hospital,
Philadelphia, Pennsylvania
  (Mechanical Ventilation, Asthma)

Sharon Buckingham, B.S.N.
Staff Nurse ICU, Huron Valley Hospital, Milford, Michigan
  (Hypertension, Cirrhosis, 2nd ed.)

Gerald A. Burns, M.S.N.
Clinical Nurse Specialist/Case Manager, Harper Hospital, Detroit, Michigan
  (Human Immunodeficiency Virus/Acquired Immunodeficiency Syndrome)

Ann Delengowski, R.N., M.S.N.
Oncology Clinical Nurse Specialist, Thomas Jefferson University Hospital,
Philadelphia, Pennsylvania
  (Leukemia, Sickle Cell Anemia, 2nd ed.)

Mary Ann Ducharme, R.N., M.S.N., C.C.R.N.
Case Manager/Clinical Nurse Specialist, Harper Hospital, Detroit, Michigan
  (Hemodynamic Monitoring, Peritoneal Dialysis)

Rita Dundon, R.N., M.S.N., C.S., O.C.N.
Clinical Nurse Specialist, Henry Ford Hospital, Detroit, Michigan
  (Cancer [Initial Diagnosis], Chemotherapy, End-Stage Cancer, Long-Term Venous Access Devices)

Doris R. Fleming, M.S.N., R.N., C.S., C.D.E.
Clinical Nurse Specialist, Harper Hospital, Detroit, Michigan
  (Diabetes Mellitus)

Andrea Sampson Haggood, M.S.N., R.N.
Clinical Nurse Specialist/Case Manager, Oncology and Otorhinolaryngology,
Harper Hospital, Detroit, Michigan
  (Tracheostomy, Neck Dissection, Laryngectomy, 2nd ed.)

Evelyn Howard, R.N., C.N.N.
Director, Renal Dialysis, St. Vincent Infirmary Medical Center, Little Rock, Arkansas
  (Acute Renal Failure, Chronic Renal Failure, 2nd ed.)

Debra J. Lynn-McHale, R.N., M.S.N., C.S., C.C.R.N.
Clinical Nurse Specialist, Surgical Cardiac Care Unit, Thomas Jefferson University
Hospital, Philadelphia, Pennsylvania
  (Coronary Artery Bypass Graft, Percutaneous Transluminal Coronary Angioplasty)

JoAnn Maklebust, M.S.N., R.N., C.S.
Clinical Nurse Specialist/Wound Care, Case Manager/General and Reconstructive Surgery,
Harper Hospital, Detroit, Michigan
(Colostomy, Ileostomy, Urostomy, Pressure Ulcers, Inflammatory Bowel Disease, Neurogenic Bladder)

Amy Ottariano, R.N., M.S.N.
Clinical Nurse Specialist, Intermediate Cardiac Care Unit, Thomas Jefferson
University Hospital, Philadelphia, Pennsylvania
(Thoracic Surgery, 2nd ed.)

Rhonda R. Panfilli, R.N., M.S.N.
Coordinator, Case Management, Grace Hospital, Detroit Medical Center,
Detroit, Michigan
(Obesity)

Gayle Vandendool Parker, R.N., B.S.N.
Nursing Practice Coordinator, London Psychiatric Hospital, London, Ontario, Canada
(Alcohol Withdrawal)

Joy Ross, R.N.
London Psychiatric Hospital, London Ontario, Canada
(Sexual Assault)

Rose B. Shaffer, R.N., M.S.N., C.C.R.N.
Clinical Nurse Specialist, Intermediate Cardiac Care Unit, Thomas Jefferson
University Hospital, Philadelphia, Pennsylvania
(Cardiac Catheterization, Pacemaker Insertion)

Ellen Stefanosky, R.N., M.S.N.
Transplant Coordinator, Thomas Jefferson University Hospital, Philadelphia, Pennsylvania
(Renal Transplant, 2nd ed.)

Patricia A. Vaccaro, R.N., M.S.N.
Clinical Nurse Facilitator, Burn Center, Lehigh Valley Hospital, Allentown, Pennsylvania
(Thermal Injuries, 2nd ed.)

Donna J. Zazworsky, R.N., M.S.
Professional Nurse Case Manager, Carondelet St. Mary's Hospital, Tucson, Arizona
(Multiple Sclerosis)

PREFACE

Nursing is primarily assisting individuals (sick or well) with those activities contributing to health, or its recovery (or to a peaceful death) that they perform unaided when they have the necessary strength, will or knowledge; nursing also helps individuals carry out prescribed therapy and to be independent of assistance as soon as possible (Henderson, 1960)

Historically, nurses have represented the core of the health care delivery system (acute, long term, and community agencies), but their image continues to be one of individuals whose actions are dependent on physician supervision. However, as Diers (1981) wrote, "Nursing is exceedingly complicated work since it involves technical skill, a great deal of formal knowledge, communication ability, use of self, timing, emotional investment, and any number of other qualities. What it also involves—and what is hidden from the public—is the complex process of thinking that leads from the knowledge to the skill, from the perception to the action, from the decision to the touch, from the observation to the diagnosis. Yet it is this process of nursing care, which is at the center of nursing's work, that is so little described . . ." (p. 1).

One way for this process of nursing work to be made visible is for every nurse to describe, discuss, and publicize the plan of nursing care. Physicians regularly and openly explain the measures they plan to the public, especially clients and families. However, nurses often fail to consistently explain their plan of care. This book provides both a framework for nurses to provide responsible nursing care and guidelines for them to document and communicate that care.

The focus of *Nursing Care Plans and Documentation* is independent nursing care—the management of client situations that the nurse can treat legally and independently. It will assist students in transferring their theoretical knowledge to clinical practice; it can help experienced nurses to provide care in a variety of unfamiliar clinical situations. This book incorporates the findings of a validation study. A description of this study (method, subjects, instrument findings) is presented in the section titled *Validation Project* (following the Preface). These findings should be very useful for practicing nurses, students of nursing, and departments of nursing.

The Bifocal Clinical Practice Model underpins this book and serves to organize the nursing care plans in Unit II. Chapter 1 describes and discusses the Bifocal Clinical Practice Model, which differentiates nursing diagnoses from other problems that nurses treat. In this chapter, nursing diagnoses and collaborative problems are explained and differentiated. The relationship of the type of diagnosis to outcome criteria and nursing interventions is also emphasized.

Efficient and appropriate documentation of nursing care is outlined in Chapter 2. Legal issues, standards, and regulatory agencies and their effect on nursing documentation are discussed. The chapter explains a documentation system from admission to discharge. Sample forms are used to emphasize efficient, professional charting. This chapter also includes a discussion of priority diagnoses and case management. The elements of critical pathways are explained with examples. Directions on how to create critical pathways using the care plans in Unit II are discussed and illustrated.

Chapter 3, new to this edition, gives an overview of the 11 steps in care planning. The chapter takes the reader through each phase of this process.

Chapter 4 explores the issues and human responses associated with illness and hospitalization. Coping strategies of the client and family are described. The chapter emphasizes the importance of assisting the client and family with end-of-life discussions whenever possible, before a crisis occurs. A discussion of Bandura's self-efficacy theory and its application to management of therapeutic regimens is also presented.

Chapter 5 focuses on the surgical experience and the related nursing care to discuss the human response to the experience. Preoperative assessment and preparation are described for preadmitted surgical clients. The nursing responsibilities in the postanesthesia recovery room are described, and the related documentation forms are included. This chapter also outlines the integration of the nursing process in caring for same-day surgery clients; again, the corresponding forms that will help the nurse to do this are included.

Unit II presents care plans that represent a compilation of the complex work of nursing in caring for individuals (and their families) experiencing medical disorders or surgical interventions or undergoing diagnostic or therapeutic procedures. It uses the nursing process to present the type of nursing care that is expected to be necessary for persons experiencing similar situations. The plans provide the nurse with a framework for providing initial, or essential, care. This is the nursing care known to be provided when a certain clinical situation is present—for example, preoperative teaching for persons awaiting surgery or the management of fatigue in individuals with arthritis. As the nurse intervenes and continues to assess, additional diagnoses, goals, and interventions can be added to the initial plan. Even though the type of care that is warranted for persons in certain clinical situations is predictable, the nurse must still assess the individual for additional responses. The fourth edition features extensive revisions or additions to the goals/outcome criteria in each care plan. When possible, research findings or the work of an expert clinician were incorporated.

The intent of this book is to assist the nurse to identify the responsible care that nurses are accountable to provide. The addition of the research findings further increases the applicability of the care plans. By using the Bifocal Clinical Practice Model, it clearly defines the scope of independent practice. The author invites comments and suggestions from readers. Correspondence can be directed to the publisher or to the author's address.

References

Diers, D. (1981). Why write? Why publish? Image, 13;991–7

Henderson, V., & Nite, G. (1960). Principles and practice of nursing (5th ed.). New York: Macmillan, p. 14.

VALIDATION PROJECT

Background

In 1984, this author published diagnostic clusters under medical and surgical conditions (Carpenito, 1984). These diagnostic clusters represented nursing diagnoses and collaborative problems described in the literature for a medical or surgical population. After the initial diagnostic clusters were created, they were reviewed by clinicians who practiced with that specific population.

Since 1984, numerous other authors (Holloway, 1988; Doenges, 1991; Sparks, 1993, Ulrich, 1994) have generated similar groupings. To date none of the clusters have been studied to determine the frequency of occurrence. In other words, are some diagnoses in the diagnostic cluster treated more frequently than others?

Reasons for Study

In the last 10 years, the health care delivery system has experienced numerous changes. Specifically, clients are in the acute care setting for a shorter length of stay. These client populations all share a high acuity. This acuity is represented with multiple nursing diagnoses and collaborative problems. However, do all these diagnoses have the same priority? Which diagnoses necessitate nursing interventions during the length of stay?

Care planning books report a varied number of diagnoses to treat under a specific condition. For example, in reviewing a care plan for an individual with a myocardial infarction, this author found the following number of diagnoses reported: Ulrich—16; Carpenito—11; Doenges—7; Holloway—4. When students review these references, how helpful are lists ranging from 4 to 16 diagnoses? How many diagnoses can nurses be accountable for during the length of stay?

The identification of nursing diagnoses and collaborative problems that nurses treat more frequently than others in certain populations can be very useful data to:

- Assist nurses with decision making
- Determine the cost of nursing services for population sets
- Plan for resources needed
- Describe the specific responsibilities of nursing

Novice nurses and students can use these data to anticipate the initial care needed. They can benefit from data reported by nurses experienced in caring for clients in that population.

These data should not eliminate an assessment of the individual to evaluate if additional nursing diagnoses or collaborative problems are present and establish priority for treatment during the hospital stay. This individual assessment will also provide information to delete or supplement the care plan found in this book. The researched data will provide a beginning focus for care.

By identifying frequently treated nursing diagnoses and collaborative problems in client populations, institutions can determine nursing costs based on nursing care provided. Nurse administrators and managers can plan for effective use of staff and resources. Knowledge of types of nursing diagnoses needing nursing interventions will also assist with matching the level of preparation of nurses with appropriate diagnoses.

To date, the nursing care of clients with medical conditions or postsurgical procedures has centered on the physician-prescribed orders. The data from this study would assist departments of nursing to emphasize the primary reason why clients stay in the acute care setting—for treatment of nursing diagnoses and collaborative problems. The purpose of this study was to identify which nursing diagnoses and collaborative problems are most frequently treated when a person is hospitalized with a specific condition.

Method

Settings and Subjects

The findings presented are based on data collected from August 1993 to March 1994. The research population consisted of registered nurses with over 2 years' experience in health care agencies in the United States and Canada. A convenience sample of 18 institutions represented five U.S. geographical regions (Northeast, Southeast, North-Midwest, Northwest, Southwest) and Ontario province in Canada. The display lists the participating institutions. The target number of R.N. responses for each condition was 10 responses for each condition from each institution. The accompanying table illustrates the demographics of the subjects.

Instrument

A graphic rating scale was developed and piloted to measure self-reported frequencies of interventions provided to clients with a specific condition. Each collaborative problem listed under the condition was accompanied by the question:

When you care for patients with this condition, how often do you monitor for this problem?
Each nursing diagnosis listed under the condition was accompanied by the question:
When you care for patients with this condition, how often do you provide interventions for this nursing diagnosis?

The respondent was asked to make an X on a frequency scale of 0 to 100%. Scoring was tabulated by summing the scores for each question and calculating the medium.

◯◯ PARTICIPATING INSTITUTIONS

Allen Memorial Hospital
1825 Logan Avenue
Waterloo, Iowa 50703

Carondelet St. Joseph's Hospital
350 N. Wilmont Road
Tucson, AZ 85711-2678

The Evanston Hospital
Burch Building
2650 Ridge Avenue
Evanston, IL 60201

Huron Valley Hospital
1601 East Commerce Road
Milford, MI 48382-9900

Lehigh Valley Hospital
Cedar Crest & I-78
Allentown, PA 18105-1556

Memorial Medical Center of Jacksonville
3625 University Blvd., South
Jacksonville, FL 32216

Presbyterian Hospital
200 Hawthorne Lane
Charlotte, NC 28233-3549

St. Francis Medical Center
211 St. Francis Drive
Cape Girardeau, MO 63701

St. Joseph Hospital
601 N. 30th Street
Omaha, NE 68131

St. Peter Community Hospital
2475 Broadway
Helena, MT 39601

San Bernardino County Medical Center
780 E. Gilbert Street
San Bernardino, CA 92415-0935

Sioux Valley Hospital
1100 South Euclid Avenue
Sioux Falls, SD 57117-5039

University of Minnesota Hospital
420 Delaware Street, S.E.
Minneapolis, MN 55455

University of New Mexico Hospital
2211 Lomas Blvd., N.E.
Albuquerque, NM 87131

Victoria Hospital
800 Commissioners Road, East
London, Canada N6A 4G5

Wills Eye Hospital
900 Walnut Street
Philadelphia, PA 19107

Wilmer Ophthalmological Institute
Johns Hopkins Hospital
Baltimore, MD 21287-9054

Winthrop-University Hospital
259 First Street
Mineola, NY 11501

Data Collection

Prior to data collection, the researcher addressed the requirements for research in the institution. These requirements varied from a review by the nursing department's research committee to a review by the institutional review board (IRB).

After the approval process was complete, each department of nursing was sent a list of the 72 conditions to be studied and asked to select only those conditions that were regularly treated in their institution. Only those questionnaires were sent to the institution. Study institutions received a packet for those selected conditions containing 10 questionnaires for each condition. Completed questionnaires were returned by the nurse respondent to the envelope and the envelope sealed by the designated distributor. Nurse respondents were given the option of putting their questionnaire in a sealed envelope prior to placing it in the larger envelope.

Since two of the study institutions did not treat ophthalmic conditions, questionnaires related to these conditions were sent to two institutions specializing in these conditions.

Findings

Of the 19 institutions that agreed to participate, 18 (including two ophthalmic institutions) returned the questionnaires. The target return was 160 questionnaires for each condition. The range of return was 29% to 70%, with the average rate of return 52.5%.

Each condition has a set of nursing diagnoses and collaborative problems with its own frequency score. The diagnoses were grouped into three ranges of frequencies: 75% to 100%—frequent; 50% to 74%—often; <50%—infrequent. Each of the 72 conditions that appear in this book has the nursing diagnoses and collaborative problems grouped according to the study findings.

Future Work

This study represents the initial step in the validation of the nursing care predicted to be needed when an individual is hospitalized for a medical or surgical condition. It is important to validate which nursing diagnoses and collaborative problems necessitate nursing interventions. Future work will include the identification of nursing interventions that have priority in treating a diagnosis, clarification of outcomes realistic for the length of stay, and evaluation and review by national groups of nurses.

References

Carpenito, L. J. (1984). *Handbook of nursing diagnosis.* Philadelphia: J. B. Lippincott.

Carpenito, L. J. (1991). *Nursing care plans and documentation.* Philadelphia: J. B. Lippincott.

Doenges, M., & Moorhouse, M. (1991). *Nurse's pocket guide: Nursing diagnoses with interventions.* Philadelphia: F. A. Davis.

Holloway, N. M. (1988). *Medical surgical care plans.* Springhouse, PA: Springhouse.

Sparks, S. M., & Taylor, C. M. (1993). *Nursing diagnoses reference manual.* Springhouse, PA: Springhouse.

Ulrich, S., Canale, S., & Wendell, S. (1994). *Medical-surgical nursing: Care planning guide.* Philadelphia: W. B. Saunders.

⚭ DEMOGRAPHICS OF RESPONDENTS

Questionnaires	
Sent	9,920
Returned	5,299
% returned	53.4%
Average Age	39
Average Years in Nursing	15
Level of Nursing Preparation	
Diploma	22.7%
AD	25.7%
BSN	36.5%
MSN	12.4%
PhD	1.5%
No indication	1.2%

Acknowledgments

The Validation Project could not have been completed without the support of the following nurses who coordinated the data collection in their institutions:

Tammy Spier, R.N., M.S.N.
Department of Nursing Services
Department of Staff Development
Allen Memorial Hospital
Waterloo, Iowa

Donna Dickinson, R.N., M.S.
Carol Mangold, R.N., M.S.N.
Carondelet St. Joseph's Hospital
Tucson, Arizona

Kathy Killman, R.N., M.S.N.
Liz Nelson, R.N., M.S.N.
The Evanston Hospital
Evanston, Illinois

Margaret Price, R.N., M.S.N.
Lynn Bobel Turbin, R.N., M.S.N.
Nancy DiJanni, R.N., M.S.N.
Huron Valley Hospital
Milford, Michigan

Pat Vaccaro, R.N., B.S.N., C.C.R.N.
Deborah Stroh, R.N.
Mary Jean Potylycki, R.N.
Carolyn Peters, R.N.
Sue DeSanto, R.N.
Christine Niznik, R.N.
Carol Saxman, R.N.
Kelly Brown, R.N.
Judy Bailey, R.N.
Nancy Root, R.N.
Cheryl Bitting, R.N.
Carol Sorrentino, R.N.
Lehigh Valley Hospital
Allentown, Pennsylvania

Loretta Baldwin, R.N., B.S.N.
Karin Prussak, R.N., M.S.N., C.C.R.N.
Bess Cullen, R.N.
Debra Goetz, R.N., M.S.N.
Susan Goucher, R.N.
Sandra Brackett, R.N., B.S.N.
Barbara Johnston, R.N., C.C.R.N.
Lisa Lauderdale, R.N.
Randy Shoemaker, R.N., C.C.R.N.
Memorial Medical Center of Jacksonville
Jacksonville, Florida

Karen Stiefel, R.N., Ph.D.
Jerre Jones, R.N., M.S.N., C.S.
Lise Heidenreich, R.N., M.S.N., F.N.P., C.S.
Christiana Redwood-Sawyerr, R.N., M.S.N.
Presbyterian Hospital
Charlotte, North Carolina

Pauline Elliott, R.N., B.S.N.
St. Francis Medical Center
Cape Girardeau, Missouri

Dena Belfiore, R.N., Ph.D.
Dianne Hayko, M.S.R.N., C.N.S.
St. Joseph Hospital
Omaha, Nebraska

Jennie Nemec, R.N., M.S.N.
St. Peter Community Hospital
Helena, Montana

Eleanor Borkowski, R.N.
Tina Buchanan, R.N.
Jill Posadas, R.N.
Deanna Stover, R.N.
Margie Bracken, R.N.
Barbara Upton, R.N.
Kathleen Powers, R.N.
Jeanie Goodwin, R.N.
San Bernardino County Medical Center
San Bernardino, California

Kathy Karpiuk, R.N., M.N.E.
Monica Mauer, R.N.
Susan Fey, R.N.
Joan Reisdorfer, R.N.
Cheryl Wilson, Health Unit Coordinator
Gail Sundet, R.N.
Pat Halverson, R.N.
Ellie Baker, R.N.
Jackie Kisecker, R.N.
Cheri Dore-Paulson, R.N.
Kay Gartner, R.N.
Vicki Tigner, R.N.
Jan Burnette, R.N.
Maggie Scherff, R.N.
Sioux Valley Hospital
Sioux Falls, South Dakota

Keith Hampton, R.N., M.S.N.
University of Minnesota Hospital
Minneapolis, Minnesota

Eva Adler, R.N., M.S.N.
Jean Giddens, R.N., M.S.N., C.S.
Dawn Roseberry, R.N., B.S.N.
University of New Mexico Hospital
Albuquerque, New Mexico

Fran Tolley, R.N., B.S.N.
Vicky Navarro, R.N., M.A.S.
Wilmer Ophthalmological Institute
Johns Hopkins Hospital
Baltimore, Maryland

Heather Boyd-Monk, R.N., M.S.N.
Wills Eye Hospital
Philadelphia, Pennsylvania

Joan Crosley, R.N., Ph.D.
Winthrop-University Hospital
Mineola, New York

Carol Wong, R.N., M.Sc.N.
Cheryl Simpson, R.N.
Victoria Hospital
London, Canada

My gratitude also extends to each of the nurses who gave their time to complete the questionnaires.

A sincere thank you to Dr. Ginny Arcangelo, Director of the Family Nurse Practitioner Program at Thomas Jefferson University in Philadelphia for her work as the methodology consultant to the project.

A study of this magnitude required over 9000 questionnaires to be produced, duplicated, and distributed. Over 100,000 data entries were made, yielding the findings found throughout this edition.

CONTENTS

S E C T I O N   3

Diagnostic and Therapeutic Procedures 921

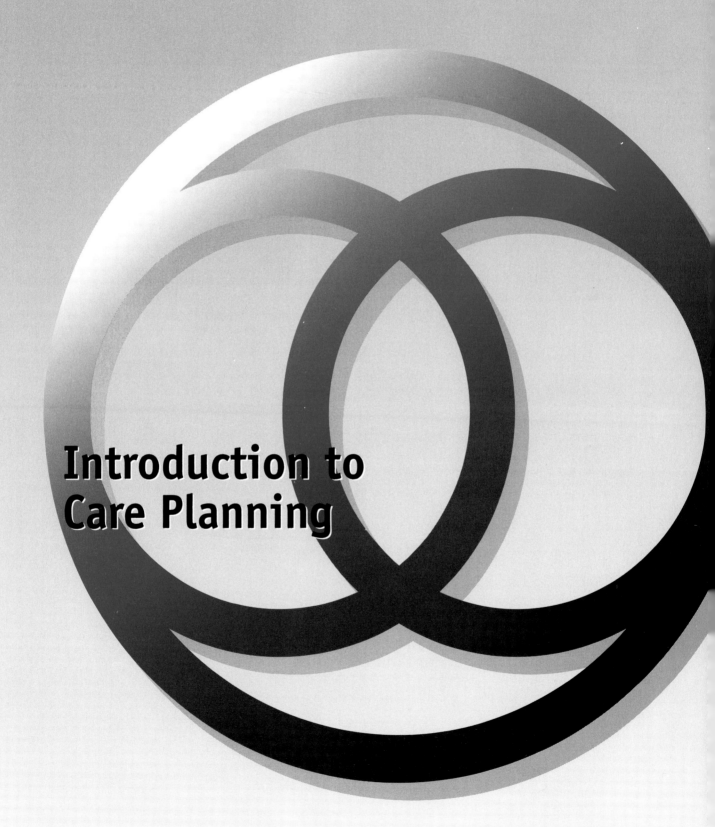

Introduction to
Care Planning

THE BIFOCAL CLINICAL PRACTICE MODEL

The classification activities of the North American Nursing Diagnosis Association (NANDA) have been instrumental in defining nursing's unique body of knowledge. This unified system of terminology

- Provides consistent language (oral and written)
- Stimulates nurses to examine new knowledge
- Establishes a system for automation and reimbursement
- Provides an educational framework
- Allows efficient information retrieval for research and quality assurance
- Provides a consistent structure for literature presentation of nursing knowledge
- Clarifies nursing as an art and a science for its members and society
- Establishes standards to which nurses are held accountable

The inside cover of this text provides a list of nursing diagnoses grouped under conditions that necessitate nursing care.

Clearly nursing diagnosis has influenced the nursing profession positively. Integration of nursing diagnosis into nursing practice, however, has proved problematic. Although references to nursing diagnosis in the literature have increased 100-fold since the first meeting in 1973 of the National Group for the Classification of Nursing Diagnosis (which later became NANDA), nurses have not seen efficient and representative applications. For example, nurses have been directed to use nursing diagnoses exclusively to describe their clinical focus. Nevertheless, nurses who strongly support nursing diagnosis often become frustrated when they try to attach a nursing diagnosis label to every facet of nursing practice. Some of the dilemmas that result from the attempt to label as nursing diagnoses all situations in which nurses intervene are as follows:

1. *Using nursing diagnoses without validation.* When the nursing diagnoses are the only labels or diagnostic statements the nurse can use, the nurse is encouraged to "change the data to fit the label," for example, using the Imbalanced Nutrition category for all clients who are given nothing-by-mouth status. Risk for Injury frequently serves as a "waste basket" diagnosis because all potentially injurious situations (e.g., bleeding) can be captured within a Risk for Injury diagnosis.
2. *Renaming medical diagnoses.* Clinical nurses know that an important component of their practice is monitoring for the onset and status of physiologic complications and initiating both nurse-prescribed and physician-prescribed interventions. Morbidity and mortality are reduced and prevented because of nursing's expert management.
   If nursing diagnoses described all situations in which nurses intervene, then clearly a vast number must be developed to describe the situations identified in the International Code of Diseases (ICD-10). Table 1.1 represents examples of misuse of nursing diagnoses and the renaming of medical diagnoses. Examination of the substitution of nursing diagnosis terminology for medical diagnoses or pathophysiology in Table 1.1 gives rise to several questions:
   - Should nursing diagnoses describe all situations in which nurses intervene?
   - If a situation is not called a nursing diagnosis, is it then less important or scientific?
   - How will it serve the profession to rename as nursing diagnoses medical diagnoses that nurses cotreat with physicians?
   - Will using the examples in Table 1.1 improve communication and clarify nursing?
3. *Omitting problem situations in documentation.* If a documentation system requires the use of nursing diagnosis exclusively and if the nurse does not choose to "change the data to fit a category" or "to rename medical diagnoses," then the nurse has no terminology to describe a critical component of nursing practice. Failure to describe these situations can seriously jeopardize nursing's effort to justify and affirm the need for professional nurses in all health care settings (Carpenito, 1983).

TABLE 1.1   Diagnostic Errors: Renaming Medical Diagnoses With Nursing Diagnosis Terminology

Medical Diagnosis	Nursing Diagnosis
Myocardial Infarction	Decreased Cardiac Output
Shock	
Adult Respiratory Distress	Impaired Gas Exchange
Chronic Obstructive Lung Disease	
Asthma	
Alzheimer's Disease	Impaired Cerebral Tissue Perfusion
Increased Intracranial Pressure	
Retinal Detachment	Disturbed Sensory Perception: Visual
Thermal Burns	Impaired Tissue Integrity
Incisions, Lacerations	Impaired Skin Integrity
Hemorrhage	Deficient Fluid Volume
Congestive Heart Failure	Excess Fluid Volume

Bifocal Clinical Practice Model

Nursing's theoretical knowledge derives from the natural, physical, and behavioral sciences, the humanities, and nursing research. Nurses can use various theories in practice including family systems, loss, growth and development, crisis intervention, and general systems theories.

The difference between nursing and the other health care disciplines is nursing's depth and breadth of focus. Certainly the nutritionist has more expertise in the field of nutrition and the pharmacist in the field of therapeutic pharmacology than any nurse. Every nurse, however, brings a knowledge of nutrition and pharmacology to client interactions. The depth of this knowledge is sufficient for many client situations; when it is insufficient, consultation is required. No other discipline has this varied knowledge, so explaining why attempts to substitute other disciplines for nursing have proved costly and ultimately unsuccessful. Figure 1.1 illustrates this varied expertise.

The Bifocal Clinical Practice Model (Carpenito, 1983) represents the situations that influence persons, groups, and communities as well as the classification of these responses from a nursing perspective. The situations are organized into five broad categories: pathophysiologic, treatment-related, personal, environmental, and maturational (Figure 1.2). Without an understanding of such situations, the nurse will be unable to diagnose responses and intervene appropriately.

Clinically these situations are important to nurses. Thus as nursing diagnoses evolved, nurses sought to substitute nursing terminology for these situations, for example, Impaired Tissue Integrity for burns and High Risk for Injury for dialysis. Nurses do not prescribe for and treat these situations (e.g., dialysis and burns). Rather they prescribe for and treat the *responses* to these situations.

The practice focus for clinical nursing is at the response level, not at the situation level. For example, a client who has sustained burns may exhibit a wide variety of responses to the burns and the treatments. Some may be predicted such as High Risk for Infection; others, such as fear of losing a job, may not be predicted. In the past, nurses focused on the nursing interventions associated with treating burns rather than on those associated with the client's responses. This resulted in nurses being described as "doers" rather than "knowers," as technicians rather than scientists.

Nursing Diagnoses and Collaborative Problems

The Bifocal Clinical Practice Model describes the two foci of clinical nursing: nursing diagnoses and collaborative problems.

> *A nursing diagnosis is a clinical judgment about individual, family, or community responses to actual or potential health problems/life processes. Nursing diagnosis provides the basis for selection of nursing interventions to achieve outcomes for which the nurse is accountable* (NANDA, 1990). *Collaborative problems are certain physiologic complications that nurses monitor to detect onset or changes of status. Nurses manage collaborative problems using physician-prescribed and nursing-prescribed interventions to minimize the complications of the events* (Carpenito, 1997). Figure 1.3 illustrates the Bifocal Clinical Practice Model.

The nurse makes independent decisions for both collaborative problems and nursing diagnoses. The difference is that in nursing diagnoses, nursing prescribes the definitive treatment to achieve the desired outcome, but in collaborative problems, prescription for definitive treatment comes from both nursing and medicine. Some physiologic complications (such as High Risk for Infection and Impaired Skin Integrity) are nursing diagnoses because nurses can order the definitive treatment. In a collaborative problem,

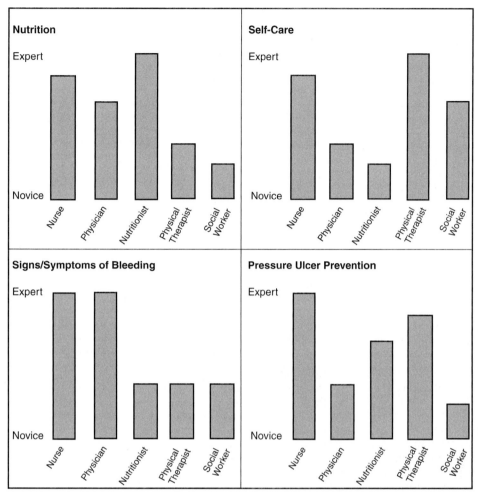

FIGURE 1.1 Knowledge of multidisciplines of selected topics

the nurse monitors for the onset and change in status of physiologic complications and manages these changes to prevent morbidity and mortality. These physiologic complications usually are related to disease, trauma, treatments, medications, or diagnostic studies. Thus collaborative problems can be labeled Potential Complication (specify), for example, Potential Complication: Hemorrhage or Potential Complication: Renal Failure.

Monitoring, however, is not the sole nursing intervention for collaborative problems. For example, in addition to monitoring a client with increased intracranial pressure, the nurse also restricts certain

Pathophysiological
Myocardial infarction
Borderline personality disorder
Burns

Treatment-related
Anticoagulants
Dialysis
Arteriogram

Personal
Dying
Divorce
Relocation

Environmental
Overcrowded school
No handrails on stairs
Rodents

Maturational
Peer pressure
Parenthood
Aging

FIGURE 1.2 Examples of pathophysiological, treatment-related, personal, environmental, and maturational situations

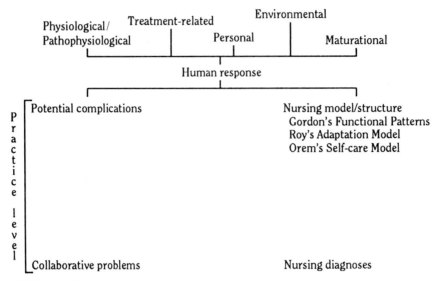

FIGURE 1.3   Bifocal clinical nursing model (© 1985, Lynda Juall Carpenito.)

activities, maintains head elevation, implements the medical regimen, and continually addresses the client's psychosocial and educational needs.

The following are some collaborative problems that commonly apply to certain situations:

Situation	Collaborative Problem
Myocardial infarction	Potential complication (PC): Dysrhythmias
Craniotomy	PC: Increased intracranial pressure
Hemodialysis	PC: Fluid/electrolyte imbalance
Surgery	PC: Hemorrhage
Cardiac catheterization	PC: Allergic reaction

If the situation calls for the nurse to monitor for a cluster or group of physiologic complications, the collaborative problems may be documented as

PC: Cardiac
or
PC: Post-op: Urinary retention
Hemorrhage
Hypovolemia
Hypoxia
Thrombophlebitis
Renal insufficiency
Paralytic ileus
Evisceration

A list of common collaborative problems grouped under conditions that necessitate nursing care appears on inside front and back covers.

All physiologic complications, however, are not collaborative problems. Nurses themselves can prevent some physiologic complications such as infections from external sources (e.g., wounds and catheters), contractures, incontinence, and pressure ulcers. Thus such complications fall into the category of nursing diagnosis.

Nursing Interventions

Nursing interventions are treatments or actions that benefit a client by presenting a problem, reducing or eliminating a problem, or promoting a healthier response. Nursing interventions can be classified as two types: nurse-prescribed or physician-prescribed. Independent interventions are nurse-prescribed; delegated interventions are physician-prescribed. Both types of interventions, however, require independent nursing judgment. By law, the nurse must determine if it is appropriate to initiate an action regardless of whether it is independent or delegated (Carpenito, 1997).

Carpenito (1987) stated that the relationship of diagnosis to interventions is a critical element in defining nursing diagnoses. Many definitions of nursing diagnoses focus on the relationship of selected interventions to the diagnoses. A certain type of intervention appears to distinguish a nursing diagnosis from a medical diagnosis or other problems that nurses treat. The type of intervention distinguishes a nursing diagnosis from a collaborative problem and also differentiates between actual risk/high risk and possible nursing diagnoses. Table 1.2 outlines definitions of each type and the corresponding intervention focus. For example, for a nursing diagnosis of Impaired Tissue Integrity related to immobility as manifested by a 2-cm epidermal lesion on the client's left heel, the nurse would order interventions to monitor the lesion and to heal it. In another client with a surgical wound, the nurse would focus on prevention of infection and promotion of healing. High Risk for Infection would better describe the situation than Impaired Tissue Integrity. Nursing diagnoses are not more important than collaborative problems, and collaborative problems are not more important than nursing diagnoses. Priorities are determined by the client's situation, not by whether it is a nursing diagnosis or a collaborative problem.

A *diagnostic cluster* represents those nursing diagnoses and collaborative problems that have a high likelihood of occurring in a client population. The nurse validates their presence in the individual client. Figure 1.4 represents the diagnostic cluster for a client after abdominal surgery. Sections 1 and 2 contain diagnostic clusters for medical and surgical conditions or goals.

Goals/Outcome Criteria

In a nursing care plan, goals (outcome criteria) are "statements describing a measurable behavior of client/family that denote a favorable status (changed or maintained) after nursing care has been delivered" (Alfaro, 1989). Outcome criteria help to determine the success or appropriateness of the nursing care plan. If the nursing care plan does not achieve a favorable status and the diagnosis is correct, the nurse must change the goal or change the plan. If neither of these options is indicated, the nurse then confers with the physician for delegated orders. Nursing diagnoses should *not* represent situations that require physician orders for treatment. Otherwise how can nurses assume accountability for diagnosis and treatment? For example, consider a client with a nursing diagnosis:

High Risk for Impaired Cerebral Tissue Perfusion related to effects of recent head injury and these goals:

The client will demonstrate continued optimal cerebral pressure as evidenced by

- Pupils equally reactive to light and accommodation
- No change in orientation or consciousness

If this client were to exhibit evidence of increased intracranial pressure, would it be appropriate for the nurse to change the goals? What changes in the nursing care plan would the nurse make to stop the cranial pressure from increasing? Actually, neither action is warranted. Rather, the nurse should confer with the physician for delegated orders to treat increased intracranial pressure. When the nurse formulates client goals or outcomes that require delegated medical orders for goal achievement, the situation is not

TABLE 1.2   Differentiation Among Types of Diagnoses

Diagnostic Statement	Corresponding Client Outcome or Nursing Goals	Focus of Intervention
Actual Diagnosis Three-part statement including nursing diagnostic label, etiology, and signs/symptoms	Change in client behavior moving toward resolution of the diagnosis or improved status	Reduce or eliminate problem
Risk/High-Risk Diagnosis Two-part statement including nursing diagnostic label and risk factors	Maintenance of present conditions	Reduce risk factors to prevent an actual problem
Possible Diagnosis Two-part statement including nursing diagnostic label and unconfirmed etiology or unconfirmed defining characteristics	Undetermined until problem is validated	Collect additional data to confirm or rule out signs/symptoms or risk factors
Collaborative Problems Potential or actual physiologic complication	Nursing goals	Determine onset or status of the problem Manage change in status

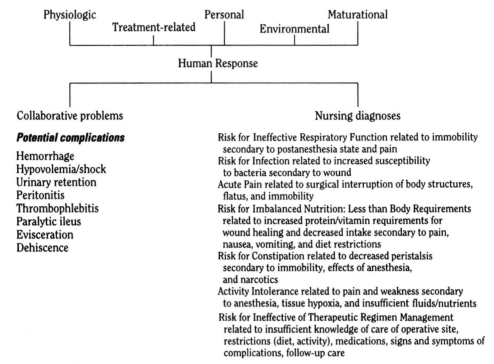

Abdominal surgery (postoperative)

FIGURE 1.4   Diagnostic cluster for client recovering from abdominal surgery

a nursing diagnosis but a collaborative problem. In this case the client's problem would be described better as a collaborative problem:

Potential Complications: Increased Intracranial Pressure and the nursing goal:
The nurse will manage and minimize changes in increased intracranial pressure

Summary

The Bifocal Clinical Practice Model provides nurses with a framework to diagnose the unique responses of a client and significant others to various situations. Clear definition of the two dimensions of nursing enhances the use and minimizes the misuse of nursing diagnoses. The Bifocal Clinical Practice Model describes the unique knowledge and focus of professional nursing.

DOCUMENTATION OF NURSING CARE

Attributes of Nursing Documentation

Historically nurses have believed that the more information a nurse has charted, the better his or her legal defense will be in any litigation. Today, however, nurses recognize that a comprehensive, streamlined documentation system actually can document more data in less time and space. Nursing documentation must be objective and comprehensive and must accurately reflect the status of the client and what has happened to him or her. If legally challenged, the nursing records represent what reasonably prudent nurses chart and should demonstrate compliance with the institution's policy.

Unfortunately most hospitals and other agencies have not examined seriously what documentation actually requires. Many nurses have been taught to write as much as possible; they operate under the philosophy "If it wasn't charted, it wasn't done." Does poor charting represent poor care? Inherent in this question are others: What is poor charting? By what standard is it poor?

If a department of nursing does not establish specific policies for charting, then the charting in question can be held to standards from another department of nursing or from expert testimony. Case law does not determine the standards for nursing documentation but instead passes a judgment regarding compliance with a standard.

The most important purpose of documentation is to communicate to other members of the health team the client's progress and condition. In addition, nursing documentation is important:

- To define the nursing focus for the client or group
- To differentiate the accountability of the nurse from that of other members of the health care team
- To provide the criteria for reviewing and evaluating care (quality improvement)
- To provide the criteria for client classification
- To provide justification for reimbursement
- To provide data for administrative and legal review
- To comply with legal, accreditation, and professional standard requirements
- To provide data for research and educational purposes

Defining documentation as always hand-written or typed as free text (in a computer) is problematic. Documentation can take the form of a standard of care, a check marked on a form, or an initial on a flow record. The accompanying policy should direct that there is to be minimal or no writing unless an unusual or unsatisfactory situation has occurred.

Assessment

In assessment—the deliberate collection of data about a client, family, or group—the nurse obtains data by interviewing, observing, and examining. The two types of assessment are the initial screening interview and focus assessment.

Initial Screening Interview

The screening interview has two parts: functional patterns and physical assessment. It focuses on determining the client's present health status and ability to function. Figure 2.1 shows a nursing admission database. Examples of specific functional pattern assessment categories are as follows:

- Ability to bathe self
- Presence of confusion
- Spiritual practices
- Ability to control urination

The physical examination uses the skills of inspection, auscultation, and palpation to assess areas such as

- Pulse
- Skin condition

**NURSING ADMISSION
DATA BASE**

Date _____ Arrival Time _____ Contact Person _____ Phone _____
ADMITTED FROM: ___ Home alone   ___Home with relative   ___Long-term care
                ___ Homeless   ___Home with_____   facility
                ___ ER   (Specify)   ___ Other _____

MODE OF ARRIVAL: ___ Wheelchair   ___ Ambulance   ___ Stretcher
REASON FOR HOSPITALIZATION: _____
_____
_____

LAST HOSPITAL ADMISSION: Date _____ Reason _____
_____

PAST MEDICAL HISTORY: _____
_____

MEDICATION (Prescription/Over-the-Counter)	DOSAGE	LAST DOSE	FREQUENCY

HEALTH MAINTENANCE–PERCEPTION PATTERN
USE OF:
Tobacco: ___None ___Quit (date) ___Pipe ___Cigar ___<1 pk/day
            ___1–2 pks/day ___>2 pks/day Pks/year history ____
Alcohol: ___None ___Type/Amount ___/day ___/wk ___/month
Other Drugs ___No ___Yes Type _____ Use _____
Allergies (drugs, food, tape, dyes): _____ Reaction _____
_____

ACTIVITY/EXERCISE PATTERN
SELF-CARE ABILITY:
  0 = Independent   1 = Assistive device   2 = Assistance from others
  3 = Assistance from person and equipment   4 = Dependent/Unable

	0	1	2	3	4
Eating/Drinking					
Bathing					
Dressing/Grooming					
Toileting					
Bed Mobility					
Transferring					
Ambulating					
Stair Climbing					
Shopping					
Cooking					
Home Maintenance					

ASSISTIVE DEVICES: ___None ___Crutches ___Bedside commode ___Walker
                    ___Cane ___ Splint/Brace ___Wheelchair ___Other___

CODE: (1) Non-applicable (2) Unable to acquire
       (3) Not a priority at this time (4) Other (specify in notes)

FIGURE 2.1 Sample admission data base (Carpenito, L. J. [2004] *Nursing diagnosis: Application to clinical practice* [10th ed.]. Philadelphia: Lippincott Williams & Wilkins.)

- Muscle strength
- Lung fields

After completing and recording the screening assessment, the nurse analyzes the data and asks questions such as the following:

- Does the client have a problem that requires nursing interventions (e.g., assistance with ambulation)?
- Is the client at risk for developing a problem (e.g., pressure ulcers)?
- Does the client's medical condition put him or her at high risk for complications (e.g., problems associated with increased blood glucose level in diabetes mellitus)?
- Do the prescribed treatments put the client at high risk for complications (e.g., phlebitis from IV therapy)?
- Is additional data collection needed?

Focus Assessment

Focus assessment involves the acquisition of selected or specific data as determined by the nurse and the client or family or as directed by the client's condition (Carpenito, 1983). The nurse can perform a focus assessment during the initial interview if the data suggest that he or she should ask additional questions. For example, on admission the nurse would question most clients about eating patterns. He or she also would ask a client with chronic obstructive pulmonary disease if dyspnea interferes with eating. This represents a focus assessment because the nurse would not ask every client if dyspnea affects food intake.

NUTRITION/METABOLIC PATTERN
Special Diet/Supplements _____
Previous Dietary Instruction: ___ Yes ___ No
Appetite: ___ Normal ___ Increased ___ Decreased ___ Decreased taste sensation
_____ ___ Nausea ___ Vomiting ___ Stomatitis
Weight Fluctuations Last 6 Months: ___ None _____ lbs. Gained/Lost
Swallowing Difficulty (Dysphagia): ___ None ___ Solids ___ Liquids
Dentures: ___ Upper (_ Partial _ Full) ___ Lower (_ Partial _ Full)
_____ With Patient ___ Yes ___ No
Historty of Skin/Healing Problems ___ None ___ Abnormal Healing ___ Rash
_____ ___ Dryness ___ Excess Perspiration

ELIMINATION PATTERN
Bowel Habits ___ # BMs/day ___ Date of last BM ___ Within normal limits
_____ ___ Constipation ___ Diarrhea ___ Incontinence
_____ ___ Ostomy: Type ___ Appliance ___ Self care ___ Yes ___ No
Bladder Habits ___ WNL ___ Frequency ___ Dysuria ___ Nocturia ___ Urgency
_____ ___ Hematuria ___ Retention
Incontinency: ___ No ___ Yes ___ Total ___ Daytime ___ Nighttime
_____ ___ Occasional ___ Difficulty delaying voiding
_____ ___ Difficulty reaching toilet
Assistive Devices: ___ Intermittent catheterization
_____ ___ Indwelling catheter ___ External catheter
_____ ___ Incontinent briefs ___ Penile implant type _____

SLEEP/REST PATTERN
Habits: ___ hrs/night ___ AM nap ___ PM nap
_____ Feel rested after sleep ___ Yes ___ No
Problems ___ None ___ Early waking ___ Insomnia ___ Nightmares

COGNITIVE–PERCEPTUAL PATTERN
Mental Status: ___ Alert ___ Receptive aphasia ___ Poor historian
_____ ___ Oriented ___ Confused ___ Combative ___ Unresponsive
Speech: ___ Normal ___ Slurred ___ Garbled ___ Expressive aphasia
_____ Spoken Language _____ Interpreter _____
Language Spoken: ___ English ___ Spanish ___ Other _____
Ability to Read English: ___ Yes ___ No _____
Ability to Communicate: ___ Yes ___ No _____
Ability to Comprehend: ___ Yes ___ No _____
Level of Anxiety: ___ Mild ___ Moderate ___ Severe ___ Panic
Interactive Skills: ___ Appropriate ___ Other _____
Hearing: ___ WNL ___ Impaired (_ Right _ Left) ___ Deaf (_ Right _ Left)
_____ ___ Hearing Aid ___ Tinnitus
Vision: ___ WNL ___ Eyeglasses ___ Contact lens
_____ ___ Impaired ___ Right ___ Left
_____ ___ Blind ___ Right ___ Left
_____ ___ Cataract ___ Right ___ Left
_____ ___ Glaucoma
_____ ___ Prosthesis ___ Right _ Left
Vertigo: ___ Yes ___ No
Discomfort/Pain: ___ None ___ Acute ___ Chronic ___ Description _____

Pain Management: _____

COPING STRESS TOLERANCE/SELF-PERCEPTION/SELF-CONCEPT PATTERN
Major concerns regarding hospitalization or illness (financial, self-care): _____

Major loss/change in past year: ___ No ___ Yes _____

Fear of violence_____ Yes_____No_____ Who_____
Outlook on future_____ (rate from 1 (poor) to 10 (very optimistic))

CODE: (1) Non-applicable (2) Unable to acquire
_____ (3) Not a priority at this time (4) Other (Specify in notes)

FIGURE 2.1 continued

(figure continues on page 12)

The nurse does certain focus assessments—such as vital signs, bowel and bladder function, and nutritional status—each shift for every client. (Section I presents a generic care plan for all hospitalized adults that includes these routine focus assessments.) The nurse determines the need for additional focus assessments based on the client's condition. For example, in a postoperative client, the nurse assesses and monitors the surgical wound and IV therapy.

Each care plan in Unit II of this book contains specific focus assessment criteria for each listed nursing diagnosis. These criteria direct the nurse to collect additional data specific to the client after the initial diagnosis is confirmed. The nurse may add these additional data to a nursing diagnosis statement as contributing factors and also may indicate that the client needs supplemental interventions. Box 2.1 shows the focus assessment criteria for a client with multiple sclerosis.

Planning

The clinical purposes of documentation are to guide the caregiver and to record the client's status or response. Directions for nursing care originate in both nursing and medicine. Interventions prescribed by physicians are transferred to various forms (e.g., Kardex or treatment and medication administration records). Nurses prescribe both routine interventions and those specific to the client. Routine or predictive nursing interventions can be found in nursing care standards. These client-specific interventions are listed in the addendum care plan.

Care plans (standards, addendum) serve the following purposes:

• They represent the priority set of diagnoses (collaborative problems or nursing diagnoses) for a client.

SEXUALITY/REPRODUCTIVE PATTERN
LMP: _____ Gravida _____ Para _____
Menstrual Problems: ____ Yes ____ No _____
Last Pap Smear: _____ Hx of abnormal PAP _____
Monthly Self-Breast/Testicular Exam: ____ Yes ____ No
Sexual Concerns R/T Illness: _____
_____

ROLE-RELATIONSHIP PATTERN
Marital status _____
Occupation: _____
Employment Status: ____ Employed ____ Short-term disability
___ Long-term disability ____ Unemployed
Support System: ____ Spouse ____ Neighbors/Friends ____ None
____ Family in same residence ____ Family in separate residence
____ Other
Family concerns regarding hospitalization: _____
_____

VALUE-BELIEF PATTERN
Religion: _____
Religious Restrictions: ____ No ____ Yes (Specify) _____
Request Chaplain Visitation at This Time: ____ Yes ____ No

PHYSICAL ASSESSMENT (Objective)
1. CLINICAL DATA
Age _____ Height _____ Weight _____ (Actual/Approximate)
Temperature _____
Pulse: ____ Strong ____ Weak ____ Regular ____ Irregular
Blood Pressure: Right Arm: ____ Left Arm ____ Sitting ____ Lying ____

2. RESPIRATORY/CIRCULATORY
Rate _____
Quality: ____ WNL ____ Shallow ____ Rapid ____ Labored ____ Other _____
Cough: ____ No ____ Yes/Describe _____
Auscultation:
Upper rt lobes ___WNL ___Decreased ___Absent ___Abnormal sounds ___
Upper lt lobes ___WNL ___Decreased ___Absent ___Abnormal sounds ___
Lower rt lobes ___WNL ___Decreased ___Absent ___Abnormal sounds ___
Lower lt lobes ___WNL ___Decreased ___Absent ___Abnormal sounds ___
Right Pedal Pulse: ____ Strong ____ Weak ____ Absent
Left Pedal Pulse ____ Strong ____ Weak ____ Absent

3. METABOLIC-INTEGUMENTARY
SKIN:
Color:___WNL ___Pale ___Cyanotic ___Ashen ___Jaundice ___Other ____
Temperature: ___WNL ____ Warm ____ Cool
Turgor: ____ WNL ____ Poor
Edema: ____ No ____ Yes/Description/location _____
Lesions: ____ None ____ Yes/Description/location _____
Bruises: ____ None ____ Yes/Description/location _____
Reddened: ____ No ____ Yes/Description/location _____
Pruritus: ____ No ____ Yes/Description/location _____
Tubes: Specify _____
Changes _____ None. If yes; description/location
MOUTH:
Gums: ____ WNL ____ White plaque ____ Lesions ____ Other _____
Teeth: ____ WNL ____ Other _____
ABDOMEN:
Bowel Sounds: ____ Present ____ Absent

4. NEURO/SENSORY
Pupils ____ Equal ____ Unequal
Left: ____ mm
Right: ____ mm
Reactive to light:
Left: ____ Yes ____ No/Specify _____
Right: ____ Yes ____ No/Specify _____
Eyes: ____ Clear ____ Draining ____ Reddened ____ Other _____

5. MUSCULAR-SKELETAL
Range of Motion: ____ Full ____ Other _____
Balance and Gait: ____ Steady ____ Unsteady
Hand Grasps: ____ Equal ____ Strong ____ Weakness/Paralysis (__ Right __Left)
Leg Muscles: ____ Equal ____ Strong ____ Weakness/Paralysis (__ Right __Left)

DISCHARGE PLANNING
Lives: Alone ____ With _____ No known residence _____
Intended Destination Post Discharge: ____ Home ____ Undetermined ____ Other ____
Previous Utilization of Community Resources:
____ Home care/Hospice ____ Adult day care ____ Church groups ____ Other ____
___Meals on Wheels ___Homemaker/Home health aide ___Community support group
Post-discharge Transportation:
____ Car ____ Ambulance ____ Bus/Taxi
____ Unable to determine at this time
Anticipated Financial Assistance Post-discharge?: ____ No ____ Yes _____
Anticipated Problems with Self-care Post-discharge?: ___No ____ Yes _____
Assistive Devices Needed Post-discharge?: ____ No ____ Yes _____
Referrals: (record date)
Discharge Coordinator _____ Home Health _____
Social Service _____ V.N.A. _____
Other Comments: _____
_____

SIGNATURE/TITLE _____ DATE _____

FIGURE 2.1 continued

⊗⊗ **BOX 2.1 SAMPLE FOCUS ASSESSMENT CRITERIA**

High Risk for Disturbed Self-Concept Related to the Effects of Prolonged Debilitating Condition on Achieving Developmental Tasks and Goals

Focus Assessment Criteria	Clinical Significance
1. Prior exposure to individuals with multiple sclerosis	1–4. This information enables the caregiver to detect patterns of response resulting from adaptation. It is helpful to note how the client's support system views the client's self-concept. Patterns can provide insight into factors that may have affected self-concept development and may be sensitive to the subtle effects of recent changes.
2. Ability to express feelings about condition	
3. Ability to share feelings with significant others	
4. Evidence of negative self-concept	
5. Participation in self-care	5,6. Participation in self-care and adaptation of goals to disability indicate attempts to cope with the changes.
6. Evidence of adapting life style to disabilities	

- They provide a "blueprint" to direct charting.
- They communicate to the nursing staff what to teach, observe, and implement.
- They provide goals/outcome criteria for reviewing and evaluating care.
- They direct specific interventions for the client, family, and other nursing staff members to implement.

To direct and evaluate nursing care effectively, the care plan should include the following:

- Diagnostic statements (collaborative problems or nursing diagnoses)
- Goals (outcome criteria) or nursing goals
- Nursing orders or interventions
- Evaluation (status of diagnosis and client progress)

Diagnostic Statements

Diagnostic statements can be either collaborative problems or nursing diagnoses. Refer to Chapter 1, The Bifocal Clinical Practice Model, for information on these two types of diagnostic statements.

Goals/Outcome Criteria

Client goals, or outcome criteria, are statements that describe a measurable behavior of the client or family, denoting a favorable status (changed or maintained) after delivery of nursing care (Alfaro, 2002). They serve as standards for measuring the care plan's effectiveness. Goals/outcome criteria for nursing diagnoses should represent favorable statuses that the client can achieve or maintain through nursing-prescribed (independent) interventions (Carpenito, 1992). If the client is not achieving goals, the nurse must reevaluate the diagnosis and revise the goals and the plan or collaborate with a physician.

When the nurse collaborates with the physician, the diagnosis is a collaborative problem not a nursing diagnosis. For example, if a client with a collaborative problem of Potential Complication: Dysrhythmia experiences premature ventricular contractions, the nurse would not change the nursing care plan but instead would initiate physician-prescribed interventions. Collaborative problems should not have client goals (outcome criteria). Any goals or outcome criteria written for collaborative problems would need to represent the criteria for evaluating both nursing and medical care. Physiologic stability is the overall goal for collaborative problems. Such measures are represented through nursing goals.

Nursing Interventions

Care plans should not contain directions for nurses regarding delegated (physician-prescribed) interventions. Instead nurses transfer physicians' orders to care and treatment records, Kardexes, and medication administration records. For this reason, the care plans presented in Unit II list only nurse-prescribed (independent) interventions. At the end of the Collaborative Problems section in each care plan, a section titled Related Physician-Prescribed Treatments provides these interventions as additional information. This chapter later explains the relationship of standards of care, physician-prescribed interventions, and critical pathways.

In the care plans, the interventions listed under nursing diagnoses generally consist of these types (Alfaro, LeFevre 2002):

- Performing activities for the client or assisting the client with activities
- Performing nursing assessments to identify new problems and to determine the status of existing problems
- Teaching the client to help him or her gain new knowledge about health or the management of a disorder
- Counseling the client to make decisions about his or her own health care
- Consulting with other health care professionals
- Performing specific actions to remove, reduce, or resolve health problems

In contrast, the interventions listed under collaborative problems focus primarily on the following:

- Monitoring for physiologic instability
- Consulting with a physician to obtain appropriate interventions
- Performing specific actions to manage and to reduce the severity of the event
- Explaining the problem and the rationale for actions

Care Planning Systems

Standards of Care

Standards of care are detailed guidelines that represent the predicted care indicated in a specific situation. Standards of care should represent the care that nurses are responsible for providing, not an ideal level of care. The nurse cannot hope to address all or even most of the problems that a client may have. Rather the nurse must select those problems that are the most serious or most important to the client. Ideal standards that are unrealistic only frustrate nurses and hold them legally accountable for care that they cannot provide. Nurses must create realistic standards based on client acuity, length of stay, and available resources.

A care planning system can contain three levels of directions:

- Level I—Generic Unit Standards of Care
- Level II—Diagnostic Cluster or Single Diagnosis Guidelines
- Level III—Addendum Care Plans

Level I Standards of Care predict the generic care that all or most individuals or families on the unit will need. Examples of generic unit standards of care are medical, surgical, oncologic, pediatric, postpartum, operating room, emergency room, mental health unit, rehabilitation unit, and newborn nursery. Figure 2.2 presents a diagnostic cluster for most hospitalized adults. The Generic Medical Care Plan at the beginning of Section 1 and the Generic Surgery Care Plan at the beginning of Section 2 are Level I standards. Because they apply to all clients, nurses do not need to write the nursing diagnoses or collaborative problems associated with the generic standard of care on an individual client's care plan. Instead, institutional policy can specify that the generic standard will be implemented for all clients. Documentation of the generic standard is discussed later in this chapter.

Level II guideline care plans contain a diagnostic cluster or a single nursing diagnosis or collaborative problem. A diagnostic cluster is a set of nursing diagnoses and collaborative problems that have been predicted to be present and of high priority for a given population. Unit II contains Level II care plans organized using diagnostic clusters. Those diagnoses indicated as primary have been reported to be managed by nurses 75% to 100% of the time. Those diagnoses that are indicated to be important are managed 50% to 74% of the time. Refer to the description of the Validation Study, p. x. Examples of Level II single-diagnosis standards are High Risk for Impaired Skin Integrity, High Risk for Violence, and PC: Fluid/Electrolyte Imbalances.

Although standards of care do not have to be part of the client's record, the record should specify what standards have been selected for the client. The problem list serves this purpose. The problem list represents the priority set of nursing diagnoses and collaborative problems for an individual client. Figure 2.3 presents a sample problem list. Next to each diagnosis, the nurse would indicate where the directions for the care can be found—on a standardized form or on the addendum plan. The nurse can use the last column to indicate the progress of the client.

Priority Set of Diagnoses

Nurses cannot address all or even most of the nursing diagnoses and collaborative problems in clients and families. Priority diagnoses are those nursing diagnoses and collaborative problems for which nurs-

Collaborative Problems
Potential Complication: Cardiovascular
Potential Complication: Respiratory

Nursing Diagnoses
Anxiety related to unfamiliar environment, routines, diagnostic tests and treatments, and loss of control
Risk for Injury related to unfamiliar environment and physical/mental limitations secondary to condition, medications, therapies, and diagnostic test
Risk for Infection related to increased microorganisms in environment, the risk of person-to-person transmission, and invasive tests and therapies
Self-Care Deficit related to sensory, cognitive, mobility, endurance, or motivation problems
Risk for Imbalanced Nutrition: Less Than Body Requirements related to decreased appetite secondary to treatments, fatigue, environment, changes in usual diet, and increased protein/vitamin requirements for healing
Risk for Constipation related to change in fluid/food intake, routine and activity level, effects of medications, and emotional stress
Disturbed Sleep Pattern related to unfamiliar or noisy environment, change in bedtime ritual, emotional stress, and change in circadian rhythm
Risk for Spiritual Distress related to separation from religious support system, lack of privacy, or inability to practice spiritual rituals
Interrupted Family Processes related to disruption of routines, change in role responsibilities, and fatigue associated with increased workload and visiting hour requirements

FIGURE 2.2   Level I diagnostic cluster for hospitalized adults

ing resources will be directed toward goal achievement. They take precedence over other nursing diagnoses/collaborative problems that may be important but not priorities (Carpenito, 1995). In acute care settings, priority diagnoses are those nursing diagnoses or collaborative problems that

1. Are associated with the primary medical or surgical condition
2. If not managed now will deter progress or negatively affect functional status

Important but nonpriority nursing diagnoses or collaborative problems need to be referred to the client for management after discharge. A referral to a community resource may be indicated. For example, the nurse can refer a woman with peripheral vascular disease who wants to quit smoking to a smoking cessation program in the community.

Addendum Care Plans

An addendum care plan represents additional interventions to be provided for the client. Nurses can add these specific interventions to a Level II guideline care plan or may associate them with additional priority nursing diagnoses or collaborative problems not included on the standardized plan.

The initial care of most hospitalized clients can be directed responsibly using standards of care. With subsequent nurse–client interactions, specific data may warrant specific addendum additions to the client's care plan to ensure holistic, empathic nursing care. Figure 2.4 presents a problem list and addendum care plan for a client recovering from gastric surgery. In addition to the diagnostic cluster in the postoperative standard of care, this client has three addendum diagnoses. High Risk for Impaired Skin Integrity is being managed with interventions from a standard for this diagnosis. Documentation will be completed each shift on the flow record. Impaired Swallowing is being treated with generic interventions and with addendum intervention specifying foods that this client can tolerate. The last diagnosis, Impaired Physical Mobility, involves only addendum interventions prescribed to increase the client's motivation and to promote correct ambulation techniques.

Nursing Problem List/Care Plan

Nursing Diagnosis/Collaborative Problem	Status	Standard	Addendum	Evaluation of Progress				

Status Code: A = Active   R = Resolved   RO = Ruled-out
Evaluation Code: S = Stable   I = Improved   *W = Worsened   *U = Unchanged   P = Progressing   *NP = Not Progressing

Addendum Care Plan

NSG DX/COLL PROB	CLIENT/NURSING GOALS	DATE/INITIALS	INTERVENTIONS

Initials/Signature			
1.	3.	5.	7.
2.	4.	6.	8.

FIGURE 2.3   Nursing problem list and care plan

Case Management

Nurse Case Managers

Every client needs his or her care managed; however, every client does *not* need a case manager (Bower, 1993). After the client populations for case management have been identified, critical pathways are developed.

Critical Pathways

The concept of critical pathways has been a well-known management tool for many years in such disciplines as economics and engineering in which they are organized as a timeline grid to monitor the progress of a project. Critical pathways in nursing were developed at the New England Medical Center in 1985 by Kathleen Bower and Karen Zander. Since then, numerous versions of critical pathways have been developed in hundreds of facilities under various names such as CareMap, critical paths, Collaborative Action Track, and Milestone Action Plans.

Nursing Problem List/ Care Plan

Nursing Diagnosis/Collaborative Problem	Status	Standard	Addendum	Evaluation of Progress				
1. STANDARD — POST-OP	A 6/8 LJC	✓		6/9 LJC *NP	6/10 JW P			
2. POT. IMPAIRED SKIN INTEGRITY RT IMMOBILITY	A 6/8 LJC			6/9 LJC S	6/10 JW S			
3. Impaired Swallowing RT Unknown etiology aEB choking with liquids	A 6/9 LJC	✓	✓	6/9 LJC P	6/10 JW P			
4. Impaired physical mobility RT fatigue, decreased motivation and uncoordinated movements 2° to Parkinson's	A 6/10 JW		✓	—	6/10 JW *NP			

Status Code: A = Active R = Resolved RO = Ruled-out
Evaluation Code: S = Stable I = Improved *W = Worsened *U = Unchanged P = Progressing *NP = Not Progressing

Addendum Care Plan

NSG DX/COLL PROB	CLIENT/NURSING GOALS	DATE/INITIALS	INTERVENTIONS
3. Impaired Swallowing	—	6/9 LJC	5. Stay with him during meals 6. Teach to moisten dry foods
4. Imp. Phys. mobility Mobility	Will walk to NSg Station with walker by 6/14	6/10 JW	1. Establish distance goal before walking 2. Talk about something interesting during walking

Initials/Signature			
1. LJC L.J. Carpenito RN	3.	5.	7.
2. JWm J. Woolsey RN	4.	6.	8.

FIGURE 2.4 Sample problem list and addendum care plan

Critical pathways "are based on the process of anticipating and describing *in advance* the care clients, within the specific case types, require and then comparing the actual status of the client to that anticipated" (Bower, 1993). They are developed on selected client populations with the participation of the disciplines involved in the care. Each discipline is asked to outline the usual anticipated care requirements and the outcomes (Bower, 1993). So before creating a critical pathway, nurses must identify their standard of care for the population. A standard of care for a population should include

1. The priority set of nursing diagnoses and collaborative problems predicted to need nursing interventions during the expected length of stay
2. Realistic, achievable outcomes
3. Realistic, pertinent interventions

Critical pathways are multidisciplinary; standards of care may or may not be. Nursing diagnoses and collaborative problems are excellent language for other disciplines such as respiratory therapy, physical therapy, social service nutritional therapy, and so on. After the standard of care is established for nursing, it could be passed on to other disciplines for addition of interventions specific to them (Carpenito, 1995). Figure 2.5 illustrates a section from a multidisciplinary care plan for a client with a fractured hip.

The additional physician orders for the client usually are not indicated on the standard of care because the problems in the standard are nursing diagnoses and collaborative problems. Physician standard orders are reflected on the critical pathway. After nursing and other disciplines have completed the standard of care, the critical pathway can be formulated.

Critical Pathway Format

Critical pathways can be developed for client populations using the medical diagnosis, the surgical or diagnostic procedure, or a therapy such as ventilator dependent or chemotherapy (Bower, 1993). The critical pathway outlines the anticipated care requirements and the outcomes to achieve within a pre-established time frame.

The outcomes identified on a critical pathway can be those linked to collaborative problems and nursing diagnoses identified for the population. Another approach is to identify the discharge criteria for the population. In either case, the client is evaluated daily for progress. Figure 2.6 represents a CareMap from the Center for Case Management, which illustrates problem statements linked with outcomes. The lower portion of the CareMap describes the staff tasks on a timeline.

Linking Standards of Care to Critical Paths

The care plans in this book represent care for a population. As a result of the validation work described on p. xiii, the nursing diagnoses and collaborative problems treated frequently by nurses have been established. These findings will assist nurses in establishing the standard from which critical pathways are derived.

The remainder of this section will outline the creation of a standard of care and critical pathway from the care plan for an individual undergoing a hip replacement. Table 2.1 illustrates the critical pathway derived from the standard of care. On the basis of the findings of the validation study, only those nursing diagnoses and collaborative problems reported to be monitored for or treated more than 75% of the time are included on the standard. In addition, outcomes that are achievable during the expected length of stay and interventions to achieve these outcomes are illustrated online.

Care Plans and Critical Paths

As discussed earlier, critical pathways offer an at-a-glance timeline to evaluate the progress of a client in a population. Critical pathways frequently do not accommodate additional nursing diagnoses or collaborative problems (addendum diagnoses) that are present and need nursing interventions. These addendum diagnoses, if not addressed, can delay client progress. For example, a woman scheduled for a hip replacement also has diabetes mellitus. This would necessitate monitoring for the collaborative problem, "PC: hypo/hyperglycemia." How will the nurse communicate this problem to other nurses with a critical path? One option is to write this additional problem under the problem list in the critical path and to insert the monitoring of blood glucose levels under the assessment section. This would work if the interventions were brief, such as "monitor blood glucose levels." However, what if this woman is also confused before surgery? This would necessitate the addition of Disturbed Thought Processes to the problem list.

Nursing Diagnosis:	*Impaired Physical Mobility related to pain, stiffness, fatigue, restrictive equipment, and prescribed activity restrictions.*
Goal:	*The client will increase activity to a level consistent with abilities*
Interventions:	

PT	1.	Establish an exercise program tailored to the client's ability.
	2.	Implement exercises at regular intervals.
PT/Nsg	3.	Teach body mechanics and transfer techniques.
PT/Nsg	4.	Encourage independence.
	5.	Teach and supervise use of ambulatory aids.

FIGURE 2.5 Sample multidisciplinary care plan for a client after a total hip replacement (Carpenito, L. J. [2004]. *Nursing diagnosis: Application to clinical practice* [10th ed.]. Philadelphia: Lippincott Williams & Wilkins.)

CareMap™: Congestive Heart Failure

Problem	Day 1 ER 1–4 hours	Day 1 Floor Telemetry or CCU 6–24 hours	Day 2 Floor	Day 3 Floor	Day 4 Floor	Day 5 Floor	Day 6 Floor
				Benchmark Quality Criteria			
1) Alteration in gas exchange/perfusion and fluid balance due to decreased cardiac output, excess fluid volume	Reduced pain from admission or pain free. Uses pain scale. O_2 sat. improved over admission baseline on O_2 therapy	Respirations equal to or less than on admission	O_2 sat = 90. Resp 20–22. Vital signs stable. Crackles at lung bases. Mild shortness of breath with activity	Does not require O_2. Vital signs stable. Crackles at base. Respirations 20–22. Mild shortness of breath with activity	Does not require O_2 (O_2 sat on room air 90%). Vital signs stable. Crackles at base. Respirations 20–22. Completes activities with no increase in respirations. No edema	Can lie in bed at baseline position. Chest X-ray clear or at baseline	No dyspnea
2) Potential for shock	No signs/symptoms of shock	No signs/symptoms of shock	No signs/symptoms of shock	No signs/symptoms of shock. Normal lab values	No signs/symptoms of shock	No signs/symptoms of shock	No signs/symptoms of shock
3) Potential for consequences of immobility and decreased activity: skin breakdown, DVT	No redness at pressure points. No falls	No redness at pressure points. No falls	Tolerate chair, washing, eating, and toileting	Has bowel movement. Up in room and bathroom with assist	Up ad lib for short periods	Activity increased to level used at home without shortness of breath	Activity increased to level used at home without shortness of breath
4) Alteration in nutritional intake due to nausea and vomiting, labored		No c/o nausea. No vomiting. Taking liquids as offered	Eating solids. Takes in 50% each meal	Taking 50% each meal	Taking 50% each meal. Weight 2 lbs. from patient's normal baseline	Taking 75% each meal	Taking 75% each meal
5) Potential for arrhythmias due to decreased cardiac output: decreased irritable foci, valve problems, decreased gas exchange	No evidence of life-threatening dysrhythmias	Normal sinus rhythm with benign ectopy	Potassium (WNL). Benign or no arrhythmias	Digoxin level DNL. Benign or no arrhythmias	Digoxin level WNL. Benign or no arrhythmias	Digoxin level WNL. Benign or no arrhythmias	Digoxin level WNL. Benign or no arrhythmias
6) Patient/family response to future treatment and hospitilization	Patient/family expressing concerns. Following directions of staff	Patient/family expressing concerns. Following directions of staff	Patient/family expressing concerns. Following directions of staff	States reasons for and cooperates with rest periods. Patient begins to assess own knowledge and ability to care for CHF at home	Patient decides if he/she wants discussion with physician about advanced directives	States plan for 1–2 days postdischarge as to meds, diet, activity, follow-up appointments. Expresses reaction to having CHF	Repeats plans. States signs and symptoms to notify physician/ER. Signs discharge consent
7) Individual problem:							

FIGURE 2.6 Sample CareMap (*From the Center for Case Management, South Natick, MA. CareMap is a registered trademark of the Center for Case Management; used with permission.*)

(figure continues on page 20)

Staff Tasks							
Assessments/Consults	Vital signs q 15 min Nursing assessments focus on lung sounds, edema, color, skin integrity, jugular vein distention Cardiac monitor Arterial line if needed Swan Ganz Intake and output	Vital signs q 15 min–1 hr Repeat nursing assessments Cardiac monitor Arterial line Swan Ganz Daily weight Intake and output	Vital signs q 4 hrs Repeat nursing assessments D/C cardiac monitor 24 hr D/C arterial and Swan Ganz Daily weight Intake and output	Vital signs q 6 hrs Repeat nursing assessments Daily weight Intake and output	Vital signs q 6 hrs Repeat nursing assessments Daily weight Intake and output Nutrition consult	Vital signs q 6 hrs Repeat Nursing assessments Daily weight Intake and output	Vital signs q 6 hrs Repeat Nursing assessments Daily weight Intake and output
Specimens/Tests	Consider TSH studies Chest X-ray EKG CPK q 8 hr x 3 ABG if pulse Ox: (range) Lytes, Na, K, Cl, CO_2 Glucose, BUN, Creatinine Digoxin: (range)	B/G	Evaluate for ECHO Lytes, BUN, Creatinine			Chest X-ray Lytes, BUN, Creatinine	
Treatments	O_2 or intubate IV or Heparin lock	O_2 IV or Heparin lock	IV or Heparin lock	DC pulse Ox if stable D/C IV or Heparin lock			
Medications	Evaluate for Digoxin Nitrodrip or paste Diuretics IV Evaluate for antiemetics Evaluate for antiarrhythmics	Evaluate for Digoxin Nitrodrip or paste Diuretics IV Evaluate for pre-load/ afterload reducers K supplements	D/C Nitrodrip or paste Diuretics IV or PO K supplements Evaluate for nicotine patch	Change to PO Digoxin PO diuretics K supplements Stool softeners Nicotine patch if consent	PO diuretics K supplements Stool softeners Nicotine patch if consent	PO diuretics K supplement Stool softeners Nicotine patch if consent	PO diuretics K supplement Stool softeners Nicotine patch if consent
Nutrition	None	Clear liquids	Cardiac, low-salt diet	Cardiac, low-salt diet	Cardiac, low-salt diet	Cardiac, low-salt diet	
Safety/Activity	Commode Bedrest with head elevated Reposition patient q 2 hrs Bedrails up Call light available	Commode Bedrest with head elevated Dangle Reposition patient q 2 hrs Enforce rest periods Bedrails up Call light available	Commode Enforce rest periods Chair with assist 1/2 hr with feet elevated Bedrails up Call light available	Bathroom privileges Chair x 3 Bedrails up Call light available	Ambulate in hall x 2 Up ad lib between rest periods Bedrails up Call light available	Encourage ADLs that approximate activities at home Bedrails up Call light available	Encourage ADLs that approximate activities at home Bedrails up Call light available
Teaching	Explain procedures Teach chest pain scale and importance of reporting	Explain course, need for energy conservation Orient to unit and routine	Clarify CHF Dx and future teaching needs Orient to unit and routine Schedule rest periods Begin medication teaching	Importance of weighing self every day Provide smoking cessation information Review energy conservation schedule	Cardiac rehab level as indicated by consult Provide smoking cessation teaching Dietary teaching	Review CHF education material with patient	Reinforce CHF teaching
Transfer/Discharge Coordination	Assess home situation: notify significant other If no arrhythmias or chest pain, transfer to floor Otherwise transfer to ICU	Screen for discharge needs Transfer to floor	Consider Home Health Care referral		Evaluate needs for diet and anti-smoking classes Physician offers discussion opportunities for advanced directives	Appointment and arrangement for follow-up care with Home Health Care nurses Contact VNA	Reinforce follow-up appointments

FIGURE 2.6 continued

TABLE 2-1. Critical Pathways for a Client Undergoing a Total Hip Replacement

Nursing Diagnosis/ Collaborative Problem	Intermediate Goals							Outcomes
	Day 1	Day 2	Day 3	Day 4	Day 5	Day 6	Day 7	Day 8
Potential complication: Fat emboli Compartmental syndrome Hemorrhage Joint displacement Sepsis Thrombosis	Nurse will manage and minimize vascular and joint complications.	→	→	→	→	→	→	State signs and symptoms that must be reported to a health care professional.
High Risk for Infection		Will exhibit wound healing free of infection	→	→	→	→	→	Demonstrate healing with evidence of intact, approximated wound edges or granulation tissue
Impaired Physical Mobility	Will relate the purpose of strengthening exercises	Will do strengthening exercises	→	Will demonstrate use of assistive device	→	→	→	Regain mobility while adhering to weight-bearing restrictions using an assistive device
Pain	Will report satisfactory relief of pain	→	Will report a lessening of pain	Will report relief from PO medications	→	→	→	Report progressive reduction of pain and an increase in activity
High Risk for Injury	Will identify factors that increase his risk of injury; will describe appropriate safety measures	→	→	→	→	→	→	Describe risk factors for injury in home
High Risk for Impaired Skin Integrity	Will demonstrate skin integrity free of pressure ulcers	→	→	→	→	→	→	Demonstrate skin integrity free of pressure ulcers
High Risk for Ineffective Therapeutic Regimen Management	Will communicate questions and concerns	→	→	→	→	Demonstrate skills needed for activities of daily living (ADLs)	→	Describe activity restrictions Describe a plan for resuming ADLs

(table continues on page 22)

TABLE 2-1. Critical Pathways for a Client Undergoing a Total Hip Replacement continued

Timeline	OR Day	POD #1	POD #2	POD #3	POD #4	POD #5	POD #6	POD #7	POD #8
Consults	OT PT Home Care								
Test	Post-op X-ray Hct; SMA6 PT/PTT	↑	↑	↑	PT/PTT	↑	↑	↑	↑
Treatments	Hemovac drain IV	↑	D/C Hemovac	↑	D/C IV D/C dressing	↑	↑	↑	D/C Staples
Medication	Antibiotic pre-op	Antibiotic IM pain meds. Anticoagulant	PO pain meds.	↑	Anticoagulant	↑	↑	↑	Prescription D/C anticoagulant
Diet	As ordered	↑	↑	↑	As ordered	↑	↑	↑	↑
Activity	Bedrest with abduction pillow; maintain alignment	OOB/chair	Weight bear as tolerated; transfer/assist Ambulate/walker	↑ ↑	Weight bear as tolerated; transfer/assist Ambulate/walker	Crutches Independent with walker	Stairs with assist	↑ ↑	↑
Assessments	Post-op assessments	Assess Ace wrap Monitor neurovascular status Monitor tissue integrity	↑	↑	Turn q 2 hrs Monitor incision Monitor neurovascular status Monitor tissue integrity	↑	↑	↑	↑
Teaching	S/S neurovascular compromise; reinforce activity and safety measures	Post-op exercises	↑	↑	Evaluate Pt/S.O. understanding	↑	↑	↑	Written instructions
Discharge Planning			Social work prn Home care prn	↑	↑				Written instructions

The interventions for this addendum diagnosis are not brief. A problem list/care plan can provide the solution. Figure 2.7 illustrates a problem list/care plan for this woman. A detailed explanation of problem lists can be found online.

Documentation and Evaluation

Care plans represent documentation of the nursing care planned for a client. They also reflect the status of the diagnosis: active, resolved, or ruled out. The documentation of care delivered and the client's status or response after care are recorded on specific forms including the following:

- Graphic records
- Flow records
- Progress notes
- Teaching records
- Discharge planning/summary

The nurse is responsible for evaluating a client's status and progress to outcome achievement daily. Evaluation of the client's status and progress is different for collaborative problems versus nursing diagnoses. For nursing diagnoses, the nurse will

- Assess the client's status.
- Compare this response to the outcome criteria.
- Conclude if the client is progressing to outcome achievement.

NURSING DIAGNOSIS/ COLLABORATIVE PROBLEM	STATUS	STANDARD	ADDENDUM	EVALUATION OF PROGRESS				
Total Hip Replacement	A	√						
PC: Hypo/Hyperglycemia	A	√						
Disturbed Thought Processes RT effects of dementia	A	√	√					

STATUS CODE: A = Active   R = Resolved   RO = Ruled-out
EVALUATION CODE: S = Stable,   I = Improved,   *W = Worsened,   U = Unchanged
    *NP = Not Progressing,   P = Progressing

Reviewed With Client/Family _9/23_, _____, _____, (Date)

ADDENDUM CARE PLAN

Nsg Dx/Coll Prob	Client/Nursing Goals	Date/Initials	Interventions
Dis thought process	Agitated episodes will diminish	LJC 9/23	1–7 STANDARD
			8. focus on decreasing fear
			9. encourage to share fears

Initials/Signature 1. LJC/ *LJ Carpenito RN*	3	5.	7.
2.	4.	6.	8.

FIGURE 2.7   Nursing problem list/care plan

The nurse can record this evaluation on a flow record as

> 7 AM–3 PM
>
> ***Comfort***
>
> ***Acute Comfort***   Report satisfaction relief from measures or on a progress note as

Sub. The medication relieved my pain well. It is easier to move and cough.
Eval. Pain controlled; continue plan.

Not all nursing diagnoses require a progress note to record evaluation. A well-designed flow record can be used.

For collaborative problems, the nurse will

- Collect selected data.
- Compare the data to the established norms.
- Judge if the data are within an acceptable range.

The nurse can record the assessment data for collaborative problems on flow records. Progress notes can be used if the findings are significant, followed by the nursing management of the situation. The last column of Figure 2.3 represents the place where the nurse can document the progress of the client for each diagnosis on the problem list. The frequency of this documentation will be determined by the institution (e.g., q 24h). If a client has not improved or has worsened and I* or N* is used. In addition, a progress note is required to record the nursing actions undertaken.

So the evaluation for nursing diagnoses is focused on progress to achievement of client outcome, whereas the evaluation for collaborative problems is focused on the client's condition compared with established norms.

Discharge Planning

Discharge planning is a systematic process of appraisal, preparation, and coordination done to facilitate provision of health care and social services before and after discharge. Discharge planning can be categorized as standard or addendum.

Standard discharge planning includes the teaching deemed necessary based on the client's specific medical or surgical condition. The standard of care usually can address the content to be taught under two nursing diagnoses: Risk for Ineffective Management of Therapeutic Regimen and Risk for Impaired Home Maintenance Management. Standard discharge planning is the responsibility of the professional nurse caring for the client or family.

Addendum discharge planning requires coordinated and collaborative action among health care providers within the institution and in the community at large. Multidisciplinary actions may be indicated. A discharge coordinator or a case manager should coordinate this type of discharge planning.

Staff nurses usually do not have the time or resources available for addendum discharge planning. However it is the staff nurse who refers high-risk clients or families to the discharge coordinator.

The goal of discharge planning is to identify the specific needs for maintaining or achieving maximum function after discharge. The discharge needs of clients and families can result in two types of nursing actions:

- Teaching the client or family how to manage the situation at home
- Referring the client or family to support services (e.g., community nurses, physical therapists, or self-help groups) for assistance with management at home

All unresolved outcome criteria on the problem list require either teaching for self-management or referrals before discharge.

Discharge planning should begin at admission. After the admission assessment, the nurse must analyze the data to identify if the client or family needs addendum discharge planning and referrals. Figure 2.8 presents questions that can help the nurse to identify high-risk clients and families. These questions can be placed either as a section at the end of the admission assessment form or as a section on a combined discharge planning and summary record as illustrated in Figure 2.1. High-risk clients and families require a referral to the discharge coordinator at admission.

Certain events that may not be predicted on admission also necessitate referral to a discharge coordinator. Some examples follow (Burgess & Raglands, 1983):

- Newly diagnosed chronic disease
- Prolonged recuperation after illness or surgery
- Complex home care regimens
- Terminal illness
- Emotional instability

I. Planning (initiate on admission)
Lives alone _____ With _____ No known residence _____
Intended destination after discharge:

  Home _____   Other _____   Undetermined _____

Anticipated caregiver: Self _____   Other _____
Prehospital functioning ability
  • Home management: Independent / Assistance needed / Dependent
  • Cooking: Independent / Assistance needed / Dependent
  • Shopping: Independent / Assistance needed / Dependent
  • Self-care: Independent / Assistance needed / Dependent

Anticipated financial assistance post discharge?   No _____   Yes _____

Anticipated problems with self-care post discharge?   No _____   Yes _____

Assistive devices needed post discharge?   No _____   Yes _____
Referrals: (record date)
  Discharge coordinator _____   Home health _____

  Social service _____   Other _____

II. Discharge Criteria and Instructions
1. Nutrition:

  _____ Explain diet to be followed upon discharge.

  Diet _____

  _____

  Restrictions _____
2. Medications:

  _____ State correct dose, time, special precautions, and side effects of medications

Name/Dose	Time(s)	Special instructions (in addition to those on container)

3. Activity

  _____ State activity restrictions

  _____ Demonstrate prescribed exercises

  _____ Demonstrate correct use of appliances/assistive devices
  ☐ Resume normal activity
  ☐ Sponge bath only   ☐ Tub bath   ☐ Shower

  ☐ Restricted activity for _____ (length of time)
    ☐ No lifting   ☐ No climbing stairs   ☐ No driving

  ☐ No sexual activity   ☐ Other _____

  _____

  _____

4. Special instructions

  _____ Correctly describe or demonstrate the prescribed treatment

  _____ State signs and symptoms that necessitate reporting

FIGURE 2.8   Discharge planning and summary record

(figure continues on page 26)

Discharge Summary

The Joint Commission on Accreditation of Healthcare Organizations (JCAHO) recommends that a discharge summary represent instructions given, referrals, client status, and the client's understanding of the instructions. The nurse can use progress notes to record this information; however, a more efficient system for recording the discharge summary can be designed. This record could be adapted with specific outcomes related to the medical or surgical condition. For example, a preprinted discharge summary record for a postoperative client could include these items:

• The client will correctly describe wound care measures.
• The client will state signs and symptoms that must be reported to a health care professional: fever, chills, redness or drainage of wound, and increasing pain.

A systematic, efficient discharge planning program can promote continuity of care by identifying a client's discharge needs early. Early identification of discharge needs also may help to eliminate unnecessary hospital days and unnecessary readmissions.

Symptoms to report: _____

_____

Other: _____

_____

_____

_____ Describe follow-up care and available community resources

☐ Appointment with _____ Date _____ Time _____

☐ Patient/Family to make appointment in _____ days/weeks

☐ Referral to _____

☐ Records sent with patient (list) _____

III. Discharge Summary

Discharge criteria met?   Yes _____   No _____

Action taken if discharge criteria not met: _____

_____

_____

_____

Discharged to _____ Date _____ Time _____

Mode of transportation _____

Accompanied by _____

Personal effects/Valuables sent home?   Yes _____   No _____

   List _____

Medications sent home from pharmacy?   Yes _____   No _____

Other comments _____

_____

_____

_____

Discharge nurse's signature _____

FIGURE 2.8 continued

Summary

The development of an efficient, professional nursing documentation system is possible within the scope of existing standards of practice. The elimination of repetitive, narrative charting on progress notes can reduce the total time spent in charting and produce a more accurate, useful representation of professional practice and client or family response. A streamlined documentation system that integrates the nursing process from admission to discharge with the designated charting requirements also presents the nurse with an optimum defense in the event of litigation proceedings and legal challenges.

11 STEPS TO CARE PLANNING

Care plans have one primary purpose: to provide directions for the nursing staff for a particular client. For students and nurses inexperienced in caring for a person with a particular condition or after a certain surgical procedure, these directions (care plan) need to be detailed. For nurses experienced in caring for people with a particular condition or after a certain surgical procedure, these directions (care plan) will be limited to only those specific interventions that are different for this particular client.

For example, a person who has diabetes mellitus is having abdominal surgery. An inexperienced nurse or student will need to refer to the generic care plan for a surgical client and an additional section on hypo/hyperglycemia (low or high blood glucose). An experienced nurse will not need to read a care plan for abdominal surgery but will need to know that the client also has diabetes and will need blood glucose monitoring. In hospitals and other health care agencies, general care plans for certain conditions or surgical procedures are usually in a computer or pre-printed to use as a reference. Other problems that are not on the general care plan are added individually.

Author's note:

Some Hospitals have Problem Lists for each Client. This Problem List would have Problems Associated with General Surgery and an Additional Problem of Hyper/Hypoglycemia.

Step 1: Assessment

If you interview your assigned client before you write your care plan, complete your assessment using the form recommended by your faculty. If you need to write a care plan before you can interview the client, go to Step 2. After you complete your assessment, circle all information that points to client strengths. Write all the strengths on an index card.

Author's note:

Strengths are Factors that will Help the Person to Recover, Cope with Stressors, and Progress to His or Her Original Health Prior to Hospitalization, Illness, or Surgery. Examples of Strengths are as Follows:
- Positive spiritual framework
- Positive support system
- Ability to perform self-care
- No eating difficulties
- Effective sleep habits
- Alert, good memory
- Financial stability
- Relaxed most of the time

Highlight all information that points to client strengths. Write all the strengths on the back of the index card.

Author's Note:

Risk Factors are Situations, Personal Characteristics, Disabilities, or Medical Conditions that can Hinder the Person's Ability to Heal, Cope with Stressors, and Progress to His or Her Original Health Prior to Hospitalization, Illness, or Surgery. Examples of Risk Factors are as Follows:

- Obesity
- Fatigue
- Limited ability to speak or understand English
- Memory problems
- Hearing problems
- Self-care problems before hospitalization
- Difficulty walking
- Financial problems
- Tobacco use
- Alcohol problem
- Moderate to high anxiety most of the time
- Frail, elderly
- Presence of chronic diseases

Arthritis	Depression
Diabetic mellitus	Cardiac disorder
HIV	Pulmonary Disease
Multiple sclerosis	

Step 2: Same Day Assessment

If you have not completed a screening assessment of your assigned client, determine the following as soon as you can by asking the client, family, or nurse assigned to your client.

- Before hospitalization:
  - Could the client perform self-care?
  - Did the client need assistance?
  - Could the client walk unassisted?
  - Did the client have memory problems?
  - Did the client have hearing problems?
  - Did the client smoke cigarettes?
- What conditions or diseases does the client have that make him or her more vulnerable to
  - Falling
  - Infection
  - Nutrition/fluid imbalances
  - Pressure ulcers
  - Severe or panic anxiety
  - Physiological instability (e.g., electrolytes, blood glucose, blood pressure, respiratory function, healing problems)
- When you meet the assigned client, determine if any of the following risk factors are present:
  - Obesity
  - Impaired ability to speak/understand English
  - Communication difficulties
  - High anxiety

Write significant data on index card. Go to Step 3.

Author's Note:

In some Nursing Programs, Students do not have the Opportunity to See or to Assess their Assigned Client Prior to the Clinical Day. Therefore they must Assess the Client on their First Clinical Day with the Client.

Step 3: Create Your Initial Care Plan

Why is your client in the hospital? Go to the index in this book and look up the medical condition or surgical procedure. If you find the condition or surgical procedure, go to Step 4.

If the condition your client is in the hospital for is not in the index, refer to the generic medical care plan at the beginning of Section I. If your client had surgery, refer to the generic surgical or ambulatory care plan at the beginning of Section 2.

Step 4: Additional Problems

If the medical condition or risk factor puts your client at high risk for a physiological complication such as electrolyte imbalances or increased intracranial pressure or for nursing diagnoses such as Impaired Skin Integrity, Risk for Infection Transmission, or Self-Care Deficit, go to the individual indexes for collaborative problems and/or nursing diagnoses. You will find the problem or nursing diagnoses there. Go to Step 5.

Author's Note:

These Individual Indexes Provide you with Numerous Options when your Assigned Client has Risk Factors and Medical Conditions that are in Addition to the Primary Reason they are Hospitalized.

Step 5: Review STANDARD Plan

- Review each section of the care plan. Review your client's risk factors on your index card.
- Review the collaborative problems listed. These are the physiological complications that you need to monitor. Do not delete any because they all relate to the condition or procedure that your client has had. You will need to add how often you should take vital signs, record intake and output, change dressings, etc. Ask the nurse you are assigned with for these times or review the Kardex, which also may have the time frames.
- Review each intervention for collaborative problems. Are any interventions unsafe or contraindicated for your client? For example if your client has edema and renal problems, the fluid requirements may be too high for him or her.

Author's Note:

Review the Collaborative Problems on the Standard plan. *Also* Review all Additional Collaborative Problems that You Found in the Separate Index that Relate to your Assigned Client.

Step 6: Review the Nursing Diagnoses on the STANDARD Plan

Review each nursing diagnosis on the plan.

- Does it apply to your assigned client?
- Does your client have any risk factors (see your index card) that could make this diagnosis worse?

An example on the Generic Medical Care Plan is *Risk for Injury related to unfamiliar environment and physical or mental limitations secondary to condition, medication, therapies, or diagnostic tests.*

Now look at your list of risk factors for your assigned client. Can any factors listed contribute to the client sustaining an injury? For example, is he or she having problems walking or seeing? Is he or she experiencing dizziness?

If your client has an unstable gait related to peripheral vascular disease (PVD), you would add the following to the diagnosis: *Risk for Injury related to unfamiliar environment and unstable gait secondary to PVD.*

Author's Note:

If you Know Your Client has PVD but You do not Know How this can Affect Functioning, Then Look Up the Diagnosis in this Book (or Another Textbook) and Review What Problems PVD Causes. Examples Include Unstable Gait, Poor Circulation to the Legs, and Risk for Injury.

Interventions

Review each intervention for each nursing diagnosis:

- Are they relevant for your client?
- Will you have time to provide them?
- Are any interventions not appropriate or contraindicated for your assigned client?
- Can you add any specific interventions?
- Do you need to modify any interventions because of risk factors (see index card)?

Author's Note:

Remember That You Cannot Individualize a Care Plan for a Client Until You Spend Time with Him or Her, but You can Add and Delete Any Inappropriate Interventions Based on Your Preclinical Knowledge of this Client (e.g., Medical Diagnosis, Coexisting Medical Conditions).

Goals/Outcome Criteria

Review the goals listed for the nursing diagnosis:

- Are they pertinent to your client?
- Can the client demonstrate achievement of the goal on the day you provide care?
- Do you need more time?

Delete goals that are inappropriate for your client. If the client will need more time to meet the goal, add "by discharge." If the client can accomplish the goal this day, write "by (insert date)" after the goal.

Hint: Faculty and references may have different words to describe goals. Ask your faculty which terminology they use.

Using the same diagnosis *Risk for Injury related to unfamiliar environment and physical or mental limitations secondary to the condition, therapies, and diagnostic tests,* consider this goal:

The client will not sustain an injury.

Indicators
- Identify factors that increase risk of injury.
- Describe appropriate safety measures.

If it is realistic for your client to achieve all the goals on the day of your care, you should add the date to all of them. If your client is confused, you can add the date to the main goal, but you would delete all the indicators because the person is confused. Or you could modify the goal by writing:

Family member will identify factors that increase the client's risk of injury.

Author's Note:

Consult with Clinical Faculty Person to Assure this is Acceptable.

Step 7: Prepare the Care Plan (Written or Printed)

You can prepare the care plan by

- Typing a care plan from this book into your word processor then deleting or adding specifics for your client (use another color for additions/deletions)
- Photocopying a care plan from this book then adding or deleting specifics for your client
- Writing the care plan

Author's Note:

Ask Your Faculty Person What Options are Acceptable. Using Different Colors or Fonts Allows Your Faculty Person to Clearly See Your Analysis. Be Prepared to Provide Rationales for Why you Added or Deleted Items.

Step 8: Initial Care Plan Completed

Now that you have a care plan of the collaborative problems and nursing diagnoses, which are associated with the primary condition for which your client was admitted? If your assigned client is a healthy adult undergoing surgery or was admitted for an acute medical problem and you have not assessed any significant risk factors in Step 1, you have completed the initial care plan. Go to Step 10.

Step 9: Additional Risk Factors

If your client has risk factors (on the index card) that you identified in Steps 1 and 2, evaluate if these risk factors make your assigned client more vulnerable to develop a problem. The following questions can help to determine if the client or family has additional diagnoses that need nursing interventions:

- Are additional collaborative problems associated with coexisting medical conditions that require monitoring (e.g., hypoglycemia)?
- Are there additional nursing diagnoses that, if not managed or prevented now, will deter recovery or affect the client's functional status (e.g., High Risk for Constipation)?
- What problems does the client perceive as priority?
- What nursing diagnoses are important but treatment for them can be delayed without compromising functional status?

You can address nursing diagnoses not on the priority list by referring the client for assistance after discharge (e.g. counseling, weight loss program).

Author's Note:

Priority Identification is a Very Important but Difficult Concept. Because of Shortened Hospital Stays and Because Many Clients have Several Chronic Diseases at Once, Nurses Cannot Address All Nursing Diagnoses for Every Client. Nurses must Focus on Those for Which the Client Would be Harmed or Not Make Progress if they were not Addressed.

Ask Your Clinical Faculty to Review Your List. Be Prepared to Provide Rationales for Your Selections.

Step 10: Evaluate the Status of Your Client (After You Provide Care)

Collaborative Problems

Review the nursing goals for the collaborative problems:

- Assess the client's status.
- Compare the data to established norms (indicators).
- Judge if the data fall within acceptable ranges.
- Conclude if the client is stable, improved, unimproved, or worse.

Is your client stable or improved?

- If yes, continue to monitor the client and to provide interventions indicated.
- If not, has there been a dramatic change (e.g., elevated blood pressure, decreased urinary output)? Have you notified the physician or advanced practice nurse? Have you increased your monitoring of the client?

Communicate your evaluations of the status of collaborative problems to your clinical faculty and to the nurse assigned to your client.

Nursing Diagnosis

Review the goals or outcome criteria for each nursing diagnosis. Did the client demonstrate or state the activity defined in the goal? If yes, then communicate (document) the achievement on your plan. If not and the client needs more time, change the target date. If time is not the issue, evaluate why the client did not achieve the goal. Was the goal

- ○ Not realistic because of other priorities
- ○ Not acceptable to the client

Author's Note:

Ask Your Clinical Faculty Person Where to Document Evaluation of Goal Achievement.

Step 11: Document the Care on the Agency's Forms, Flow Records, and Progress Notes

Author's Note:

Ask Your Clinical Faculty Person Where You Should Document Your Evaluation of the Client After You have Provided Care.

THE ILL ADULT: ISSUES AND RESPONSES

Illness, trauma, hospitalization, diagnostic studies, and treatments can precipitate various client responses. Depending on the situation, the client's individual personality, and other factors, these responses may include the following:

- Fear
- Anxiety
- Anger
- Denial
- Grief
- Apathy
- Confusion
- Hopelessness
- Loss of control

The nurse, as the primary presence 24 hours a day and as the practitioner of the science and art of nursing, represents the optimal health care provider for an ill client and his or her support persons (family members or significant others).

According to Henderson and Nite (1960), "Nursing is primarily assisting individuals (sick or well) with those activities contributing to health or its recovery (or to a peaceful death) that they perform unaided when they have the necessary strength, will, or knowledge." Nursing also helps clients to carry out prescribed therapy and to become independent of assistance as soon as possible (Henderson & Nite, 1960).

Stress and Adaptation

According to Hoskins (1988), "Stress is a state produced by a change in the environment that is perceived as challenging, threatening or damaging to the person's dynamic equilibrium." Lazarus and Folkman (1980) have developed a theory of stress that focuses on the interaction or transaction between the person and the external environment. Lazarus and Monat (1977) describe coping as the psychological and behavioral activities done to master, tolerate, or minimize external or internal demands and conflicts. According to Miller (1995), individuals "who have a rigid set or narrow range of coping skills are at more risk for impaired coping because different types of coping strategies are effective in different situations."

Every person has a concept of self that encompasses feelings about self-worth, attractiveness, lovability, and capabilities. Everyone also has implicit or explicit goals. Illness, other disruptions of health, and associated treatments can negatively affect a person's self-concept and ability to achieve goals. These negative effects are losses, which precipitate grieving. The extent of a person's grief response is directly related to the extent of interference in goal-directed activity and the significance of the goal.

Coping Strategies

Adaptive and effective coping strategies produce these results (Visotsky, 1961):

- Distress is kept at or returned to a manageable level.
- Hope is maintained or renewed.
- Positive self-esteem is maintained or restored.
- Cooperative relationships are maintained.

Cohen and Lazarus (1983) have described five modes of coping:

- Information seeking
- Direct action
- Inhibition of actions
- Intrapsychic processes
- Turning to others for support.

Table 4.1 presents examples of these five modes.

Information Seeking

A person attempting to cope with a disturbing or unfamiliar situation often seeks out knowledge to help in managing the situation. Many nurses assume that a client always needs to know as much information as possible about his or her condition and treatments. In reality, according to Burckhardt (1987), "sometimes little attention is paid to whether the patient is seeking information and, if so, what information is most valuable." Burckhardt goes on to state that some clients may need to be allowed *not* to acquire information. However if a client's lack of information for self-care is seen as detrimental, the nurse must continue to supervise the client or initiate a referral so that the client can be supervised.

In today's health care delivery system, interaction time between nurses and clients has been reduced as a direct result of reduced lengths of hospital stays. To facilitate the coping strategy of information-seeking despite decreased interaction time, the nurse can provide the client and family with opportunities to acquire information in the following ways:

- By creating and distributing printed material
- By developing audio or visual programs
- By providing information on community groups or commercial products that provide relevant information
- By directing them to call the unit with questions

Direct Action

This coping strategy incorporates any change or effort (except cognitive) that a person does to manage a situation. For example, having an ample supply of work- or leisure-related items when traveling by

TABLE 4.1   Emotion-Focused Behaviors Versus Problem-Focused Behaviors

	Description	Advantages/Disadvantages
Emotion-Focused Behaviors		
Intrapsychic processes		
Minimization	Reduces the seriousness of the event or problem	Provides time for appraisal and adjustment
Projection, displacement, suppression of anger	Directs anger to a less threatening person or object	Suppressed anger may increase stress
Anticipatory preparation	Rehearsal of possible consequences of behavior in stressful situations	Provides opportunity to prepare for worst; becomes dysfunctional when it produces unmanageable stress
Attribution	Finds personal meaning in the problem situation (e.g., religious faith)	Offers consolation, becomes dysfunctional when self-responsibility is lost
Problem-Focused Behaviors		
Goal setting	Setting time limitations on behaviors	May increase stress if unrealistic
Information seeking	Learning all about the problem	Reinforces self-control
Direct action or mastery	Learning new skills	Facilitates self-esteem by providing control
Help seeking	Sharing feelings with others for support	Provides an emotional release and comfort; if excessive, may alienate others
Inhibition of action	Eliminating an action	May increase stress if action is valued

air or waiting for an appointment can help to reduce the frustration associated with delays. Initiation of a regular exercise program is another example of direct action.

Inhibition of Action

Effective coping commonly requires avoiding or limiting certain situations or actions. This strategy sometimes can cause problems. A person has to weigh the advantages and disadvantages of each action. In some cases, coping that protects or enhances physical health but compromises self-esteem can have more detrimental effects. For example, a person with Parkinson's disease may be safer using a wheelchair than a walker; however, if embarrassment and loss of control result from wheelchair use, the outcome may be decreased mobility and social isolation.

Sometimes well-intentioned family members may inhibit the actions of the ill person without evaluating the other losses that coexist with the loss of these actions. For example, prohibiting an elderly woman from continuing to host Thanksgiving dinner may damage her self-esteem and reduce her perception of her purpose in life. Instead it may be more constructive to allow her to supervise the meal preparation.

Intrapsychic Processes

The coping strategies involved in intrapsychic processes represent attempts to manage a stressful situation through the cognitive activities of defense mechanism, such as denial, avoidance, or rationalization, or stress reduction strategies such as thought-stopping or relaxation.

These coping activities provide the person with much-needed control over the emotions of fear and anxiety. Although some health care professionals view defense mechanisms as pathologic (Burckhardt, 1987), in most cases these mechanisms actually are constructive. If, however, the person does not use any other coping strategy (i.e., information seeking, direct action, or support seeking) then defense mechanisms may produce unsatisfactory or destructive outcomes. If a person delays dealing with a situation or retreats, this may be seen as maladaptive when actually it may give the person a reprieve for internal readjustment.

For example, anger is often perceived as negative. Anger can, however, energize behavior, assist with expression of negative feelings, and help the person to defend against a threat (Taylor, Baird, Malone, & McCorkle, 1993). The nurse must proceed cautiously when determining how much time a client or family needs for internal readjustment. Reduced lengths of stay often propel nurses to push clients faster than their coping abilities can adapt. Again, it may be more constructive to provide clients and families with community resources that they can contact after internal readjustment has been achieved.

Turning to Others

This coping response involves a client's social network and social support. *Social network* is defined as the structural interrelationship of the client's family, friends, neighbors, co-workers, and others who provide support; *social support* is the psychological and tangible aid provided by the social network. House (1981) has defined four basic types of social support:

- Emotional
- Appraisal
- Informational
- Instrumental

Table 4.2 lists characteristics of these four types.

The nurse assesses and evaluates the client's perception that he or she received enough support and the extent to which the client can return support to others—a quality known as *reciprocity*. Reciprocity is crucial to balanced, healthy relationships. According to Tilden and Weinert (1987), "ill persons, unlike healthy people, who can terminate relationships that fail to satisfy their needs, often are locked into unsatisfactory relationships." In an ill client, impaired ability to reciprocate often leads to feelings of depression, dependency, and low self-esteem. Moreover caregiver burnout can result from "one-way giving," particularly when caring for a chronically ill person (Tilden & Weinert, 1987). The nurse may be able to help a client to identify effective ways of reciprocating. For example, an ill client may not be able to cook but can offer to peel or chop vegetables.

Coping with Chronic Illness

Chronic illness is the number one health problem in the United States. More than 30 million Americans have chronic disabilities, and over 15 million have limited ability for independent self-care (Larkin,

TABLE 4.2   Types of Social Support

Type of Support	Effect
Emotional support	Communicates concern, trust, caring, liking, or love
Appraisal support	Communicates respect and affirms self-worth
Informational support	Communicates useful advice and information for problem solving
Instrumental support	Provides assistance (besides cognitive) or tangible goods (e.g., money or help with chores)

1987). In American culture, the ability to be productive is a highly valued trait. Vitality, productivity, and success often are linked; thus chronic illness assaults a person's core values.

According to Burckhardt (1987), "persons with chronic illness face permanent changes in life style, threats to dignity and self-esteem, disruption of normal life-transitions, and decreasing resources." The nurse must assist an ill client's family in recognizing and agreeing on how chronic illness has affected the family system and individual members. Open dialogue about the influences of the chronic illness may help to preserve family relationships. Failure to acknowledge the effects and changes likely will lead to destruction and dissolution of the family system.

Social supports can buffer stress and reduce adverse health effects (Broadhead, Kaplan, & James, 1983). Unfortunately chronic illness can negatively influence social supports and networks (Table 4.3).

As discussed earlier, chronic illness presents a unique and often frustrating challenge for clients, support networks, and health care professionals. Responses to the losses associated with the experience of illness and its aftermath can include denial, anger, fear, anxiety, guilt, and sadness.

Denial

To cope with a difficult situation, sometimes a person disavows or minimizes the seriousness of the situation and the feelings connected to it. In many cases, denial is a useful and healthy way to deal with a problematic situation because it provides the time needed to regain and maintain emotional equilibrium. However, denial can be harmful if it leads to detrimental outcomes, e.g., refusal of appropriate treatment or drug abuse.

Anger

Anger can be an appropriate response to an unacceptable situation. Unfortunately, direct expressions of anger usually are considered inappropriate and commonly evoke feelings of guilt afterward. But a person who habitually suppresses angry feelings cultivates hostility. As a result of the person's inability or unwillingness to express anger, conflicts remain unresolved; unresolved conflicts can lead to depression.

Nurses, like others, typically are uncomfortable with clients' expressions of anger. However anger may be a productive response for a client in a vulnerable position. A person typically expresses anger to those he or she deems least likely to retaliate or to be least important; thus nurses are often the tar-

TABLE 4.3   Effects of Chronic Illness on Social Supports and Social Networks

Resulting Factors (Contributory/Risk Factors)	Resulting Nursing Diagnoses (Possible, Actual, Potential)
Decreased mobility Loss of control of bodily functions Fatigue Loss of employment Avoidance by others Fluctuations in functioning Anger, depression, self-preoccupation	Self-Care Deficits Social Isolation Impaired Social Interactions Fatigue
Changes in family functioning 　Role reversal 　Financial burden 　Reduced free time 　Avoidance of social functions 　Reduced reciprocity	Caregiver Role Strain Interrupted Family Processes Ineffective Coping (family, individual)

get of the anger of clients or their families (just as nurses may use peers or family as targets for their anger at hospital administration or the "system"). A nurse may deal with an angry client by avoiding him or her. In most persons, this avoidance is commonly seen as a benign response; for a nurse, however, avoidance is a malignant response because it results in reducing or withholding nursing care.

To deal effectively with an angry client, the nurse must first examine her or his feelings about and responses to angry behavior. Did the nurse witness anger as a child? Was she or he allowed to express anger as a child? Next the nurse should examine the client's or family's anger by asking herself or himself these questions:

- What could be the source(s) of the anger? Loss of control? Fear? Embarrassment?
- Is this the client's or family's usual response to stress?
- Is the anger serving a useful purpose?

When intervening with an angry client, the nurse may find it productive to give the client a direct message that he or she has a right to be angry (if appropriate) but that screaming, verbal abuse, obscene language, and physical violence are not acceptable. Helping a client to express anger without alienation is a difficult but productive strategy. Communicating the message that "if I were in your position or situation, I would be angry too; however, screaming at me will not reduce your anger or contribute to finding satisfying options" validates that the client has a right to feel anger but not to express it in a hurtful manner.

Anxiety

Anxiety is a state in which a person experiences feelings of uneasiness or apprehension and activation of the autonomic nervous system in response to a vague, nonspecific threat. Anxiety differs from fear in that an anxious person cannot identify the threat, whereas a fearful person can. Anxiety can occur without fear; however, fear usually does not occur without anxiety (Carpenito-Moyet, 2004).

Feelings of uneasiness, dread, and inadequacy accompany anxiety. The response to a threat may range from mild anxiety to panic. The four degrees of anxiety—mild, moderate, severe, and panic—are differentiated in Box 4.1. Mild anxiety has been described as normal anxiety, moderate anxiety as chronic anxiety, and severe anxiety as acute anxiety. Mild anxiety is necessary for a person to function and respond effectively to the environment and events.

Management of Therapeutic Regimen

Successful management of the therapeutic regimen requires a person to initiate one or more activities or life-style changes (Bandura, 1982). These activities can be as simple as blood pressure monitoring or as complex as home dialysis. Activities or life-style changes treat, prevent, or monitor problems. Box 4.2 illustrates examples of activities for each of the three types.

Bandura (1982) described self-efficacy theory as an individual's evaluation of his or her capabilities to manage stressful situations or to change behaviors to manage the situation. Successful management depends on outcome expectancy and self-efficacy expectancy. Outcome expectancy is the belief that a behavior change will improve the situation. Self-efficacy is the belief that one can make the behavior change (Bandura, 1982).

Individuals with a history of coping successfully in a similar situation have higher self-efficacy than those who were unsuccessful. In addition to a history of successful coping, three other factors that promote positive self-efficacy are:

- Witnessing others successfully coping
- Others believing that the individual can successfully cope or manage
- Not experiencing high autonomic arousal in response to the situation

Addressing the preceding three factors, nurses can initiate related interventions to promote positive self-efficacy. Box 4.3 illustrates interventions to promote positive self-efficacy.

End-of-Life Decisions

Families and health care providers experience intense stress when faced with decisions regarding either initiation or discontinuation of life support systems or other medical interventions that prolong life (Johnson and Justin, 1988). Additional conflicts arise if the client's wishes are unknown, especially if the family disagrees with the decisions of health care providers or vice versa. For this reason, clients

---

⊗ BOX 4.1 TYPES OF ANXIETY

Mild Anxiety

- Heightened perception and attention; alertness
- Ability to deal with problems
- Ability to integrate past, present, and future experiences
- Use of learning and consensual validation
- Mild tension-relieving behaviors (nail biting, hair twisting)
- Sleeplessness

Moderate Anxiety

- Slightly narrowed perception; selective inattention that can be directed
- Slight difficulty concentrating; learning requires more effort
- View of present experiences in terms of past
- Possible failure to notice what is happening in a peripheral situation; some difficulty adapting and analyzing
- Voice/pitch changes
- Increased respiratory and heart rates
- Tremors, shakiness

Severe Anxiety

- Distorted perception; focus on scattered details; inability to attend to more even when instructed
- Severely impaired learning; high distractibility and inability to concentrate
- View of present experiences in terms of past; almost cannot understand current situation
- Poor function; communication difficult to understand
- Hyperventilation, tachycardia, headache, dizziness, nausea
- Complete self-absorption

Panic

- Irrational reasoning; focuses on blown-up detail
- Inability to learn
- Inability to integrate experiences; focus only on present; inability to see or understand situation; lapses in recall of thoughts
- Inability to function; usually increased motor activity or unpredictable responses to minor stimuli; communication not understandable
- Feelings of impending doom (dyspnea, dizziness/faintness, palpitations, trembling, choking, paresthesia, hot/cold flashes, sweating)
- Thoughts related to loss of control, death, illness

(Carpenito-Moyet, L. J. [2004]. *Nursing diagnosis: Application to clinical practice*
[10th ed.]. Philadelphia: Lippincott Williams & Wilkins)

and families should be encouraged to discuss and record their directions to guide possible future clinical decision making (Johnson & Justin, 1988).

The nurse should instruct a client and family members to provide the following information (Carpenito, 1999):

- Person(s) to contact in an emergency
- Person the client trusts most with personal decisions
- Person(s) who will be consulted for decisions if the client becomes mentally incompetent
- Preference to die at home, in the hospital, or no preference
- Desire to sign a living will
- Decision on organ donation
- Funeral arrangements: burial or cremation
- Circumstances, if any, in which information should be withheld from the client

All decisions made should be documented. One copy should be given to the person designated as the decision maker if the client becomes incompetent or unable to make decisions, and the other copy should be retained in a safe deposit box.

BOX 4.2 EXAMPLES OF ACTIVITIES TO MANAGE THERAPEUTIC REGIMEN

Treatment

Wound care
Medications
Range-of-motion exercises
Low-salt diet

Preventive

Balanced diet
Exercise program
Dental hygiene

Monitoring

Blood pressure
Foot assessment
Urine testing

A living will is a document that reflects a person's desires or choices should terminal illness occur. Living wills do not apply to initial treatment decisions; they apply only to situations in which no reasonable possibility of recovery exists. Many states have laws governing living wills; however, all are not necessarily legally binding. Nurses should be familiar with their state's laws regarding living wills. To obtain a copy of your state's living will, write to the Society for the Right to Die, 250 West 57th Street, New York, NY 10107.

Legal and Ethical Accountability

Health care raises conflicts for both clients and health care providers. Often nurses experience conflict when it is unclear to whom they are accountable. Nursing accountability involves both legal and ethical obligations for the nurse. Legally nurses are accountable to state regulations known as nurse practice acts. Nurse practice acts vary greatly from state to state; some specify that nurses address diagnosis and

 BOX 4.3 INTERVENTIONS TO PROMOTE POSITIVE SELF-EFFICACY

1. Explore with person(s) past successful management of problems.
2. Emphasize past successful coping.
3. Tell stories of other "successes."
4. If appropriate, encourage opportunities to witness others successfully coping in a similar situation.
5. Encourage participation in self-help groups.
6. If high autonomic response (e.g., rapid pulse, diaphoresis) is reducing feeling of confidence, teach short-term anxiety interrupters (Grainger, 1990).
   a. Look up.
   b. Control breathing.
   c. Lower shoulders.
   d. Slow thoughts.
   e. Alter voice.
   f. Give self directions (out loud if possible).
   g. Exercise.
   h. "Scruff your face"—change facial expression.
   i. Change perspective: imagine watching the situation from a distance.

(Carpenito-Moyet, L. J. [2004]. *Nursing diagnosis: Application to clinical practice*
[10th ed.]. Philadelphia: Lippincott Williams & Wilkins)

> ⊙⊙ **BOX 4.4 AMERICAN NURSES ASSOCIATION CODE OF ETHICS FOR NURSES**
>
> 1. The nurse, in all professional relationships, practices with compassion and respect for the inherent dignity, worth, and uniqueness of every individual, unrestricted by considerations of social or economic status, personal attributes, or the nature of health problems.
> 2. The nurse's primary commitment is to the patient, whether an individual, family, group, or community.
> 3. The nurse promotes, advocates for, and strives to protect the health, safety, and rights of the patient.
> 4. The nurse is responsible and accountable for individual nursing practice and determines the appropriate delegation of tasks consistent with the nurse's obligation to provide optimum patient care.
> 5. The nurse owes the same duties to self as to others, including the responsibility to preserve integrity and safety, to maintain competence, and to continue personal and professional growth.
> 6. The nurse participates in establishing, maintaining, and improving health care environments and conditions of employment conducive to the provision of quality health care and consistent with the values of the profession through individual and collective action.
> 7. The nurse participates in the advancement of the profession through contributions to practice, education, administration, and knowledge development.
> 8. The nurse collaborates with other health professionals and the public in promoting community, national, and international efforts to meet health needs.
> 9. The profession of nursing, as represented by associations and their members, is responsible for articulating nursing values, for maintaining the integrity of the profession and its practice, and for shaping social policy.

American Nurses Publishing, 2001

case planning. Unfortunately nurses sometimes allow their practice to be sanctioned by other members of the health care team even when these practices are within the legal boundaries of the applicable nurse practice act.

Besides legal considerations, most situations also involve ethical implications. According to Carpenito and Duespohl (1985), ethical behavior is "a moral obligation, as opposed to a legal one imposed by the law." Carpenito and Duespohl stated the following:

> Whereas the professional nurse is held accountable to the law for providing safe nursing care to the consumer, ethical accountability is a personal responsibility that nurses and all other health professionals must accept. Protecting the rights of the client who has entered the health care system is a responsibility the professional nurse shares with others in the medical professions. As the client's advocate, the professional nurse is obligated to coordinate the health services provided to the client by all members of the health team. Every professional nurse has an ethical obligation to place the client's best interest first.

Many state nurse practice acts state specifically that the nurse is ethically accountable to the health care consumer. The American Nurses Association's code of ethics for nurses (Box 4.4) has been used to revoke the nursing licenses of nurses who have behaved in direct contradiction to its precepts.

Summary

Like other stressors that affect lives and life events, illness, trauma, and hospitalization have the potential to leave the involved parties (clients and families or significant others) disorganized and devastated. However, they may also provide an opportunity for increased growth and cohesiveness. The nurse can be instrumental in directing clients and families to paths of mutual support and individual autonomy.

RESPONSE TO THE SURGICAL EXPERIENCE

A planned trauma, surgery evokes a range of physiologic and psychological responses in a client that are based on personal and unique past experiences, coping patterns, strengths, and limitations. Most clients and their families view any surgery, regardless of its complexity, as a major event, and they react with some degree of anxiety and fear.

Perioperative nursing is the term used to describe the nursing responsibilities associated with the preoperative, intraoperative, postanesthesia recovery, and postoperative surgical phases. Throughout the perioperative period, the nurse applies the nursing process to identify the client's positive functioning, altered functioning, and potential for altered functioning. The nursing responsibilities for each phase (Box 5.1) focus on specific actual or potential health problems.

Preoperative Assessment

The nursing history and physical assessment of a preoperative client focus on present status and the potential for complications. Because all clients receive a nursing assessment on admission, these criteria can be integrated into the general nursing interview. (See Figure 2.1, Nursing Admission Data Base.)

In addition to the general data collected on admission, the nurse caring for a client in any phase of the perioperative period completes focus assessments—acquisition of selected or specific data as determined by the nurse and the client or family or as directed by the client's condition. The nurse who assesses a new postoperative client's condition (e.g., vital signs, incision, hydration, comfort) is performing a focus assessment. Preoperative focus assessments involve evaluating certain factors that can influence the client's risk for intraoperative or postoperative complications:

- Client's understanding of events
- Impairments
- Acute or chronic conditions
- Client's previous surgical experience
- Nutritional status
- Fluid and electrolyte status
- Risk for infection
- Emotional status

Communication, Cognitive, Mobility Status

Preoperatively the nurse must assess the client's ability to process information and to communicate questions and needs. Assessment of preoperative mobility limitations can help the nurse to determine if special positioning techniques are needed intraoperatively.

Understanding Events

The surgeon is responsible for explaining the nature of the operation, any alternative options, the expected results, and the possible complications. The surgeon obtains two consents—one for the procedure and one for anesthesia. The nurse is responsible for determining the client's understanding of the information then notifying the surgeon if more information is needed for a valid informed consent.

Acute or Chronic Condition

To compensate for the effects of surgical trauma and anesthesia, the human body needs optimal respiratory, circulatory, cardiac, renal, hepatic, and hematopoietic functions. Any condition that interferes with any of these systems' functions (e.g., diabetes mellitus, congestive heart failure, chronic obstructive pulmonary disease, anemia, cirrhosis, renal failure, lupus erythematosus, substance abuse [alcohol drugs]) compromises recovery. In addition to preexisting medical conditions, advanced age, obesity, and alcohol abuse also make a client more vulnerable to complications as outlined in Table 5.1.

BOX 5.1 FOCUS OF NURSING CARE IN THE PERIOPERATIVE PERIOD

Preoperative Phase

Preoperative assessment
Preoperative teaching
Preparation for transfer to operating room
Psychological support
Support of significant other

Intraoperative Phase

Environmental safety
Asepsis control
Physiologic monitoring
Psychological support (preinduction)
Transfer to postanesthesia recovery room

Postanesthesia Recovery Phase

Physiologic monitoring (cardiac, respiratory, circulatory, renal, neurologic)
Psychological support
Environmental safety
Comfort measures
Stability for transfer to unit

Postoperative Phase

Physiologic monitoring
Psychological support
Comfort measures
Support of significant other
Physiologic equilibrium (nutrition, fluid, elimination)
Mobilization
Wound healing
Discharge teaching

The increased incidence of latex allergies from 1988 to 1992 and the report of 1,000 systematic allergic reactions to latex with 15 deaths necessitates identification of persons at high risk. Box 5.2 outlines the assessment. High-risk individuals should be placed under latex precaution protocol (e.g., latex-free vials, syringes, gloves, ID bracelets, etc.).

Previous Surgical Experience

The nurse must ask the client and family specific questions regarding past surgical experiences. The information obtained is used to promote comfort (physical and psychological) and to prevent serious complications.

To detect a possible predisposition to malignant hyperthermia, the nurse should ask, "Has a doctor or a nurse ever mentioned to you or a family member that you had difficulty with anesthesia—excessive somnolence, vomiting, allergic reaction, or hyperthermia?" and "Has a family member experienced difficulty with anesthesia?" Malignant hyperthermia—a life-threatening syndrome occurring during surgery predominantly in apparently healthy children and young adults—is associated with a hereditary predisposition and the use of muscle relaxants and inhalation anesthetics. Incidence was previously 80% but now it has a reduced rate of 10% (Malignant Hyperthermia Association of United States [MHAUS], 1992).

Nutritional Status

The client's preoperative nutritional status directly influences his or her response to surgical trauma and anesthesia. After any major wound from either trauma or surgery, the body must build and repair tissue and protect itself from infection. To facilitate these processes, the client must increase protein—carbohydrate intake sufficiently to prevent negative nitrogen balance, hypoalbuminemia, and weight loss. Malnourished states result from inadequate intake, compromised metabolic function, or increased metabolic demands. Healthy clients can tolerate short periods of negative nitrogen balance postoperatively,

TABLE 5.1   Intraoperative and Postoperative Implications of Preexisting Compromised Functions

Condition	Associated Compromised Functions	Intraoperative Implications	Postoperative Implications
Advanced age	↑ Arterial thickening	Cardiac failure ———————→	
	↑ Peripheral resistance ——————————————→		Thrombosis
	↓ Ability to increase cardiac output	Hypotension/shock ———————→	
	↓ Lung capacity	Hypoxia	Pneumonia, atelectasis
	↑ Residual volume	Electrolyte imbalances ———→	
	↓ Cough reflex ———————————————————→		Respiratory infection
	↓ Renal blood flow	Shock	
	↓ Glomerular filtration	Impaired ability to excrete anesthetics ———→	
	Enlarged prostate ———————————————→		Urinary retention
	↓ Gastric motility ————————————————→		Paralytic ileus, constipation
	↑ Bone resorption	Fractures ———————————→	
	Impaired ability to regulate temperature	Hypothermia	Hypo/hyperthermia
	↓ Sound transmission	Difficulty hearing ————————→	
	↓ Lens elasticity ————————————————→		Risk for falls
	↓ Hepatic function	↓ Excretion of medications = ↑ toxicity	Impaired protein synthesis ↓ phagocytosis
Obesity	Excess of adipose tissue (vascularity)	Larger incision	Delayed healing
	Impaired mobility	Prolonged anesthesia time	Dehiscence/evisceration
	↓ Efficiency of respiratory muscles	↑ Risk of injury	Thrombosis
		Hypoventilation	Respiratory infection
	↓ Gastric emptying time ———————————→		Aspiration, pneumonia
Alcoholism	↓ Hepatic function	↓ Excretion of medications = ↑ toxicity	Malnourishment
	↓ Phagocytosis ————————————————→		Delayed healing
	Impaired protein synthesis	Cross-tolerance to anesthetics	Cross-tolerance to analgesics
	↓ Adrenocortical response ————————————→		Withdrawal symptoms

---

 BOX 5.2 CASE FINDING: HIGH-RISK INDIVIDUAL FOR LATEX SENSITIVITY

Allergic History

Asthma, eczema, hay fever, food allergy (especially banana, avocado, potato, and tomato)

Surgical History

Multiple surgeries, multiple urinary catheterizations, urticaria or angioedema or respiration distress during surgery, reactions during dental or radiological procedures

Occupational History

Latex exposure, work-related symptoms of cutaneous dermatitis, eczema, and urticaria, upper respiratory symptoms, rhinorrhea, pruritus, sneezing, or lower respiratory symptoms, cough, wheeze, shortness of breath

    Local or systemic symptoms with the use of household gloves, balloons, condoms, diaphragms, or touching poinsettia plants

    Gender—75% are female

(From Jackson, D. [1995], Latex allergy and anaphylaxis: What to do. *Journal of Intravenous Nursing,* 18; 33–52; and Williams, G. D. C. [1997]. Preoperative assessment and health history interview, *Nursing Clinics of North America; 32*[2]; 395–416.)

but clients who are malnourished before surgery are at high risk for infections, sepsis, and evisceration (Summer & Ebbert, 1992). Preoperatively the nurse should identify those clients who are malnourished and those who are at higher risk for postoperative nutritional compromise. The nurse then can consult with the nutritionist and the physician for preoperative treatment to correct nutritional deficits.

Fluid and Electrolyte Status

A client with a fluid and electrolyte imbalance is prone to complications of shock, hypotension, hypoxia, and dysrhythmias both intraoperatively and postoperatively. Fluid volume fluctuations result from decreased fluid intake or abnormal fluid loss, both of which occur in surgical trauma. Box 5.3 lists factors that decrease fluid intake and increase fluid loss.

The nurse can assess a client's daily fluid balance by evaluating the following:

- Daily weights
- Intake and output
- Urine specific gravity (in adults under age 65)
- Condition of mucous membranes (in infants and children)

Additional parameters assessed when monitoring fluid and electrolyte status include these:

- Central venous pressure
- Pulmonary arterial pressure
- Serum electrolytes
- Hemoglobin and hematocrit
- Blood urea nitrogen
- Creatinine

Adults with no preexisting fluid and electrolyte problem usually can compensate for the losses associated with surgery. However, clients of advanced age and those with cirrhosis, cancer, chronic pulmonary disease, diabetes mellitus, renal disorders, adrenal or thyroid dysfunction, or cardiovascular disorders or those on corticosteroid therapy may be unable to compensate.

Infection Risk

Skin is the first line of defense for prevention of infection. Because surgery reduces this defense, theoretically all surgical clients are at risk for infections. Routine nursing interventions prevent contamination of the wound and, if healthy, the client's defenses will prevent infection. Any factor that delays healing will increase the risk for infection. The following factors have been identified to contribute to delayed wound healing: malnourishment, diabetes mellitus, fever, dry wound surface, steroids, anemia, radiation, and chemotherapy. Nursing interventions focus on factors that can be improved such as nutritional status, glucose control, hydration, and smoking reduction (temporary).

 BOX 5.3 FACTORS THAT DECREASE FLUID INTAKE AND INCREASE FLUID LOSS

Decreased Fluid Intake

Nothing by mouth
Nausea/vomiting
Imposed fluid restrictions
Fatigue, pain

Increased Fluid Loss

Vomiting
Blood loss
Burns
Fever
Ascites
Abnormal drainage (wound, drains)
Diarrhea
Diuretics
Bowel preparations (enema, medications)

Emotional Status

A client's, family's, and significant other's responses to anticipated surgery depend on the following:

- Past experiences
- Usual coping strategies
- Significance of the surgery
- Support system (quality and availability)

Most clients anticipating surgery experience anxiety and fear. The uncertainties of surgery produce the anxiety; anticipated pain, incisions, and immobility can produce fear. Anxiety has been classified as mild, moderate, severe, and panic. (See Table 4.4 for more information.)

Anxiety can be differentiated into *state anxiety* and *trait anxiety*. *State anxiety* is the response to a stressful situation; *trait anxiety* refers to the variable interpretations persons make of threatening situations (Spielberger & Sarason, 1975). It is expected that clients and their families would have state anxiety. To help assuage this anxiety, the nurse should explore with the client and family their fears and concerns. Besides identifying sources of anxiety, the nurse also should assess possible avenues of support or comfort by asking questions such as "What would provide you with more comfort before surgery?" and "What do you usually do when you are under stress?"

Moderate anxiety is expected before surgery. Usually clients with moderate anxiety are willing to share their concerns. Clients who demonstrate panic anxiety or verbalize that they will die in the operating room present a serious situation clinically. When faced with such a client, the nurse should consult with the physician, who may want to consider postponing surgery.

Clients who are suffering, either physically or emotionally, can be best aided by a nonjudgmental listener who encourages them to express their feelings and conveys that it is acceptable to have such emotions. This behavior demonstrates sincerity and warmth to the client.

To communicate effectively, a nurse must first acknowledge and accept her or his own personal vulnerability. As human beings, nurses feel the emotions of sadness, fear, and frustration. To deny the existence of these feelings is to deny one's own humanity. The nurse has a responsibility to encourage clients to share, to indicate that she or he accepts clients' responses to situations, and to convey that she or he is emotionally involved. This emotional involvement is often quite difficult for nurses to incorporate into their nursing practice; however, pride and personal satisfaction soon replace all personal discomfort as nurses realize they make a positive difference in clients' surgical experiences.

A client who is suffering tends to respond positively to a nurse who accepts his or her response. For example, explaining that fear before surgery is normal to a client experiencing fear usually is comforting; sharing with a grieving family that you understand their loss does not eliminate the loss but does convey support. The ability to communicate effectively does not come automatically; it is a planned and learned art involving practice and caring.

Preoperative Teaching

Preoperative teaching is defined as the supportive and educational actions that the nurse takes to assist a surgical client in promoting his or her own health before and after surgery. The client's requirements for nursing assistance lie in the areas of decision making, acquisition of knowledge and skills, and behavioral changes (Williams, 1997).

Preoperative teaching should be a combination of emotional support and information giving (Felton, 1992; Williams, 1997). Studies have shown that clients who receive structured information regarding what they will feel, see, hear, and smell in addition to what will happen report less anxiety during surgical procedures (Johnson, 1978; Felton, 1992; King & Tarsitano, 1982). For example, explaining the sensations involved in intravenous catheter insertion rather than limiting the instruction to "an IV will be in your arm" helps to reduce the client's anxiety associated with unexpected sensations.

The advent of new, more effective instructional technology and the reduced lengths of stay require that the nurse use a variety of strategies to achieve outcome criteria. Retention of information is increased when the teaching–learning process involves a variety of senses. The client's active involvement and provisions for practice also enhance learning; for example, it helps to encourage the client to practice coughing, deep breathing, and leg exercises during the teaching sessions.

Many of these strategies can be used in group classes. Group sessions are time- and cost-effective by allowing one nurse to provide general information to a group of clients experiencing a similar event (e.g., new diagnosis of diabetes mellitus, upcoming coronary surgery). They also provide an opportunity for clients and families to share their concerns. Many people find it comforting to know that others are undergoing a similar experience.

At these sessions, the nurses can do the following:

- Elicit questions and concerns
- Evaluate achievement of outcome criteria
- Provide additional information

Providing the client with instruction and opportunities to practice preoperatively can enhance his or her participation in postoperative care. Moreover, family members who are involved in preoperative teaching sessions can later be enlisted to coach the client in necessary postoperative care measures such as coughing and deep breathing exercises.

Today most clients are admitted the day of surgery and have reduced lengths of stay; this minimizes the time available for client teaching. In response to increasing time constraints, nursing departments have developed various simple, quick teaching programs aimed at ensuring positive outcome criteria; for example, brochures on postoperative care routines for a specific type of surgery and group classes for same-day surgery clients held the week before surgery is scheduled.

Preoperative Nursing Record

Figure 5.1 presents a preoperative assessment/care plan that the nurse completes the evening before surgery or, if this is not possible, on the morning of surgery. This form also can be used in a same-day surgical setting. This record helps the nurse to collect essential preoperative data. Section I outlines specific areas concerning medical and surgical history, informed consent, and laboratory or diagnostic studies. Section II is a combination of assessment and plan of care. Content areas relating to present status and risk factors are specified in the left-hand column. If the data indicate no anticipated problems or identify no specific risk factors, they are recorded in the assessment column only. If the data present a problem or a risk factor for a potential problem, they are recorded under the diagnosis/plan column and the diagnostic statement is checked as are the contributing or risk factors. If the nurse has identified additional contributing or risk factors, they can be written in. The diagnoses identified on this form are both nursing diagnoses and collaborative problems.

Each nursing diagnosis or collaborative problem identified has corresponding standards of care that specifically direct the nurse to reduce or eliminate, monitor, or report the problem. These standards of care are in addition to the generic standards of care that have been identified by the American Association of Operating Room Nurses (AAORN). Under this standard, the only documentation required is if an unusual response is observed (item 13).

Policies that require nurses to copy from standards of care further reduce the nurse–client interaction time. Copy from a printed sheet does not produce an individualized plan; rather, it would be more prudent to require only specific interactions to be handwritten. Space is provided under each diagnosis on the assessment form so that the nurse can add any additional interventions beyond the standard when indicated. Figure 5.2 illustrates some additional interventions added for a client by the nurse prior to surgery. Any additional interventions provided by the nurse but not identified preoperatively should be recorded on the progress or nurse's notes not on the care plan. Remember that a care plan is written only if another nurse will be responsible for providing the care; a nurse should not write a care plan just for herself or himself to follow.

If the nurse has not identified any specific diagnoses, she or he places a checkmark before this statement at the end of the form:

Problems requiring addendum nursing interventions are not present at this time. Follow standard of care for perioperative nursing care.

The nurse completing the preoperative section then signs in the space indicated. When a nurse cannot visit all postoperative clients, she or he should select certain clients according to preoperative assessment findings, with clients having problems or risk factors validated before surgery receiving top priority. During the postoperative visit, the nurse assesses whether the interventions provided have prevented or reduced the problems.

The Postanesthesia Recovery Period

Surgical trauma and anesthesia disrupt all major body system functions but most clients have the compensatory capability to restore homeostasis. However, certain clients are at greater risk for ineffective compensation for the adverse effects of surgery and anesthesia on cardiac, circulatory, respiratory, and other functions (Box 5.4). During the immediate postoperative period, a client is extremely vulnerable to physiologic complications resulting from the effects of anesthetics on respiratory and circulatory function.

Section I Peroperative Phase

Date _____

Diagnosis _____

_____

Surgeon _____
Procedure scheduled and date_____
Age_____ Weight _____ Height _____
I.D. Band on Yes_____ No_____
H & P done Yes_____ No_____
Medical clearance Yes_____ No_____
Pre-op instruction done Bedside_____ Group _____
Consent signed
    Scheduled procedure Yes_____ No_____
    Blood Yes_____ No_____
    Other Yes_____ No_____
    (specify) _____
_____ Chart incomplete   _____Patient not available for visit

Lab/Diagnostic Studies

	Normal	Abnormal	No Results	Not Ordered
Hct				
HgB				
K				
Na				
PT/PTT				
Calcium				
RPR				
HIV				
Cultures				
Glucose				
Chest X-ray				
EKG				
Type and cross units				
Urinalysis				
Other				

Medical Problems and Surgical History

Previous surgical experience? Yes_____ No_____
    Specify:_____
Past problems with anesthesia? Individual Yes_____No_____Unknown _____
                                Family   Yes_____ No_____ Unknown _____
Existing medical problems: (check)
_____ Diabetes   _____Cardiac disease_____Arthritis
_____ Hypertension _____Cancer   _____Respiratory
_____ Hematologic _____Hepatic   _____AIDS
_____ Seizures   _____CVA   _____Renal
_____ Other _____

Section II Peroperative Nursing Record

ASSESSMENT	DIAGNOSIS/PLAN
I. Ability to Communicate Verbal ☐ Appropriate	Impaired Verbal Communication related to ☐ Inability to speak secondary to (specify)_____ ☐ Inability to communicate in English
Language spoken ☐ English ☐ Spanish ☐ Other (specify)_____	Impaired communication related to ☐ Deafness
Hearing ☐ Appropriate	☐ Impaired hearing ☐ Diminished level of consciousness

FIGURE 5.1 Preoperative nursing assessment/care plan

(figure continues on page 48)

Throughout the client's stay in the postanesthesia recovery room (PAR), the nurse should monitor the client at least every 15 to 20 minutes.

Level I Standards of Care should include the nursing diagnoses and collaborative problems present in most clients in PAR. Table 5.2 lists the collaborative problems and nursing diagnoses commonly seen in postsurgical clients in PAR. The nurse should record assessments and usual interventions on the PAR flow record. Unusual data or events will be recorded on the progress note.

Level II standards in the PAR would refer to additional standard care needed after a specific surgery (e.g., mastectomy). Level II standards could also address a single diagnosis. For example, if the preoperative assessment indicates that a client recovering from a hip-pinning operation has a nursing diagnosis of Disturbed Thought Processes related to unknown etiology (as manifested by repetitive questions of "Where am I?" or "Why am I here?"), the PAR nurse would continually need to orient the client to the environment and to the reasons for the hip pain. The standardized care plan for Altered Thought Processes

ASSESSMENT	DIAGNOSIS/PLAN
II. Risks for Injury	
1. Level of consciousness	High Risk for Injury related to
☐ Alert	☐ Confusion
	☐ Drowsiness
2. Weight _____ Height _____	☐ Nonresponsive state
☐ Within normal limits (WNL) within 15% of ideal wt.	
	High Risk for Injury: Fall related to
3. Allergies (latex, chemicals, tape, meds)	☐ Obesity > 15%
☐ None reported	
	☐ Drug allergy (specify) _____
4. Therapeutic devices	
☐ None present	☐ IV, Foley, drains, casts (circle or specify)
5. Skin integrity	Impaired Skin Integrity related to
☐ Presence of lesions/edema	
☐ None	☐ Lesions ☐ Edema
☐ Deferred	(specify size and location) _____
☐ Allergies (refer to 3)	High Risk for Impaired Skin Integrity related to
☐ None reported	☐ Allergy to metal, chemicals, cleansers, adhesives, latex (circle or
	specify) _____
☐ Weight	
☐ Within 15% of ideal weight	☐ Cachexia
	☐ Obesity
☐ Circulatory status	Anxiety related to
☐ WNL	☐ Lack of understanding of (specify) _____
6. Understanding of surgical experience	Anxiety/fear:
☐ Satisfactory	☐ Moderate } related to impending surgical experience and:
☐ Unable to evaluate	☐ Severe
	☐ First surgical experience
7. Emotional status	☐ History of negative surgical experience (own, relative, specify)
☐ Anxiety	_____
☐ Mild	☐ Specify _____
8. Risk for hemorrhage	Potential Complication: Hemorrhage
☐ History of hematologic disorder	
☐ None reported	☐ History of hematologic disorder (specify) _____
☐ Presence of medications that increase risk	☐ Aspirin or NSAID therapy
☐ None	☐ Anticoagulants
	☐ None
9. History of:	
☐ Substance use:	Potential Complication: Cardiac, Hepatic, Respiratory, Hemorrhage
☐ Alcohol use	☐ Alcohol use
☐ None reported	Drinks day/wk
☐ Smoking	☐ pk/day
☐ None reported	
☐ <1/2 pk/day	☐ (Specify)
☐ Street drugs	Support System
☐ None reported	☐ Unavailable
	☐ No support system
☐ Anesthesia problems (individual, family)	
☐ None reported	☐ (Specify)
	☐ Problems requiring addendum nursing interventions are not present
10. Support system	at this time. Follow standard of care for perioperative nursing care.
☐ Available identity: _____	
☐ Can be notified at no. _____	
	_____RN
11. Other problems	
☐ None identified	

FIGURE 5.1 continued

would contain the usual nursing interventions indicated. Interventions for specific nursing diagnoses should be recorded, as should the client's status.

Figure 5.3 illustrates how the nurse can record nursing diagnoses and collaborative problems that frequently occur in the PAR, and Figure 5.4 presents a nursing record form for documenting the client's status and nursing interventions in the PAR.

Before discharge or transfer from the PAR to the nursing unit, the client must meet preestablished criteria. The criteria used in many PAR discharge protocols include those listed below:

• Ability to turn head
• Extubated with clear airway
• Conscious, easily awakened
• Vital signs stable (blood pressure within 20 mm Hg of client's baseline)
• Dry, intact dressing
• Urine output at least 30 mL/hr
• Patent, functioning drains, tubes, and intravenous lines
• Anesthesiologist's approval for discharge (Summer & Ebbert, 1992)

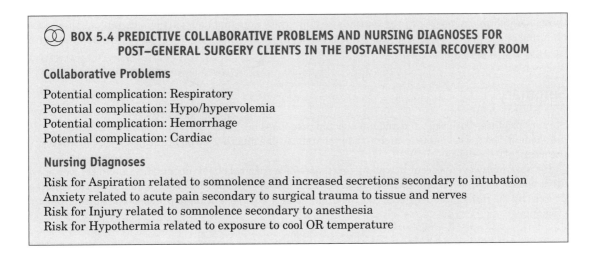

ASSESSMENT	DIAGNOSIS/PLAN

I. Ability to Communicate
Verbal
☒ Appropriate
 	
Language spoken
☒ English
☐ Spanish
☐ Other (specify) _____
 	
Hearing
☐ Appropriate
 	
II. Risks for Injury
  1. Level of consciousness
     ☒ Alert
 	
  2. Weight _140_ Height _5'6"_
     ☒ Within normal limits (WNL) within 15% of ideal wt.
  3. Allergies
     ☒ None reported
 	
  4. Therapeutic devices
     ☐ None present
 	
  5. Skin integrity
     Presence of lesions/edema
     ☒ None
       ☐ Deferred
 	
     Allergies (refer to 3)
     ☒ None reported
 	
     Weight
     ☐ within 15% of ideal weight
	Impaired Verbal Communication related to
	☐ Inability to speak secondary to (specify) _____
	☐ Inability to communicate in English
	
	Impaired communication related to
	☐ Deafness
	☒ Impaired hearing
	☐ Diminished level of consciousness
	  Speak into left ear.
	
	Potential for Injury related to
	☐ Confusion
	☐ Drowsiness
	☐ Nonresponsive state
	
	Potential for Injury: Fall related to
	☐ Obesity > 15%
	
	☐ Drug allergy (specify) _____
	
	☒ⓘⓥ Foley, drains, casts (circle or specify) _____
	Impaired Skin Integrity related to
	
	☐ Lesions ☐ Edema
	  (specify size and location) _____
	Potential Impaired Skin Integrity related to
	☐ Allergy to metal, chemicals, cleansers, adhesives (circle or
	  specify) _____
	
	☐ Cachexia
	☐ Obesity

FIGURE 5.2 Preoperative nursing record

Exceptions for these discharge criteria can be made if the transfer is to intensive care or if the surgeon or anesthesiologist has evaluated the client and approved discharge.

Same-Day Surgery

In same-day surgery (also known as outpatient or ambulatory surgery), the client is admitted the morning of surgery and discharged when stable later that day to recover at home. For this reason, departments of nursing and selected nursing areas must have systems in place to address the nursing process efficiently even when client contact time is limited. A nurse's accountability for assessment, diagnosis, plan-

---

○○ **BOX 5.4 PREDICTIVE COLLABORATIVE PROBLEMS AND NURSING DIAGNOSES FOR POST–GENERAL SURGERY CLIENTS IN THE POSTANESTHESIA RECOVERY ROOM**

Collaborative Problems

Potential complication: Respiratory
Potential complication: Hypo/hypervolemia
Potential complication: Hemorrhage
Potential complication: Cardiac

Nursing Diagnoses

Risk for Aspiration related to somnolence and increased secretions secondary to intubation
Anxiety related to acute pain secondary to surgical trauma to tissue and nerves
Risk for Injury related to somnolence secondary to anesthesia
Risk for Hypothermia related to exposure to cool OR temperature

TABLE 5.2 Adverse Consequences of Surgery and Anesthesia and Factors That Interfere With Compensatory Mechanisms

Consequences	Factors That Impair Ability to Compensate	Results
Nothing by mouth	Elderly/very young Malnourished Dehydrated Diabetes mellitus	Hypovolemia Shock Hypoglycemia
Blood loss	Same as NPO, plus: Coagulation disorders Aspirin Anticoagulants Antiplatelets Tobacco use	 Hemorrhage
Biotransformation of anesthetic compounds	Renal disorders Hepatic disorders Elderly Alcohol or drug abuse	Drug toxicity
Myocardial depression	Uncompensated heart disease Hypertension	Dysrhythmias Hypotension Shock
Hypotension	Coronary artery disease Monoamine oxidase inhibitors Phenothiazines	Shock Stroke
Respiratory depression	Chronic obstructive pulmonary disease History of smoking Congestive heart failure Obesity Upper respiratory infection Diuretics "Mycin" medications	Hypoxia Apnea

ning, implementation, and evaluation does not diminish merely because the client is not hospitalized the day before surgery. As discussed earlier, there are several options available (video, telephone, interview, and group classes). If assessment has been conducted by telephone or mail, the nurse still must assess certain areas on the morning of surgery. Figure 5.5 presents a short-stay nursing record. On this record, Section I includes the areas to be assessed before surgery; Section II is designated for postoperative care and status documentation. The nurse should also complete a preoperative diagnosis summary record (Fig. 5.6). This summary record also can be used for clients coming from in-house units. All this information should be communicated to the operating room/PAR staff.

Because another shift will not care for a same-day surgery client, writing an individualized care plan is unnecessary. Instead care plans in short-stay units can be standardized. Appendix III presents a generic Level I standard of care for same-day surgical clients. The nurse documents delivery of care primarily on a flow record. If the client has additional diagnoses or interventions to address, the nurse records these addendum diagnoses or interventions as a progress note, not as a part of a care plan. Discharge planning should be addressed in the standardized care plan under the diagnosis Risk for Ineffective Therapeutic Regimen Management.

Summary

Surgery produces both expected and unexpected responses in clients. Through vigilant assessment, the nurse identifies those clients at high risk for complications and those who are responding negatively to the surgical experience.

Because many events occur in a short time span for a surgical client, documentation in the perioperative phases must be concise but specific. The described documentation reflects the use of the nursing process by the nurse preoperatively and postoperatively with attention to professional standards and efficiency.

High Risk for Aspiration related to: ☐ Anesthesia   ☐ Surgery
Data: ☐ Airway in place   ☐ Uncuffed ET   ☐ Deflated ET Cuff
Intervention: ☐ Close observation   ☐ Removal of airway/ET tube   ☐ Position on side: ☐ (L)   ☐ (R)
Evaluation: ☐ Pulse oximeter readings   ☐ ABGs   ☐ Lung Sounds   ☐ Chest   RN: _____

PC: Cardiac   ☐ Dysrhythmia   ☐ COPD/CHF   ☐ Hyper/Hypotension
Data: ☐ ECG monitor   ☐ Swan-Ganz   ☐ Dyspnea   ☐ Tachycardia   ☐ Bradycardia
              ☐ Hypotension   ☐ Hypertension   ☐ Abnormal lung sounds
Intervention: ☐ Adjust IV rate   ☐ Analgesic given ☐ HOB → ☐ Notify MD   ☐ Trendelenberg
Evaluation: ☐ BP > 90 systolic ☐ Stable cardiac rhythm/rate   ☐ Pre- and post-op SPO₂ within 2–3 percentage points
                                                                                 RN: _____

FIGURE 5.3 Documentation example for postanesthesia care unit (*Developed by Ceciliu A. Cathey, RN, and nursing staff in PACU, St. Cloud Hospital, St. Cloud, Minnesota; reprinted with permission.*)

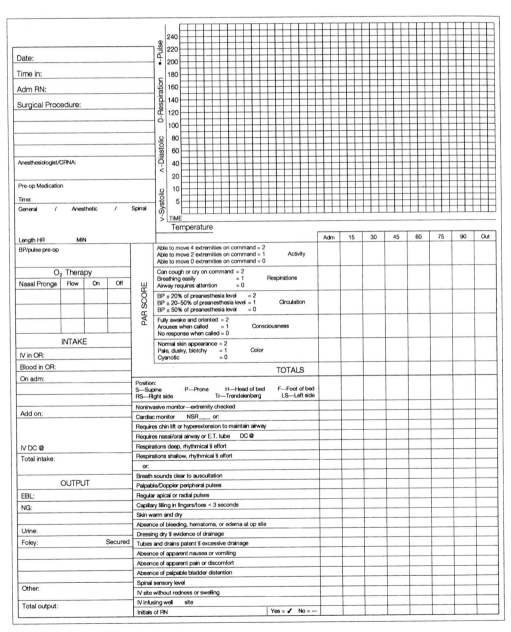

FIGURE 5.4 Sample PAR nursing record

(figure continues on page 52)

Initials | Signatures

Laboratory Reports:

Allergies:

Isolation required: ______ Yes ______ No

Medications | Time | Initials

Care classification: ☐ Emergency after hours

I-Requires one RN for 50% of stay (1:2)

II-Requires one RN for ↑50% of stay (1:1)

III-Requires ↑one RN for 50% of stay (2:1)

Anesthesiologist:

Discharge: Yes = ✔ No = —

Discharge criteria met: ______

Instructed to deep breath/cough: ______

Instructed to stay in bed and call for assistance: ______

Instructed to call for pain/nausea medication: ______

Instructed on food/fluid intake: ______

Appears to understand: ______

Family member/friend present: ______

Special instructions: ______

Side rails up: ______ Bed in low position: ______

Call light within range: ______

Dentures: ______

Vital signs on arrival to unit: ______

Transferred to care of: ______

Time: ______ PACU Nurse: ______

Signature receiving nurse: ______

FIGURE 5.4 continued

Section I: Preoperative

Date: _____

Time of Arrival on Unit:

_____ A.M.
P.M.

Via: □ Ambulatory
    □ Wheelchair
    □ Stretcher

Accompanied by:
□ Member of family
□ Friend
□ Unaccompanied

Name and phone number of person driving client home
Name: _____
Phone no.: _____
Waiting room: _____ Yes _____ No

Patient Has?

	No	Yes			
Hearing aid	□	□	Dentures		
Eye glasses	□	□	None	□	
Contact lenses	□	□	Partial	□	
Artificial eye	□	□	Upper	□	
Prosthesis	□	□	Lower	□	
Wig or hair piece	□	□	Denture cup	□	
			Removed	□	

Medical Problems and Surgical History

Previous surgical experience? Yes _____ No _____
Specify: _____

Past problems with anesthesia? Individual Yes _____ No _____
Family Yes _____ No _____

Existing medical problems: (Circle)
_____ Diabetes   _____ Cardiac disease   _____ Arthritis   _____ Seizures   _____ Pregnancy
_____ Hypertension   _____ Cancer   _____ Respiratory   _____ CVA
_____ Hematologic   _____ Liver   _____ AIDS   _____ Renal
_____ Other _____

Allergies (tape, chemicals, latex, meds)   Medications (Include time of last dose.)
_____   _____
_____   _____
_____   _____

□ No known allergies

Vital signs: Temperature _____   Respiration _____
BP _____   Pulse _____   Height _____   Weight _____ Actual/Reported

Diet: A.M.   Skin:
Last solid food _____   P.M.   No   Yes
                                     A.M.   Rash   □   □   _____
Last liquids _____   P.M.   Bruises   □   □   _____
                                               Cuts   □   □   _____
                                               Scars   □   □   _____
                                               Lesions   □   □   _____
                                               Other   □   □   _____

Abnormal lab work _____ No _____ Yes Called to _____

Abnormal X-ray results _____ No _____ Yes Called to _____

Pre-op teaching done _____ Video _____ Printed _____ Bedside
Operative permit signed _____ Yes _____ No
Identification band on _____ Yes _____ No
PAT studies done _____ Yes _____ No
H & P done _____ Yes _____ No

Time	Premedication given	Site	By

FIGURE 5.5   Same-day surgery nursing record

(figure continues on page 54)

NOTES:

_____

_____

_____

_____

_____

_____

_____ R.N.
Signature of Admitting Nurse

Section II: Postoperative

Graphic Chart

Name: _____

Time: _____

260												
240												
RESP ○ 220												
200												
180												
PULSE. 160												
140												
120												
DIAS ∧ 100												
80												
60												
SYST ∨ 40												
20												
TEMP												
URINE												
STOOLS												

Date _____ Time _____ A.M. P.M.

Operation _____

Dressings _____

Other _____

Medications given:

Time	Medication	Site	By

Nourishment _____
Amt _____
Tolerated _____ Yes _____ No

Activity tolerated
_____ HOB 60° _____ Time
_____ Dangle _____ Time
_____ OOB chair _____ Time

Section III: Discharge Summary

Discharge Status:

BP _____ Pulse _____ Respiration _____ Temperature _____
IV D/c'd: Time _____ Amt absorbed _____
Voided _____ Yes _____ No
Dressing intact/dry _____ Yes _____ No
Pain tolerable _____ Yes _____ No
Prescriptions given _____ No _____ Yes List: _____
General instruction sheets given _____ Client _____ Other _____
_____ Instruction sheet given _____ Client _____ Other _____
Instructed to call for appointment _____ Yes _____ No
Accompanied by _____ Family _____ Friend _____ Unaccompanied in taxi

Notes: (Unusual events, interactions)

_____

_____

_____

_____

Discharged by _____ R.N.

FIGURE 5.5 continued

ASSESSMENT	DIAGNOSIS/PLAN
Impaired Communication related to ☐ Deafness ☐ Impaired hearing ☐ Diminished level of consciousness ☐ Inability to speak secondary to (specify)_____ ☐ Inability to communicate in English	Potential Complication: Hemorrhage ☐ History of hematologic disorder (specify) ☐ Aspirin therapy ☐ Anticoagulants ☐ None
High Risk for Infection Transmission related to ☐ HIV positive ☐ Hepatitis: Type_____ ☐ Other_____	Potential Complication: Cardiac, Hepatic, Respiratory, Hemorrhage ☐ Alcohol use _____ Drinks day/wk ☐ Smoking _____ pk/day ☐ Street drugs (specify)_____
High Risk for Injury related to ☐ Confusion ☐ Drowsiness ☐ Nonresponsive state ☐ Obesity > 15% ☐ IV, Foley, drains, casts (circle or specify)_____	Support System ☐ Unavailable ☐ No support system (Specify)_____
Impaired Skin Integrity related to ☐ Lesions ☐ Edema (specify size and location)_____	Allergies ☐ None reported ☐ Unable to determine ☐ List:_____
High Risk for Impaired Skin Integrity related to ☐ Allergy to metal, chemicals, cleansers, adhesives, latex (circle or specify)_____ ☐ Cachexia ☐ Obesity ☐ ↓Circulation secondary to (specify)_____	Other Significant Data/Comments _____ _____ _____ _____ _____
Anxiety related to ☐ Lack of understanding of (specify)_____	_____ _____
Anxiety/Fear: ☐ Moderate ☐ Severe ☐ First surgical experience ☐ History of negative surgical experience (own, relative, specify) _____ ☐ Specify_____	☐ Problems requiring addendum nursing interventions are not present at this time. Follow standard of care for perioperative nursing care. R.N.

FIGURE 5.6 Preoperative diagnosis summary record

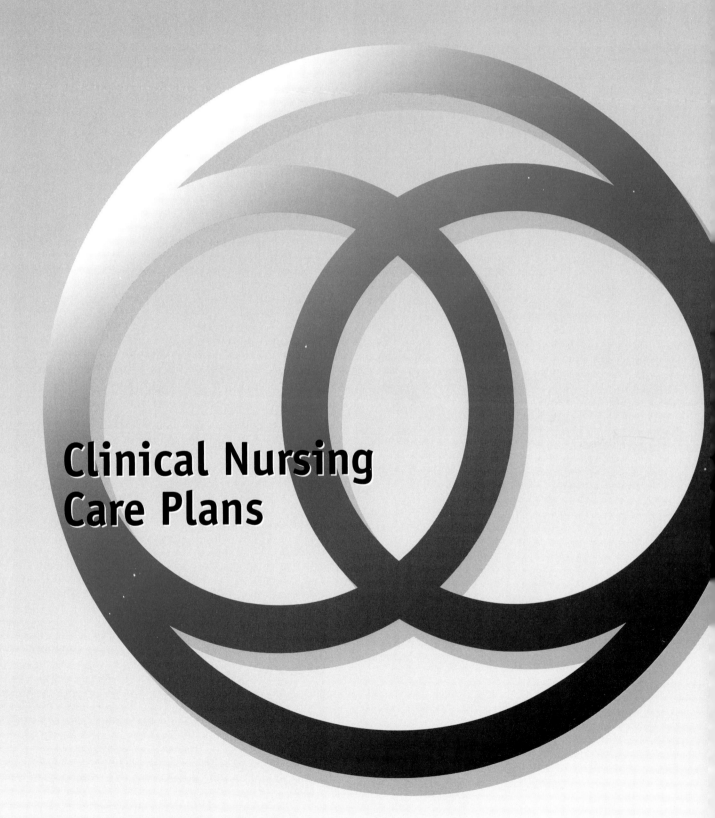

Clinical Nursing
Care Plans

Unit II comprises care plans for 79 clinical situations. The 44 care plans in Section 1 focus on persons experiencing medical conditions; the 23 care plans in Section 2 discuss people experiencing surgery; and the 12 care plans in Section 3 address people undergoing diagnostic studies or therapeutic procedures. These care plans represent the nursing diagnoses and collaborative problems known to occur frequently in these clinical situations and to be of significant importance. Data collected about a specific client must confirm the diagnosis.

Components of Each Care Plan

Definition

Each care plan begins with a description of the clinical situation. This information highlights certain aspects of the condition or situation or summarizes a knowledge base for the reader.

Time Frame

A client's response to certain situations or conditions can vary depending on when the event occurs in the health–illness continuum. For example, a client with newly diagnosed diabetes mellitus will have different responses than a client with an exacerbation. Therefore each care plan designates a time frame. The focus of the care plans in this book is the initial diagnosis. The nurse also can use the care plan if a client is readmitted for the same condition; however, the nurse will need to reevaluate the client and his or her needs.

Diagnostic Cluster

A diagnostic cluster represents a set of collaborative problems and nursing diagnoses predicted to be present and of significant importance in a selected clinical situation. Clients can experience, of course, many collaborative problems and nursing diagnoses. The diagnostic cluster represents those with high predictability. As discussed previously under the validation project section, this edition contains the results of a multi-site validation project. Nurses were asked to identify which nursing diagnoses and collaborative problems are treated most frequently. These findings are reported in the care plans of the 70 conditions studied. However the client may have additional nursing diagnoses or collaborative problems not listed in the diagnostic cluster for a given situation. Therefore these diagnostic clusters serve to assist the nurse in creating the initial care plan. As the nurse interacts with and assesses the client, he or she can add more specific diagnoses, goals, and interventions.

In addition, collaborative problems and nursing diagnoses not detailed in the care plan are listed under the heading "Refer to." These are included in the diagnostic cluster to give the nurse a complete picture of clinical care.

Discharge Criteria

Discharge criteria are the desired behaviors to maintain or to achieve maximum functioning after discharge. The discharge needs of clients and families can necessitate two types of nursing actions: teaching the client and family to manage the situation at home and referring the client and family to agencies for assistance with continuing care and management at home. The discharge criteria cited in each care plan represent those that a staff nurse can usually achieve with a client or family during a typical length of stay.

Many of the care plans use the nursing diagnosis "High Risk for Ineffective Therapeutic Regimen Management related to insufficient knowledge of _____" or "High Risk for Impaired Home Maintenance related to _____." These two diagnoses apply to a client or family at risk for problems after discharge. The plan of care for these diagnoses aims to prevent them. For these two diagnoses then, the discharge criteria also represent the goals. In other words, the goals—measurable behaviors that represent a favorable status—are the client meeting discharge criteria. Therefore no goals are cited for these two diagnoses. The nurse is referred instead to the discharge criteria.

Collaborative Problems

Each care plan describes and discusses nursing care for one or more physiologic complications that the nurse jointly treats with medicine. These collaborative problems have both physician- and nursing-prescribed interventions associated with them. The independent nursing interventions consist of monitoring the client for the onset of the complication or for an occurring complication's status. Other independent nursing interventions may include positioning, activity restrictions, etc. Keep in mind that collaborative problems are not physiologic nursing diagnoses. Physiologic nursing diagnoses that nurses independently treat are listed in the care plan as nursing diagnoses, e.g., Impaired Skin Integrity.

You will note that collaborative problems do not have client goals. Client goals are not useful in assisting the nurse to evaluate the effectiveness of nursing interventions for collaborative problems. For example, consider the collaborative problem "Potential Complication: Increased intracranial pressure." Appropriate goals might be as follows: The client will be alert and oriented, and the pupils will be equal and react to light accommodation. If the client's sensorium changes and the pupils respond sluggishly to light, will these data accurately evaluate the effectiveness of nursing care? The answer, of course, is no. The data evaluate the client's clinical status, which is the result of many factors.

Goals are used to assist the nurse in evaluating whether to continue, revise, or discontinue the care plan. The goals in the above example clearly do not serve this purpose. They set forth monitoring criteria that the nurse can add to the care plan as established norms for evaluating the client's condition (e.g., normal range for urine output, blood pressure, serum potassium). These are clearly not *client* goals. Certain nursing goals will serve to evaluate the effectiveness of nursing actions for collaborative problems, because nurses are accountable for detecting early changes in physiologic status and managing these episodes. Thus collaborative problems on the care plans in Unit II will have associated *nursing* goals. Refer to Chapter 1 of this book and to Chapter 2 in Carpenito (2003) for a more thorough discussion of collaborative problems.

Related Physician-Prescribed Interventions

This section is provided as reference material. It outlines physician-prescribed interventions for the specific condition or situation. These interventions have established systems for delivery and communication, e.g., physician order forms. Physician-prescribed interventions do not treat nursing diagnoses. Along with nursing-prescribed interventions, they do treat collaborative problems.

Nursing Diagnoses

Each care plan has at least two actual or high-risk nursing diagnoses. Keep in mind that the nurse should have validation for the diagnosis before initiating the care plan. Appropriate major signs and symptoms validate actual nursing diagnoses. Appropriate risk factors validate high-risk nursing diagnoses.

Focus Assessment Criteria

Each nursing diagnosis section begins with focus assessment criteria that direct the nurse's assessment toward specific data collection. These data will help to better evaluate the client's present status or response. A discussion of and rationale for this clinical significance accompany each assessment criterion.

Goals

The goals outlined for each nursing diagnosis consist of measurable behaviors of the client or family that represent a favorable status. Because a high-risk nursing diagnosis represents a situation that a nurse can prevent, the goals for that diagnosis represent a health status that the nurse will aim to maintain, thereby preventing the situation. The following is an example of a high-risk nursing diagnosis and its corresponding goal:

High Risk for Impaired Skin Integrity related to immobility
Goal: The client will demonstrate continued intact tissue.

If the goals are associated with an *actual* nursing diagnosis, they represent a behavior or status that the nurse will assist the client to achieve. The following is an example of an actual nursing diagnosis and its corresponding goal:

Impaired Skin Integrity related to immobility
Goal: The client will demonstrate evidence of granulation tissue.

Rationales

A supporting rationale is presented for each nursing intervention for both collaborative problems and nursing diagnoses. The rationale explains why the intervention is appropriate and why it will produce the desired response. Rationales may be scientific principles derived from the natural, physical, and behavioral sciences or they may be drawn from the humanities and nursing research. The rationales for client teaching interventions also include why the teaching is needed and why the specific content is taught.

Some topics in nursing are well studied whereas others have had little or no research. When possible, references no older than 5 years are used. A reference that is 5 or more years older is used because it is a classic or represents the most recent source on the subject.

Documentation

Each nursing diagnosis or collaborative problem section ends with a list of where and how the nurse will most appropriately document the care given. For some diagnoses, responsible documentation is recorded on a flow record, e.g., vital signs or urine output. For others, the nurse records a progress note. Teaching can be recorded on a teaching flow record or on a discharge summary record. The department of nursing determines policies for documentation. This section can serve to assist departments of nursing in formulating their documentation policies. It is unnecessary to record a progress or nursing note for every diagnosis on the care plan. Flow records can be used to document such routine or standard care as repetitive assessment results and even interventions.

Addendum Diagnoses

Frequently the nurse will identify and validate the presence of a high-risk or actual diagnosis that is not included in the given care plan for the situation or diagnostic cluster. The nurse can refer to the index of nursing diagnoses and collaborative problems in the back of this book to retrieve information about the identified diagnosis. For example, Mr. Jamie has had a myocardial infarction: the nurse initiates the care plan for an individual experiencing an MI. In addition, Mr. Jamie is immobile. The nurse can find "Disuse Syndrome" in the index and retrieve the information about that diagnosis. Then the diagnosis, goals, and interventions can be added as additional or addendum diagnoses.

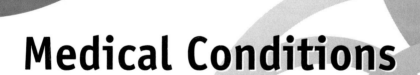

Medical Conditions

GENERIC MEDICAL CARE PLAN FOR THE HOSPITALIZED ADULT CLIENT

This care plan (Level I) presents nursing diagnoses and collaborative problems that commonly apply to clients (and their significant others) undergoing hospitalization for any medical disorder. Nursing diagnoses and collaborative problems specific to a disorder are presented in the care plan (Level II) for that disorder.

 DIAGNOSTIC CLUSTER

Collaborative Problems

PC: Cardiovascular Dysfunction
PC: Respiratory Insufficiency

Nursing Diagnoses

Anxiety related to unfamiliar environment, routines, diagnostic tests, treatments, and loss of control

Risk for Injury related to unfamiliar environment and physical and mental limitations secondary to condition, medications, therapies, and diagnostic tests

Risk for Infection related to increased microorganisms in environment, risk of person-to-person transmission, and invasive tests and therapies

(Specify) Self-Care Deficit related to sensory, cognitive, mobility, endurance, or motivation problems

Risk for Imbalanced Nutrition: Less Than Body Requirements related to decreased appetite secondary to treatments, fatigue, environment, and changes in usual diet, and to increased protein and vitamin requirements for healing

Risk for Constipation related to change in fluid and food intake, routine, and activity level; effects of medications; and emotional stress

Risk for Impaired Skin Integrity R/T prolonged pressure on tissues associated with decreased mobility, increased fragility of the skin associated with dependent edema, decreased tissue perfusion, malnutrition and urinary/fecal incontinence

Disturbed Sleep Pattern related to unfamiliar, noisy environment, change in bedtime ritual, emotional stress, and change in circadian rhythm

Risk for Spiritual Distress related to separation from religious support system, lack of privacy, or inability to practice spiritual rituals

Interrupted Family Processes related to disruption of routines, change in role responsibilities, and fatigue associated with increased workload and visiting hour requirements

Risk for Ineffective Therapeutic Regimen Management related to complexity and cost of therapeutic regimen, complexity of health care system, shortened length of stay, insufficient knowledge of treatment and barriers to comprehensive secondary to language barriers, cognitive deficits, hearing and/or visual impairment, anxiety and lack of motivation

---

Discharge Criteria

Specific discharge criteria vary depending on the client's condition. Generally, all diagnoses in the above diagnostic cluster should be resolved before discharge.

Collaborative Problems

PC: Cardiovascular Dysfunction

PC: Respiratory Insufficiency

Nursing Goal

The nurse will detect early signs and symptoms of (a) cardiovascular dysfunction and (b) respiratory insufficiency and will intervene collaboratively to stabilize the client.

Indicators

- Calm, alert, oriented (a, b)
- Respirations 16–20 beats/min (b)
- Respirations relaxed and rhythmic (b)
- Breath sounds present all lobes (b)
- No rales or wheezing (b)
- Pulse 60–100 beats/min (a, b)
- BP >90/60, <140/90 mm Hg (a, b)
- Capillary refill < 3 seconds (a)
- Peripheral pulses full, equal (a)
- Skin warm and dry (a, b)
- Temperature 98.5–99°F (a, b)

Interventions	Rationales
1. Monitor cardiovascular status:	1. Physiologic mechanisms governing cardio-vascular function are very sensitive to any changes in body function, making changes in cardiovascular status important clinical indicators.
a. Radial pulse (rate and rhythm)	a. Pulse monitoring provides data to detect cardiac dysrhythmias, blood volume changes, and circulatory impairment.
b. Apical pulse (rate and rhythm)	b. Apical pulse monitoring is indicated if the client's peripheral pulses are irregular, weak, or extremely rapid.
c. Blood pressure	c. Blood pressure represents the force that the blood exerts against the arterial walls. Hypertension (systolic pressure > 140 mm Hg, diastolic pressure > 85 mm Hg) may indicate increased peripheral resistance, cardiac output, blood volume, or blood viscosity. Hypotension can result from significant blood or fluid loss, decreased cardiac output, and certain medications.
d. Skin (color, temperature, moisture) and temperature e. Pulse oximetry	d. Skin assessment provides information evaluating circulation, body temperature and hydration status.

2. Monitor respiratory status:
   a. Rate
   b. Rhythm
   c. Breath sounds
	2. Respiratory assessment provides essential data for evaluating the effectiveness of breathing and detecting adventitious or abnormal sounds, which may indicate airway moisture, narrowing, or obstruction.

Related Physician-Prescribed Interventions

Dependent on the underlying pathology

 Documentation

Flow records
  Pulse rate and rhythm
  Blood pressure
  Respiratory assessment
Progress notes
  Abnormal findings
  Interventions

Nursing Diagnoses

Anxiety Related to Unfamiliar Environment, Routines, Diagnostic Tests, Treatments, and Loss of Control

Focus Assessment Criteria	Clinical Significance
1. Physical condition	1. Pain, fatigue, dyspnea, or other symptoms can increase a client's anxiety and hinder his or her motivation to learn, ability to concentrate, and retention of learning.

2. Sensory status:
  a. Vision
  b. Hearing
 	
3. Intelligence and learning ability:
  a. Education
  b. Occupation
  c. Learning disabilities
  d. Language difficulties
	2,3. Impaired hearing, vision, cognition, or memory; a learning disability; or a language barrier can interfere with communication and learning. A client with any such problem needs alternative client teaching techniques.

4. Anxiety level: mild, moderate, severe, panic	4. Extreme anxiety impairs a client's learning and coping abilities.
5. Past experience with hospitalization	5. This influences a client's expectations and perceptions of his or her hospital stay, both positively and negatively.
6. Specific stressors; nature of concerns	6. Every client experiences some emotional reaction to illness and hospitalization. The nature and degree of this reaction depends on how the client perceives his or her situation and its anticipated effects—physical, psychological, financial, social, occupational, and spiritual.
7. Support system: availability and quality	7. Adequate support from family, friends, and other sources can provide comfort and help the client maintain self-esteem. Poor support can increase stress and impair the client's coping ability.

Goal

The client will communicate feelings regarding the condition and hospitalization.

Indicators

- Verbalize, if asked, what to expect regarding routines and procedures.
- Explain restrictions.

Interventions	Rationales
1. Introduce yourself and other members of the healthcare team, and orient the client to the room (e.g., bed controls, call bell, bathroom).	1. A smooth, professional admission process and warm introduction can put a client at ease and set a positive tone for his or her hospital stay.

2. Explain hospital policies and routines:
  a. Visiting hours
  b. Mealtimes and availability of snacks
  c. Vital sign monitoring
  d. Availability of newspapers
  e. Television rental and operation
  f. Storage of valuables
  g. Telephone use
  h. Smoking policy
  i. Policy for off-unit trips
 	
3. Determine the client's knowledge of his or her condition, its prognosis, and treatment measures. Reinforce and supplement the physician's explanations as necessary.
	2,3. Providing accurate information can help decrease the client's anxiety associated with the unknown and unfamiliar.

4. Explain any scheduled diagnostic tests, covering the following:
  a. Description
  b. Purpose
  c. Pre-test routines
  d. Who will perform the procedure and where
  e. Expected sensations
  f. Post-test routines
  g. Availability of results
 	
5. Discuss all prescribed medications:
  a. Name and type
  b. Purpose
  c. Dosage
  d. Special precautions
  e. Side effects
 	
6. Explain any prescribed diet:
  a. Purpose
  b. Duration
  c. Allowed and prohibited foods
	4–6. Teaching the client about tests and treatment measures can help decrease his or her fear and anxiety associated with the unknown and improve his or her sense of control over the situation.

7. Provide the client with opportunities to make decisions about his or her care, whenever possible.	7. Participating in decision-making can help give a client a sense of control, which enhances his or her coping ability. Perception of loss of control can result in a sense of powerlessness, then hopelessness.

(continues on page 69)

Interventions continued	Rationales continued
8. Provide reassurance and comfort. Spend time with the client, encourage him or her to share feelings and concerns, listen attentively, and convey empathy and understanding.	8. Providing emotional support and encouraging sharing may help a client clarify and verbalize his or her fears, allowing the nurse to get realistic feedback and reassurance.
9. Correct any misconceptions and inaccurate information the client may express.	9. A common contributing factor to fear and anxiety is incomplete or inaccurate information; providing adequate, accurate information can help allay client fears.
10. Allow the client's support people to share their fears and concerns, and encourage them in providing meaningful and productive support.	10. Supporting the client's support people can enhance their ability to help the client.

Documentation

Progress notes
  Unusual responses or situations
Multidisciplinary client education record
  Client's knowledge/information provided related to diagnosis, treatment and hospital routine

Risk for Injury Related to Unfamiliar Environment and Physical or Mental Limitations Secondary to the Condition, Medications, Therapies, and Diagnostic Tests

Focus Assessment Criteria	Clinical Significance
1. Vision and hearing 2. Mental status 3. Mobility	1–3. An unfamiliar environment and problem with vision, orientation, mobility, and fatigue can increase a client's risk of falling.

Goal

The client will not injure self during hospital stay.

Indicators

• Identify factors that increase risk of injury.
• Describe appropriate safety measures.

Interventions	Rationales
1. Orient the client to his or her environment (e.g., location of bathroom, bed controls, call bell). Leave a light on in the bathroom at night.	1. Orientation helps provide familiarity; a light at night helps the client find his or her way safely.

(continues on page 70)

Interventions continued	Rationales continued
2. Instruct the client to wear slippers with non-skid soles and to avoid newly washed floors.	2. These precautions can help prevent foot injuries and falls from slipping.
3. Teach him or her to keep the bed in the low position with side rails up at night.	3. The low position makes it easier for the client to get in and out of bed.
4. Make sure that the telephone, eyeglasses, and frequently used personal belongings are within easy reach.	4. Keeping objects at hand helps prevent falls from overreaching and overextending.
5. Instruct the client to request assistance whenever he needs it.	5. Getting needed help with ambulation and other activities reduces a client's risk of injury.
6. Explain the hospital's smoking policy.	6. The hospital is a non-smoking institution.
7. For an uncooperative, high-risk client, consult with the physician for a 24-hour sitter or restraints, as indicated.	7. In some cases, extra measures are necessary to ensure a client's safety and prevent injury to him or her and others.

Documentation
Progress notes
Multidisciplinary client education record
Client teaching
Response to teaching

Risk for Infection Related to Increased Microorganisms in the Environment, Risk of Person-to-Person Transmission, and Invasive Tests or Therapies

Focus Assessment Criteria	Clinical Significance
1. Personal hygiene	1. Poor personal hygiene encourages a microorganism population, increasing the risk of infection.
2. Nutritional status	2. Poor nutritional status increases a client's susceptibility to infection by impairing the phagocytic defense mechanism.
3. History of invasive tests or therapies (e.g., IV lines, indwelling urinary catheter)	3. Invasive tests or therapies can introduce microorganisms into the body.

Goal
The client will describe or demonstrate appropriate precautions to prevent infection.

Interventions	Rationales
1. Teach the client to wash his or her hands regularly, especially before meals and after toileting.	1. Proper handwashing deters the spread of microorganisms.
2. Teach the client to avoid coughing, sneezing or breathing on others and to use disposable tissues.	2. These techniques help prevent infection transmission through airborne droplets.
3. Follow institutional policies for IV and indwelling urinary catheter insertion and care.	3. Proper insertion and care reduce the risk of inflammation and infection.
4. Teach a client undergoing IV therapy not to bump or disturb the IV catheterization site.	4. Movement of the device can cause tissue trauma and possible inflammation.
5. Teach a client with an indwelling catheter in place to do the following: a. Avoid pressure on the catheter. b. Wipe from front to back after a bowel movement.	5. Catheter movement can cause tissue trauma, predisposing to inflammation. Feces can readily contaminate an indwelling catheter.
6. Instruct the client to watch for and report immediately any signs and symptoms of inflammation: a. Redness or pain at the catheter insertion site b. Bladder spasms and cloudy urine, for a client with an indwelling urinary catheter c. Feelings of warmth and malaise	6. Nosocomial infections occur in 5–6% of all hospitalized clients. Early detection enables prompt intervention to prevent serious complications and a prolonged hospital stay.

 Documentation

Flow records
  Catheter and insertion site care
Progress notes
  Abnormal findings
Multidisciplinary client education record

(Specify) Self-Care Deficit Related to Sensory, Cognitive, Mobility, Endurance, or Motivational Problems

Focus Assessment Criteria	Clinical Significance
1. Self-feeding ability 2. Self-bathing and grooming abilities 3. Self-dressing ability 4. Self-toileting ability 5. Motivation for self-care 6. Endurance	1–6. Assessing the client's abilities helps the nurse determine what assistance the client needs to achieve the greatest level of independence possible.

Goal

The client will perform self-care activities (feeding, toileting, dressing, grooming, bathing) with assistance as needed.

Indicators

* Demonstrate optimal hygiene after care is provided.
* Describe restrictions or precautions needed.

Interventions	Rationales

1. Promote the client's maximum involvement in self-feeding:
  a. Determine the client's favorite foods and provide them, when possible.
  b. As feasible, arrange for meals to be served in a pleasant, relaxed, familiar setting without too many distractions.
  c. Ensure good oral hygiene before and after meals.
  d. Encourage the client to wear his or her dentures and eyeglasses when eating, as appropriate.
  e. Have the client sit upright in a chair at a table, if possible. If not, position him or her as close to upright as he can be.
  f. Provide some social contact during meals.
  g. Encourage a client who has trouble handling utensils to eat "finger foods" (bread, sandwiches, fruit, nuts).
  h. Provide needed adaptive devices for eating such as a plate guard, suction device under the plate or bowl, padded-handle utensils, wrist or hand splints with clamp, special drinking cup.
  i. Assist with meal setup as needed—open containers, napkins and condiment packages, cut meat, and butter bread.
  j. Arrange foods so the client can eat them easily.
 	
2. Promote the client's maximum involvement in bathing.
  a. Encourage and help set up a regular schedule for bathing.
  b. Keep the bathroom and bath water warm.
  c. Ensure privacy.
  d. Provide needed adaptive equipment, such as bath board, tub chair or stool, washing mitts, hand-held shower spray.
  e. Make sure the call bell is within easy reach of a client bathing alone.
	1–4. Enhancing a client's self-care abilities can increase his or her sense of control and independence, promoting overall well-being.

(continues on page 73)

Interventions continued	**Rationales** continued

3. Promote or provide assistance with grooming and dressing:
  a. Deodorant application
  b. Cosmetic application
  c. Hair care: shampooing and styling
  d. Shaving and beard care
  e. Nail and foot care
 	
4. Promote the client's maximum involvement in toileting activities.
  a. Evaluate his or her ability to move to and use the toilet unassisted.
  b. Provide assistance and supervision only as needed.
  c. Provide needed adaptive devices, e.g., commode chair, spill-proof urinal, fracture bedpan, raised toilet seat, support rails.
  d. Whenever possible, encourage a regular elimination routine using the toilet and avoiding a bedpan or urinal.	

🕭 Documentation

Flow records
Assistance needed for self-care

Risk for Imbalanced Nutrition: Less Than Body Requirements Related to Decreased Appetite Secondary to Treatments, Fatigue, Environment, and Changes in Usual Diet, and to Increased Protein and Vitamin Requirements for Healing

Focus Assessment Criteria	**Clinical Significance**
1. Usual dietary patterns (24-hour diet recall); caloric intake and types of foods	1. A 24-hour diet recall provides data to evaluate the quality of the client's diet and identify the need for modifications and teaching.
2. Height, daily weight	2. Daily weighing provides data to evaluate nitrogen balance; rapid weight gain can indicate edema.

3. Presence of the following:
  a. Bowel sounds
  b. Nausea and vomiting
  c. Flatus
	3. Certain conditions and medications and prolonged immobility can disturb gastrointestinal (GI) function.

Goal

The client will ingest daily nutritional requirements in accordance with activity level, metabolic needs, and restrictions.

dicators
Relate the importance of good nutrition.
Relate restrictions if any.

Interventions	Rationales
1. Explain the need for adequate consumption of carbohydrates, fats, protein, vitamins, minerals, and fluids.	1. During illness, good nutrition can reduce the risk of complications and speed recovery (Salmond, 1980).
2. Consult with a nutritionist to establish appropriate daily caloric and food type requirements for the client.	2. Consultation can help ensure a diet that provides optimal caloric and nutrient intake.
3. Discuss with the client possible causes of his or her decreased appetite.	3. Factors such as pain, fatigue, analgesic use, and immobility can contribute to anorexia. Identifying a possible cause enables interventions to eliminate or minimize it.
4. Encourage the client to rest before meals.	4. Fatigue further reduces an anorexic client's desire and ability to eat.
5. Offer frequent small meals instead of a few large ones.	5. Even distribution of total daily caloric intake throughout the day helps prevent gastric distention, possibly increasing appetite.
6. Restrict liquids with meals and avoid fluids 1 hour before and after meals.	6. These fluid restrictions help prevent gastric distention.
7. Encourage and help the client to maintain good oral hygiene.	7. Poor oral hygiene leads to bad odor and taste, which can diminish appetite.
8. Arrange to have high-calorie and high-protein foods served at the times that the client usually feels most like eating.	8. This measure increases the likelihood of the client's consuming adequate calories and protein.
9. Take steps to promote appetite: a. Determine the client's food preferences and arrange to have those foods provided, as appropriate. b. Eliminate any offensive odors and sights from the eating area. c. Control any pain or nausea before meals.	9. These measures can improve appetite and lead to increased intake.

(continues on page 75)

Interventions continued	Rationales continued
d. Encourage the client's support persons to bring allowed foods from home, if possible. e. Provide a relaxed atmosphere and some socialization during meals.	
10. Give the client printed materials outlining a nutritious diet that includes the following: a. High intake of complex carbohydrates and fiber b. Decreased intake of sugar, simple carbohydrates, salt, cholesterol, total fat, and saturated fats c. Alcohol use only in moderation d. Proper caloric intake to maintain ideal weight e. Approximately 10 cups of water daily, unless contraindicated	10. Today, diet planning focuses on avoiding nutritional excesses. Reducing fats, salt, and sugar can reduce the risk of heart disease, diabetes, certain cancers, and hypertension.

Documentation

Flow records
    Dietary intake
    Daily weight
Multidisciplinary client education record
    Diet instruction
    Use of assistive devices

Risk for Constipation Related to Change in Fluid or Food Intake, Routine, or Activity Level; Effects of Medications; and Emotional Stress

Focus Assessment Criteria	Clinical Significance
1. Pre-hospitalization elimination patterns	1. These data help the nurse evaluate whether the client had any elimination problem before admission.
2. Laxative or enema use	2. Excessive use of these substances could cause constipation.
3. Character of bowel sounds, presence and degree of abdominal distension	3. Assessment helps the nurse monitor for the return of peristalsis, if absent.

Goal

The client will maintain pre-hospitalization bowel patterns.

Indicators

- State importance of fluids, fiber, and activity.
- Report difficulty promptly.

Interventions	Rationales
1. Auscultate bowel sounds.	1. Bowel sounds indicate the nature of peristaltic activity.
2. Implement measures to promote a balanced diet that promotes regular elimination: a. Encourage increased intake of high-fiber foods, such as fresh fruit with skin, bran, nuts and seeds, whole-grain breads and cereals, cooked fruits and vegetables, and fruit juices. (Note: If the client's diet is low in fiber, introduce fiber slowly to reduce irritation to the bowel.) b. Discuss the client's dietary preferences and plan diet modifications to accommodate them, whenever possible. c. Encourage the client to eat approximately 800 grams of fruits and vegetables—the equivalent of about four pieces of fresh fruit and a large salad—daily to promote regular bowel movements.	2. A well-balanced diet high in fiber content stimulates peristalsis and regular elimination.
3. Promote adequate daily fluid intake: a. Encourage intake of at least two liters (8 to 10 glasses) per day, unless contraindicated. b. Identify and accommodate fluid preferences, whenever possible. c. Set up a schedule for regular fluid intake.	3. Adequate fluid intake helps maintain proper stool consistency in the bowel and aids regular elimination.
4. Establish a regular routine for elimination: a. Identify the client's usual elimination pattern before the onset of constipation. b. Review the client's daily routine to find an optimal time for elimination, and schedule adequate time. c. Suggest that he attempt defecation about 1 hour following meals; instruct him or her to remain on the toilet for a sufficient length of time.	4. Devising a routine for elimination based on the body's natural circadian rhythms can help stimulate regular defecation.
5. Attempt to simulate the client's home environment for elimination: a. Have the client use the toilet rather than a bedpan or commode, if possible. Offer a bedpan or commode only when necessary.	5. A sense of normalcy and familiarity can help reduce embarrassment and promote relaxation, which may aid defecation.

(continues on page 77)

Interventions continued	Rationales continued
b. Assist the client into proper position on the toilet, bedpan, or commode, as necessary. c. Provide privacy during elimination attempts—close the bathroom door or draw curtains around the bed, play the television or radio to mask sounds, use a room deodorizer. d. Provide adequate comfort, reading material as a diversion, and a call bell for safety reasons.	
6. Teach the client to assume an optimal position on the toilet or commode (sitting upright, leaning forward slightly) or bedpan (head of bed elevated to put the client in high Fowler's position or at permitted elevation); assist him or her in assuming this position as necessary.	6. Proper positioning takes full advantage of abdominal muscle action and the force of gravity to promote defecation.
7. Explain how physical activity affects daily elimination. Encourage and, as necessary, assist with regular ambulation, unless contraindicated.	7. Regular physical activity aids elimination by improving abdominal muscle tone and stimulating appetite and peristalsis.

 Documentation

Flow records
    Bowel movements
    Bowel sounds
Multidisciplinary client education record
    Instructions for obtaining regular elimination pattern

Risk for Impaired Skin Integrity Related to Prolonged Pressure on Tissues Associated with Decreased Mobility, Increased Fragility of the Skin Associated with Dependent Edema, Decreased Tissue Perfusion, Malnutrition, Urinary/Fecal Incontinence

Goal

The client will maintain present intact skin/tissue.

Indicators

- No redness (erythema)
- Relate risk factors to skin/tissue trauma.

Interventions	Rationales
1. Skin assessment a. *Assessment.* All clients will be assessed upon admission for risk factors that pre-	1. To prevent pressure ulcers, individuals at risk must be identified so that risk factors can be reduced through intervention.

(continues on page 78)

Interventions continued	**Rationales** continued
dispose to skin breakdown. These risk factors include, but are not limited to, the following: • Altered level of consciousness • Poor nutrition/hydration • Impaired mobility • Impaired sensation (paralysis) • Incontinence • Multisystem failure • Steroid or immunosuppressive therapy • Age over 65 b. *Inspection.* Upon admission, bony prominences and skin folds will be inspected for evidence of redness or skin breakdown. c. *Documentation.* Within 8 hours of admission, document the following information on skin section of Nursing Admission History: • Indicate whether client is at risk for breakdown/risk factors present by checking appropriate boxes. • Describe existing areas of breakdown and indicate location on body.	

2. Prevention protocol
  a. Pressure relief
    • Change client's position when in bed at least every 2 hours around the clock. Use large and small shifts of weight.
    • Post position change schedule ("turn clock") at bedside.
    • Utilize prevention mode on specialty beds.
    • Use foam with cushion in chair; no donuts.
 	
  b. Limit shearing forces/friction
    • Keep head of bed at or below 30 degrees whenever possible.
	• The critical time period for tissue changes due to pressure is between 1 and 2 hours, after which irreversible changes can occur.
	
	• The "turn clock" alerts caregiver to recommended position changes and appropriate time intervals for turning.
	
	• The risk of developing a pressure ulcer can be diminished by reducing the mechanical loading on the tissue. This can be accomplished by using pressure-reducing devices. Donuts are known to cause venous congestion and edema. A study of at-risk clients found that ring cushions are more likely to cause pressure ulcers than prevent them (AHCPR, 1992). The donut relieves pressure in one area but increases pressure in the surrounding areas.
	• Clinically, shear is exerted on the body when the head of the bed is elevated. In this position, the skin and superficial fascia remain fixed against the bed linens while the deep fascia and skeleton slide down toward the foot of the bed. As a

(continues on page 79)

Interventions continued	**Rationales** continued
	result of shear, blood vessels in the sacral area are likely to become twisted and distorted and tissue may become ischemic and necrotic (Porth, 1998).
• Avoid dragging client in bed. Use lift sheet or overhead trapeze.	• Friction injuries to the skin occur when it moves across a coarse surface such as bed linens. Most friction injuries can be avoided by using appropriate techniques when moving individuals so that their skin is never dragged across the linens.
• Use elbow protectors. Remove to inspect every shift. • Apply transparent film dressing (Tegaderm) over bony prominences as appropriate.	• Voluntary and involuntary movements by the individuals themselves can lead to friction injuries, especially on elbows and heels. Any agent that eliminates this contact or decreases the friction between the skin and the linens will reduce the potential for injury.
c. Nutritional assessment • Monitor intake and consider consultation with physician/dietary if the client: Eats less than 50% of meals for three or more days Is NPO or on a clear liquid diet for 5 days Has a serum albumin of <3.5 • Place on intake and output. If intake is less than 2000 cc/24 hours, force fluids unless contraindicated. • Record actual weight on admission and weekly thereafter. • Request multivitamin/mineral supplement and/or dietary supplements (Burnshakes, Ensure) if indicated. • Assess lab values: CBC Albumin Hemoglobin/hematocrit	c. Nutritional deficit is a known risk factor for the development of pressure ulcers. Poor general nutrition is frequently associated with loss of weight and muscle atrophy. The reduction in subcutaneous tissue and muscle reduces the mechanical padding between the skin and underlying bony prominences and increases susceptibility to pressure ulcers. Poor nutrition also leads to decreased resistance to infection and interferes with wound healing.
d. Skin care* • Inspect skin at least daily during bath for reddened areas or breakdown. Check bony prominences for redness with each position change.	• Skin inspection is fundamental to any plan for preventing pressure ulcers. Skin inspection provides the information essential for designing interventions to reduce risk and for evaluating the outcomes of those interventions.
• Keep skin clean and dry. Gently apply moisturizers such as Eucerin, Lubriderm, or Sween Cream as needed.	• For maximum skin vitality, metabolic wastes and environmental contaminants that accumulate on the skin should be removed frequently. It is prudent to treat clinical signs and symptoms of dry skin with a topical moisturizer.
• Avoid massage over bony prominences.	• There is research evidence to suggest that massage over bony prominences may be harmful (AHCPR, 1992).

(continues on page 80)

Interventions continued	Rationales continued

e. Incontinence care
• Assess the cause of incontinence:
  History of incontinence
  Change in medications
  Antibiotic therapy
  Client disoriented at night
• Maintain skin as dry as possible.
  Have call light within reach.
  Check client for incontinence every
    1–2 hours.
  Take client to bathroom or offer
    bed pan every 2 hours while awake
    and h.s.
  If diapers are used, check every
    2 hours and prn for wetness.
  If chux are used, place chux inside lift
    sheet, never in direct contact with
    the client's skin.
	• Moist skin due to incontinence leads to maceration; which can make the skin more susceptible to injury. Moisture from incontinence of urine or feces also reduces the resistance of the skin to bacteria. Bacteria and toxins in the stool increase the risk of skin breakdown.

Cleanse perineal area after each incontinent episode, followed by the application of a moisture barrier ointment (Desitin, Vaseline, A & D Ointment, BAZA.)	Chux hold moisture next to the skin. They are not absorbent and serve only as "bed protectors." Never use chux unless they are covered with smooth linen to absorb moisture. A moisture barrier is a petrolatum-based ointment that repels urine and fecal material and moisturizes the skin to assist in healing reddened, irritated areas resulting from incontinence.

Disturbed Sleep Pattern Related to an Unfamiliar, Noisy Environment, a Change in Bedtime Ritual, Emotional Stress, and a Change in Circadian Rhythm

Focus Assessment Criteria	Clinical Significance
1. Usual sleep requirements	1. Sleep requirements vary among clients depending on age, life style, activity level, stress, and other factors.
2. Usual bedtime routines, environment, position	2. Bedtime rituals may aid relaxation and promote sleep.
3. Quality of sleep	3. Only the client can subjectively evaluate the quality of sleep and his or her satisfaction or dissatisfaction with that quality.

Goal

The client will report a satisfactory balance of rest and activity.

Indicators

• Complete at least four sleep cycles (100 minutes) undisturbed.
• State factors that increase or decrease the quality of sleep.

Interventions	Rationales
1. Discuss the reasons for differing individual sleep requirements, including age, life style, activity level, and other possible factors.	1. Although many believe that a person needs 8 hours of sleep each night, no scientific evidence supports this. Individual sleep requirements vary greatly. Generally, a person who can relax and rest easily requires less sleep to feel refreshed. With age, total sleep time usually decreases—especially Stage IV sleep—and Stage I sleep increases.
2. Institute measures to promote relaxation: a. Maintain a dark, quiet environment. b. Allow the client to choose pillows, linens, and covers as appropriate. c. Provide a regular bedtime ritual. d. Ensure good room ventilation. e. Close the door, if desired.	2. Sleep is difficult without relaxation. The unfamiliar hospital environment can hinder relaxation.
3. Schedule procedures to minimize the times you need to wake the client at night. If possible, plan for at least 2-hour periods of uninterrupted sleep.	3. In order to feel rested, a person usually must complete an entire sleep cycle (70 to 100 minutes) four or five times a night.
4. Explain the need to avoid sedative and hypnotic drugs.	4. These medications begin to lose their effectiveness after a week of use, requiring increased dosages and leading to the risk of dependence.
5. Assist with usual bedtime routines as necessary, such as personal hygiene, snack, or music for relaxation.	5. A familiar bedtime ritual may promote relaxation and sleep.
6. Teach the client sleep-promoting measures: a. Eating a high-protein snack (such as cheese or milk) before bedtime b. Avoiding caffeine c. Attempting to sleep only when feeling sleepy d. Trying to maintain consistent nightly sleep habits	6. These practices may help promote sleep. a. Digested protein produces tryptophan, which has a sedative effect. b. Caffeine stimulates metabolism and deters relaxation. c. Frustration may result if the client attempts to sleep when not sleepy or relaxed. d. Irregular sleeping patterns can disrupt normal circadian rhythms, possibly leading to sleep difficulties.
7. Explain the importance of regular exercise in promoting good sleep.	7. Regular exercise not only increases endurance and enhances the ability to tolerate psychological stress, but also promotes relaxation.

Documentation

Progress notes
Reports of unsatisfactory sleep

Risk for Spiritual Distress Related to Separation from Religious Support System, Lack of Privacy, or Inability to Practice Spiritual Rituals

Focus Assessment Criteria	Clinical Significance
1. Religious beliefs and ability to worship 2. Access to religious leader or group	1,2. A client's religious beliefs and practices can be a source of comfort and strength.
3. Emotional response to inability to practice religious or spiritual rituals or separation from spiritual support system, e.g., calmness, anger, guilt, self-hatred, sadness	3. Certain religious or spiritual beliefs and practices may conflict with prevalent health-care practices and may be prohibited.

Goal

The client will maintain usual spiritual practices not detrimental to health.

Indicators

- Ask for assistance as needed.
- Relate support from staff as needed.

Interventions	Rationales
1. Explore whether the client desires to engage in an allowable religious or spiritual practice or ritual. If so, provide opportunities for him or her to do so.	1. For a client who places a high value on prayer or other spiritual practices, these practices can provide meaning and purpose and can be a source of comfort and strength.
2. Express your understanding and acceptance of the importance of the client's religious or spiritual beliefs and practices.	2. Conveying a nonjudgmental attitude may help reduce the client's uneasiness about expressing his or her belief and practices.
3. Provide privacy and quiet for spiritual rituals, as the client desires and as practicable.	3. Privacy and quiet provide an environment that enables reflection and contemplation.
4. If you wish, offer to pray with the client or read from a religious text.	4. The nurse—even one who does not subscribe to the same religious beliefs or values of the client—can still help him or her meet his or her spiritual needs.
5. Offer to contact a religious leader or hospital clergy to arrange for a visit. Explain available services, e.g., hospital chapel, Bible.	5. These measures can help the client maintain spiritual ties and practice important rituals.

(continues on page 83)

Interventions continued	Rationales continued
6. Explore whether any usual hospital practices conflict with the client's beliefs, e.g., diet, hygiene, treatments. If so, try to accommodate the client's beliefs to the extent that policy and safety allow.	6. Many religions prohibit certain behaviors; complying with restrictions may be an important part of the client's worship.

 Documentation

Progress notes
  Spiritual concerns

Interrupted Family Processes Related to Disruption of Routines, Changes in Role Responsibilities, and Fatigue Associated with Increased Workload, and Visiting Hour Requirements

Focus Assessment Criteria	Clinical Significance
1. Understanding of condition 2. Usual family coping patterns 3. Current response 4. Available resources 5. Cultural/religious beliefs	1–5. The family unit is a system based on interdependent members and patterns that provide structure and support. Hospitalization can disrupt these patterns, leading to family dysfunction.

Goal

The client and family members will verbalize feelings regarding the diagnosis and hospitalization.

Indicators

* Identify signs of family dysfunction.
* Identify appropriate resources to seek when needed.

Interventions	Rationales
1. Approach the family and attempt to create a private and supportive environment.	1. Approaching a family communicates a sense of caring and concern.
2. Provide accurate information, using simple terms.	2. Moderate or high anxiety impairs the ability to process information. Simple explanations impart useful information most effectively.
3. Explore the family members' perceptions of the situation.	3. Evaluating family members' understanding can help identify any learning needs they may have.

(continues on page 84)

Interventions continued	**Rationales** continued
4. Assess their current emotional response—guilt, anger, blame, grief—to the stresses of hospitalization.	4. A family member's response to another member's illness is influenced by the extent to which the illness interferes with his or her goal-directed activity, the significance of the goal interfered with, and the quality of the relationship.
5. Observe the dynamics of client–family interaction during visitations. Evaluate the following: a. Apparent desire for visit b. Effects of visit c. Interactions d. Physical contact	5. These observations provide information regarding family roles and interrelationships and the quality of support family members provide for each other.
6. Determine whether the family's current coping mechanism is effective.	6. Illness of a family member may necessitate significant role changes, putting a family at high risk for maladaptation.
7. Promote family strengths: a. Involve family members in caring for the client. b. Acknowledge their assistance. c. Encourage a sense of humor and perspective.	7. These measures may help maintain an existing family structure, allowing it to function as a supportive unit.
8. As appropriate, assist the family in reorganizing roles at home, resetting priorities, and reallocating responsibilities.	8. Reordering priorities may help reduce stress and maintain family integrity.
9. Warn family members to be prepared for signs of depression, anxiety, anger, and dependency in the client and other family members.	9. Anticipatory guidance can alert family members to impending problems, enabling intervention to prevent the problems from occurring.
10. Encourage and help the family to call on their social network (friends, relatives, church members) for support.	10. Adequate support can eliminate or minimize family members' feelings that they must "go it alone."
11. Emphasize the need for family members to address their own physical and psychological needs. To provide time for this, suggest measures such as these: a. Taking a break and having someone else visit the client for a change b. Calling the unit for a status report rather than traveling to the hospital every day	11. A family member who ignores his or her own needs for sleep, relaxation, or nutrition and changes his or her usual health practices for the worse impairs his or her own effectiveness as a support person.

(continues on page 85)

Interventions continued	Rationales continued
12. If the family becomes overwhelmed, help them to prioritize their duties and problems and to act accordingly.	12. Prioritizing can help a family under stress focus on and problem-solve those situations requiring immediate attention.
13. At the appropriate time, have family members list perceived problems and concerns. Then develop a plan of action to address each item.	13. Addressing each problem separately allows the family to identify resources and reduce feelings of being overwhelmed.
14. Encourage the family to continue their usual method of decision-making, including the client when appropriate.	14. Joint decision-making reduces the client's feelings of dependency and reinforces that continued support is available.
15. As possible, adjust visiting hours to accommodate family schedules.	15. This measure may help promote regular visitation, which can help maintain family integrity.

16. Identify any dysfunctional coping mechanisms:
a. Substance abuse
b. Continued denial
c. Exploitation of one or more family members
d. Separation or avoidance
e. Assess for domestic abuse/violence
 • Definition of domestic abuse/violence
  Any person who has been physically, emotionally, or sexually abused by an intimate partner or former intimate partner
  Involves infliction or threat of infliction of any bodily injury; harmful physical contact; the destruction of property or threat thereof as a method of coercion, control, revenge, or punishment
 • Subcategories of domestic abuse/violence
  Physical
  Sexual
  Harassment
  Intimidation of a dependent
  Interference with personal liberty or willful deprivation
 • High risk indicators for suspected abuse: Should you notice any of the following indicators in combination with each other, it may warrant a
	16. Families with a history of unsuccessful coping may need additional resources. Families with unresolved conflicts prior to a member's hospitalization are at high risk.

(continues on page 86)

Interventions continued	**Rationales** continued
referral to either the Medical Social Work Department (clients admitted to medical units) or Crisis Intervention.	
Physical indicators: Physician's exam reveals that the client has injuries the spouse/ intimate partner/client had not divulged Too many "unexplained" injuries or explanations inconsistent with injuries Over time, explanations for injuries become inconsistent Prolonged interval between trauma or illness and presentation for medical care Conflicting or implausible accounts regarding injuries or incidents History of MD shopping or ER shopping	
Social indicators: Age Young (chronologically or developmentally) Older Spouse/intimate partner is forced by circumstances to care for client who is unwanted Spouse/intimate partner inappropriately will not allow you to interview client alone despite explanation Client/spouse/intimate partner socially isolated or alienated Client/spouse/intimate partner demonstrates poor self-image Financial difficulties Client claims to have been abused	
Behavioral indicators: Client/spouse/intimate partner presents vague explanation regarding injuries with implausible stories Client/spouse/intimate partner is very evasive in providing explanations Client has difficulty maintaining eye contact and appears shameful about injuries Client appears very fearful, possibly trembling Client expresses ambivalence regarding relationship with spouse/ intimate partner	

(continues on page 87)

Interventions continued	Rationales continued
Client quickly blames himself/ herself for injuries Client is very passive or withdrawn Spouse/intimate partner appears "overprotective" Client appears fearful of spouse/ intimate partner Refer for counseling if necessary.	
17. Direct the family to community agencies and other sources of emotional and financial assistance, as needed.	17. Additional resources may be needed to help with management at home.
18. As appropriate, explore whether the client and family have discussed end-of-life decisions; if not, encourage them to do so.	18. Intense stress is experienced when families and health care providers are faced with decisions regarding either initiation or discontinuation of life-support systems or other medical interventions that prolong life, e.g., nasogastric tube feeding. If the client's wishes are unknown, additional conflicts arise—especially if the family disagrees with decisions made by the health care providers, or vice versa.
19. When appropriate, instruct the client or family members to provide the following information: a. Person to contact in the event of emergency b. Person whom the client trusts with personal decisions c. Decision whether to maintain life support if the client were to become mentally incompetent d. Any preference for dying at home or in the hospital e. Desire to sign a living will f. Decision on organ donation g. Funeral arrangements; burial, cremation	19. During an episode of acute illness, these discussions may not be appropriate. Clients and families should be encouraged to discuss their directions to be used to guide future clinical decisions, and their decisions should be documented. One copy should be given to the person designated as the decision-maker in the event the client becomes incapacitated or incompetent, with another copy retained in a safe deposit box and one copy on the chart.

🌐 Documentation

Progress notes
  Interactions with family
Assessment of family functioning
End-of-life decisions, if known
  Advance directive in chart

Risk for Ineffective Therapeutic Regimen Management Related to Complexity and Cost of Therapeutic Regimen, Complexity of Health Care System, Insufficient Knowledge of Treatment, and Barriers to Comprehension Secondary to Language Barriers, Cognitive Deficits, Hearing and/or Visual Impairment, Anxiety, and Lack of Motivation

Focus Assessment Criteria	Clinical Significance
1. Physical condition	1. Pain, fatigue, dyspnea, or other symptoms can interfere with client's motivation and ability to learn.

2. Sensory status
3. Intelligence and learning ability:
  a. Education
  b. Learning disabilities
  c. Language difficulties
	2,3. Impaired hearing, vision, cognition, or memory, a learning disability, or a language barrier can interfere with communication and learning. A client with any such problem needs alternative teaching techniques.

4. Anxiety level; mild, moderate, severe, panic	4. Extreme anxiety impairs a client's learning and coping abilities.
5. Specific stressors, nature of concerns	5. Every client experiences some emotional reaction to illness. The nature and degree of this reaction depends on how the client perceives his situation and its anticipated effects—physical, psychological, financial, social, occupational, and spiritual. Negative emotional reactions can interfere with motivation and ability to learn.
6. Support system: availability and quality	6. Adequate support from family, friends, and other sources can provide comfort and help maintain self-esteem. Poor support can increase stress and impair client's ability to maintain a home care regimen.

Goal

The client or primary care giver will describe disease process, causes and factors contributing to symptoms, and the regimen for disease or symptom control.

Indicators

- Relate the intent to practice health behaviors needed or desired for recovery from illness/symptom management and prevention of recurrence or complications.
- Describe signs and symptoms that need reporting.

Interventions	Rationales
1. Determine the client's knowledge of his condition, prognosis, and treatment mea-	1. Assessing the client's level of knowledge will assist in the development of an indi-

(continues on page 89)

Interventions continued	**Rationales** continued
sures. Reinforce and supplement the physician's explanations as necessary.	vidualized learning program. Providing accurate information can decrease the client's anxiety associated with the unknown and unfamiliar.
2. Identify factors that influence learning.	2. The client's ability to learn will be affected by a number of variables that need to be considered. Denial of illness, lack of financial resources, and depression may affect the client's ability and motivation to learn. Cognitive changes associated with this might influence the client's ability to learn new information.
3. Provide the client and family with information about how to utilize the health care system (billing and payment, making appointments, follow-up care, resources available, etc.).	3. Information on how to "work the system" will help the client and family to feel more comfortable and more in control of client's health care. This will positively influence compliance with the health care regimen.
4. Explain and discuss with client and family/caregiver (when possible): a. Disease process b. Treatment regimen (medications, diet, procedures, exercises, equipment use) c. Rationale for regimen d. Side effects of regimen e. Life style changes needed f. Follow-up care needed g. Signs or symptoms of complications h. Resources, support available i. Home environment alterations needed	4. Depending on client's physical and cognitive limitations, it may be necessary to provide the family/caregiver with the necessary information for managing the treatment regimen. In order to assist the client with post-discharge care, the client needs information about the disease process, treatment regimen, symptoms of complications, etc., as well as resources available for assistance.
5. Promote a positive attitude and active participation of the client and family. a. Solicit expression of feelings, concerns and questions from client and family. b. Encourage client and family to seek information and make informed decisions. c. Explain responsibilities of client/family and how these can be assumed.	5. Active participation in the treatment regimen helps the client and family feel more in control of the illness, which enhances the effective management of the therapeutic regimen.
6. Ensure that the client with visual and/or hearing impairments has glasses and a hearing aid available and uses them during teaching sessions. Provide adequate lighting and a quiet place for teaching sessions. Provide written teaching materials in the client's first language when possible.	6. Vision and hearing aids, adequate lighting, written materials in client's primary language, etc., will help to compensate for barriers to learning. Decreasing external stimuli will assist the client to correctly perceive what is being said.

(continues on page 90)

Interventions continued	Rationales continued

7. Explain that changes in life style and needed learning will take time to integrate.
  a. Provide printed material (in client's primary language when possible).
  b. Explain whom to contact with questions.
  c. Identify referrals or community services needed for follow-up.
	7. Explaining that changes are expected to take time to integrate will provide reassurance for the client that he or she does not have to make changes all at once. Support and reassurance will assist the client with compliance. Providing information about available resources also helps the client to feel supported in his or her efforts.

 Documentation

Progress notes
  Specific discharge needs and plans
Discharge instructions
  Referrals made
Multidisciplinary client education record
  Client and family teaching about disease, plan of treatment, referrals, etc.

Cardiovascular and Peripheral Vascular Disorders

CONGESTIVE HEART FAILURE

Congestive heart failure (CHF) is a syndrome that occurs when the heart cannot pump sufficient blood to meet the tissues' metabolic and oxygen needs. Symptoms vary depending on whether CHF is left-sided, right-sided, or both. Left-sided failure is caused by decreased contractile force of the left ventricle and manifests as pulmonary congestion/edema and decreased cardiac output. It can result from hypertension, myocardial ischemia/infarction, and aortic or mitral valve disease. Right-sided failure is caused by decreased right-ventricle contractile force and manifests as systemic venous congestion and peripheral edema. It can result from pulmonary disease, pericarditis, tricuspid/pulmonary stenosis, acute pulmonary embolus, or most often left-sided failure. The 6-year mortality rate is 85% for men and 67% for women (Dahl & Penque, 2000).

Time Frame
- Initial diagnosis (nonintensive care unit or intensive care unit)
- Exacerbation of chronic condition

◯◯ DIAGNOSTIC CLUSTER

Collaborative Problems	Refer to
▲ PC: Hypoxia	
△ PC: Deep Vein Thrombosis	Myocardial Infarction
△ PC: Cardiogenic Shock	Myocardial Infarction
* PC: Dysrhythmias	
* PC: Multiple Organ Failure	
PC: Hepatic Insufficiency	Cirrhosis

Nursing Diagnoses	Refer to
▲ Activity Intolerance related to insufficient oxygen for activities of daily living	Chronic Obstructive Pulmonary Disease
▲ Anxiety related to breathlessness	Chronic Obstructive Pulmonary Disease
△ Imbalanced Nutrition: Less Than Body Requirements related to nausea; anorexia secondary to venous congestion of gastrointestinal tract and fatigue	Chronic Obstructive Pulmonary Disease
△ Impaired Peripheral Tissue Perfusion related to venous congestion secondary to right-sided heart failure	Cirrhosis

(continues on page 94)

Nursing Diagnoses continued	Refer to continued
△ Disturbed Sleep Pattern related to nocturnal dyspnea and inability to assume usual sleep position	Chronic Obstructive Pulmonary Disease
△ Powerlessness related to progressive nature of condition	Chronic Obstructive Pulmonary Disease
△ High Risk for Ineffective Therapeutic Regimen Management related to lack of knowledge of low-salt diet, drug therapy (diuretic, digitalis vasodilators), activity program, signs and symptoms of complications	
* High Risk for Impaired Skin Integrity related to edema and decreased tissue perfusion	Deep Vein Thrombosis

▲ This diagnosis was reported to be monitored for or managed frequently (75%–100%).
△ This diagnosis was reported to be monitored for or managed often (50%–74%).
* This diagnosis was not included in the validation study.

Discharge Criteria

Before discharge, the client or family will

1. Describe the rationales for prescribed treatments.
2. Demonstrate the ability to count pulse rate correctly.
3. State the causes of symptoms and describe their management.
4. State the signs and symptoms that must be reported to a health care professional.

Collaborative Problems

Potential Complication: Hypoxia

Nursing Goal

The nurse will detect early signs of hypoxia and collaboratively intervene to stabilize the client.

Indicators
- Serum pH 7.35–7.45
- Serum PCO_2 35–45 mm Hg
- Regular pulse rate and rhythm (60–100 beats/minute)
- Respirations 16–20 per minute
- Blood pressure < 140/90 mm Hg, > 90/60 mm Hg
- Urine output > 30ml/hour

Interventions	Rationales

1. Monitor for signs and symptoms of hypoxia:
  a. Increased and irregular pulse rate
  b. Increased respiratory rate
  c. Decreased urine output (< 30 mL/hr)
	1. Decreased cardiac output leads to insufficient oxygenated blood to meet the tissues' metabolic needs. Decreased circulating volume/cardiac output can cause hypo-

(continues on page 95)

Interventions continued	Rationales continued

d. Changes in mentation, restlessness
   e. Cool, moist, cyanotic, mottled skin
   f. Decreased capillary refill time
	perfusion of the kidneys and decreased tissue perfusion with a compensatory response of decreased circulation to extremities and increased pulse and respiratory rates. Changes in mentation may result from cerebral hypoperfusion. Vasoconstriction and venous congestion in dependent areas (e.g., limbs) produce changes in skin and pulses.

2. Use a pulse oximeter.	2. It is an accurate, noninvasive monitor of oxygen concentrations.

3. Monitor for signs and symptoms of acute pulmonary edema:
   a. Severe dyspnea with use of accessory muscles
   b. Tachycardia
   c. Adventitious breath sounds
   d. Persistent cough
   e. Productive cough with frothy sputum
   f. Cyanosis
   g. Diaphoresis
	3. Circulatory overload can result from the reduced size of the pulmonary vascular bed. Hypoxia causes increased capillary permeability that, in turn, causes fluid to enter pulmonary tissue, producing the signs and symptoms of pulmonary edema.

4. Cautiously administer intravenous (IV) fluids. Consult with physician if the ordered rate plus the PO intake exceeds 2–2.5l/24 hr. Be sure to include additional IV fluids (e.g., antibiotics) when calculating the hourly allocation.	4. Failure to regulate IV fluids carefully can cause circulatory overload.
5. Assist client with measures to conserve strength such as resting before and after activities (e.g., meals).	5. Adequate rest reduces oxygen consumption and decreases the risk of hypoxia.

▼ Related Physician-Prescribed Interventions

Medications. Digitalis glycosides, diuretics, potassium supplements, vasodilators, morphine, angiotensin-converting enzyme (ACE) inhibitors, sympathomimetics, anticoagulants, nitrates, sedatives, aspirin (low-dose), beta blockers, serum atrial natriuretic peptides, serum brain natriuretic peptides

Intravenous Therapy. Nonsaline solutions with replacement electrolytes

Laboratory Studies. Electrolytes; blood urea nitrogen (BUN); creatinine; liver function studies (serum glutamic-oxaloacetic transaminase, lactate dehydrogenase); coagulation studies; arterial blood gas analysis; hemoglobin and hematocrit

Diagnostic Studies. Chest X-ray film, ECG, hemodynamic monitoring, transthoracic echocardiography, radionuclide ventriculography, cardiac catheterization, PAP monitoring, nuclear imaging scan, echocardiography, exercise stress testing

Therapies. Emergency protocols (cardiac shock, dysrhythmias); fluid restrictions; sodium-restricted diet; oxygen via cannula/mask; intra-aortic balloon pump; fluid removal by hemodialysis or ultrafiltration; inotropic therapy; rotating tourniquets (in extreme cases); pacemaker insertion (in selected cases); rehabilitation therapy; anti-embolism stockings

Documentation

Flow records
  Vital signs
  Intake and output
  Assessment data
Pulse oximeter
Progress notes
  Change in physiological status
  Interventions
  Client response to interventions

Nursing Diagnoses

High Risk for Ineffective Therapeutic Regimen Management Related to Insufficient Knowledge of Low-Salt Diet, Activity Program, Drug Therapy (Diuretics, Digitalis, Vasodilators), and Signs and Symptoms of Complications

Focus Assessment Criteria	Clinical Significance
Readiness and ability to learn and retain information	A client or family who does not achieve goals for learning will require a referral for assistance postdischarge.

Goal

The goals for this diagnosis represent those associated with discharge planning. Refer to discharge criteria.

Interventions	Rationales
1. Teach client and family about CHF and its causes.	1. Teaching reinforces the need to comply with prescribed treatments (diet, activity, and medications).

2. Explain the importance of nonpharmacologic interventions:
  a. Relaxation strategies
  b. Self-monitoring
  c. Exercise training
	2. Outcome studies have shown multimodal nonpharmacologic therapy to significantly improve functional capacity, body weight, and mood (Sullivan & Hawthorne, 1996).

3. Explain the need to adhere to a low-sodium (<2 gm a day) and fluid-restricted diet (2 liters a day) as prescribed. Consult with a nutritionist as necessary.	3. Excess sodium intake increases fluid retention, which in turn increases vascular volume and cardiac workload.
4. Explain the actions of prescribed medications: typically digitalis preparations, vasodilators, and diuretics. Digitalis increases the heart's stroke volume, which reduces congestion and diastolic pressure. Diuretics decrease the reabsorption of electrolytes, particularly sodium, thus	4. Such explanations can help increase client compliance and reduce errors in self-administration.

(continues on page 97)

Interventions continued	**Rationales** continued
promoting water loss. Vasodilators reduce preload and afterload, thus improving cardiac performance.	
5. Teach client how to count his or her pulse rate.	5. Pulse-taking can detect an irregular rhythm or a high (>120) or low (<60) rate, which may indicate a drug side effect or disease complication.
6. Teach client to weigh himself or herself daily and to report a gain of 3 or more lbs.	6. Daily weights can help to detect fluid retention early, enabling prompt treatment to prevent pulmonary congestion.
7. Explain the need to increase activity gradually and to rest if dyspnea and fatigue occur.	7. Regular exercise, such as walking, can improve circulation and increase cardiac stroke volume and cardiac output. Dyspnea and fatigue indicate hypoxemia resulting from overexertion.
8. Explain the effects of smoking and obesity on cardiac function. Refer client to appropriate services.	8. Nicotine is a powerful vasoconstrictor. Obesity causes compression of vessels, leading to peripheral resistance, which increases cardiac workload.
9. Instruct client and family to report the following signs and symptoms to a health care professional: a. Loss of appetite b. Visual disturbances c. Shortness of breath d. Persistent cough e. Edema in the ankles and feet f. Muscle weakness or cramping g. Chest pain h. Increased fatigue	9. Early detection and prompt intervention can reduce the risk of severe drug side effects or worsening CHF. a,b. These are common side effects of digitalis. c,d. These indicate worsening CHF. e. Edema indicates circulatory overload secondary to decreased cardiac output. f. These may indicate hypokalemia secondary to increased potassium excretion from diuretic therapy. g,h. These indicate worsening CHF.
10. Provide information about or initiate referrals to community resources (e.g., American Heart Association, home health agencies).	10. They may provide client and family with needed assistance in home management and self-care.

Documentation

Discharge summary record
  Client teaching
  Outcome achievement or status
  Referrals if indicated

For critical paths on CHF, visit http://connection.lww.com.

DEEP VENOUS THROMBOSIS

Deep vein thrombosis (DVT) is a clot in the deep veins of the legs or pelvis. Predisposing causes are Virchow's triad (venous statis, hypercoagulability, endothelial injury with inflammation to the vessel lining), antithrombin III deficiency, protein S and protein C deficiency, dysfibrinogenemia, thrombocytosis, systemic lupus erythematosus, and polycythemia vera (Eftychiou, 1996). Risk factors include prolonged immobility, debilitating chronic disease (e.g., cancer, CHF), pelvic or lower-extremity surgery, obesity, oral contraceptive use, and varicose veins (Eftychiou, 1996).

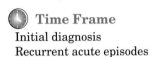 Time Frame

Initial diagnosis
Recurrent acute episodes

DIAGNOSTIC CLUSTER	
Collaborative Problems	**Refer to**
▲ PC: Pulmonary Embolism	
▲ PC: Chronic Leg Edema	
Nursing Diagnoses	**Refer to**
▲ Pain related to impaired circulation	
▲ High Risk for Impaired Skin Integrity related to chronic ankle edema	
△ High Risk for Ineffective Therapeutic Regimen Management related to lack of knowledge of prevention of recurrence of deep vein thrombosis and signs and symptoms of complications	
△ High Risk for Ineffective Respiratory Function related to immobility	Immobility or Unconsciousness
△ High Risk for Constipation related to decreased peristalsis secondary to immobility	Immobility or Unconsciousness

▲ This diagnosis was reported to be monitored for or managed frequently (75%–100%).
△ This diagnosis was reported to be monitored for or managed often (50%–74%).

Related Care Plan

Anticoagulant Therapy

Discharge Criteria

Before discharge, the client or family will do the following:

1. Identify factors that contribute to thrombosis recurrence.
2. Relate the signs and symptoms that must be reported to a health care professional.
3. Verbalize intent to implement life style changes.

Collaborative Problems

Potential Complication: Pulmonary Embolism

Potential Complication: Chronic Leg Edema

Nursing Goal

The nurse will detect early signs/symptoms of pulmonary embolism and vascular alterations and collaboratively manage to stabilize the client.

Indicators
- No chest pain
- Respirations 16–20 beats/min
- Clear breath sounds
- Heart rate 60–100 breaths/min
- Temperature 98–99.5°F
- Normal sinus rhythm

Interventions	Rationales
1. Monitor respiratory function.	1. Assessment should establish a baseline for subsequent comparisons to detect any changes.
2. If the client is on anticoagulant therapy, monitor prothrombin time (PT) with ratio (INR), partial thromboplastin time (APTT), and platelets.	2. Anticoagulant therapy can cause thrombocytopenia. PT and APTT values greater than two times normal (control) can produce bleeding and hemorrhage.
3. Instruct client to maintain strict bed rest with the legs elevated above the heart.	3. The recumbent position promotes venous drainage.
4. Explain the rationale for anticoagulant therapy and for immobilization.	4. The client's understanding of the need for treatments may improve compliance.
5. Avoid massaging the affected extremity.	5. Massage may dislodge the clot.
6. Instruct the client to report (and save) any pink-tinged sputum.	6. Blood-tinged sputum may indicate pulmonary bleeding.
7. Monitor for signs and symptoms of pulmonary embolism (Eftychiou, 1996):	7. a,b. The clot causes obstruction with increased resistance to pulmonary

(continues on page 100)

Interventions continued	**Rationales** continued
a. Symptoms • Dyspnea • Pleuritic chest pain • Anxiety/apprehension • Cough • Hemoptysis • Diaphoresis b. Signs • Tachypnea (>16 breaths/min) • Tachycardia (>100 beats/min) • Fever (>99.5, deg.F) • Crackles, wheezes, ↓BS • Accentuated S_2 and P_2 heart sounds • Thrombophlebitis	blood flow, which can progress to right ventricular failure. These effects produce hypoxia with a tachypnea response. The local obstruction produces an inflammatory response (e.g., cough, fever, pain, diaphoresis) (Eftychiou, 1996).
8. Instruct client to report any change in breathing or sudden feelings of apprehension immediately.	8. Early reporting enables prompt evaluation and treatment.
9. Monitor leg edema, pain, and inflammation. Measure leg circumference 10 cm below and above knee. Report any increases immediately.	9. These measures help to track the progression of the clot and inflammation (Caswell, 1993).
10. If you suspect an increase in the thrombosis, consult physician or nurse practitioner for a venous Doppler examination done by the vascular laboratory.	10. Propagation of a thrombosis from the calf to the thigh increases the risk of a pulmonary embolus; Doppler exam can detect thrombosis propagation.
11. Prepare client for insertion of a vena caval filter if thrombosis continues to propagate during heparin therapy.	11. Occasionally a venous thrombosis continues to propagate despite heparin therapy, e.g., if a malignancy alters the clotting mechanism. The only way to prevent the clot from traversing the vena cava to the lungs is to provide a mechanical barrier such as a vena cava filter (Caswell, 1993).
12. Refer to anticoagulant care plan. If elastic support stockings are ordered, remove and reapply every 8 hours. Inspect skin during changes.	12. Compression stockings promote venous return and reduce chronic leg edema (Byrne, 2002).

▼ Related Physician-Prescribed Interventions

Medications. Warfarin, analgesics, antipyretics, low-molecular weight heparin

Intravenous Therapy. Continuous or intermittent intravenous

Laboratory Studies. CBC, cardiac isoenzymes, INR, arterial blood gases, PT/APPT, SMA7

Diagnostic Studies. Ultrasound; noninvasive vascular studies (Doppler, oscillometry, plethysmography); ventilation/scan perfusion (V/Q scan); contrast venography; chest X-ray; ECG

Therapies. Compression stockings, elastic support hose, moist heat

🔖 Documentation

Flow records
    Position in bed and activity restrictions
    Leg measurements and changes in measurement, color, or pain
Progress notes
    Client teaching

Nursing Diagnoses

Pain Related to Impaired Circulation

Focus Assessment Criteria	Clinical Significance

1. Pain
    a. Description
    b. Location
    c. Duration
    d. Intensity (0 -10)
    e. Aggravating factors
    f. Alleviating factors
    g. Accompanying signs and symptoms
	1. Baseline assessment of pain enables evaluation of the client's response to pain relief measures.

Goal

The client will report a decrease in pain after pain relief measures.

Indicators

- Report factors that increase pain.
- Demonstrates a relaxed mode.

Interventions	Rationales
1. Elevate the affected leg higher than the heart.	1. Venous pain usually is aggravated with leg in the dependent position and is slightly relieved with the leg elevated to promote venous return.

2. Explain the need to avoid
    a. Aspirin
    b. Medications containing aspirin, e.g., Bismuth, Pepto-Bismol, Alka-Seltzer, some cold and allergy remedies
    c. Nonsteroidal anti-inflammatory medications, e.g., Advil, Midol, Motrin, Indocin, Feldene
	2. These products interfere with plasma platelet coagulation (Kelsey, 1993).

3. Refer to the General Surgery care plan, Appendix II, for additional interventions for pain.	

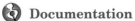 **Documentation**

Medication administration record
  Type, route, dosage of all medications
Progress notes
  Response to pain relief measures

High Risk for Impaired Skin Integrity Related to Chronic Ankle Edema

Focus Assessment Criteria	Clinical Significance
1. Client's understanding of DVT and sequela	1. The client's understanding of possible complications may encourage compliance with restrictions and exercises.
2. Condition of skin on ankles	2. Baseline assessment enables detection of any changes in status.

Goal

The client will demonstrate intact skin integrity.

Indicators

• Explain rationale for interventions.
• Demonstrate no erythema, blanching, or ulceration.

Interventions	Rationales
1. Teach client about the vulnerability of the skin on the ankles to the effects of chronic venous insufficiency.	1. Postphlebitic syndrome, caused by incompetent valves in deep veins, results in edema, altered pigmentation, and stasis dermatitis.
2. Teach client to avoid situations that impede leg circulation (e.g., sitting for long periods).	2. Impeded leg circulation can promote recurrence of DVT.
3. Teach client to perform leg exercises every hour, when possible.	3. Leg exercises promote the muscle pumping effect on the deep veins, which improves venous return.
4. If ankle edema occurs, encourage the use of elastic stockings for support.	4. Elastic stockings reduce venous pooling by exerting even pressure over the leg and increase flow to deeper veins by reducing the caliber of the superficial veins.
5. Teach the client to report any ankle injury or lesion immediately.	5. Decreased circulation can cause a minor injury to become serious.
6. Instruct client to report history of thrombosis at all future hospitalizations.	6. A high-risk client should alert nursing and medical staff so preventive measures can be initiated.

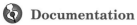 **Documentation**

Flow record
    Present condition of ankles
    Client teaching
    Client's response to teaching

High Risk for Ineffective Therapeutic Regimen Management Related to Lack of Knowledge of Prevention of Recurrence of Deep Vein Thrombosis and Signs and Symptoms of Complications

Focus Assessment Criteria	Clinical Significance
1. Knowledge of the pathology of DVT and preventive measures	1. This assessment guides client and family teaching.
2. Readiness and ability to retain information	2. A client or family who does not achieve goals for learning requires a referral for assistance postdischarge.

Goal

The goals for this diagnosis represent those associated with discharge planning. Refer to the discharge criteria.

Interventions	Rationales

1. Explain relevant venous anatomy and physiology including
  a. Leg vein anatomy
  b. Function of venous valves
  c. Importance of muscle pumping action
	1,2. This teaching helps reinforce the need to comply with instructions (restrictions, exercises).

2. Teach the pathophysiology of DVT including
  a. Effect of thrombosis on valves
  b. Hydrostatic pressure in venous system
  c. Pressure transmitted to capillary system
  d. Pressure in subcutaneous tissue	

3. Teach preventive measures:
 	
  a. Initiating a regular exercise program (e.g., walking or swimming)
  b. Avoiding immobility
  c. Elevating the legs whenever possible
 	
  d. Using elastic support stockings (*Note:* These stockings should be checked by a health care professional to ensure proper fit.)
	3. These measures can help to prevent subsequent episodes of DVT.
	  a. Exercise increases muscle tone and promotes the pumping effect on veins.
	  b. Immobility increases venous stasis.
	  c. Elevation reduces venous pooling and promotes venous return.
	  d. The use of over-the-counter support stockings is controversial; improperly fitted stockings may produce a tourniquet effect.

(continues on page 104)

Interventions continued	Rationales continued
e. Using extra means of support if exposed to additional risk, e.g., ace wraps or compression pump if prolonged immobility is necessary	e. External elastic compression or a compression pump can provide the external pressure during a long period of immobility and help to prevent venous pooling.
4. If the client is being discharged on anticoagulant therapy, refer to the Anticoagulant Therapy care plan for more information.	4. Low-dose heparin therapy has been shown to be of value by preventing DVT in clients for whom it is not contraindicated.
5. Explain the need to do the following: a. Maintain a fluid intake of 2,500 mL a day unless contraindicated. b. Stop smoking. c. Maintain ideal weight. d. Avoid garters, girdles, and knee-high over-the-counter (OTC) stockings.	5. These practices help to decrease risk of recurrence (Caswell, 1993). a. Adequate hydration prevents increased blood viscosity. b. Nicotine is a potent vasoconstrictor. c. Obesity increases compression of vessels and causes hypercoagulability. d. Garters, girdles, and knee-high stockings constrict vessels, causing venous pooling.
6. Teach the client and family to watch for and promptly report these symptoms: a. Diminished sensation in legs or feet b. Coldness or bluish color in legs or feet c. Increased swelling or pain in legs or feet d. Sudden chest pain or dyspnea	6. Early detection enables prompt intervention to prevent serious complications. a,b,c. These changes in the legs and feet may point to an extension of the clot with resulting compromised circulation and inflammation. d. Sudden chest pain or dyspnea may indicate a pulmonary embolism.
7. Instruct client and family to advise health care providers of the history of deep vein thrombosis (DVT), e.g., before surgery.	7. Persons with previous DVT are at four times greater risk for developing new DVT (Carroll, 1993).
8. Explain post thrombotic syndrome a. Pain, fatigue b. Heaviness in leg c. Pigmentation d. Spider veins e. Ulceration f. Edema of leg	8. Post thrombotic syndrome refers to persistent symptoms after the acute episode. These symptoms can persist for 2 to 5 years (New options for deep vein thrombosis, 1998).

 Documentation

Discharge summary record
   Client teaching
   Outcome achievement or status

HYPERTENSION

The Joint National Committee on Detection, evaluation and Treatment of High Blood Pressure (JNC, 1997) has classified the disease into four stages:

Blood pressure for adults 18 years of age and older:

Normal: Systolic, <130 mm Hg
             Diastolic, <85 mm Hg
Abnormal: Systolic, 130 to 139 mm Hg
             Diastolic, 85 to 89 mm Hg
Stage 1:   Systolic, 140 to 159 mm Hg
             Diastolic, 90 to 99 mm Hg
Stage 2:   Systolic, 160 to 179 mm Hg
             Diastolic, 100 to 109 mm Hg
Stage 3:   Systolic, 180 or greater
             Diastolic, 100 or greater

Hypertension is the major cause of coronary heart disease, cerebrovascular accident, and renal failure. Sustained hypertension and accompanying increased peripheral resistance cause a disruption in the vascular endothelium, forcing plasma and lipoproteins into the vessel's intimal and subintimal layers and causing plaque formation (atherosclerosis). Increased pressure also causes hyperplasia of smooth muscle, which scars the intima and results in thickened vessels with narrowed lumina (Woods, Sivarajan, Froelicher & Motzer, 2000). Elevated systemic blood pressure increases the work of the left ventricle, leading to hypertrophy and increased myocardial oxygen demand (Copestead, 1995).

 Time Frame

Initial diagnosis

 DIAGNOSTIC CLUSTER*

Collaborative Problems

- Potential Complication: Vascular Insufficiency

Nursing Diagnoses

- High Risk for Noncompliance related to negative side effects of prescribed therapy versus the belief that treatment is not needed without the presence of symptoms
- High Risk for Ineffective Therapeutic Regimen Management related to lack of knowledge of condition, diet restrictions, medications, risk factors, and follow-up care

---

* This medical condition was not included in the validation study.

Discharge Criteria

Before discharge, the client will

1. Demonstrate blood pressure self-measurement.
2. Identify risk factors for hypertension.
3. Explain the action, dosage, side effects, and precautions for all prescribed medications.
4. Verbalize dietary factors associated with hypertension.

5. Relate an intent to comply with life style changes and prescriptions postdischarge.
6. Describe the signs and symptoms that must be reported to a health care professional.

Collaborative Problems

Potential Complication: Vascular Insufficiency

Nursing Goal

The nurse will detect early signs and symptoms of vascular insufficiency and collaboratively intervene to stabilize client.

Indicators
- No new visual defects
- Oriented
- Equal strength upper/lower extremities
- Serum protein

Interventions	Rationales
1. Monitor for evidence of tissue ischemia:	1. Hypertension adversely affects the entire cardiovascular system. Chronic increases in perfusion pressure result in hypertrophy of vascular smooth muscle and increased collagen concentration. The changes reduce the size of the lumen of the vessel, changes in vessel's shape and cyclospasm of the vessel cells. The results are plaque formation from increased adherence of monocytes to the endothelium. The increase in the wall to lumen ratio in the arteries causes greater vessel resistance and a reduced ability to dilate in response to increased metabolic need for oxygen (Porth, 2002).
a. Visual defects including blurring, spots, and loss of visual acuity	a. Evidence of blood vessel damage in the retina indicates similar damage elsewhere in the vascular system
b. Cerebrovascular deficits • Orientation or memory deficits • Weakness • Paralysis • Mobility, speech, or sensory deficits	b. In the brain, sustained hypertension causes progressive cerebral arteriosclerosis and ischemia. Interruption of cerebral blood supply caused by cerebral artery occlusion or rupture results in sensory and motor deficits.
c. Renal insufficiency • Decreased serum protein level • Sustained elevated urine specific gravity • Elevated urine sodium levels • Sustained insufficient urine output (<30 mL/hr) • Increased BUN, serum creatinine, potassium, phosphorus, and ammonia levels; decreased creatinine clearance	c. With decreased blood supply to the nephrons, the kidney loses some ability to concentrate and form normal urine. (Porth, 2002) • Further structural abnormalities may cause the vessels to become more permeable and allow leakage of protein into the renal tubules. • Decreased ability of the renal tubules to reabsorb electrolytes causes increased urine sodium levels and increased urine specific gravity.

(continues on page 107)

Interventions continued	Rationales continued
	• Decreased glomerular filtration rate eventually causes insufficient urine output and stimulates renin production, which results in increased blood pressure in an attempt to increase blood flow to the kidneys. • Decreased renal function impairs the excretion of urea and creatinine in the urine, thus elevating BUN and creatinine levels.
d. Cardiac insufficiency • Substernal discomfort	d. Microvascular coronary atherosclerotic plaques or vasospasm reduce the caliber of vessel and its ability to oxygenate tissue (Porth, 2002).

 Related Physician-Prescribed Interventions

Medications. Diuretics, calcium-channel blockers, beta-adrenergic inhibitors, adrenergic inhibitors, angiotensin II receptor blockers, vasodilators, angiotensin-converting enzyme inhibitors, lipid-lowering agents

Intravenous Therapy. Not indicated

Laboratory Studies. Hemoglobin/hematocrit, serum cholesterol, triglycerides; thyroid studies; urinalysis, BUN/creatinine clearance; 24-hr urine for vanillylmandelic acid (VMA), catecholamine; aldosterone (serum, urine); uric acid; serum glucose/fasting; urine steroids; serum potassium, calcium

Diagnostic Studies. ECG, chest X-ray film, renal scan

Therapies. Sodium-restricted diet, decreased fat diet

Documentation

Graphic/flow record
  Vital signs
  Intake and output
  Laboratory values
Progress notes
  Status of client
  Unusual events
  Changes in behavior

Nursing Diagnoses

High Risk for Noncompliance Related to Negative Side Effects of Prescribed Therapy Versus the Belief that Treatment is not Needed Without the Presence of Symptoms

Focus Assessment Criteria	Clinical Significance
Client's perception of hypertension	The client's understanding of the seriousness of hypertension is critical to compliance. Compliance should be viewed on a continuum rather than as separate states of compliance or noncompliance (Blevins & Lubkin, 1995).

Goal

The client will

1. Verbalize feelings related to following the prescribed regimen.
2. Identify sources of support for assisting with compliance.
3. Verbalize the potential complications of noncompliance.

Interventions	Rationales

1. Identify any factors that may predict client noncompliance such as these:
  a. Lack of knowledge
  b. Noncompliance in the hospital
  c. Failure to perceive the seriousness or chronicity of hypertension
  d. Belief that the condition will go away
  e. Belief that the condition is hopeless
	1. Estimates are that 40% to 50% of clients with hypertension withdraw from treatment programs within the first year. Identifying any barriers to compliance enables the nurse to plan interventions to eliminate these problems and improve compliance (Miller, Wikoff & Hiatt, 1992).

2. Emphasize to the client the potentially life-threatening consequences of noncompliance. (Refer to Collaborative Problems for more information.)	2. This emphasis may encourage the client to comply with treatment by pointing out the seriousness of hypertension.
3. Point out that blood pressure elevation typically produces no symptoms.	3. Absence of symptoms often encourages noncompliance.
4. Discuss the likely effects of a future stroke, renal failure, or coronary disease on significant others (spouse, children, grandchildren)	4. This discussion may encourage compliance by emphasizing the potential impact of the client's hypertension on his significant others.
5. Include the client's significant others in teaching sessions whenever possible.	5. Significant others also should understand the possible consequences of noncompliance; this encourages them to assist the client to comply with treatment (Miller et al., 1992).
6. Emphasize to the client that ultimately it is his or her choice whether or not to comply with the treatment plan.	6. Helping the client to understand that he or she is responsible for compliance may enhance the client's sense of control and self-determination; this may help to improve compliance.
7. Instruct the client to check or have someone else check his blood pressure at least once a week and to keep an accurate record of readings.	7. Weekly blood pressure readings are needed to evaluate the client's response to treatments and life-style changes.

(continues on page 109)

Interventions continued	Rationales continued
8. Explain the possible side effects of anti-hypertensive medications (e.g., impotence, decreased libido, vertigo); instruct the client to consult the physician for alternative medications should these side effects occur.	8. A client who experiences these side effects may be tempted to discontinue medication therapy on his own.
9. If the cost of antihypertensive medications is a burden for the client, consult with social services.	9. The client may require financial assistance to prevent noncompliance due to financial reasons.

 Documentation
Discharge summary record
    Client teaching
    Response to interventions

High Risk for Ineffective Therapeutic Regimen Management Related to Lack of Knowledge of Condition, Diet Restrictions, Medications, Risk Factors, and Follow-up Care

Focus Assessment Criteria	Clinical Significance
1. Client's ability and readiness to retain information	1. A client or family who does not achieve learning goals requires a referral for assistance postdischarge.

Goal

The goals for this diagnosis represent those associated with discharge planning. Refer to discharge criteria.

Interventions	Rationales

1. Discuss blood pressure concepts using terminology the client and significant other(s) can understand:
  a. Normal values
  b. Effects of sustained high blood pressure on the brain, heart, kidneys, and eyes
  c. Control versus cure
	1. Risk of stroke rises directly with a person's blood pressure (both systolic and diastolic). The reported decline in strokes coincides with the aggressive treatment and effective control of hypertension during the past several years (American Heart Association, 1989).

2. Teach the client blood pressure self-measurement, or teach significant other(s) how to measure the client's blood pressure.	2. Self-monitoring is more convenient and may improve compliance.

(continues on page 110)

Interventions continued	**Rationales** continued
3. Discuss life-style modifications that can reduce hypertension (National High Blood Pressure Education Program [NHBPEP], 1997).	3. Life-style modifications have proved to eliminate hypertension in some persons without the use of medications (NHBPEP, 1997).
a. Achieve weight loss to within 10% of ideal weight.	a. Obesity increases peripheral resistance and cardiac workload that raise blood pressure (Cunningham, 1992).
b. Limit alcohol intake daily (2 oz liquor, 8 oz wine, or 24 oz beer).	b. Alcohol is a vasodilator causing rebound vasoconstriction that has been associated with increased blood pressure (Cunningham, 1992).
c. Engage in regular exercise (30–45 minutes) three to five times a week.	c. Regular exercise increases peripheral blood flow and muscle and cardiac efficiency. The results are a more effective cardiovascular system (NHBPEP, 1997).
d. Reduce sodium intake to 4.6 g of sodium chloride.	d. Sodium controls water distribution throughout the body. An increase in sodium causes an increase in water, thus increasing circulating volume and raising blood pressure. (Muntzel & Drueke, 1992).
e. Stop smoking.	e. Tobacco acts as a vasoconstrictor, which raises blood pressure (Cunningham, 1992).
f. Reduce saturated fat and cholesterol to <30% of dietary intake.	f. A high-fat diet contributes to plaque formation and narrowing vessels (Cunningham, 1992).
g. Ensure the daily allowance of calcium, potassium, and magnesium in diet.	g. These elements maintain the cardiovascular and muscular systems.

4. Provide client or significant other(s) with medication guidelines and drug information cards for all prescribed medications. Explain the following:
   a. Dosage
   b. Action
   c. Side effects
   d. Precautions
	4. This teaching conveys to the client which side effects should be reported and precautions that should be taken.

5. Alert client and significant other(s) to OTC medications that are contraindicated such as these:
   a. High-sodium medications (Maalox, Bromoseltzer, Rolaids)
   b. Decongestants, e.g., Vicks Formula 44
   c. Laxatives, e.g., Phospho-soda
	5. OTC medications commonly are viewed as harmless, when in fact many can cause complications.
	   a. High-sodium content medications promote water retention.
	   b. Decongestants act as vasoconstrictors that raise blood pressure.
	   c. Some laxatives contain high levels of sodium.

6. Stress the importance of follow-up care.	6. Follow-up care can help to detect complications.

(continues on page 111)

Interventions continued	Rationales continued

7. Teach the client and significant other(s) to report these symptoms:
  a. Headaches, especially on awakening
  b. Chest pain
  c. Shortness of breath
  d. Weight gain or edema
  e. Changes in vision
  f. Frequent nosebleeds
  g. Side effects of medications
	7. These signs and symptoms may indicate elevated blood pressure or other cardio-vascular complications.

 Documentation

Discharge summary record
  Status of goal attainment
  Status at discharge
  Discharge instructions
  Referrals

MYOCARDIAL INFARCTION

Myocardial infarction (MI) is the death of myocardial tissue resulting from impaired myocardial coronary blood flow. The cause of inadequate blood flow most commonly is narrowing or occlusion of the coronary artery resulting from atherosclerosis or decreased coronary blood flow from shock or hemorrhage.

Time Frame
Initial diagnosis
Postintensive care
Recurrent episodes

DIAGNOSTIC CLUSTER

Collaborative Problems

▲ PC: Dysrhythmias
▲ PC: Cardiogenic Shock
▲ PC: Congestive Heart Failure
▲ PC: Thromboembolism
▲ PC: Recurrent Myocardial Infarction
* PC: Pericarditis
* PC: Pericardial Tamponade/Rupture
* PC: Structural Defects
* PC: Extension of Infarct

Nursing Diagnoses

▲ Anxiety/Fear (individual, family) related to unfamiliar situation status, unpredictable nature of condition, negative effect on life style, fear of death, possible sexual dysfunction
▲ Pain related to cardiac tissue ischemia or inflammation
▲ Activity Intolerance related to insufficient oxygenation for activities of daily living (ADLs) secondary to cardiac tissue ischemia, prolonged immobility, narcotics or medications
△ Grieving related to actual or perceived losses secondary to cardiac condition
△ High Risk for Ineffective Therapeutic Regimen Management related to lack of knowledge of hospital routines, procedures, equipment, treatments, conditions, medications, diet, activity progression, signs and symptoms of complications, reduction of risks, follow-up care, community resources

---

▲ This diagnosis was reported to be monitored for or managed frequently (75%–100%).
△ This diagnosis was reported to be monitored for or managed often (50%–74%).
* This diagnosis was not included in the validation study.

Discharge Criteria

Before discharge, the client or family will

1. State the cause of cardiac pain and the rationales for medication therapy and activity and dietary restrictions.
2. Demonstrate accuracy in taking pulse.
3. Identify modifiable personal risk factors.
4. Describe at-home activity restrictions.

5. Describe self-administration of daily and PRN medications.
6. Describe signs and symptoms that must be reported to a health care professional.
7. Verbalize the follow-up care needed and the community resources available.
8. Describe appropriate actions to take in the event of problems.

Collaborative Problems

Potential Complication: Dysrhythmias

Potential Complication: Cardiogenic Shock

Potential Complication: CHF

Potential Complication: Thromboembolism

Potential Complication: Recurrent MI

Potential Complication: Pericarditis

Potential Complication: Pericardial Tamponade/Rupture

Potential Complication: Structural Defects

Nursing Goal

The nurse will detect for early signs and symptoms of cardiac and vascular alterations and collaboratively intervene to stabilize the client.

Indicators

- Oxygen saturation >95% (pulse oximeter)
- Normal sinus rhythm
- No life-threatening dysrhythmias
- No chest pain
- Pulse: regular rhythm, rate 60–100 beats/min
- Respirations 16–20 breaths/min
- Blood pressure > 90/60, < 140/90 mm Hg
- Urine output > 30 ml/hour
- Serum pH 7.35–7.45
- Serum PCO_2 35–45 mm Hg

Interventions	Rationales
1. Per protocol, initiate pharmacologic reperfusion therapy (e.g., thrombolytics).	1. These agents restore full blood flow through the blocked artery.
2. Maintain continuous EKG, BIP, and pulse oximetry monitoring. Report changes.	2. Continuous monitoring allows for early detection of complications.
3. Administer medications as indicated and continue to monitor for side effects. Consult pharmaceutical reference for specifics.	3. Multiple classes of medications (e.g., nitrates, beta blockers, analgesics) are used.
4. Monitor for signs and symptoms of dysrhythmias:	4. Myocardial ischemia results from reduced oxygen to myocardial tissue. Ischemic

(continues on page 114)

Interventions continued	**Rationales** continued
a. Abnormal rate, rhythm b. Palpitations, syncope c. Hemodynamic compromise (i.e., hypotension) d. Cardiac emergencies (arrest, ventricular fibrillation)	tissue is electrically unstable causing dysrhythmias, such as premature ventricular contractions, that can lead to ventricular fibrillation and death. Dysrhythmias can result from reperfusion of ischemic tissue secondary to thrombolytics.
5. Maintain oxygen therapy as prescribed. Evaluate pulse oximeter readings.	5. Supplemental oxygen therapy increases the circulating oxygen available to myocardial tissue. Pulse oximeter readings should be >95%.
6. Monitor for signs and symptoms of cardiogenic shock: a. Tachycardia b. Urine output <30 mL/hr c. Restlessness, agitation, change in mentation d. Tachypnea e. Diminished peripheral pulses f. Cool, pale, or cyanotic skin g. MAP <60 mm Hg h. Cardiac index <2.0 L i. Increased systemic vascular resistance	6. Cardiogenic shock results most often from loss of viable myocardium and impaired contractility. This manifests as decreased stroke volume and cardiac output. The compensatory response to decreased circulatory volume aims to increase blood oxygen levels by increasing heart and respiratory rates and to decrease circulation to extremities (marked by decreased pulses and cool skin). Diminished oxygen to the brain causes changes in mentation.
7. Monitor for signs and symptoms of CHF and decreased cardiac output: a. Gradual increase in heart rate b. Increased shortness of breath c. Adventitious breath sounds d. Decreased systolic blood pressure e. Presence of or increase in S_3 or S_4 gallop f. Peripheral edema g. Distended neck veins	7. Myocardial ischemia causes CHF. Ischemia reduces the ability of the left ventricle to eject blood, thus decreasing cardiac output and increasing pulmonary vascular congestion. Fluid enters pulmonary tissue causing rales, productive cough, cyanosis, and possibly signs and symptoms of respiratory distress.
8. Monitor for signs and symptoms of thromboembolism: a. Diminished or no peripheral pulses b. Unusual warmth/redness or cyanosis/coolness c. Leg pain localized to calf area	8. Prolonged bed rest, increased blood viscosity and coagulability, and decreased cardiac output contribute to thrombus formation. a. Insufficient circulation causes pain and diminished peripheral pulse. b. Unusual warmth and redness point to inflammation; coolness and cyanosis indicate vascular obstruction. c. Leg pain results from tissue hypoxia.

(continues on page 115)

Interventions continued	Rationales continued
d. Sudden severe chest pain, increased dyspnea e. Positive Homans' sign	d. Obstruction to pulmonary circulation causes sudden chest pain and dyspnea. e. In a positive Homans' sign, dorsiflexion of the foot causes pain as a result of insufficient circulation.

9. Monitor for signs and symptoms of pericarditis:
  a. Chest pain influenced by change in respiration or position
  b. Pericardial rub
  c. Temperature elevation >101°
  d. Diffuse ST segment electrocardiogram (ECG) changes
	9. Pericarditis is inflammation of the pericardial sac. Damage to the epicardium causes it to become rough, which tends to irritate and inflame the pericardium.

10. Monitor for signs and symptoms of pericardial tamponade/cardiac rupture:
  a. Hypotension
  b. Distended neck veins
  c. Tachycardia
  d. Pulsus paradoxus
  e. Equalization of cardiac pressures
  f. Narrowed pulse pressure
  g. Muffled heart tones
  h. Electrical alternans
	10. Cardiac tamponade results from accumulation of fluid in the pericardial space, causing impaired cardiac function and decreased cardiac output. Cardiac rupture occurs most often from 3 to 10 days after MI, resulting from leukocyte scavenger cells removing necrotic debris, which thins the myocardial wall. The onset is sudden with bleeding into the pericardial sac (Dahlen & Roberts, 1996).

11. Monitor for signs and symptoms of structural defects:
  a. Severe chest pain
  b. Syncope
  c. Hypotension
  d. Loud holosystolic murmur
  e. CHF
  f. Left-to-right shunt
	11. Ventricular aneurysm, ventricular septal defect, and papillary muscle rupture all result from ischemia or necrosis to the structures.

12. Monitor for signs and symptoms of recurrent MI:
  a. Classic symptoms: Sudden, severe chest pain with nausea/vomiting and diaphoresis; pain may or may not radiate
  b. Increased dyspnea
  c. Increased ST elevation and abnormal Q waves on ECG
	12. These signs and symptoms indicate myocardial tissue deterioration with increasing hypoxia.

13. Apply below-knee antiembolic stockings. 14. Progressive activity after chest pain is controlled; involve client in cardiac rehabilitation.	13,14. These measures actively promote venous return.

Related Physician-Prescribed Interventions

Medications. Vasodilators, antianginals, antidysrhythmics, beta-blockers, stool softeners, angiotensin-converting enzyme (ACE) inhibitors, anticoagulants, analgesics, diuretics, sedatives/hypnotics, thrombolytics, inotropic therapy (selected cases), nitrates, aspirin, antiplatelets

Intravenous Therapy. IV access for medication administration, IV access for blood sampling

Laboratory Studies. Arterial blood gas analysis, electrolytes, cholesterol, white blood count, tri-glycerides, sedimentation rate, coagulation studies, chemistry profile, creatinine kinase, MB isoenzyme, troponin I, troponin T, myoglobin, CK-MB isoforms

Diagnostic Studies. ECG, stress test, chest X-ray film, cardiac catheterization, echocardiogram, digital subtraction angiography, nuclear imaging studies, thallium scans, magnetic resonance imaging, thoracic electrical bioimpedance (IEB), SvO_2 monitoring, hemodynamic monitoring

Therapies. Oxygen via cannula; pacemaker insertion (selected cases); therapeutic diet (low-salt, low-saturated fats, low-cholesterol); cardiac rehabilitation program; pulse oximetry

Interventional Therapies. Percutaneous transluminal coronary angioplasty, intracoronary stents, atherectomy, intra-aortic balloon pump

Documentation

Graphic/flow record
 Vital signs
 Intake and output
 Rhythm strips
Progress notes
 Status of client
 Unusual events

Nursing Diagnoses

Anxiety/Fear (individual, family) Related to Unfamiliar Situation, Unpredictable Nature of Condition, Fear of Death, Negative Effects on Life Style, or Possible Sexual Dysfunctions

Focus Assessment Criteria	Clinical Significance
1. Anxiety level	1,2. All people experience some type of emotional reaction post-MI. Perception of the effects of MI (financial, physical, psychological, spiritual, and social) determine the nature and extent of the reaction.
2. Present coping response (client and family): a. Denial b. Anger c. Depression d. Guilt	

Goal

The client or family will relate increased psychological and physiologic comfort.

Indicators
- Verbalize fears related to the disorder.
- Share concerns about the disorder's effects on normal functioning, role responsibilities, and life style.
- Use one relaxation technique.

Interventions	Rationales

1. Assist client to reduce anxiety:
  a. Provide reassurance and comfort.
  b. Convey understanding and empathy. Do not avoid questions.
  c. Encourage client to verbalize any fears and concerns regarding MI and its treatment.
  d. Identify and support effective coping mechanisms.
	1. An anxious client has a narrowed perceptual field and diminished ability to learn. He or she may experience symptoms caused by increased muscle tension and disrupted sleep patterns. Anxiety tends to feed on itself, trapping the client in a spiral of increasing anxiety, tension, and emotional and physical pain.

2. Assess client's anxiety level. Plan teaching when level is low or moderate.	2. Some fears are based on inaccuracies; accurate information can relieve them. A client with severe or panic anxiety does not retain learning.
3. Encourage family and friends to verbalize fears and concerns.	3. Verbalization allows sharing and provides the nurse with an opportunity to correct misconceptions.
4. Provide client and family valid reassurance; reinforce positive coping behavior.	4. Praising effective coping can reinforce future positive coping responses.
5. Encourage client to use relaxation techniques such as guided imagery and relaxation breathing.	5. They enhance the client's sense of control over the body's response to stress.
6. Contact the physician immediately if the client's anxiety is at severe or panic level. Sedate if necessary.	6. Severe anxiety interferes with learning and compliance and also increases heart rate.
7. Refer also to the nursing diagnosis Anxiety in the Generic Care Plan, for general assessment and interventions.	

 Documentation

Progress notes
  Present emotional status
  Response to interventions

Pain Related to Cardiac Tissue Ischemia or Inflammation

Focus Assessment Criteria	Clinical Significance
1. Site, onset, precipitating factors, description of pain (e.g., crushing, radiating, constricting). 2. Associated behaviors such as restlessness	1,2. Decreased oxygen to myocardial tissue results in cardiac pain. Narrowed or blocked coronary arteries cause hypoxia. Treatment focuses on reducing pain, decreasing energy expenditure, and dilating the coronary arteries.

Goal

The client will report satisfactory control of chest pain within an appropriate time frame.

Indicators

- Report pain relief after pain relief measures.
- Demonstrate a relaxed mode.

Interventions	Rationales
1. Instruct client to report any pain episode immediately.	1. Less pain medication generally is required if administered early. Acute intervention can prevent further ischemia or injury.
2. Administer analgesics (e.g., nitrates) per physician's order. Document administration and the degree of relief the client experiences.	2. Severe, persistent pain unrelieved by analgesics may indicate impending or extending infarction.
3. Instruct client to rest during a pain episode.	3. Activity increases oxygen demand, which can exacerbate cardiac pain.
4. Reduce environmental distractions as much as possible.	4. Environmental stimulation can increase heart rate and may exacerbate myocardial tissue hypoxia, which increases pain.
5. After acute pain passes, explain its cause and possible precipitating factors (physical and emotional).	5. Calm explanation may reduce the client's stress associated with fear of the unknown.
6. Obtain and evaluate a 12-lead ECG and rhythm strip during pain episodes. Notify physician.	6. Cardiac monitoring may help to differentiate variant angina from extension of the infarction.
7. Explain and assist with alternative pain relief measures: a. Positioning b. Distraction (activities, breathing exercises) c. Massage d. Relaxation exercises	7. These measures can help to prevent painful stimuli from reaching higher brain centers by replacing the painful stimuli with another stimulus. Relaxation reduces muscle tension, decreases heart rate, may improve stroke volume, and enhances the client's sense of control over the pain.

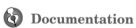 **Documentation**

Graphic/flow record
   Medication administration
Progress notes
   Unsatisfactory pain relief
   Status of pain

Activity Intolerance Related to Insufficient Oxygenation for ADLs Secondary to Cardiac Tissue Ischemia, Prolonged Immobility, Narcotics or Medications

Focus Assessment Criteria	Clinical Significance
1. Degree of activity progression 2. Physiological response to activity	1,2. A client post-MI must be monitored carefully to determine the rate at which activity can safely progress.

Goal

The client will

- Identify factors that increase cardiac workload.
- Demonstrate cardiac tolerance (marked by stable pulse, respirations, and blood pressure) to activity increases.
- Identify methods to reduce activity intolerance.

Interventions	Rationales
1. Increase client's activity each shift, as indicated: 　a. Allow client's legs to dangle first while supporting client from the side. 　b. Increase gradual progression of activity. 　c. Allow client to set his or her rate of ambulation. Provide adequate rest periods. 　d. Set an increased ambulation distance goal for each shift as agreed on by the client. 　e. Increase activity when pain is at a minimum or after pain relief measures take effect. 　f. Increase client's self-care activities from partial to complete self-care, as indicated.	1. Gradual activity progression, directed by the client's tolerance, enhances physiologic functioning and reduces cardiac tissue hypoxia.
2. Monitor vital signs: 　a. Before ambulation 　b. During ambulation 　c. Immediately after activity 　d. If pulse rate is 20–30 beats above the baseline at the end of ambulation, monitor vital signs at 1-, 2-, and 3-minute checks.	2. Tolerance to increased activity depends on the client's ability to adapt to the accompanying physiologic requirements. Adaptation requires optimal cardiovascular, pulmonary, neurologic, and musculoskeletal function. The expected immediate physiological responses to activity include the following: 　a. Increased pulse rate and strength 　b. Increased systolic blood pressure 　c. Increased respiratory rate and depth After 3 minutes, pulse should return to within 10 beats/min of the client's resting pulse rate.
3. Assess for abnormal responses to increased activity:	3. Abnormal responses indicate intolerance to increased activity.

(continues on page 120)

Interventions continued	**Rationales** continued
a. Tachycardia (20–30 beats above baseline) b. Decreased or no change in systolic blood pressure c. Excessive increase or decrease in respiratory rate d. Failure of pulse to return to near resting rate within 3 minutes after activity e. Confusion, vertigo, uncoordinated movements f. Chest pain g. Change in rhythm/ECG pattern h. Dizziness/syncope	
4. Plan adequate rest periods according to the client's daily schedule.	4. Rest provides the body with intervals of low energy expenditure.
5. Identify and acknowledge the client's progress.	5. Providing incentive can promote a positive attitude and decrease frustration associated with dependency.
6. Take steps to increase the quality and quantity of the client's sleep and rest periods. Make provisions for at least 2 hours of uninterrupted sleep at night.	6. A person must complete an entire sleep cycle (70–100 minutes) to feel rested.
7. Instruct client how to monitor his or her physiologic response to activities post-discharge.	7. This self-monitoring can detect early signs and symptoms of hypoxia.
8. Teach client how to conserve energy during ADLs, at work, and during recreational activities: a. Explain the need for rest periods both before and after certain activities. b. Instruct client to stop an activity if fatigue or other signs of cardiac hypoxia occur. c. Instruct client to consult with the physician or nurse practitioner before increasing activity after discharge.	8. Energy conservation prevents oxygen requirements from exceeding a level that the heart can meet.

 Documentation

Graphic/flow record
    Vital signs
    Ambulation (time, amount)
Progress notes
    Abnormal or unexpected response to increased activity

Grieving Related to Actual or Perceived Losses Secondary to Cardiac Condition

Focus Assessment Criteria	Clinical Significance
1. Signs and symptoms of grief reaction such as crying, anxiety, fear, withdrawal, restlessness, decreased appetite, and decreased independence in activities	1. Losses related to function, livelihood, and possibly life invariably provoke grief. This response can be profound depending on how the client perceives the condition to interfere with personal goals.

Goals

The client will

- Express grief.
- Describe the meaning of loss.
- Report an intent to discuss feelings with significant others.

Interventions	Rationales
1. Provide client opportunities to express feelings: a. Discuss the loss openly. b. Explain that grief is a normal reaction to a loss. c. Explore the client's perception of the loss.	1. Frequent contact by the nurse indicates acceptance and may facilitate trust. Open communication can help the client to work through the grieving process.
2. Encourage client to use coping strategies that have helped in the past.	2. This strategy helps the client to refocus on problem-solving and enhances his or her sense of control.
3. Promote grief work—the adaptive process of mourning—with each response. a. Denial: • Explain the presence of denial in the client or a family member to the other members. • Do not push the person to move past denial without emotional readiness. b. Isolation: • Convey acceptance by allowing expressions of grief. • Encourage open, honest communication to promote sharing. • Reinforce the person's sense of self-worth by allowing privacy when desired. • Encourage a gradual return to social activities (e.g., support groups, church activities, etc.).	3. Responses to grief vary. To intervene appropriately, the nurse must recognize and accept each client's individual response.

(continues on page 122)

Interventions continued	**Rationales** continued
c. Depression: • Reinforce the person's sense of self-esteem. • Identify the level of depression and tailor your approach accordingly. • Use empathetic sharing; acknowledge the grief (e.g., "It must be very difficult for you."). • Identify any signs of suicidal ideation or behavior (e.g., frequent statements of intent, revealed plan). d. Anger: • Encourage verbalization of anger. • Explain to other family members that the person's anger is an attempt to control his or her environment more closely because of the inability to control the loss. e. Guilt: • Acknowledge the person's expressed self-view. • Encourage the person to focus on positive aspects. • Avoid arguing with the person about what he or she should have done differently. f. Fear: • Focus on the present reality, and maintain a safe and secure environment. • Help the person to explore reasons for his or her fears. g. Rejection: • Reassure the person by explaining that this response is normal. • Explain this response to other family members. h. Hysteria: • Reduce environmental stressors (e.g., limit staff, minimize external noise). • Provide a safe, private area to display grief in his or her own fashion.	
4. Promote family cohesiveness: a. Support the family at its level of functioning. b. Encourage family members to evaluate their feelings and to support one another.	4. A grieving person often isolates himself or herself physically and especially emotionally. Repression of feelings interferes with family relationships.

 Documentation

Progress notes
  Present emotional status
  Interventions
  Client's and family's response to interventions

High Risk for Ineffective Therapeutic Regimen Management Related to Lack of Knowledge of Condition, Hospital Routines (Procedures, Equipment), Treatments, Medications, Diet, Activity Progression, Signs and Symptoms of Complications, Reduction of Risks, Follow-Up Care, and Community Resources

Focus Assessment Criteria	Clinical Significance
1. Client's knowledge of and experience with cardiac disorders	1. Knowledge and personal experiences can deter or improve compliance.
2. Readiness and ability to learn	2. A client who does not achieve goals for learning requires a referral for assistance postdischarge.

Goal

The goals for this diagnosis represent those associated with discharge planning. Refer to discharge criteria.

Interventions	Rationales
1. Explain the pathophysiology of MI using teaching aids appropriate for client's educational level (e.g., pictures, models, written materials).	1. Such explanations reinforce the need to comply with instructions on diet, exercise, and other aspects of the treatment regimen.
2. Explain risk factors for MI that can be eliminated or modified: a. Obesity b. Tobacco use c. Diet high in fat or sodium d. Sedentary life style e. Excessive alcohol intake f. Hypertension	2. Focusing on controllable factors can reduce the client's feelings of powerlessness. a. Obesity increases peripheral resistance and cardiac workload. Fifty percent of coronary artery disease in women is attributed to overweight (Reeves, 1997). Refer to the obesity care plan. b. Smoking unfavorably alters lipid levels. It impairs oxygen transport while increasing oxygen demand (Porth, 2002). c. A high-fat diet contributes to plaque formation in arteries; excessive sodium intake increases water retention. d. A sedentary life style leads to poor collateral circulation and predisposes the client to other risk factors. e. Alcohol is a potent vasodilator; subsequent vasoconstriction increases cardiac workload. f. Hypertension with increased peripheral resistance damages the arterial intima, which contributes to arteriosclerosis.

(continues on page 124)

Interventions continued	**Rationales** continued
g. Oral contraceptives	g. Oral contraceptives alter blood coagulation, platelet function, and fibrinolytic activity, thereby affecting the integrity of the endothelium.
h. Diabetes	h. Elevated glucose levels damage the arterial intima.
3. Teach client the importance of stress management through relaxation techniques and regular, appropriate exercise.	3. Although the exact effect of stress on CAD is unclear, release of catecholamines elevates systolic blood pressure, increases cardiac workload, induces lipolysis, and promotes platelet clumping (Porth, 2002).
4. Teach client how to assess radial pulse and instruct him or her to report any of the following: a. Dyspnea b. Chest pain unrelieved by nitroglycerin c. Unexplained weight gain or edema d. Unusual weakness, fatigue e. Irregular pulse or any unusual change	4. These signs and symptoms may indicate myocardial ischemia and vascular congestion (edema) secondary to decreased cardiac output.
5. Instruct client to report side effects of prescribed medications; these may include diuretics, digitalis, beta-adrenergic blocking agents, ACE inhibitors, or aspirin.	5. Recognizing and promptly reporting medication side effects can help to prevent serious complications (e.g., hypokalemia, hypotension).
6. Reinforce physician's explanation for the prescribed therapeutic diet. Consult with a dietitian if indicated.	6. Repetitive explanations may help to improve compliance with the therapeutic diet as well as promote understanding.
7. Explain the need for activity restrictions and how activity should progress gradually. Instruct client to a. Increase activity gradually. b. Avoid isometric exercises and lifting objects weighing more than 30 lb. c. Avoid jogging, heavy exercise, and sports until the physician advises otherwise. d. Consult with the physician on when to resume work, driving, sexual activity, recreational activities, and travel. e. Take frequent 15- to 20-minute rest periods, four to six times a day for 1 to 2 months. f. Perform activities at a moderate, comfortable pace; if fatigue occurs, stop and rest 15 minutes then continue.	7. Increasing activity gradually allows cardiac tissue to heal and accommodate increased demands. Overexertion increases oxygen consumption and cardiac workload.

(continues on page 125)

Interventions continued	**Rationales** continued

8. When the physician allows the client to resume sexual activity, teach the client to do the following:
  a. Avoid sexual activity in extremes of temperature, immediately after meals (wait 2 hours), when intoxicated, when fatigued, with an unfamiliar partner or in an unfamiliar environment, and with anal stimulation.
  b. Rest before engaging in sexual activity. (mornings are the best time) and after activity
  c. Terminate sexual activity if chest pain or dyspnea occurs.
  d. Take nitroglycerin before sexual activity, if prescribed.
  e. Use usual positions unless they increase exertion.
	8. To meet the increased myocardial oxygen demands resulting from sexual activity, the client should avoid all situations that cause vasoconstriction and vasodilation, which lead to anal stimulation and decrease heart rate.

9. Reinforce the necessity of follow-up care.	9. Proper follow-up is essential to evaluate if and when progression of activities is advisable.
10. Provide information on community resources such as the American Heart Association, self-help groups, counseling, and cardiac rehabilitation groups.	10. Such resources can provide additional support, information, and follow-up assistance that the client and family may need postdischarge.

 Documentation

Discharge summary record
    Discharge instructions
    Follow-up instructions
    Status at discharge (pain, activity, wound)
    Achievement of goals (individual or family)

PERIPHERAL ARTERIAL DISEASE (ATHEROSCLEROSIS)

Atherosclerosis obliterans, a progressive disease, is the leading cause of obstructive arterial disease of the extremities in people older than 30 years. At least 95% of arterial occlusive disease is atherosclerotic in origin.

The World Health Organization describes atherosclerosis as "a variable combination of changes in the intima of arteries, consisting of the focal accumulation of lipids, complex carbohydrates, blood and blood products, fibrous tissue, and calcium deposits and associated with medial changes." It is characterized by specific changes in the arterial wall as well as the development of an intraluminal plaque. Atherosclerosis can lead to myocardial infarction, renal hypertension, stroke, and amputation.

The known risk factors for atherosclerosis include hyperlipidemia, smoking history, hypertension, diabetes mellitus, and a family history of strokes or heart attacks especially at an early age. Altering modifiable risk factors has been shown to reduce significantly the chances of progressing to the morbid consequences of this disease. Teaching the risk factors and modifying behaviors that reduce risk factors are important components of nursing interventions for atherosclerotic disease.

 Time Frame

Initial diagnosis

 DIAGNOSTIC CLUSTER*

Collaborative Problems

PC: Stroke
PC: Ischemic Ulcers
PC: Acute Arterial Thrombosis
PC: Hypertension (refer to Hypertension)

Nursing Diagnoses

Activity Intolerance related to claudication
High Risk for Injury related to effects of orthostatic hypotension
High Risk for Ineffective Therapeutic Regimen Management related to lack of knowledge of condition, management of claudication, risk factors, foot care, and treatment plan

---

* This medical condition was not included in the validation study.

Discharge Criteria

Before discharge, the client or family will

1. List common risk factors for atherosclerosis.
2. State specific activities to manage claudication.
3. Describe principles and steps of proper foot care.
4. Describe any life style changes indicated (e.g., cessation of smoking, low-fat diet, regular exercise program).
5. State goal to lower low-density lipoprotein (LDL) cholesterol to less than 160 mg/dL, or less than 130 mg/dL if coronary heart disease or two risk factors are present.
6. Relate the signs and symptoms that must be reported to a health care professional.
7. Identify community resources available for assistance.

Collaborative Problems

Potential Complication: Stroke

Potential Complication: Ischemic Ulcers

Potential Complication: Acute Arterial Thrombosis

Nursing Goal

The nurse will detect early signs/symptoms of cardiovascular complications and collaboratively intervene to stabilize the client.

Indicators

- BP >90/60, < 140/90 mm Hg
- Oriented and alert
- Palpable peripheral pulses
- Warm, dry skin
- Intact motor/sensation of extremities

Interventions	Rationales
1. Teach the client about the signs and symptoms of transient ischemic attack (TIA) and the importance of reporting to the physician if they occur. a. Dizziness, loss of balance, or fainting b. Changes in sensation or motor control in arms or legs c. Numbness in face d. Speech changes e. Visual changes or loss of vision f. Temporary loss of memory	1. The risk of stroke increases in clients who have had a TIA. Disruption of cerebral circulation can result in motor or sensory deficits.
2. Assess for ischemic ulcers in extremities. Report ulcers or darkened spots of skin to the physician.	2. Atherosclerosis causing arterial stenosis and subsequent decreased tissue perfusion interferes with and may prevent healing of skin ulcers. Darkened spots of skin distal to arterial stenosis may indicate tissue infarctions related to ischemia.
3. Reinforce teaching of foot care. (Refer to the nursing diagnosis High Risk for Ineffective Management of Therapeutic Regimen for more information.)	3. Protection from skin loss may preserve tissue by preventing access to infective agents.
4. Monitor peripheral circulation (pulses, sensation, skin color). Report any changes immediately.	4. In acute arterial thrombosis, loss of sensation distal to the thrombosis occurs first with accompanying ischemic pain. This may be followed by a decrease in motor function.

▼ **Related Physician-Prescribed Interventions**

Specific interventions also depend on how atherosclerosis affects circulation and renal, cerebral, and cardiac functions.

Refer to specific care plan (e.g., Hypertension, Renal Failure) for more information.

Medications. Vasodilators, adrenergic blocking agents

Intravenous Therapy. Not indicated

Laboratory Studies. Cholesterol/triglycerides

Diagnostic Studies. Doppler ultrasonic flow, oscillometry, exercise test

Therapies. Angioplasty (selected), arterial reconstruction, pentoxifylline, aspirin, lipid-lowering agents, antiplatelet agents, hemoglobin/hematocrit, angiography, plethysmography, low-salt diet, saturated fats, cholesterol

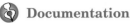 **Documentation**

Flow record
   Assessment results
Progress notes
   Changes in condition

Nursing Diagnoses

Activity Intolerance Related to Claudication

Focus Assessment Criteria	Clinical Significance

1. Client's daily activity:
  a. Need for ambulation for employment, e.g., mail carrier
  b. Sources of relaxation, daily activities
	1. This assessment determines the extent to which the condition affects the client's life style.

2. Degree of activity necessary to cause claudication:
  a. Walking distance at a certain pace
  b. Duration exercise
	2. Depending on the extent of circulatory compromise, the client may be taught measures to allow maximum tissue perfusion and prevent any further compromise.

3. Client's learned behavior to reduce or eliminate symptoms	3. Conservative self-care management may increase the time that the client is able to deal with the condition before seeking an operation.
4. Presence of obesity or tobacco use	4. Obesity increases peripheral vascular resistance and smoking causes vaso-constriction, both of which reduce circulation to the legs.

Goal

The client will progress activity to (specify level of activity desired).

Indicators

- Identify activities that cause claudication.
- State why pain occurs with activity.
- Develop a plan to increase activity and decrease claudication.

Interventions	Rationales
1. Teach client about the physiology of blood supply in relation to activity and the pathophysiology of claudication.	1. The client's understanding of the condition may promote compliance with restrictions and the exercise program.
2. Reassure client that activity does not harm the claudicating tissue.	2. The client may be tempted to discontinue activity when pain occurs in an attempt to avoid further injury.

3. Plan activities to include a scheduled ambulation time (Burch, 1991):
  a. Institute a daily walking regimen of at least 30 minutes.
  b. Teach client to "walk into" the pain, to pause when claudication occurs, and then to continue as soon as discomfort disappears.
  c. Start slowly.
  d. Emphasize that the action of walking is important, not the speed or distance.
	3. A regimented exercise program can help to develop collateral blood flow and ameliorate claudication.

4. Have client keep a continuous written record of actual activities and distances. Review to evaluate progress.	4. Self-reports of activity have low reliability.

5. Provide information on pentoxifylline (Trental) or Cilostazol (Pletal), if prescribed by the physician. Explain the following:
  a. Drug action
  b. The drug does not reduce the need for other activities to reduce risk factors.
  c. An immediate effect should not be expected because it takes from 4 to 6 weeks of therapy to determine effectiveness.
	5. These medications reportedly improve red blood cell flexibility, decrease platelet aggregation, and improve vascular vasodilatation (Kupecz, 2000).

 Documentation

Discharge summary record
  Client teaching
  Outcome achievement or status
  Referrals

High Risk for Injury Related to Effects of Orthostatic Hypotension

Focus Assessment Criteria	Clinical Significance
1. History of dizziness, lightheadedness, falling, medication use (e.g., vasodilators, antihistamines), other medical conditions	1. Clinical disorders and pharmacologic agents may be associated with orthostatic hypotension (Miller, 2004).

(continues on page 130)

Focus Assessment Criteria continued	Clinical Significance continued
2. Bilateral brachial blood pressure (blood pressure taken in the supine position followed immediately by blood pressure taken in the standing position). *Note:* If brachial pressures differ, use the arm with the higher pressure.	2. A significant difference between the supine and standing blood pressure readings confirms orthostatic hypotension (Miller, 2004).

Goal

The client will relate fewer episodes of dizziness.

Indicators

* State the relationship of blood pressure changes to symptoms.
* State activities that cause orthostatic hypotension.
* Plan activities to reduce symptoms of orthostatic hypotension.

Interventions	Rationales
1. Teach client about the nature of orthostatic hypotension and its probable causes. Explain that the change to an upright position normally causes a decrease in venous return and cardiac output (caused by venous pooling) of 500 mL to 1 liter of blood in the legs. The corresponding drop in blood pressure stimulates baroreceptors, causing venous and arterial constriction and an increase in heart rate through increased sympathetic activity.	1. Understanding orthostatic hypotension may help the client to modify behavior to reduce the frequency and severity of episodes.
2. If brachial pressures differ between arms, explain the need to use one arm consistently for blood pressure measurement.	2. Use of the arm with the higher pressure gives a more accurate assessment of the mean blood pressure.
3. Instruct client to avoid prolonged bed rest and to rise from the supine to the standing position in stages, first with one leg dependent, then the other.	3. Prolonged bed rest increases venous pooling. Gradual position change allows the body to compensate for venous pooling.
4. Teach to maintain adequate hydration especially in summer months or in hot, dry climates.	4. Adequate hydration is necessary to prevent decreased circulating volume.
5. Refer to a physician if you suspect that a prescribed medication may be responsible for the symptoms.	5. Certain medications—e.g., vasodilators, antihistamines—can precipitate orthostatic hypotension.

(continues on page 131)

Interventions continued	Rationales continued

6. Teach to prevent postprandial hypotension (Miller, 2004):
  a. Take hypertensive medications after meals.
  b. Eat small, frequent meals.
  c. Remain seated or lie down after meals.
  d. Avoid excessive alcohol intake.
	6. Studies have shown a blood pressure reduction of 20 mm Hg within 1 hour of eating the morning or noon meal in healthy, older adults. This is thought to be due to impaired baroreflex compensatory response to splanchnic blood pooling during digestion (Miller, 2004).

7. Instruct client to avoid hot baths or showers.	7. External heat may dilate the superficial vessels sufficiently to shunt blood from the brain, causing neurologic symptoms.
8. If a pressure (40–50 mm Hg) support garment (waist-high stocking) is prescribed, teach the client how to use it properly. Instruct the client to put on the garment early in the day and to avoid sitting while wearing it.	8. This device reduces venous pooling by applying constant pressure over the leg surface. Elastic compression garments are easier to put on in the morning before gravity causes increased edema. Bending at the groin and the knee causes garment constriction and increases pressure.
9. Teach client to sleep with pillows under the head.	9. Decreasing the contrast between the supine and upright positions helps to decrease the amount of intravascular fluid shift with position changes.

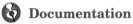 **Documentation**

Progress notes
  Episodes of vertigo
  Client teaching and response
  Application of support garment

High Risk for Ineffective Therapeutic Regimen Management Related to Lack of Knowledge of Condition, Management of Claudication, Risk Factors, Foot Care, and Treatment Plan

Focus Assessment Criteria	Clinical Significance
1. Readiness and ability to retain learning	1. A client or family that does not achieve learning goals requires a referral for assistance postdischarge.
2. History of claudication and distance the client can walk before onset	2. Claudication is disabling when it restricts life style or earning ability.

Goal

The outcome criteria for this diagnosis represent those associated with discharge planning. Refer to the discharge criteria.

Interventions	Rationales
1. Explain atherosclerosis and its effects on cardiac, circulatory, renal, and neurologic functions.	1. Health education offers clients some control over the direction of their disease (Edelman & Mandle, 1998).
2. Briefly explain the relationship of certain risk factors to the development of atherosclerosis: a. Smoking • Vasoconstriction • Decreased blood oxygenation • Elevated blood pressure • Increased lipidemia • Increased platelet aggregation b. Hypertension • Constant trauma of pressure causes vessel lining damage, which promotes plaque formation and narrowing. c. Hyperlipidemia • Promotes atherosclerosis d. Sedentary life style • Decreases muscle tone and strength • Decreases circulation e. Excess weight (>10% of ideal) • Fatty tissue increases peripheral resistance. • Fatty tissue is less vascular.	2a. The effects of nicotine on the cardiovascular system contribute to coronary artery disease, stroke, hypertension, and peripheral vascular disease (Havranek, 1999). b. Changes in arterial walls increase the incidence of stroke and coronary artery disease (Porth, 2002). c. High circulating lipids increase the risk of coronary heart disease, peripheral vascular disease, and stroke (Havranek, 1999). d. Lack of exercise inhibits the pumping action of muscles that enhance circulation. With peripheral vascular disease, exercise promotes collateral circulation (Havranek, 1999). e. Overweight status increases cardiac work load, thus causing hypertension (Cunningham, 1992).
3. Encourage client to share feelings, concerns, and understanding of risk factors, disease process, and effects on life.	3. This dialogue will provide data to assist with goal setting (Maves, 1992).
4. Assist client to select life-style behaviors that he or she chooses to change (Burch, 1991). a. Avoid multiple changes. b. Consider personal abilities, resources, and overall health. c. Be realistic and optimistic.	4. The older client may have life-style patterns of inactivity, smoking, and high-fat diet.
5. Assist to set goal(s) and the steps to achieve them (e.g., will walk 30 minutes daily.) a. Will walk 10 minutes daily. b. Will walk 10 minutes daily and 20 minutes three times a week. c. Will walk 20 minutes daily. d. Will walk 2 minutes daily and 30 minutes three times a week.	5. Attaining short-term goals can foster motivation to continue the process (Edelman & Mandle, 1998).

(continues on page 133)

Interventions continued	Rationales continued
6. Suggest a method to self-monitor progress (e.g., graph, checklist).	6. A structured monitoring system increases client involvement beyond the goal-setting stage (Maves, 1992).
7. Provide specific information to achieve selected goals (e.g., self-help programs, referrals, techniques).	7. The educational program should not overload the client.
8. If appropriate, refer to Obesity Care Plan for additional interventions in weight loss and exercise.	
9. Explain the risks that atherosclerotic disease poses to feet: a. Diabetes-related peripheral neuropathy and microvascular disease b. Pressure ulcers	9. Understanding may encourage compliance with necessary life-style changes. a. Diabetes accelerates the atherosclerotic process. Diabetic neuropathy prevents the client from feeling ischemic or injured areas (Helt, 1991). b. Healing of open lesions requires approximately 10 times the blood supply necessary to keep live tissue intact (Sieggreen, 1987).
10. Teach foot care measures. a. Daily inspection • Use a mirror. • Look for corns, calluses, bunions, scratches, redness, and blisters. • If vision is poor, have a family member or other person inspect the feet. b. Daily washing • Use warm, not hot, water. (Check the water temperature with the hand or elbow before immersing feet.) • Avoid prolonged soaking. • Dry well especially between the toes c. Proper foot hygiene • Cut nails straight across; use an emery board to smooth edges. • Avoid using any chemicals on corns or calluses. • Avoid using antiseptics such as iodine. • If feet are dry, apply a thin coat of lotion. Avoid getting lotion between the toes.	a. Daily foot care can reduce tissue damage and help to prevent or detect early further injury and infection (Helt, 1991). b. • This will prevent burning insensitive tissue. • This can macerate tissue. They can cause an injury that will not heal. These can damage healthy tissue.
11. Teach client to a. Avoid hot water bottles and heating pads. b. Wear wool socks to warm feet at night.	11. These precautions help to reduce the risk of injury (Helt, 1991).

(continues on page 134)

Interventions continued	Rationales continued
c. Wear warm foot covering before going out in cold weather (wool socks and lined boots). d. Avoid walking barefoot.	
12. Instruct client to wear well-fitting leather shoes (may require shoes made with extra depth), to always wear socks with shoes, to avoid sandals with straps between the toes, and to inspect the insides of shoes daily for worn areas, protruding nails, or other objects.	12. Well-fitting shoes help to prevent injury to skin and underlying tissue (Helt, 1991).
13. Teach client to a. Wear socks that fit well. b. Avoid socks with elastic bands. c. Avoid sock garters. d. Avoid crossing the legs.	13. Tight garments and certain leg positions constrict leg vessels, which further reduces circulation (Helt, 1991).
14. Emphasize the importance of visiting a podiatrist for nail/callus/corn care if client has poor vision or any difficulty with self-care.	14. The client may require assistance with foot care to ensure adequate care and prevent self-inflicted injuries (Helt, 1991).
15. Explain that if client cannot inspect his or her feet, he or she should arrange for another person to inspect them regularly.	15. Daily inspection helps to ensure early detection of skin or tissue damage (Helt, 1991).
16. Advise client to consult with primary care provider regarding the advantages of daily use of aspirin, Vitamin E (400 mg), and folate (400 ng).	16. Some evidence supports that these may prevent ischemic cardiac events (Clinical Evidence, 2002).
17. Identify available community resources.	17. They can assist with weight loss, smoking cessation, diet, and exercise programs.

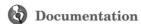 **Documentation**

Discharge summary record
    Client teaching
    Outcome achievement or status
    Referrals when indicated

Respiratory Disorders

ASTHMA

Asthma is a disorder of airway inflammation and bronchial hyperactivity characterized symptomatically by cough, chest tightness, shortness of breath, and wheezing as a result of decreased airflow. More than 12 million people in the United States have asthma. Exposure to common aeroallergens (e.g., animal dander, tobacco smoke, dust, molds) can trigger an acute episode. Many people ignore the seriousness of this disease. Frequent hospitalizations result from disregarding the warning signs of impending asthma attacks and noncompliance with the therapeutic regimen. Status asthmaticus refers to a severe case of asthma that does not respond to conventional treatment. This life-threatening situation requires prompt action.

 Time Frame

Acute episode

⚭ DIAGNOSTIC CLUSTER

Collaborative Problems

▲ PC: Hypoxemia
△ PC: Acute Respiratory Failure
△ PC: Status Asthmaticus

Nursing Diagnoses	Refer to
▲ Ineffective Airway Clearance related to increased mucous production, tenacious secretions, and bronchospasm	
△ High Risk for Ineffective Therapeutic Regimen Management related to lack of knowledge of condition, treatment, prevention of infection, breathing exercises, risk factors, and signs and symptoms of impending attack	
△ Anxiety related to breathlessness and fear of suffocation	Chronic Obstructive Pulmonary Disease
* Powerlessness related to feeling of loss of control and restrictions that this condition places on life style	Chronic Obstructive Pulmonary Disease
* High Risk for Ineffective Breathing Pattern related to increased work of breathing, hypoxemia, agitation, and impending respiratory failure	Mechanical Ventilation

---

▲ This diagnosis was reported to be monitored for or managed frequently (75%–100%).
△ This diagnosis was reported to be monitored for or managed often (50%–74%).
* This diagnosis was not included in the validation study.

Collaborative Problems

Potential Complication: Hypoxemia

Potential Complication: Respiratory Failure

Potential Complication: Status Asthmaticus

Nursing Goal

The nurse will detect early signs/symptoms of hypoxemia and respiratory failure and collaboratively intervene to stabilize client.

Indicators

- Serum pH 7.35–7.45
- Serum PCO_2 35–45 mm Hg
- Pulse: regular rhythm, rate 60–100 beats/min
- Blood pressure: > 90/60, < 140–90 mm Hg
- Urine output > 30 ml/hour
- Alert, oriented
- No abnormal breath sounds
- Oxygen saturation >95% (pulse oximetry)

Interventions	Rationales
1. Obtain a thorough history from either the client or family.	1. History taking is an essential factor in the treatment of asthma. Points to focus on are: What triggered the event? What methods have been used to alleviate the symptoms? Did they work? What medications are generally prescribed? What stimulants exacerbate the asthma? How long did the client wait before seeking treatment?
2. Monitor for signs and symptoms of acid-base imbalance: a. Initially pH >7.45, PCO_2 <35 mm Hg (alkalemia); look for decompensation: pH <7.35, PCO_2 >45 mm Hg (acidemia).	a. Acid-base analysis helps to evaluate gas exchange in the lungs. Anxiety and air hunger will lead to an increase in the respiratory rate. In severe cases, a decreased PO_2 will lead to hypoxemia. Respiratory alkalosis will be exhibited. In status asthmaticus, the client will tire, and air trapping will worsen. Acid–base results will return to baseline, which is an ominous sign. The PCO_2 will then rise quickly. Respiratory acidosis and failure will result. Intubation will be required (Porth, 2002).
b. Increased/decreased blood pressure c. Monitor intake and output. d. Cool, pale, cyanotic skin	b,c,d. First the client will have an elevated blood pressure resulting from anxiety and feelings of air hunger. As the client's condition and air trapping worsen, pressure in the thoracic cavity

(continues on page 139)

Interventions continued	**Rationales** continued
	will increase which decreases venous return. Thus the client will exhibit a decrease in blood pressure and the signs and symptoms of decreased cardiac output.
e. Tachypnea and dyspnea at rest. Respiratory rate >20 breaths/min.	e. The client experiences dyspnea because of narrowed passages and air trapping related to bronchospasms (Orsi, 1991).
f. Evaluate overall appearance.	f. The client, often sitting while leaning forward, may appear anxious, diaphoretic, and restless. The client may appear to be air gulping. Also an increased anteroposterior diameter and a lowered diaphragm will be noted because of hyperinflation of the lungs. As the work of breathing increases, use of shoulder, neck, and intercostal muscles will be evident.
g. Abnormal breath sounds	g. Auscultation of the chest is often misleading. Initially wheezing may be heard throughout all lung fields during both phases of respiration. As airflow becomes restricted because of severe obstruction and mucous secretion, breath sounds become diminished or absent. This is a sign of impending respiratory failure.
h. Cough	h. For some persons with asthma, cough may be their only symptom. Spasmodic contractions of the bronchi produce the cough (Schumann, 1995).
i. Changes in mental status	i. The client is often anxious and restless. However changes in mentation reflect changes in oxygenation. Confusion, agitation, and lethargy are signs of imminent respiratory failure.
3. Administer O_2 via nasal cannula.	3. Hypoxemia is common due to ventilation/perfusion disturbances. Air trapping and increased respiratory rate impede gas exchange. PO_2 <60 mm Hg requires supplemental oxygen. Administration of O_2 via nasal cannula is preferred to reduce the client's feelings of suffocation. In severe cases, intubation and mechanical ventilation may be required.
4. Administer intravenous hydration.	4. Excess mucus production is common. Adequate hydration prevents dehydration and enhances clearance of secretions. Daily intake of 2 to 4 L is recommended.

(continues on page 140)

Interventions continued	**Rationales** continued
5. Obtain sputum specimen.	5. Sputum is generally clear, mucoid, or white during exacerbation of asthma. Discoloration of sputum is indicative of infection. Administration of antihistamines and decongestants is common to decrease mucus production.
6. Assess pulmonary function.	6. Examining pulmonary function aids in determining the degree of destruction and responsiveness to treatment. Forced expiratory volume (FEV-1) measures the force of exhaled air. An FEV-1 <1,000 mL or 25% of the client's normal predicted value indicates a severe obstruction. Pulsus paradoxes (a decrease in the systolic blood pressure 12 mm Hg during inspiration) is associated with the work of breathing and is assessed to determine responsiveness to treatment. A decrease in pulsus paradoxes reflects favorable responsiveness to treatment.
7. Identify and eliminate stimulants.	7. Irritants such as smoke, pollen, and dusts may exacerbate asthma. Avoidance of stimulants should be stressed.
8. Administer sedatives as ordered.	8. Clients are often anxious, which often intensifies the situation. Sedatives aid in minimizing anxiety and decreasing the respiratory rate. A decreased respiratory rate increases exhalation, enhancing gas exchange and correcting respiratory alkalosis.
9. Monitor for status asthmaticus: • Labored breathing • Prolonged exhalation • Engorged neck veins • Wheezing	9. Status asthmaticus does not respond to conventional therapy. As status asthmaticus worsens, the $PaCO_2$ increases and pH falls. The extent of wheezing does not indicate the severity of the attack (Porth, 2002).
10. Evaluate level of hypoxia with arterial blood gases and (PCO_2, PaO_2, pH, SaO_2) pulse oximetry.	10. As ventilation perfusion abnormality results in hypoxemia and respiratory allealosis then followed by respiratory acidosis. (Porth, 2002)

11. Initiate treatment:
  a. O_2 low-flow humidified oxygen with venturi mask or nasal catheter
  b. Nebulizer treatment with Albuterol
	a. Oxygen therapy is needed to treat dyspnea, central cyanosis, and hypoxemia.
	b. The Nebulizer disperses a bronchodilator into microscopic particles that reach the lungs with inhalations.

(continues on page 141)

Interventions continued	Rationales continued
c. Intravenous fluids	c. Fluid intake is critical to prevent dehydration and to facilitate expectoration by liquifying secretions
d. Corticosteroids	d. Corticosteroids are administered parenterally to reduce the inflammation of the airways.
e. Possible mechanical ventilation	e. Respiratory acidosis is tiring; mechanical ventilation may be required. (Refer to Care Plan for Mechanical Ventilation if needed.)
12. Provide a quiet environment and eliminate respiratory irritants (flowers, perfumes, odors of cleaning agents, tobacco smoke [direct or on clothes]).	12. Irritants will aggravate an already compromised respiratory status.

Related Physician-Prescribed Interventions

Medications. Beta$_2$ agonists (short or long acting) (inhaled, oral), glucosteroids (inhaled, oral, intravenous in acute stages), cromolyn sodium (nonsteroidal anti-inflammatory drug), antimicrobials, sympathomimetics, sedatives, theophylline, leukotriene synthesis inhibitors and receptor antagonist, anti-IgE antibody therapy, PDE inhibitors

Intravenous Therapy. 2 to 4 L/day

Laboratory Studies. Arterial blood gases analysis, sputum culture, electrolytes, serum IgE levels CBC with differential

Diagnostic Studies. Pulmonary function tests, chest X-rays, electrocardiogram, allergy skin testing, incentive spirometry, x-ray or MRI of sinuses

Therapies. Oxygen therapies, high-flow nebulizers, chest physiotherapy

Nursing Diagnoses

Ineffective Airway Clearance Related to Increased Mucus Production, Tenacious Secretions, and Bronchospasm

Focus Assessment Criteria	Clinical Significance
1. Ability to maintain position that increases air exchange	1. A nonupright position causes abdominal organs to shift to the chest, preventing sufficient lung expansion to produce an effective cough.
2. Cough (productive, painful, effective)	2. The cough must be effective to remove secretions.
3. Sputum (color, character, amount, odor)	3. The secretions must be sufficiently liquid to enable expulsion.

Goal

The client will not experience aspirations.

Indicators

- Assume comfortable position that facilitates increased air exchange.
- Demonstrate effective coughing.
- Relate strategies to decrease tenacious secretions.

Interventions	Rationales

1. Instruct the client on the proper method of controlled coughing:
  a. Breathe deeply and slowly while sitting up as high as possible.
 	
  b. Use diaphragmatic breathing.
 	
  c. Hold the breath for 3 to 5 seconds, then slowly exhale as much as possible through the mouth. (The lower rib cage and abdomen should sink down.)
  d. Take a second breath, hold, and cough from the chest (not from the back of the mouth or throat) using two short, forceful coughs.
  e. Demonstrate pursed-lip breathing.
	1. Uncontrolled coughing is tiring and ineffective, leading to frustration.
	  a. Sitting high shifts the abdominal organs away from the lungs, enabling greater expansion.
	  b. Diaphragmatic breathing reduces the respiratory rate and increases alveolar ventilation.
	  c,d. Increasing the air volume in lungs promotes expulsion of secretions.
	
	  e. Pursed-lip breathing prolongs exhalation to decrease air trapping.

2. Teach the client measures to reduce the viscosity of secretions:
  a. Maintain adequate hydration: Increase fluid intake 2 to 4 L/day if not contraindicated by decreased cardiac output or renal disease.
  b. Maintain adequate humidity of inspired air.
  c. Avoid environmental stimulants.
	2. Thick secretions are difficult to expectorate and can cause mucus plugs, which can lead to atelectasis.

3. Auscultate the lungs before and after treatment.	3. This assessment helps to evaluate treatment effectiveness.
4. Encourage or provide good mouth care.	4. Good oral hygiene promotes a sense of well-being and prevents mouth odor.

 Documentation

Progress notes
  Effective of cough
  Description of sputum
  Lung assessment

High Risk for Ineffective Therapeutic Regimen Management Related to Lack of Knowledge of Condition, Treatment, Prevention of Infection, Breathing Exercises, Risk Factors, and Signs and Symptoms of Impending Attack

Focus Assessment Criteria	Clinical Significance
1. Readiness and ability to learn and retain information	1. Clients with asthma must learn to live with a chronic disease. The client needs to learn individual coping strategies to maintain compliance with the long-term treatment goals of asthma. A client who does not achieve goals for learning requires a referral for assistance postdischarge.

Goal

The goals for this diagnosis represent those associated with discharge planning. Refer to discharge criteria.

Interventions	Rationales
1. Help client to formulate and accept realistic short- and long-term goals.	1. This may help the client to realize his or her control over life and make choices to improve quality of life.
2. Teach about the diagnosis and treatment regimen.	2. Understanding may help to encourage compliance and participation in self-care.
3. Teach measures to manage asthma and prevent hospitalizations. a. Eat a well-balanced diet. b. Take sufficient rest periods. c. Gradually increase activity. d. Avoid exposure to the following: • Smoke • Dust • Severe air pollution • Extremely cold or warm temperatures	a,b,c. These practices promote overall good health and increase the resistance to infection. d. Exposure to these respiratory irritants can cause bronchospasm and increase mucus production. Smoking destroys the ciliary cleansing mechanism of the respiratory tract. Heat raises body temperature and increases the body's oxygen requirements, possibly exacerbating symptoms.
4. Teach and have the client demonstrate breathing exercises. a. Use incentive spirometer.	4. Clients experiencing asthma frequently become anxious and assume an ineffective breathing pattern. Decreasing the work of breathing using positioning and effective breathing patterns may lessen the episode and prevent hospitalizations. a. Incentive spirometry encourages deep, sustained inspiratory efforts.

(continues on page 144)

Interventions continued	**Rationales** continued
b. Assume a leaning forward position.	b. Leaning forward enhances diaphragmatic excursions and diminishes the use of accessory muscles.
c. Use pursed-lip breathing.	c. Pursed-lip breathing prolongs exhalation, which prevents air trapping and air gulping.
5. Explain the hazards of infection and ways to reduce the risk: a. Avoid contact with infected persons. b. Receive immunization against influenza and bacterial pneumonia. c. Take antibiotics as prescribed if sputum becomes yellow or green. d. Adhere to medications and hydration schedule.	5. Upper respiratory infections (URI) are associated with asthma. Viral infections are the most common culprit. It is thought that the URI causes inflammation of the bronchial tree, leading to bronchoconstriction and air trapping.
6. Instruct the client to report the following: a. Change in sputum characteristics or failure of sputum to return to usual color after 3 days of antibiotic therapy b. Elevated temperature c. Increase in cough, weakness, or shortness of breath d. Weight gain or swelling in ankles and feet	a. Sputum changes may indicate an infection or resistance of the infective organism to the prescribed antibiotic. b. Circulating pathogens stimulate the hypothalamus to elevate body temperature. c. Hypoxia is chronic; exacerbations must be detected early to prevent complications. d. These signs may indicate fluid retention secondary to pulmonary arterial hypertension and decreased cardiac output.
7. Seek medical attention if asthma is not relieved after using method outlined in the client therapeutic regimen.	7. Unrelieved symptoms of asthma may lead to status asthmaticus. It is documented that clients with asthma repeatedly ignore the warning signs and seek medical attention when the case becomes life-threatening.
8. Teach and observe the proper use of a hand-held nebulizer and inhalers. a. For inhalers: • Shake canister. • Blow out air. • Put inhaler to mouth, release medication, and breathe in deeply. • Hold breath for 10 seconds; then exhale slowly. • Wait 1 minute and repeat. • Rinse mouth if using a corticosteroid inhaler. • Add a spacer if needed.	8. Accurate instructions can help to prevent medication overdose. Improper use of inhalers has been outlined as an antecedent of asthma. Clients tend to overuse inhalers, which leads to inhaler ineffectiveness.

(continues on page 145)

Interventions continued	**Rationales** continued

b. For nebulizer:
  • Follow directions for assembly.
  • Using mouthpiece or mask slowly. Take deep breaths and slowly exhale.
  • When mist is gone, stop treatment.	

9. Develop an exercise routine.	9. Exercise increases the client's stamina. Warn the client that improper exercise may also trigger asthma. Instruct the client to avoid exercising in extreme hot or cold weather. Wearing a paper mask may reduce the sensitivity to stimulants. Emphasize the importance of a cool-down period. Suggest swimming and exercising indoors to avoid exposure to stimulants.

10. Enlist client to create a management plan:
  a. Instruct client to keep a diary of peak flows for 7 days (every morning and at bedtime).
  b. If beta-antagonist inhaler is needed, measure peak flow before and after using and document.
  c. Determine the individual's personal best peak flow.
  d. Calculate zones for management:
    • Green: 80–100% of personal best
    • Yellow: 50–80% of personal best
    • Red: Below 50%
  e. Instruct what to do in response to peak flow in yellow:
    • Beta$_2$-Antagonist inhaler: Call primary provider if incomplete response.
  f. Instruct client to go to emergency room if response to initial therapy or if peak flow is <50% of baseline (red zone).
	10. Unrelieved asthma symptoms may lead to status asthmaticus. It is documented that clients with asthma repeatedly ignore the warning signs and seek medical attention when the case becomes life threatening (Spector & Nicklas, 1995).

11. Instruct client to reduce irritants at home (Jablonski, 2001):
  a. Eliminate smoking and smoke on clothes around the affected person.
  b. Remove carpets from bedroom.
  c. Avoid pets in home (at least keep them out of bedroom).
  d. Vacuum and dust regularly when affected person is not present.
  e. Avoid people with colds and perfume.
  f. Reduce exposure to high ozone levels and high humidity.
	11. These are known triggers.

(continues on page 146)

Interventions continued	Rationales continued
g. Eliminate insects and mold in home.	
h. Avoid food containing metabisulfate preservatives (e.g., beer, wine, deli meats).	
i. Caution client about use of aspirin, nonsteroidal anti-inflammatory drugs, and ophthalmic beta-antagonists.	
12. Instruct on use of inhalers:	12.
a. Use controller medications (oral, inhalers) every day (e.g., inhaled steroids, leukotriene-receptor antagonists).	a,b. Proper use of inhalers will promote control.
b. Use quick-relief or rescuer inhaler as needed.	
c. If you use the rescuer inhaler more than twice a week or waken with symptoms of asthma more than twice a month, call your primary health care provider.	c. Asthma is not under control; a reevaluation is needed.

 Documentation

Discharge summary record
   Client teaching
   Outcome achievement or status
   Referrals if indicated

CHRONIC OBSTRUCTIVE PULMONARY DISEASE

Chronic obstructive pulmonary disease (COPD) refers to a group of disorders that cause airway obstruction including chronic bronchitis, emphysema, bronchiectasis, and asthma.

Chronic bronchitis and bronchiectasis are characterized by excessive bronchial mucus production and cough caused by chronic inflammation of the bronchioles and hypertrophy and hyperplasia of the mucous glands. In emphysema, airway obstruction is caused by hyperinflation of the alveoli, loss of lung tissue elasticity, and narrowing of small airways. Asthma is characterized by narrowing of the bronchial airways.

COPD most commonly results from chronic irritation by chemical irritants (industrial, tobacco), air pollution, or recurrent respiratory tract infections. Acute exacerbations are usually due to infection or exposure to allergens and pollutants.

 Time Frame

Acute episode (nonintensive care)

 DIAGNOSTIC CLUSTER

Collaborative Problems

▲ PC: Hypoxemia
▲ PC: Right-Sided Heart Failure

Nursing Diagnoses

▲ Ineffective Airway Clearance related to excessive and tenacious secretions
▲ Activity Intolerance related to fatigue and inadequate oxygenation for activities
▲ Anxiety related to breathlessness and fear of suffocation
△ Powerlessness related to feelings of loss of control and lifestyle restrictions
△ Disturbed Sleep Pattern related to cough, inability to assume recumbent position, environmental stimuli
△ High Risk for Imbalanced Nutrition: Less Than Body Requirements related to anorexia secondary to dyspnea, halitosis, and fatigue (refer to Pressure Ulcers)
▲ High Risk for Ineffective Therapeutic Regimen Management related to lack of knowledge of condition, treatments, prevention of infection, breathing exercises, risk factors, signs and symptoms of complications

---

▲ This diagnosis was reported to be monitored for or managed frequently (75%–100%).
△ This diagnosis was reported to be monitored for or managed often (50%–74%).

Discharge Criteria

Before discharge, the client or family will

1. Identify long- and short-term goals to modify risk factors (e.g., diet, smoking, exercise).
2. Identify adjustments needed to maintain self-care.
3. State how to prevent further pulmonary deterioration.
4. State signs and symptoms that must be reported to a health care professional.
5. Identify community resources that can provide assistance with home management

Collaborative Problems

Potential Complication: Hypoxemia

Potential Complication: Right-Sided Heart Failure

Nursing Goal

The nurse will detect early signs/symptoms of hypoxia and heart failure and collaboratively intervene to stabilize client.

Indicators

- Serum pH 7.35–7.45
- Serum PCO_2 35–45 mm Hg
- Pulse: regular rhythm and rate 60–100 beats/min
- Respirations 16–20 breaths/min
- Blood pressure <140/90, >90/60 mm Hg
- Urine output >30 ml/hour

Interventions	Rationales
1. Monitor for signs of acid–base imbalance: a. Arterial blood gas (ABG) analysis: pH < 7.35 and PCO_2 > 46 mm Hg	1. a. ABG analysis helps to evaluate gas exchange in the lungs. In mild to moderate COPD, the client may have a normal $PaCO_2$ level because of chemoreceptors in the medulla responding to increased $PaCO_2$ by increasing ventilation. In severe COPD, the client cannot sustain this increased ventilation and the $PaCO_2$ value increases.
b. Increased and irregular pulse c. Increased respiratory rate followed by decreased rate	b,c. Respiratory acidosis develops owing to excessive CO_2 retention. The client with respiratory acidosis from chronic disease at first increases heart rate and respiration in an attempt to compensate for decreased oxygenation. After a while, the client breathes more slowly and with prolonged expiration. Eventually his respiratory center may stop responding to the higher CO_2 levels, and breathing may stop abruptly.
d. Changes in mentation	d. Changes in mentation result from cerebral tissue hypoxia.
e. Decreased urine output (<30 mL/hr) f. Cool, pale, or cyanotic skin	e,f. The compensatory response to decreased circulatory oxygen is to increase blood oxygen by increasing heart and respiratory rates and to decrease circulation to the kidneys and to the extremities (marked by decreased pulses and skin changes).

(continues on page 149)

Interventions continued	Rationales continued
2. Administer low flow (2 L/min) of oxygen as needed through a cannula.	2. This measure increases circulating oxygen levels. Higher flow rates increase carbon dioxide retention. The use of a cannula rather than a mask reduces the client's fears of suffocation.
3. Obtain a sputum sample for culture and sensitivity.	3. Sputum culture and sensitivity determine if an infection is contributing to symptoms.
4. Eliminate smoke and strong odors in the client's room.	4. Irritants to the respiratory tract can exacerbate symptoms.
5. Monitor electrocardiogram (ECG) for dysrhythmias secondary to altered arterial blood gases (ABGs).	5. ABG alterations may precipitate cardiac dysrhythmias.
6. Monitor for signs of right-sided congestive heart failure: a. Elevated diastolic pressure b. Distended neck veins c. Peripheral edema d. Elevated central venous pressure (CVP).	6. The combination of arterial hypoxemia and respiratory acidosis acts locally as a strong vasoconstrictor of pulmonary vessels. This leads to pulmonary arterial hypertension, increased right ventricular systolic pressure, and eventually right ventricular hypertrophy and failure.
7. Refer to the Congestive Heart Failure care plan for additional interventions if right-sided failure occurs.	
8. Refer to thoracotomy if surgery is planned.	

Related Physician-Prescribed Interventions

Medications. Methylxanthines (IV), anticholinergics (inhaled), bronchodilators (inhaled), adrenergics, corticosteroids (oral, inhaled, V), antimicrobials, sympathomimetics (inhaled), antitussives (nonnarcotic)

Intravenous Therapy. Variable depending on mode of medication administration

Laboratory Studies. ABG analysis, electrolytes, serum albumin, liver function studies, sputum culture, complete blood count (CBC) with differential

Diagnostic Studies. Chest X-ray film, pulmonary function tests, bronchography, stress test

Therapies. Intermittent positive-pressure breathing (IPPB), chest physiotherapy, low oxygen through a cannula, ultrasonic nebulizer

Documentation

Flow record
  Vital signs
  Intake and output
  Assessment data
Progress notes
  Change in status
  Interventions
  Client's response to interventions

Nursing Diagnoses

Ineffective Airway Clearance Related to Excessive and Tenacious Secretions

Focus Assessment Criteria	Clinical Significance
1. Ability to maintain upright position	1. A nonupright position causes abdominal organs to shift to the chest, preventing sufficient lung expansion to produce an effective cough.
2. Cough (productive, painful, effective)	2. The cough must be effective to remove secretions.
3. Sputum (color, character, amount, odor)	3. The secretions must be sufficiently liquid to enable expulsion.

Goal

The client will not experience aspiration.

Indicators

• Demonstrate effective coughing and increased air exchange in lungs.
• Relate strategies to decrease tenacious secretions.

Interventions	Rationales
1. Instruct the client on the proper method of controlled coughing: a. Breathe deeply and slowly while sitting up as high as possible. b. Use diaphragmatic breathing. c. Hold the breath for 3 to 5 seconds then slowly exhale as much as possible through the mouth. (The lower rib cage and abdomen should sink down.) d. Take a second breath, hold, and cough from the chest (not from the back of the mouth or throat) using two short, forceful coughs.	1. Uncontrolled coughing is tiring and ineffective, leading to frustration. a. Sitting high shifts the abdominal organs away from the lungs, enabling greater expansion. b. Diaphragmatic breathing reduces the respiratory rate and increases alveolar ventilation. c,d. Increasing the volume of air in lungs promotes expulsion of secretions.

(continues on page 151)

Interventions continued	Rationales continued

2. Teach the client measures to reduce the viscosity of secretions:
  a. Maintain adequate hydration; increase fluid intake to 2 to 3 quarts a day if not contraindicated by decreased cardiac output or renal disease.
  b. Maintain adequate humidity of inspired air.
	2. Thick secretions are difficult to expectorate and can cause mucus plugs, which can lead to atelectasis.

3. Auscultate the lungs before and after the client coughs.	3. This assessment helps to evaluate the effectiveness of the client's cough effort.
4. Encourage or provide good mouth care after coughing.	4. Good oral hygiene promotes a sense of well-being and prevents mouth odor.

 Documentation
Progress notes
  Effectiveness of cough
  Description of sputum

Activity Intolerance Related to Fatigue and Inadequate Oxygenation for Activities

Focus Assessment Criteria	Clinical Significance
1. Tolerance to activities of daily living (ADLs) and physiologic response to activity, i.e., pulse rate, blood pressure, respirations 2. Aggravating factors (environmental or emotional)	1,2. Activity tolerance hinges on the client's ability to adapt to the physiologic requirements of increased activity. Adaptation requires optimal cardiopulmonary, vascular, neurological, and musculoskeletal functions.

Goal
The client will progress activity to (specify level of activity).

Indicators
- Demonstrate methods of effective coughing, breathing, and conserving energy.
- Identify a realistic activity level to achieve or maintain.

Interventions	Rationales

1. Explain activities and factors that increase oxygen demand:
  a. Smoking
  b. Extremes in temperature
  c. Excessive weight
  d. Stress
	1. Smoking, extremes in temperature, and stress cause vasoconstriction, which increases cardiac workload and oxygen requirements. Excess weight increases peripheral resistance, which also increases cardiac workload.

(continues on page 152)

Interventions continued	Rationales continued

2. Provide the client with ideas for conserving energy:
  a. Sit whenever possible when performing ADLs, e.g., on a stool when showering.
  b. Pace activities throughout the day.
  c. Schedule adequate rest periods.
  d. Alternate easy and hard tasks throughout the day.
	2. Excessive energy expenditure can be prevented by pacing activities and allowing sufficient time to recuperate between activities.

3. Gradually increase the client's daily activities as tolerance increases.	3. Sustained moderate breathlessness from supervised exercise improves accessory muscle strength and respiratory function.
4. Teach the client effective breathing techniques such as diaphragmatic and pursed-lip breathing.	4. Diaphragmatic breathing deters the shallow, rapid, inefficient breathing that usually accompanies COPD. Pursed-lip breathing slows expiration, keeps alveoli inflated longer, and provides some control over dyspnea.
5. Teach the importance of supporting arm weight.	5. When arms are not supported, the respiratory muscles are required to perform dual roles: increase respirations and stabilize the chest wall in support of arm weight and activity (Bauldoff, Hoffman, Sciurba & Zullo, 1996).
6. Teach how to increase unsupported arm endurance with lower-extremity exercises performed during the exhalatory phase of respiration.	6. Increasing endurance will improve metabolic function of trained extremity and respiratory muscles and reduced dyspnea with longer endurance limits (Bauldoff et al., 1996).
7. Maintain supplemental oxygen therapy as needed.	7. Supplemental oxygen increases circulating oxygen levels and improves activity tolerance.
8. Provide emotional support and encouragement.	8. Fear of breathlessness may impede increased activity.

9. After activity, assess for abnormal responses to increased activity:
  a. Decreased pulse rate
  b. Decreased or unchanged systolic blood pressure
  c. Excessively increased or decreased respiratory rate
	9. Intolerance to activity can be assessed by valuating cardiac, circulatory, and respiratory statuses.

(continues on page 153)

Interventions continued	**Rationales** continued
d. Failure of pulse to return to near resting rate within 3 minutes after activity e. Confusion, vertigo, uncoordinated movements	
10. Plan adequate rest periods according to the client's daily schedule.	10. Rest periods allow the body a period of low energy expenditure, which increases activity tolerance.
11. Evaluate client's nutritional status.	11. The increased work of breathing causes decreased appetite and intake. Increased CHO intake increases CO_2 production. Decreased intake causes an energy deficit. Energy deficit causes malnutrition and muscle wasting, which decreases diaphragm and muscle strength.
12. Explain the effects of malnutrition. a. Higher mortality b. Depressed immune system c. Decreased muscle strength of diaphragm and chest wall d. Decreased surfactant production	 a. Clients with significant weight loss have higher mortality rates then those with normal weight (Hunter & King, 2001). b. Depressed immune system will reduce ability to fight infection (Hunter & King, 2001). c. These effects will reduce inspiratory and expiratory volumes and the ability to cough effectively (Hunter & King, 2001). d. Inadequate surfactant will increase alveolar surface tension, making inflation more difficult (DeLetter, 1991).
13. Assess for problems associated with eating. a. Breathing competing with eating b. Abdominal gas c. Grocery shopping d. Meal preparation	13. Identification of barriers to proper nutrition can prevent or reduce malnutrition.
14. Teach strategies to increase nutritional status. a. Eat a diet high in lipid/proteins and low in carbohydrates. b. Avoid foods high in fat and calories. c. Prepare meals in advance. d. Sit at table when preparing food. e. Have a large fluid intake (2,000–2,500 mL) daily. f. Avoid milk, chocolates, and other foods that increase viscosity of saliva.	 a. CHO digestion produces more carbon dioxide. Protein is essential for healing. b. They offer the client little benefit. c. Client can rest before warming meal. d. Sitting will reduce energy expenditure. e. This reduces viscosity of secretions and choking sensations. f. Secretions that can be expectorated will lessen anorexia.

(continues on page 154)

Interventions continued	Rationales continued
g. Avoid caffeine and alcohol.	g. These act as diuretics.
h. Reduce amount of liquids at meals.	h. This will reduce bloating and volume of material in stomach.
i. Avoid dry and hot foods.	i. These will irritate throat and stimulate coughing.
j. Eat four to six small meals.	j. These will irritate throat and stimulate coughing.

Documentation

Progress notes
  Activity level
  Physiologic response to activity (vital signs)

Anxiety Related to Breathlessness and Fear of Suffocation

Focus Assessment Criteria	Clinical Significance
1. Anxiety level	1. Anxiety increases respiratory and heart rates, resulting in increased oxygen requirements.
2. Knowledge of breathing techniques	2. This assessment guides client teaching.

Goal

The client will verbalize increased psychological and physiologic comfort.

Indicators

- Verbalize feelings of anxiety.
- Demonstrate breathing techniques to decrease dyspnea.

Interventions	Rationales
1. Provide a quiet, calm environment when the client is experiencing breathlessness.	1. Reducing external stimuli promotes relaxation.
2. Do not leave the client alone during periods of acute breathlessness.	2. The client needs reassurance that help is available if needed.
3. Acknowledge fear and give positive reinforcement for efforts. Acknowledge when dyspnea is worse than usual.	3. Fear triggers dyspnea and dyspnea increases fear. Clients report this lessened their fear and breathing difficulty.

(continues on page 155)

Interventions continued	Rationales continued
4. Acknowledge feelings of helplessness. Avoid suggesting "take control" or "relax."	4. Clients report that nurses who focus on the client's failure to maintain control increase feelings of helplessness (DeVito, 1990).
5. Provide assistance with all tasks during acute episodes of shortness of breath.	5. The client will not be capable of performing activities that they usually do.
6. During acute episode do not discuss preventive measures.	6. Teaching is warranted when client is less dyspneic.
7. Demonstrate breathing techniques and have the client initiate the technique with the nurse.	7. Role modeling breathing techniques for the client to copy will reduce the need to spend energy in concentration.
8. During nonacute episodes teach relaxation techniques, e.g., tapes, guided imagery.	8. Relaxation techniques have been shown to decrease anxiety, dyspnea, and airway obstruction.
9. During periods of acute breathlessness do the following: a. Open curtains and doors. b. Eliminate unnecessary equipment. c. Limit visitors. d. Eliminate smoke and odors.	9. These measures may help reduce feelings of suffocation.
10. Encourage the client to use breathing techniques especially during times of increased anxiety. Coach client through the breathing exercises.	10. Concentrating on diaphragmatic or pursed-lip breathing slows the respiratory rate and gives client a sense of control.

 Documentation

Progress notes
  Acute anxiety episodes
  Interventions
  Client's response to interventions

Powerlessness Related to Feelings of Loss of Control and Life Style Restrictions

Focus Assessment Criteria	Clinical Significance
1. Understanding of disease process 2. Perception of control 3. Effects on life style	1,2,3. A client's response to loss of control depends on the meaning of the loss, individual coping patterns, personal characteristics, and responses of others.

Goal

The client will verbalize ability to influence situations and outcomes.

Indicators

- Identify personal strengths.
- Identify factors that he or she can control.

Interventions	Rationales
1. Explore the effects of the condition on the following: a. Client's occupation b. Leisure and recreational activities c. Role responsibilities d. Relationships	1. Illness can negatively affect the client's self-concept and ability to achieve goals. Specifically in COPD, dyspnea can interfere with the client's ability to work and play.
2. Determine the client's usual response to problems.	2. To plan effective interventions, the nurse must determine if the client usually seeks to change her or his own behaviors to control problems or if she or he expects others or external factors to control problems.
3. Allow client to share his or her losses. a. Life style b. Independence c. Roles	3. Clients with severe COPD experience the formal loss of self. Former self-image changes negatively because of a restricted life style, social isolation, unmet expectations, and dependence on others (Kersten, 1990).
4. Help client to identify personal strengths and assets.	4. Individuals with chronic illness need to be assisted not to see themselves as helpless victims. Persons with a sense of hope, self-control, direction, purpose, and identity are better able to meet the challenges of their disease.
5. Assist in identifying energy patterns and in scheduling activities around these patterns.	5. A review of the client's daily schedule can help the nurse and client to plan activities that promote feelings of self-worth and dignity and to schedule appropriate rest periods to prevent exhaustion.
6. Discuss the need to accept help from others and to delegate some tasks.	6. Client may need assistance to prevent exhaustion and hypoxia.
7. Help client to seek support from other sources, e.g., self-help groups, support groups.	7. Client may benefit from opportunities to share similar experiences and problem solving with others in the same situation.

(continues on page 157)

Interventions continued	Rationales continued
8. Encourage client to make decisions that might increase ability to cope.	8. Self-concept can be enhanced when clients actively engage in decisions regarding health and life style (Lee, Graydon & Ross, 1991).
9. Help client to establish a goal, determine alternatives, and select the best action for self.	9. Setting realistic goals can increase motivation and hope.
10. With clients with severe disease, avoid emphasizing what caused their disease (e.g., smoking).	10. Research has shown that 75% of clients with COPD do not think about the cause of their illness. Persons who do not engage in causal thinking may be in denial. This denial may produce a feeling of control, enabling them to be more functional. Contemplating causes may produce feelings of powerlessness, depression, and decreased functional status (Weaver & Narsavage, 1992).

 Documentation
Progress notes
  Interactions with the client

Disturbed Sleep Pattern Related to Cough, Inability to Assume Recumbent Position, Environmental Stimuli

Focus Assessment Criteria	Clinical Significance
1. Usual sleep requirements	1. Sleep requirements vary with age, life style, activity, and stress level.
2. Usual bedtime routines, environment, and sleeping position	2. Bedtime rituals, a familiar environment, and comfortable positioning help relaxation and promote sleep.
3. Quantity and quality of sleep	3. Only the client can determine his or her satisfaction with quantity and quality of sleep.

Goals
The client will report a satisfactory balance of rest and activity.

Indicators
• Describe factors that inhibit sleep.
• Identify techniques to induce sleep.

Interventions	Rationales
1. Explain the sleep cycle and its significance: a. Stage I: Transitional stage between wakefulness and sleep (5% of total sleep) b. Stage II: Asleep but easily aroused (50%–55% of total sleep) c. Stage III: Deeper sleep; arousal is more difficult (10% of total sleep) d. Stage IV: Deepest sleep; metabolism and brain waves slow (10% of total sleep).	1. A person typically goes through four or five complete sleep cycles each night. If the person awakens during a sleep cycle, he or she may not feel rested in the morning.
2. Discuss individual differences in sleep requirements based on these factors: a. Age b. Activity level c. Life style d. Stress level	2. The usual recommendation of 8 hours of sleep every night actually has no scientific basis. A person who can relax and rest easily requires less sleep to feel refreshed. With aging, total sleep time generally decreases, especially Stage IV sleep, and Stage I sleep time increases.
3. Promote relaxation: a. Provide a dark, quiet environment. b. Allow choices regarding pillows, linens, covers. c. Provide comforting bedtime rituals as necessary. d. Ensure good room ventilation. e. Close the room door if the client desires.	3. Sleep is difficult until relaxation is attained. The hospital environment can impair relaxation.
4. Plan procedures to limit sleep disturbances. Allow the client at least 2-hour segments of uninterrupted sleep.	4. Generally a person must complete an entire sleep cycle (70–100 minutes) four to five times a night to feel rested (Cohen & Merrit, 1992).
5. Explain why hypnotics or sedatives should be avoided.	5. These medications lose their effectiveness after a week; increasing dosages carries the risk of dependence.
6. If desired, elevate the head of the bed on 10-inch blocks or use a gatch with pillows under the arms.	6. This can enhance relaxation and sleep by giving the lungs more room for expansion through reducing upward pressure of abdominal organs.
7. Take measures to control coughing: a. Avoid giving the client cold or hot liquids at bedtime. b. Consult the physician for antitussives if indicated.	7. These measures help to prevent cough stimulation and disruption of sleep.

(continues on page 159)

Interventions continued	Rationales continued

8. Teach the client measures to promote sleep:
  a. Eat a high-protein snack before bed-time, e.g., cheese, milk.
  b. Avoid caffeine.
 	
  c. Attempt to sleep only when feeling sleepy.
 	
  d. If sleeping difficulty occurs, leave the bedroom and engage in a quiet activity, such as reading, in another room.
  e. Try to maintain the same sleep habits 7 days a week.
	a. Digested protein produces tryptophan, which has a sedating effect.
	  b. Caffeine stimulates metabolism and deters relaxation.
	  c. Frustration increases if sleep is attempted when not sleepy or relaxed.
	  d. The bedroom should be reserved specifically for sleep.
	
	  e. Irregular retiring and arising patterns can disrupt the biological clock, which exacerbates sleep difficulties.

9. Assist with a usual bedtime routine, e.g., personal hygiene, snack, music.	9. Following a familiar bedtime routine may help to promote relaxation and aid sleep.

 Documentation

Progress notes
  Sleep patterns (amount, awakenings)
  Client's evaluation of sleep quantity and quality

High Risk for Ineffective Therapeutic Regimen Management Related to Lack of Knowledge of Condition, Treatments, Prevention of Infection, Breathing Exercises, Risk Factors, Signs and Symptoms of Complications

Focus Assessment Criteria	Clinical Significance
1. Readiness and ability to learn and retain information	1. Episodes of cerebral hypoxia can prevent retention of learning. A client who does not achieve goals for learning requires a referral for assistance postdischarge.

Goal

The goals for this diagnosis represent those associated with discharge planning. Refer to discharge criteria.

Interventions	Rationales
1. Help the client to formulate and accept realistic short- and long-term goals.	1. This may help the client to realize that he or she has much control over his or her life and can make choices to improve quality of life.
2. Teach about the diagnosis and the treatment regimen.	2. Understanding may help to encourage compliance and participation in self-care.

(continues on page 160)

Interventions continued	**Rationales** continued
3. Teach measures to help control dyspnea and infections: a. Eat a well-balanced diet.	a. Weight loss and malnutrition decrease chances of survival (Hunter & King, 2001).

b. Take sufficient rest periods.
  c. Gradually increase activity.
  d. Increase fluids unless contraindicated.
  e. Avoid exposure to the following:
    • Smoke
    • Dust
    • Severe air pollution (rush hour traffic)
    • Extremely cold or warm temperatures
	b,c,d. These practices promote overall good health and increase resistance to infection.
	e. Exposure to these respiratory irritants can cause bronchospasm and increased mucus production. Smoking destroys the ciliary cleansing mechanism of the respiratory tract. Heat raises body temperature and increases the body's oxygen requirements, possibly exacerbating symptoms.

4. Teach and have the client demonstrate breathing exercises (Pederson, 1992):
 	
  a. Incentive spirometer
 	
  b. Diaphragm exercise: Place fingers on the lower ribs; inhale, pushing out against light pressure of fingers.
  c. Lung apex exercises: Apply light pressure just below the clavicle as you inhale. While exhaling, apply pressure to the sternum with the heel of your hand.
  d. Posterior lung exercises: Lie on your side, and have someone else place both hands over your lower thorax and apply pressure as you exhale.
  e. Lateral lower rib area exercises: Exhale completely, then have another person apply pressure to the lower rib cage area with both hands as you inhale. During exhalation, tighten the abdomen as the other person again applies pressure.
	4. A client with COPD typically breathes shallowly from the upper chest. Breathing exercises increase alveolar ventilation and reduce respiratory rate.
	a. Incentive spirometry encourages deep, sustained inspiratory efforts.
	b. Expanding and contracting the diaphragm muscle can help to strengthen it.
	c. Counterpressure forces the client to breathe harder, which strengthens muscles and aerates lung apexes.
	
	d. Adequate fluids will liquefy secretion.
	
	e. Breathing against gravity and counterpressure strengthens respiratory muscles. Complete exhalation promotes maximum expansion of the rib cage.

5. Teach and evaluate the technique of postural drainage:
  a. Assume a dependent position to drain the involved lung area, using pillows or a reclining chair.
  b. Cough and expectorate secretions while in the dependent position.
  c. Hold the position for 10 to 15 minutes.
	5. The force of gravity helps to loosen and drain secretions.

(continues on page 161)

Interventions continued	**Rationales** continued
6. Advise the client not to perform breathing exercises shortly before or after eating.	6. The exertion associated with breathing exercises may reduce appetite. Performing the exercises after eating may cause vomiting.
7. Explain the hazards of infection and ways to reduce the risk: a. Avoid contact with infected persons. b. Receive immunization against influenza and bacterial pneumonia. c. Take antibiotics as prescribed if sputum becomes yellow or green. d. Adhere to chest physiotherapy, medications, and hydration schedule. e. Cleanse all equipment well.	7. A client with COPD is prone to infection due to inadequate primary defenses, i.e., decreased ciliary action and stasis of secretions. Minor respiratory infections can cause serious problems in a client with COPD. Chronic debilitation and retention of secretions (which provide a medium for microorganism growth) put the client at high risk for complications.
8. Instruct the client to report the following: a. Change in sputum characteristics or failure of sputum to return to usual color after 3 days of antibiotic therapy b. Elevated temperature c. Increase in cough, weakness, or shortness of breath d. Increased confusion or drowsiness e. Weight loss f. Weight gain or swelling in ankles and feet	a. Sputum changes may indicate an infection or resistance of the infective organism to the prescribed antibiotic. b. Circulating pathogens stimulate the hypothalamus to elevate body temperature. c. Hypoxia is chronic; exacerbations must be detected early to prevent complications. d. Cerebral hypoxia can produce confusion or drowsiness. e. Inadequate intake can result from dyspnea, fatigue, medication side effects, and anorexia secondary to hypoxia and sputum production. f. These signs may indicate fluid retention secondary to pulmonary arterial hypertension and decreased cardiac output.
9. Teach and observe use of a hand-held nebulizer or metered dose inhaler and oxygen therapy. a. Hand washing b. Assembling equipment, supplies c. Using correct dose of medication d. Correct positioning e. Proper cleaning of equipment after use	9. Accurate instructions can help to prevent medication overdose or infections, and increase effectiveness of treatments.
10. Teach methods to conserve energy. See the nursing diagnosis Fatigue in the Inflammatory Joint Disease care plan for more information.	10. Energy conservation helps prevent exhaustion and exacerbation of hypoxia.

(continues on page 162)

Interventions continued	Rationales continued
11. Consult with primary care provider for possible referral to physical therapy strength and endurance training.	11. Increased strength and endurance of upper arms can decrease dyssynchronous breathing and fatigue and increase over-all quality of life (Bauldoff et al., 1996).
12. Explain the effects of smoking on progression of disease and mortality. Explain the benefits of quitting.	12. The mortality rate for 60-year-old smokers with chronic bronchitis is four times higher then for 60-year-old non-smoking asthmatics.
13. Discuss various available methods to quit smoking • Individual/group counseling • Self-help materials/written, audio, video • Nicotine replacement therapy • Bupropion (Zyban)	13. All these methods have been found to be effective (Best Practice, 2001).
14. Provide information about or initiate referrals to community resources such as the American Lung Association, self-help groups, Meals-on-Wheels, and home health agencies.	14. These resources can provide the client with needed assistance with home management and self-care.

 Documentation

Discharge summary record
  Client teaching
  Outcome achievement or status
  Referrals if indicated

PNEUMONIA

An inflammatory process of the lung parenchyma usually in the bronchioles and alveolar sacs, pneumonia can be caused by bacteria, viruses, fungi, parasites, chemical inhalation, aspiration of gastric contents, or fluid accumulation in lung bases. Pneumonia is the most common infectious cause of death in the United States. One-fourth to one-third of clients hospitalized with pneumococcal pneumonia develop bacteremia. About 50% of all pneumococcal pneumonias occur in people older than 60 years. Community-acquired pneumonia is the leading cause of death from infectious disease in the United States (King & Pippin, 1997).

 Time Frame
Acute episode

⊕ DIAGNOSTIC CLUSTER

Collaborative Problems

▲ PC: Respiratory Insufficiency
PC: Septic Shock
PC: Paralytic Ileus

Nursing Diagnoses	Refer to
▲ Activity Intolerance related to insufficient oxygenation for ADL	COPD
▲ Ineffective Airway Clearance related to pain, increased tracheobronchial secretions, and fatigue	COPD
△ High Risk for Impaired Oral Mucous Membrane related to mouth breathing, frequent expectorations, and decreased fluid intake secondary to malaise	
△ High Risk for Imbalanced Nutrition: Less than Body Requirements related to anorexia, dyspnea, and abdominal distention secondary to air swallowing	Cirrhosis
△ High Risk for Ineffective Therapeutic Regimen Management related to lack of knowledge of condition, infection transmission, prevention of recurrence, diet, signs and symptoms of recurrence, and follow-up care	

▲ This diagnosis was reported to be monitored for or managed frequently (75%–100%).
△ This diagnosis was reported to be monitored for or managed often (50%–74%).

Discharge Criteria

Before discharge, the client or family will

1. Describe how to prevent infection transmission.
2. Describe rest and nutritional requirements.
3. Describe methods to reduce the risk of recurrence.
4. State signs and symptoms that must be reported to a health care professional.

Collaborative Problems

Potential Complication: Respiratory Insufficiency

Potential Complication: Septic Shock

Potential Complication: Paralytic Ileus

Nursing Goal

The nurse will detect early signs/symptoms of hypoxia and septic shock and collaboratively intervene to stabilize client.

Indicators

- Temperature 98–99.5°F
- Pulse regular rhythm rate 60–100 per minute
- Blood pressure >90/60, <140/90
- Urine output >30ml/hour
- Bowel sounds detected
- Alert

Interventions	Rationales

1. Closely monitor high-risk individuals (King & Pippin, 1997):
  • Age >65
  • Unstable vital signs (heart rate >140 beats/minute, systolic BP <90mm Hg, respiratory rate >30 per min)
  • Altered mental status
  • PO$_2$ <60mm Hg
  • Severe underlying disease (COPD, DM, liver disease, heart failure, renal failure)
  • Immunocompromised state (HIV, cancer, history of corticosteroid use)
  • Complicated pneumonia
  • Severe electrolyte, hematologic, or metabolic abnormality
	1. These factors further compromise hypoxemia and increase mortality rates (King & Pippin, 1997).

2. Monitor for signs and symptoms of hyperthermia:
  a. Fever of 103°F or above
  b. Chills
  c. Tachycardia
  d. Signs of shock: restlessness or lethargy, confusion, decreased systolic blood pressure
	2. Bacteria can act as a pyrogen by raising the hypothalamic thermostat through the production of endogenous pyrogens, which may mediate through prostaglandins. Chills can occur when the temperature set-point of the hypothalamus changes rapidly. High fever increases metabolic needs and oxygen consumption. The impaired respiratory system cannot compensate, and tissue hypoxia results (Porth, 2002).

(continues on page 165)

Interventions continued	**Rationales** continued
3. Provide cooling measures (e.g., reduced clothing and bed linen, tepid baths, increased fluids, hypothermia blanket).	3. Reduced body temperature is necessary to lower metabolic rate and reduce oxygen consumption.
4. Obtain sputum for Gram stain and cultures and blood cultures.	4. Cultures help to identify specific causative organism and sensitive or resistant antibiotics.

5. Monitor respiratory status and assess for signs and symptoms of hypoxia:
  a. Increased respiratory rate
  b. Fever, chills (sudden or insidious)
  c. Productive cough
  d. Diminished or absent breath sounds
  e. Pleuritic pain
  f. Tachycardia
  g. Marked dyspnea
  h. Cyanosis
	5. Tracheobronchial inflammation, impaired alveolar capillary membrane function, edema, fever, and increased sputum production disrupt respiratory function and alter the blood's oxygen-carrying capacity. Reduced chest wall compliance in older adults also affects the quality of respiratory effort. In older adults, tachypnea > 26 respirations/min is one of the earliest signs of pneumonia and often occurs 3 to 4 days before a confirmed diagnosis. Delirium or mental status changes are often seen early in pneumonia in older clients (Brown, 1993). Sputum specimens often are contaminated with oropharyngeal secretions and may not identify the causative organism. Specimens that have more than 25 polymorphonuclear leukocytes and less than 10 squamous epithelial cells per low-power field are considered to be adequate specimens (Marrie, 1992).

6. Monitor for signs and symptoms of septic shock:
  a. Subnormal body temperature
  b. Hypotension
  c. Decreased level of consciousness
  d. Weak, rapid pulse
  e. Rapid, shallow respirations
  f. Cold, clammy skin
  g. Oliguria
	6. Septic shock may develop in a client with pneumonia if treatment is delayed or if the causative organism is very virulent and drug resistant. An older client has an increased risk of other complicating illnesses and may exhibit only subtle signs of septic shock (Ely, 1991).

7. Monitor for signs and symptoms of paralytic ileus:
  a. No bowel movements
  b. No bowel sounds
  c. Abdominal rigidity and distention
  d. Nausea and vomiting
	7. Paralytic ileus can result from anorexia and decreased food intake or from increased insensible fluid loss related to hyperthermia and hyperventilation. Abdominal distention is aggravated by "air hunger"—mouth breathing resulting from hypoxia (Leedom, 1988).

(continues on page 166)

Interventions continued	Rationales continued
8. Administer cough suppressants or expectorants as ordered by the physician.	8. Dry, hacking cough interferes with sleep and saps energy. Cough suppressants should be used judiciously, however, because complete depression of the cough reflex can cause atelectasis by preventing the movement of tracheobronchial secretions.
9. Initiate antibiotics as prescribed. Consult pharmacological reference for specifics.	9. Current pharmacological references provide information regarding action, administration, cautions, and side effects.
10. Maintain oxygen therapy as prescribed and monitor its effectiveness.	10. Oxygen therapy may help to prevent restlessness if the client is becoming dyspneic and it also may help to prevent pulmonary edema. Because the client is no longer gasping for air, the risk of abdominal distention is decreased. Frequent ABG analysis is essential to detect depressed ventilatory drive.
11. Provide respiratory physiotherapy (e.g., percussion, postural drainage) to move thick, tenacious secretions along the tracheobronchial trees.	11. Exudate in the alveoli and bronchospasms caused by an increase in bronchopulmonary secretions can decrease ventilatory effort and impair gas exchange.

 Related Physician-Prescribed Interventions

Medications. Antimicrobials, analgesics (non-narcotic), bronchodilators, mucolytics, expectorants

Intravenous Therapy. Supplemental as needed

Laboratory Studies. ABG analysis, serologic tests, sputum cultures/Gram stain, sedimentation rate, complete blood count, electrolytes, thoracentesis

Diagnostic Studies. Chest X-ray film, pulse oximeter, protected specimen brush (PSB), bronchoalveolar lavage (BAL)

Therapies. Continuous positive airway pressure (CPAP), ultrasonic nebulizer, oxygen via cannula

 Documentation

Medication administration record
   Type, dosage, routes of all medications
Flow record
   Vital signs
   Assessments
Progress notes
   Cooling measures employed
   Effects on temperature

Nursing Diagnoses

High Risk for Impaired Oral Mucous Membrane Related to Mouth Breathing, Frequent Expectorations, and Decreased Fluid Intake Secondary to Malaise

Focus Assessment Criteria	Clinical Significance
1. Overall condition and moisture of the oral cavity and lips	1. These assessment data serve as a baseline for continuous evaluation.
2. Ability to perform oral care	2. The client may need assistance in performing essential oral care.
3. Hydration status	3. Dehydrated oral mucosa is more vulnerable to injury.

Goal

The client will exhibit intact, moist oral mucous membranes.

Indicators
- Describe factors that increase oral injury.
- Relate the techniques of optimal oral hygiene.

Interventions	Rationales
1. Discuss importance of frequent oral hygiene.	1. It removes microorganisms that decrease the risk of infection.
2. Encourage frequent rinsing of the mouth with water; discourage mouth breathing.	2. Dry oral mucosa causes discomfort and increases the risk of breakdown and infection. Mouth breathing causes loss of oral moisture.
3. Teach client to avoid lemon-glycerin swabs and mouthwashes containing alcohol.	3. These agents dry mucous membranes.
4. Monitor hydration status: a. Oral intake b. Parenteral therapy c. Intake and output d. Urine specific gravity	4. Proper hydration must be maintained to liquefy secretions and prevent drying of oral mucosa.
5. If the mouth or lips are sore, instruct client to avoid acidic and very hot or cold foods.	5. These foods can irritate oral mucosa.

(continues on page 168)

Interventions continued	Rationales continued
6. Encourage client to avoid alcohol and tobacco use.	6. Alcohol and tobacco can irritate oral mucosa.
7. Encourage client to lubricate the lips every 2 hours or as needed.	7. Proper lip care replaces moisture and reduces cracking.

Documentation

Flow record
   Oral Assessment
   Oral care
Discharge summary record
   Client teaching

High Risk for Ineffective Therapeutic Regimen Management Related to Lack of Knowledge of Condition, Infection Transmission, Prevention of Recurrence, Diet, Signs and Symptoms of Recurrence, and Follow-up Care

Focus Assessment Criteria	Clinical Significance
1. Readiness and ability to learn and retain information.	1. Malaise and other factors may impede the ability to learn. If learning goals are not achieved, a referral may be needed for postdischarge assistance.

Goal

The goals for this diagnosis represent those associated with discharge planning. Refer to the discharge criteria.

Interventions	Rationales
1. Explain the pathophysiology of pneumonia using teaching aids (e.g., illustrations, models) appropriate for the client's or family's educational level.	1. Understanding the disease process and its possible complications may encourage the client's compliance with the therapeutic regimen.

2. Explain measures to prevent the spread of infection:
  a. Cover the nose and mouth when sneezing or coughing.
  b. Dispose of used tissues in a paper bag; when the bag is half full, close it securely and place it in a larger disposal unit.
  c. Wash hands frequently.
	2. Although pneumococcal pneumonia is not highly communicable, during the acute phase the client should refrain from visiting with persons predisposed to pneumonia, e.g., elderly or seriously ill persons, those with sickle cell disease, postsurgical patients, or persons with chronic respiratory disease.

(continues on page 169)

Interventions continued	**Rationales** continued
3. Explain measures to prevent recurrence:	3. A client with pneumonia commonly has an underlying chronic disease; impaired host defenses increase the risk of recurrence.
a. Complete the entire course of prescribed antibiotic therapy and report any side effects.	a. If there is no response to treatment within 24 to 48 hours, a reevaluation should be initiated. Possibly there has been an inaccurate diagnosis, the causative organism is resistant to prescribed antibiotic, or dosage has to be adjusted. More invasive techniques for obtaining respiratory secretions for culture may be required. The possibility of infection in the pleural space or the presence of an obstructive lesion, particularly in smokers, should be considered (LaForce, 1992). Because most clients notice a decrease in symptoms after 72 hours of treatment, they sometimes do not recognize the importance of continuing the antibiotic as prescribed. The course of medication is usually 7 to 14 days but may be as long as 21 days depending on severity of illness, presence of underlying disease, and patient response. Antibiotics should be continued until completed and a follow-up X-ray film confirms that infection has subsided.
b. Keep scheduled, follow-up medical appointments.	b. Even though clinical signs may be absent, particularly in older clients, a chest X-ray film is necessary to confirm absence of pneumonia. This also allows further evaluation, as some clients with lung cancer initially present with pneumonia. In the older patient, initial chest X-rays may indicate progression of the pneumonia; however, this is usually a reflection of better hydration. The follow-up X-ray films take longer to show resolution, often showing opacities far beyond 14 weeks. In younger individuals, complete resolution is usually seen in 4 to 8 weeks (Marrie, 1992).
c. Continue deep breathing exercises for 6 to 8 weeks during the convalescent period.	c. Deep breathing increases alveolar expansion and thus facilitates movement of secretions from the tracheobronchial tree with coughing. Routine planned deep breathing and coughing sessions increase vital capacity and pulmonary compliance. Sometimes dry cough occurs with chest wall pain related to myalgias of the intercostal muscles so increased efforts must be made to encourage regular lung expansion. A pillow may be used to splint the chest wall while coughing.

(continues on page 170)

Interventions continued	Rationales continued
d. Plan rest periods during morning and afternoon.	d. Increased metabolism results from hyperthermia and from the body's defense mechanisms for fighting infection. More energy is expended as the lungs work harder to perfuse the tissues of the body adequately. These factors result in increased physical fatigue.
e. Obtain influenza and pneumococcal immunizations if the client has a chronic respiratory condition, is elderly, or is immunosuppressed.	e. Because bacterial pneumonia may occur as a complication of influenza, yearly influenza immunization is recommended for at-risk groups. Those individuals are (1) adults with chronic disorders of the pulmonary or cardiovascular systems, (2) residents of nursing homes or other chronic care facilities that house individuals with chronic medical conditions, (3) persons age 65 or older, (4) adults requiring regular medical follow-up or hospitalization during previous year because of chronic metabolic diseases, renal dysfunction, hemoglobinopathies, or immunosuppression. The currently used pneumococcal vaccine (Pneumovax) confers a very high rate of immunity because it contains 23 of the most common pneumococcal organisms that protect against types that cause 85% of bacteremia infections. Current studies identify if more than one pneumococcal immunization is necessary. Current recommendations are that individuals who are at high risk for sepsis-related complications such as asplenics or those who are nephrotic or immunosuppressed should be vaccinated every 6 years. (Arcangelo & Peterson, 2001). Otherwise, Pneumovax should be administered only on a one-time basis.
4. Encourage adequate hydration with intake of 3000 mL per day if not contraindicated.	4. Insensible fluid losses from hyperthermia and productive cough predispose the client to dehydration, particularly an elderly client.
5. Encourage adequate, nutritious food intake and use of high-protein supplements if necessary.	5. Increased metabolism raises the client's calorie requirements; however, dyspnea and anorexia sometimes prevent adequate caloric intake. High-protein supplements provide increased calories and fluids if anorexia and fatigue from eating interfere with food intake.

(continues on page 171)

Interventions continued	Rationales continued
6. Encourage client to avoid smoking.	6. Chronic smoking destroys the tracheo-bronchial ciliary action, the lungs' first defense against infection. It also inhibits alveolar macrophage function and irritates the bronchial mucosa.
7. Instruct client and family to report any signs or symptoms after initiation of treatment (e.g., thickening of respiratory secretions, return or persistence of fever, increased chest pain, malaise).	7. Pneumonia may be resistant to the prescribed antibiotic, or secondary infection with organisms not susceptible to prescribed antibiotic may have occurred.
8. Position client to minimize aspiration.	8. Approximately 50% of healthy individuals aspirate during sleep with minimal problems. In recently hospitalized individuals, there is increased chance of oropharyngeal colonization. Hydrochloric acid protects against pneumonia from aspiration; however, antacids, by changing the pH of the stomach contents, increase the risk of nosocomial pneumonia. Sucralfate and other agents that do not alter normal gastric pH reduce the risk of nosocomial pneumonia with aspiration. Individuals at increased risk of aspiration are those with impaired pulmonary defenses, such as those on O_2 therapy, steroids, antibiotics, and tracheal suctioning, as well as those suffering from alcoholism and diabetes. Also, individuals receiving tube feedings, even in the jejunum, and receiving sedatives are at risk (Scheld & Mandell, 1991).
9. Encourage the client to avoid factors that lower resistance to pneumonia— e.g., overexertion, chilling, and excessive alcohol intake—particularly during the convalescent period.	9. A client who has had one episode of pneumonia is at increased risk for recurrence. Any upper respiratory infection may lead to bacterial invasion in the lower respiratory tract.

 Documentation

Graphic/flow record
   Discharge instructions
   Follow-up instructions
Progress notes
   Status at discharge
   Outcome achievement or status

For a Care map on pneumonia, visit http://connection.lww.com

Metabolic and Endocrine Disorders

CIRRHOSIS

A set of changes in liver tissue characterized by the nodular regeneration of parenchymal cells and scar tissue formation, cirrhosis is divided into three types: (1) Laennec's portal cirrhosis, which results from chronic alcohol toxicity and the accompanying malnutrition; (2) postnecrotic cirrhosis, which involves scar tissue resulting from viral hepatitis; and (3) biliary cirrhosis, in which scarring results from chronic biliary obstruction. In all types, the fibrosis or scarring interferes with normal liver function and portal blood flow. Impaired portal blood flow causes venous congestion in the spleen and gastrointestinal (GI) tract.

 Time Frame

Initial diagnosis
Recurrent acute episodes

⊚ **DIAGNOSTIC CLUSTER**

Collaborative Problems

▲ PC: Hemorrhage
▲ PC: Medication Toxicity (opiates, short-acting
        barbiturates, major tranquilizers)
△ PC: Metabolic Disorders
△ PC: Portal Systemic Encephalopathy
△ PC: Renal Insufficiency

Nursing Diagnoses	**Refer to**
▲ Imbalanced Nutrition: Less Than Body Requirements related to anorexia, impaired protein, fat, glucose metabolism, and impaired storage of vitamins (A, C, K, D, E)	
▲ Impaired Comfort related to pruritus secondary to accumulation of bilirubin pigment and bile salts	
▲ Excess Fluid Volume related to portal hypertension, lowered plasma colloidal osmotic pressure, and sodium retention	
▲ Pain related to liver enlargement and ascites (Pancreatitis)	

(continues on page 176)

Nursing Diagnoses continued	Refer to continued
▲ High Risk for Ineffective Therapeutic Regimen Management related to lack of knowledge of pharmacologic contraindications, nutritional requirements, signs and symptoms of complications, and risks of alcohol ingestion	
▲ Diarrhea related to excessive secretion of fats in stool secondary to liver dysfunction	Pancreatitis
▲ High Risk for Infection related to leukopenia secondary to enlarged, overactive spleen and hypoproteinemia	Leukemia

▲ This diagnosis was reported to be monitored for or managed frequently (75%–100%).
△ This diagnosis was reported to be monitored for or managed often (50%–74%).

Discharge Criteria

Before discharge, the client or family will

1. Describe the causes of cirrhosis.
2. Describe activity restrictions and nutritional requirements.
3. State actions that reduce anorexia, edema, and pruritus at home.
4. State the signs and symptoms that must be reported to a health care professional.

Collaborative Problems

Potential Complication: Hemorrhage

Potential Complication: Metabolic Disorders

Potential Complication: Portal Systemic Encephalopathy

Potential Complication: Medication Toxicity

Potential Complication: Renal Insufficiency

Nursing Goal

The nurse will monitor to detect early signs/symptoms of (a) hemorrhage, (b) metabolic disorders, (c) encephalopathy, (d) renal insufficiency, and (e) medication toxicities and collaboratively intervene to stabilize the client.

Indicators
- BP > 90/60, < 140/90 mm Hg
- Heart rate 60–100 beats/min
- Respirations 16–20 breaths/min
- Hemoglobin
  - Male 14–18 g/dL
  - Female 12–16 g/dL
- Hematocrit, a
  - Male 42–52%
  - Female 37–47%

- Stools negative occult blood (a)
- Prothrombin time 11–12.5 seconds (a)
- Electrolytes within normal range (b)
- Serum pH 7.35–7.45 (a, b, c)
- Serum PCO_2 35–45 mm Hg (b, c)
- Oxygen saturation >95% (pulse oximeter) (a, b, c)
- Alert, oriented (a, b, c)
- Urine output >30 ml/1 hour (a, b, d)
- Urine specific gravity 1.005–1.030 (b, d)
- Sodium 135–145 mEq/L (b, d)
- Creatinine 0.7–1.4 mg/dL (b, d)
- Albumin 3.5–5.0 m/U/ml (b, d)
- Prealbumin 16–40 m/U/ml (b, d)
- Blood urea nitrogen 5–25 mg/dl

Interventions	Rationales
1. Monitor for hemorrhage by assessing the following: a. Vital signs b. Hematocrit and hemoglobin c. Stools, for occult blood d. Prothrombin time	1. The liver has a central role in hemostasis. Decreased platelet count results from impaired production of new platelets from the bone marrow. Decreased clearance of old platelets by the reticuloendothelial system also results. In addition, the synthesis of coagulation factors (II, V, VII, IX, and X) is impaired, resulting in bleeding. Most frequent site is upper GI tract. Other sites are nasopharynx, lungs, retroperitoneum, kidneys, intracranial and skin puncture sites (McEwen, 1996).
2. Monitor for bleeding from esophageal varices: a. Hematemesis (vomiting blood) b. Melena (black, sticky stools)	2. One-third of clients with cirrhosis and varices experience bleeding. Varices are dilated tortuous veins in the lower esophagus. Portal hypertension caused by obstruction of the portal venous system results in increased pressure on the vessels in the esophagus, making them fragile (Porth, 2002).
3. Teach the client to report unusual bleeding (e.g., in the mouth after brushing teeth) and ecchymotic areas.	3. Mucous membranes are more prone to injury because of their great surface vascularity.
4. Monitor for signs and symptoms of (refer to index under each electrolyte for specific signs and symptoms): a. Hypoglycemia	4. a. Hypoglycemia is caused by loss of glycogen stores in liver from damaged cells and decreased serum concentrations of glucose, insulin, and growth hormones (McEwen, 1996).

(continues on page 178)

Interventions continued	**Rationales** continued
b. Hyponatremia	b. Reduced capacity of kidneys to excrete water results in dilutional hyponatremia (McEwen, 1996).
c. Hypokalemia	c. Potassium losses are from vomiting, nasogastric suctioning, diuretics, or excessive renal losses (McEwen, 1996).
d. Hypocalcemia	d. Hypomagnesemia or pancreatitis can decrease calcium levels (McEwen, 1996).
e. Hypomagnesemia	e. The loss of potassium ions causes the proportional loss of magnesium ions (McEwen, 1996).
f. Hypophosphatemia	f. Increased phosphate loss, transcellular shifts, and decreased phosphate intake contribute to hypophosphatemia (McEwen, 1996).
5. Monitor for acid–base disturbances.	5. Hepatocellular necrosis can result in accumulation of organic anions resulting in metabolic acidosis. Persons with ascites often have metabolic alkalosis from increased bicarbonate levels resulting from increased sodium/hydrogen exchange in distal tubule (Porth, 2002).
6. Monitor for portal systemic encephalopathy by assessing the following: a. General behavior b. Orientation to time and place c. Speech patterns	6. Profound liver failure results in accumulation of ammonia and other identical toxic metabolites in the blood. The blood-brain barrier permeability increases, and both toxins and plasma proteins leak from capillaries to the extracellular space, causing cerebral edema (McEwen, 1996).
7. Assess for side effects of medications. 8. Avoid administering medications that can impair liver function (e.g., narcotics, sedatives, tranquilizers, lipid-lowering agents, hypoglycemic agents).	7,8. Liver dysfunction results in decreased metabolism of certain medications, which increases the risk of toxicity from high drug blood levels. Some drugs increase liver dysfunction.
9. Monitor for renal failure by assessing the following: a. Intake and output b. Urine specific gravity c. Laboratory values: serum sodium, creatinine, pre-albumin	9. Obstructed hepatic blood flow results in decreased blood to the kidneys, which impairs glomerular filtration and leads to fluid retention and decreased urinary output.
10. Monitor for hypertension.	10. Fluid retention and overload can cause hypertension.

(continues on page 179)

Interventions continued	Rationales continued
11. Teach the client and family to report signs and symptoms of complications:	11. Early detection allows prompt intervention to help prevent progression of complications.
a. Increased abdominal girth	a. Increased abdominal girth may indicate worsening portal hypertension.
b. Rapid weight loss or gain	b. Rapid weight loss points to negative nitrogen balance; weight gain, to fluid retention.
c. Bleeding	c. Bleeding indicates decreased prothrombin time and clotting factors.
d. Tremors	d. Tremors result from impaired neurotransmission due to failure of the liver to detoxify enzymes that act as false neurotransmitters.
e. Confusion	e. Confusion results from cerebral hypoxia caused by high serum ammonia levels due to the liver's impaired ability to convert ammonia to urea.

▼ Related Physician-Prescribed Interventions

Medications. Vitamin/mineral supplement, lactulose, digestive enzymes, potassium-sparing diuretics, vasodilators, electrolyte replacements

Intravenous Therapy. Hyperalimentation

Laboratory Studies. Blood urea nitrogen (BUN); serum bilirubin, albumin, prealbumin; serum ammonia; serum glutamic-oxaloacetic transaminase (SGOT), serum glutamic-pyruvic transaminase, lactate dehydrogenase (LDH); serum glucose; electrolytes; urine urobilinogen; alkaline phosphatase; aspartate aminotransferase (AST); IgA, IgG; alanine aminotransferase (ALT); CBC; prothrombin time

Diagnostic Studies. Liver scan, percutaneous transhepatic cholangiography, liver biopsy, chest X-ray film, esophagogastroduodenoscopy, upper GI series, CT Scan

Therapies. Diet (high-calorie, low-fat, moderate-protein, low-salt); oxygen via cannula; fluid restrictions; paracentesis; enteral feedings

⟳ Documentation

Flow records
  Weight
  Vital signs
  Stools for occult blood
  Abdominal girth
  Urine specific gravity
  Intake and output
Progress notes
  Evidence of bleeding
  Evidence of tremors or confusion

Nursing Diagnoses

Imbalanced Nutrition: Less Than Body Requirements Related to Anorexia, Impaired Protein, Fat, and Glucose Metabolism, and Impaired Storage of Vitamins (A, C, K, D, E)

Focus Assessment Criteria	Clinical Significance
1. Intake (caloric count, type of food, supplements)	1. Intake must be evaluated because of the effects of cirrhosis on metabolism, vitamin storage, and appetite.
2. Weight (daily)	2. Daily weights are indicated to evaluate nitrogen balance.
3. Abdominal girth (daily)	3. Hepatic congestion causes ascites, which can be evaluated by abdominal girth measurements.
4. Laboratory values: serum albumin and protein levels	4. A decrease in plasma proteins results from decreased hepatic synthesis of plasma proteins.

Goal

1. The client will describe the reasons for nutritional problems.
2. The client will relate which foods are high in protein and calories.
3. The client will gain weight (specify amount) without increased edema.
4. The client will explain the rationale for sodium restrictions.

Interventions	Rationales
1. Discuss the causes of anorexia, dyspepsia, and nausea. Explain that obstructed hepatic blood flow causes GI vascular congestion, (which results in gastritis and diarrhea or constipation), and that impaired liver function causes metabolic disturbances (fluid, electrolyte, glucose metabolism), resulting in anorexia and fatigue (Caregaro et al., 1996).	1. Helping the client to understand the condition can reduce anxiety and may help to improve compliance.
2. Teach and assist the client to rest before meals.	2. Fatigue further decreases the desire to eat.
3. Offer frequent small feedings (six per day plus snacks).	3. Increased intra-abdominal pressure from ascites compresses the GI tract and reduces its capacity.
4. Restrict liquids with meals and avoid fluids 1 hour before and after meals.	4. Fluids can overdistend the stomach, decreasing appetite and intake.

(continues on page 181)

Interventions continued	**Rationales** continued
5. Maintain good oral hygiene (brush teeth, rinse mouth) before and after ingestion of food.	5. Accumulation of food particles in the mouth can contribute to foul odors and taste that diminish appetite.
6. Arrange to have foods with the highest protein/calorie content served at the time the client feels most like eating.	6. This increases the likelihood of the client consuming adequate amounts of protein and calories.

7. Teach the client measures to reduce nausea (Rhodes, 1990):
  a. If possible, avoid the smell of food preparation, and try eating cold foods that have less odor.
  b. Loosen clothing when eating.
  c. Sit in fresh air when eating.
  d. Avoid lying down flat for at least 2 hours after eating. (A client who must rest should sit or recline so his head is at least 4 inches higher than his feet.)
	7. Venous congestion in the GI tract predisposes client to nausea (McEwen, 1996).

8. Limit foods and fluids high in fat.	8. Impaired bile flow results in malabsorption of fats.

9. Explain the need to increase intake of foods high in the following elements:
  a. Vitamin B$_{12}$ (eggs, chicken, shellfish)
  b. Folic acid (green leafy vegetables, whole grains, meat)
  c. Thiamine (legumes, beans, oranges)
  d. Iron (organ meats, dried fruit, green vegetables, whole grains)
	9. Vitamin intake must be increased to compensate for decreased metabolism and vitamin storage due to liver tissue damage.

10. Teach client the need to take water-soluble forms of fat-soluble vitamins (A, D, and E).	10. Impaired bile flow interferes with absorption of fat-soluble vitamins.
11. Explain the risks of alcohol ingestion.	11. Alcohol is toxic to the liver and decreases appetite, contributing to inadequate intake.
12. Consult with the physician if the client does not consume sufficient nutrients.	12. High-protein supplements, total parenteral nutrition, or tube feedings may be needed.

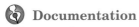 **Documentation**

Flow records
  Weight
  Intake (type, amount)
  Abdominal girth

Impaired Comfort Related to Pruritus Secondary to Accumulation of Bilirubin Pigment and Bile Salts

Focus Assessment Criteria	Clinical Significance
1. Skin condition 2. Factors that aggravate or relieve pruritus	1,2. Obstruction of bile flow causes deposition of bile salts in the skin where they act as an irritant and cause itching (Porth, 2002).

Goal
The client will verbalize decreased pruritus.

Indicators
- Describe factors that increase pruritus.
- Describe factors that improve pruritus.

Interventions	Rationales

1. Maintain hygiene without causing dry skin:
  a. Give frequent baths using cool water and mild soap (castile, lanolin) or a soap substitute.
  b. Blot skin dry; do not rub.
	1. Dryness increases skin sensitivity by stimulating nerve endings.

2. Prevent excessive warmth by maintaining cool room temperatures and low humidity, using light covers with a bed cradle, and avoiding overdressing.	2. Excessive warmth aggravates pruritus by increasing sensitivity through vasodilation.
3. Advise against scratching; explain the scratch-itch-scratch cycle. Instruct the client to apply firm pressure to pruritic areas instead of scratching.	3. Scratching stimulates histamine release, which produces more pruritus.
4. Consult with the physician for a pharmacologic treatment (e.g., antihistamines, antipruritic lotions) if necessary.	4. If pruritus is unrelieved or if the skin is excoriated from scratching, topical or systemic medications are indicated.
5. Keep room cool and with humidity at 30% to 40%.	5. Coolness will reduce vasodilatation, and humidity will reduce dryness.

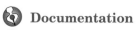 **Documentation**

Progress notes
  Unrelieved pruritus
  Excoriated skin

Excess Fluid Volume Related to Portal Hypertension, Lowered Plasma Colloidal Osmotic Pressure, and Sodium Retention

Focus Assessment Criteria	Clinical Significance
1. Diet (sodium and protein content)	1. A diet high in sodium and low in protein can contribute to edema formation.
2. Presence of edema	2. A baseline assessment of edema enables ongoing assessment for changes.

Goal

1. The client will relate actions that decrease fluid retention.
2. The client will list foods high in sodium.

Interventions	Rationales
1. Assess the client's diet for inadequate protein or excessive sodium intake. 2. Encourage the client to decrease salt intake. Teach the client to take the following actions: 　a. Read food labels for sodium content. 　b. Avoid convenience foods, canned foods, and frozen foods. 　c. Cook without salt and use spices (e.g., lemon, basil, tarragon, mint) to add flavor. 　d. Use vinegar in place of salt to flavor soups, stews, etc. (e.g., 2–3 teaspoons of vinegar to 4–6 quarts according to taste).	1,2. Decreased renal flow results in increased aldosterone and antidiuretic hormone secretion, causing water and sodium retention and potassium excretion.
3. Ascertain with the physician if the client may use a salt substitute. Avoid substitutes containing ammonium.	3. Ammonium elevates serum ammonia levels and may contribute to hepatic coma.
4. Take measures to protect edematous skin from injury: 　a. Inspect the skin for redness and blanching. 　b. Reduce pressure on skin, e.g., pad chairs and footstools. 　c. Prevent dry skin by using soap sparingly, rinsing off soap completely, and using a lotion to moisten skin.	4. Edematous skin is taut and easily injured. Dry skin is more vulnerable to breakdown and injury.

 Documentation

Progress notes
　Presence of edema

High Risk for Ineffective Therapeutic Regimen Management Related to Lack of Knowledge of Pharmacologic Contraindications, Nutritional Requirements, Signs and Symptoms of Complications, and Risks of Alcohol Ingestion

Focus Assessment Criteria	Clinical Significance
Client's or family's readiness and ability to learn and retain information	A client or family that does not achieve the goals for learning requires a referral for assistance postdischarge.

Goal

The goals for this diagnosis represent those associated with discharge planning. Refer to the discharge criteria.

Interventions	Rationales
1. Teach the client or family about the condition and its causes and treatments.	1. This teaching reinforces the need to comply with the therapeutic regimen including diet and activity restrictions.
2. Explain portal system encephalopathy to the family. Teach them to observe for and report any confusion, tremors, night wandering, or personality changes.	2. Family members typically first note the development of encephalopathy.
3. Explain the need for adequate rest and avoidance of strenuous activity.	3. As the liver repairs itself, physical activity depletes the body of the energy needed for healing. Adequate rest is needed to prevent relapse.
4. Explain the need for a diet high in protein and calories and low in salt. (Refer to the nursing diagnosis Altered Nutrition in the index for specific interventions.)	4. Protein and caloric requirements are greater when tissue is healing.
5. Explain the hazards of certain medications, including narcotics, sedatives, tranquilizers, and ammonia products.	5. Impaired liver function slows metabolism of some drugs, causing levels to accumulate, increasing toxicity.

6. Teach the client or family to watch for and report signs and symptoms of complications:
 	
  a. Bleeding (gums, stools)
	6. Progressive liver failure affects hematopoietic function and electrolyte and fluid balance, causing potentially serious complications that require prompt intervention.
	  a. Bleeding indicates decreased platelets and clotting factors.

(continues on page 185)

Interventions continued	Rationales continued
b. Hypokalemia (muscle cramps, nausea, vomiting)	b. Hypokalemia results from over-production of aldosterone, which causes sodium and water retention and potassium excretion.
c. Confusion, altered speech patterns, fluctuating moods, and personality changes	c. Confusion and altered speech patterns result from cerebral hypoxia because of high serum ammonia levels caused by the liver's impaired ability to convert ammonia to urea.
d. Increasing severity of symptoms	d. Exacerbation of symptoms indicates progressive liver damage.
e. Rapid weight loss or gain	e. Rapid weight loss points to negative nitrogen balance; weight gain, to fluid retention.
7. Explain the need to avoid alcohol.	7. Alcohol increases hepatic irritation and may interfere with recovery.
8. Stress the importance of follow-up care and laboratory studies.	8. Timely follow-up enables evaluation of liver function and early detection of relapse or recurrence.

 Documentation

Flow records
   Client teaching
   Referrals when indicated
Progress notes
   Unachieved outcomes

DIABETES MELLITUS

Diabetes mellitus is a chronic disease of abnormal metabolism requiring lifelong treatment with diet, exercise, and medication. There are three clinical subclasses of diabetes: type 1, type 2, and other types (gestational diabetes, glucose intolerance, and secondary diabetes). The diagnosis of diabetes is based on two fasting plasma glucose measurements greater than or equal to 126 mg/dL. Although the etiology, clinical course, and treatment differ, the common denominator of all types is glucose intolerance. Type 1 diabetes is characterized by acute onset. Clients with type 1 diabetes are usually young and thin, always require insulin treatment, and account for 10% of known cases in the United States. Type 2 affects 90% of people with diabetes and has an insidious onset. Usual clients are older, obese and usually have a positive family history of the disease. Diabetes affects all body systems because clients are susceptible to the chronic complications of the disease—specifically retinopathy, nephropathy, neuropathy, and vascular disease (American Diabetes Association [ADA], 1997).

DIAGNOSTIC CLUSTER

Collaborative Problems

▲ PC: Diabetes Ketoacidosis (DKA)
▲ PC: Hypoglycemia
▲ PC: Infections
▲ PC: Vascular Disease
▲ PC: Neuropathy
▲ PC: Hyperosmolar, Hyperglycemic, Nonketotic (HHNK) Coma
▲ PC: Retinopathy
▲ PC: Nephropathy

Nursing Diagnoses

▲ Imbalanced Nutrition: More Than Body Requirements related to intake in excess of activity expenditures, lack of knowledge, or ineffective coping
▲ Fear (client, family) related to diagnosis of diabetes, insulin injections, and the risk of acute and chronic complications of diabetes
▲ Risk for Ineffective Coping (client, family) related to the chronicity of diabetes, the complexity of care regimens, and an uncertain future
△ Risk for Injury related to severe episodes of hypoglycemia, diminished visual acuity, and decrease tactile sensation
  Risk for Ineffective Sexuality Patterns (male) related to erectile difficulty secondary to peripheral neuropathy and/or psychological stressors associated with diabetes
  Risk for Sexual Dysfunction (female) related to frequent genitourinary, physical, and psychological stressors, infections
△ Risk for Noncompliance related to the complexity and chronicity of the prescribed regimen
△ Risk for Ineffective Management of Therapeutic Regimen related to insufficient knowledge of diabetes, self-monitoring of blood glucose, medications, ADA exchange, diet, hypoglycemia, weight control, sick day care, exercise, foot care, s/s of complications, and the need for comprehensive diabetes outpatient education

---

▲ This diagnosis was reported to be monitored for or managed frequently (75%–100%).
△ This diagnosis was reported to be monitored for or managed often (50%–74%).

Discharge Criteria

Before discharge, the client or family will

1. Define diabetes as a chronic disease requiring lifelong treatment with food, exercise, and often medication.
2. Consult with a dietitian for an individualized ADA meal plan.
3. State the relationship of food and exercise to blood glucose (BG) and hemoglobin A1C levels.
4. State the effects of weight loss on BG control with type 2 diabetes.
5. Describe self-care measures that may prevent or decrease progression of chronic complications.
6. State the value of monitoring BG and a plan to obtain supplies and begin testing BG.
7. Explain the importance of foot care.
8. Agree to attend comprehensive outpatient diabetes education program.
9. Agree to home care referral for diabetes education and self-care management.

For Clients Requiring Medications

Oral Agents

1. State name, dose, action, and time to take diabetes medications.
2. State risk of hypoglycemia with delayed meals or increased activities.
3. State s/s and treatment of hypoglycemia.
4. State intent to wear diabetes identification.

Insulin

1. Demonstrate technique for administration of insulin.
2. State brand, type, onset, peak, duration, and dose of insulin.
3. State recommendations for site rotation, storage of insulin, and disposal of syringes.
4. State s/s and treatment of hypoglycemia.
5. State intent to wear diabetes identification.
6. Describe self-care measures during illness.

Collaborative Problems

Potential Complication: Diabetic Ketoacidosis (DKA)

Potential Complication: Hypoglycemia

Potential Complication: Infections

Potential Complication: Vascular Disease

Potential Complication: Neuropathy

Potential Complication: Hyperosmolar Hyperglycemia Nonketotic (HHNK) Coma

Potential Complication: Retinopathy

Potential Complication: Nephropathy

Nursing Goal

The nurse will monitor for early signs and symptoms of (a) diabetic ketoacidosis; (b) hyperosmolar hyperglycemia (nonketotic); (c) hypoglycemia; (d) infections; (e) vascular, (f) neurological, (g) retinal, and (h) renal complications and collaboratively intervene to stabilize.

Indicators
- pH 7.35–7.45, *a, b*
- Fasting blood glucose 70–115 mg/dL, *a, b, c*
- No ketones in urine, *a, b*
- Serum sodium 1.35–1.45 mEq/L, *a, b, h*
- Serum phosphates, 1.8–2.6 m Osm/kg, *a, b, h*
- Serum osmolality, 280–295 m Osm/kg, *a, b, h*
- BP <90/160 or >140/190 mm Hg, *e*

- , oriented (a, b, e, f)
- 60–100 beats/min (e)
- ations 16–20 breaths/min (a, b, e)
- ry refill <3 seconds (e)
- ral pulse, equal, full (e)
- dry skin (a, b, e)
- ge of vision (f, g)
- don reflexes intact (f)
- unds, present (f)
- od cells 300–10,800 mm (d)
- tein-negative (h)
- e 0.7–1.4 mg/dL (h)
- a nitrogen 5–25mg/dL (h)

Interventions	Rationales
1. Monitor for s/s of DKA: a. Recent illness/infection b. BG >300 mg/dL c. Moderate/large ketones d. Anorexia, nausea, vomiting, abdominal pain e. Kussmaul's respirations (deep, nonlabored) f. pH <7.35 g. Decreased sodium, potassium, phosphates h. Dehydration	1. When insulin is not available, BG levels rise and the body metabolizes fat for energy-producing ketone bodies. Excessive ketone bodies cause headaches, nausea, vomiting, and abdominal pain. Increased respiratory rate and depth helps CO_2 excretion and reduces acidosis. Glucose inhibits water reabsorption in the renal glomerulus, leading to osmotic diuresis with loss of water, sodium, potassium, and phosphates. DKA occurs in Type 1 diabetes (Porte & Sherwin, 1997).
2. Monitor for s/s of HHNK coma: a. Blood glucose 600 to 2,000 mg/dL b. Severe dehydration c. Serum osmolality >350 mOsm/kg d. Hypotension e. Altered sensorium	2. HHNK coma is a state of marked dehydration and excessive hyperglycemia and occurs in Type 2 diabetes. Ketones are not present. Glucose inhibits water reabsorption in the renal glomerulus, leading to osmotic diuresis with loss of water, sodium, potassium, and phosphates. Cerebral impairment is due to intracellular dehydration (Porte & Sherwin, 1997).
3. Monitor cardiac status: a. Vital signs b. Skin color c. Capillary refill d. Peripheral pulses e. Serum potassium	3. Severe dehydration may cause reduced cardiac output and compensatory vasoconstriction. Cardiac dysrhythmias may result from potassium imbalances (Kahn & Weir, 1994).
4. Monitor for s/s of hypoglycemia: a. Blood glucose <70 mg/dL b. Pale, moist, cool skin c. Tachycardia, diaphoresis	4. Hypoglycemia may be caused by too much insulin, too little food, or physical activity. When blood glucose falls rapidly, the sympathetic system is stimulated to

(continues on page 189)

Interventions continued	**Rationales** continued
d. Jitteriness, irritability e. Incoordination f. Drowsiness g. Hypoglycemia unawareness	produce adrenaline, which causes diaphoresis, cool skin, tachycardia, and jitteriness (ADA, 1997; Hass, 1993). Hypoglycemia unawareness is a defect in the body's defense system that impairs the ability to feel the warning symptoms usually associated with hypoglycemia. Such a client may progress from alertness to unconsciousness rapidly (Hass, 1993).

5. Monitor for s/s of infection:
  a. Upper respiratory tract infection
  b. Urinary tract infection
  c. External otitis
  d. Red, painful, or warm skin
  e. Furunculosis
  f. Carbuncles
	5. Increased glucose in epidermis and urine promotes bacterial growth. The early diagnosis and treatment of infection in a patient with diabetes is necessary because infection is a leading cause of metabolic abnormalities (Guthrie & Guthrie, 1997).

6. Assess for risk factors and monitor for s/s of macrovascular complications:
  a. Family history of heart disease
  b. Male over age 40
  c. Cigarette smoker
  d. Hypertension
  e. Hyperlipidemia
  f. Obesity
  g. Uncontrolled diabetes
	6. Diabetes is associated with severe degenerative vascular changes. Lesions of the blood vessels strike at an earlier age and tend to produce more severe pathologic changes. Early atherosclerotic changes are probably caused by high blood glucose and lipid levels characteristic of persistent hyperglycemia. Atherosclerosis leads to premature coronary artery disease.

7. Monitor for s/s of retinopathy:
  a. Blurred vision
  b. Black spots
  c. "Cobwebs"
  d. Sudden loss of vision
	7. Retinopathy does not cause visual symptoms until a fairly advanced stage, usually macular edema or proliferative retinopathy, has occurred. Five thousand new cases of blindness related to diabetes occur annually in the United States. The incidence and severity of retinopathy are thought to be related to the duration and the degree of control of blood glucose (ADA, 1997).

8. Teach the client to have an annual ophthalmologic examination.	8. Early detection of retinopathy can successfully be treated with laser therapy (Davidson, 1998).

9. Monitor for s/s of peripheral neuropathy:
  a. Uncontrolled diabetes
  b. Diagnosis of diabetes >10 years
  c. Pain
	9,10. Among the most common and perplexing complications of diabetes, neuropathy is one of the earliest complications and may even be present on diagnosis.

(continues on page 190)

Interventions continued	**Rationales** continued
d. Decreased sensation e. Decreased deep tendon response (Achilles and patella) f. Decreased vibratory sense g. Charcot's foot ulcer h. Decreased proprioception i. Paresthesia	Sensory symptoms usually predominate and include numbness, tingling, pain, or loss of sensation. Current treatments include improved control of blood glucose and use of antidepressant drugs as well as aldose reductase inhibitors (ADA, 1997).
10. Monitor for s/s of automatic neuropathy: a. Uncontrolled diabetes b. Diagnosis of diabetes >10 years. c. Orthostatic hypotension d. Impotence e. Abnormal sweating f. Bladder paralysis g. Nocturnal diarrhea h. Gastroparesis	
11. Monitor for s/s of nephropathy: a. Uncontrolled diabetes b. Diabetes ≥10 years c. Hypertension d. Proteinuria, bacteriuria, casts e. Elevated white blood cell (WBC) f. Abnormal BUN and creatinine	11. In nephropathy, the capillary basement membrane thickens owing to chronic filtering of high glucose. The membrane becomes more permeable, causing increased loss of blood proteins in urine. Increased filtration requirements increase the pressure in renal blood vessels, contributing to sclerosis (Porte & Sherwin, 1997).
12. Monitor for proteinuria: a. Consult with physician to order a 24-hour urine test.	12. Clinical manifestations of nephropathy occur late in the disease. Proteinuria is the first sign of the disorder. A 24-hour urine test is more sensitive than a urinalysis to the presence of microalbumin. Alert the physician of decreased kidney function. When decreased kidney function is identified early, more aggressive therapy may be initiated (DeGrott, 1995).
13. Instruct the client on the importance of controlling blood pressure.	13. Blood pressure control is the most important therapy to prevent or ameliorate renal damage (ADA, 1997).
14. Teach the client about the risk factors that may precipitate renal damage: a. Uncontrolled blood glucose b. Hypertension c. Neurogenic bladder d. Urethral instrumentation e. Urinary tract infection f. Nephrotoxic drugs	14. Making the client aware of risk factors may help to reduce renal impairment.

Related Physician-Prescribed Interventions

Medications

Oral: Sulfonylureas, biguanides, thiazolidinediones, alpha-glucosidase inhibitors, meglitinide combination agents

Insulin: Regular, intermediate, long-acting, combination (NPH & regular)

Other: Angiotensin-converting enzyme inhibitors (ACE inhibitors)

Intravenous Therapy. For DKA and HHNKC

Laboratory Studies. Blood glucose (BG), plasma acetone/urine ketones, serum osmolality, electrolytes, oral glucose tolerance test (OGTT), glycosylated hemoglobin (Hb A, C), fructosamine

Diagnostic Studies. Fasting blood glucose >126 mg/dL × 2; RBG >200 mg/dL + s/s; OGTT >200 mg/dL at 2 hr + 1 other sample. Adults age 45 years or older should be tested every 3 years; those with increased risk, more frequently (ADA, 1997). Not all pregnant women should be screened for diabetes. Testing does not need to be performed in women at low risk.

Therapies. Self-monitoring blood glucose (SMBG), pancreas transplant, ADA meal plan, exercise

Documentation

Flow records
   Vital signs
   Blood glucose Hgb A, C
   Glycosylated hemoglobin lipids
   BUN/creatinine
Date last eye exam
Date last 24-hr urine test
Progress notes
   Client complications
   Abnormal labs
   Episodes hypoglycemia
   Changes in medications

Nursing Diagnoses

Imbalanced Nutrition: More Than Body Requirements Related to Intake in Excess of Activity Expenditures, Lack of Knowledge, or Ineffective Coping

Focus Assessment Criteria	Clinical Significance

1. Height, weight, age, and sex
2. Occupation, educational level, economic level, and cultural heritage
3. Nutritional history and current meal plan
4. History of weight loss or weight gain
5. Social history:
  a. Resistance associated with obesity
  b. Person who shops
  c. Cooking facilities at home
  d. Meals eaten away from home
  e. Person who prepares meals
  f. If the client lives or eats alone
  g. Available support systems
6. Exercise regimen:
  a. Frequency of exercise
  b. Type of exercise
  c. Employment activity
7. A 3- to 5-day food intake diary
	1–11. The primary goal in type 2 diabetes management is weight reduction. Moderate weight loss (10–20 lbs) may improve the abnormalities of glucose intolerance, insulin secretion, and insulin use. The client's experiences, beliefs, and activities have a profound influence on eating behaviors and exercise. Behavior modification may help the client to achieve long-term success. Without significant alterations in life style, resumption of previous eating habits and return of obesity invariably occurs (Powers, 1996).

(continues on page 192)

Focus Assessment Criteria continued	Clinical Significance continued
8. Emotional connotation of food to the client 9. Client's motivation to follow the pre- scribed meal plan 10. Client's attitudes, beliefs, and behaviors related to eating and exercise 11. Laboratory results: BG, glycosylated hemoglobin level	

Goal

The client will relate the intent to modify diet to lose weight.

Indicators

• State an intent to follow a prescribed meal plan in which caloric intake is sufficient to decrease weight.
• Verbalize the value of decreasing weight related to control of blood glucose.

Interventions	Rationales
1. Refer to the Obesity care plan for specific interventions and rationales.	

Documentation

Flow records
  Height, weight, BG
Progress notes
  Nutritional history
  Written contract stating specific goals and rewards
  Graphs showing weight loss or weight gain

Fear (Client, Family) Related to Diagnosis of Diabetes, Insulin Injections, and the Risk of Acute and Chronic Complications of Diabetes

Focus Assessment Criteria	Clinical Significance

1. Client's level of anxiety:
  a. Mild anxiety
  b. Moderate anxiety
  c. Severe anxiety
  d. Panic anxiety
	1. Anxiety varies depending on how the client perceives the severity of the disease, the presence of complications, ability to cope, and available support systems (Wysocki, 1997).

2. Client's stressors 3. Client's past experiences related to diabetes 4. Client's specific concerns or fears	2–4. A client with diabetes typically is justifi-ably afraid of pain, complications, and dependency. The client may be able to express some fears and not others or may not share any feelings (Wysocki, 1997).
5. Available support systems	5. Support is needed; sources may be family, friends, and health care professionals (Feste, 1987).

Goal
The client will relate increased psychological and physiologic comfort.

Indicators
- Effectively communicate feelings regarding the diagnosis of diabetes.
- Identify two methods to cope with diabetes.

Interventions	Rationales
1. Assist the client in reducing anxiety: a. Encourage the client to verbalize fears and concerns. b. Convey a sense of understanding and empathy. c. Actively listen to client's concerns. d. Identify and support effective coping mechanisms.	1. An anxious client has narrowed perceptual field and impaired ability to learn. Anxiety tends to feed on itself, catching the client in a spiral of anxiety and emotional and physical pain (Wysocki, 1997).
2. Provide current information on the disease process, risk of complications, and self-treatment options.	2. A person with diabetes needs support from health care professionals, peers, and family. Lack of support increases anxiety and fear (Feste, 1987).
3. Encourage family and friends to verbalize their fears. Involve them in teaching sessions.	
4. Encourage the client to practice relaxation techniques.	
5. Refer for professional counseling	

 Documentation

Progress notes
Present emotional status
Response to nursing actions
Participation in self-care

High Risk for Ineffective Coping (Client, Family) Related to the Chronicity of Diabetes, the Complexity of Care Regimens, and an Uncertain Future

Focus Assessment Criteria	Clinical Significance

1. Life event changes
 2. Emotional resources
   a. Social integration
   b. Ability to solve problems
   c. Values and beliefs
   d. Goals, hopes, and desires
	1–5. Chronic disease affects the emotional composition of the client and all significant others. Emotional stress is a significant factor in metabolic homeostasis. A thorough psychosocial assessment is the first

(continues on page 194)

Focus Assessment Criteria continued	Clinical Significance continued

3. External resources
  a. Peers, friends, family
  b. Financial resources
  c. Educational level
4. Life style (effects on or changes in)
5. Communication skills
	step in developing an individualized and effective care plan (Feste, 1987).

Goal

The client will make decisions and follow through with appropriate actions to cope effectively.

Interventions	Rationales

1. Explore with the client and significant others the actual or perceived effects of diabetes on:
  a. Finances
  b. Occupation (sick time)
  c. Life style
  d. Energy level
  e. Relationships
	1. Common frustrations associated with diabetes stem from problems involving the disease itself, the treatment regimen, and the health care system. Recognizing that these problems are common indicates a need to use anticipatory guidance to prevent the associated frustrations (Hass, 1993).

2. Assist the client and significant others in identifying previous coping strategies that proved successful.	2. Coping methods vary. Some people avoid the situation; others confront it, seek more information, or rely on religious beliefs for support (Wysocki, 1997).
3. Encourage the client to participate in the plan of care.	3. The client's participation in self-care indicates attempts to cope with the diabetes positively.
4. Encourage the client to discuss plans to incorporate diabetes into his/her life style.	4. Evidence that the client will pursue his goals and maintain his or her life style reflects positive adjustment and self-esteem.
5. Encourage strong family support.	5. Family support is a significant contributing factor to a client's acceptance of diabetes.
6. Provide an environment in which the client may function independently.	6. Self-care reduces feelings of dependency and loss of control.
7. Encourage the client to join support groups.	7. Sharing with persons in a similar situation may provide opportunities for mutual support and problem solving (Feste, 1987).

(continues on page 195)

Interventions continued	Rationales continued
8. Encourage the client to subscribe to journals (e.g., *Diabetes Forecast* or *Diabetes Self-Management*). Give the client a list of resources including outpatient diabetes education programs support groups, organizations, books, and suppliers of diabetes products.	8. Clients vary in the resources they have available. Making use of available resources improves the client's ability to cope (Wysocki, 1997).

Documentation

Progress notes
  Interactions
  Participation in self-care
  Referrals

High Risk for Injury Related to Episodes of Hypoglycemia, Diminished Visual Acuity, and Decreased Tactile Sensation

Focus Assessment Criteria	Clinical Significance

1. Onset, severity, and frequency of hypoglycemia
  a. Mild hypoglycemia (50–60 mg/dL)
  b. Moderate hypoglycemia (≤50 mg/dL)
  c. Severe hypoglycemia (≤40 mg/dL)
2. Does patient live alone?
	1,2. Severe hypoglycemia symptoms can precipitate falling. Low BG is caused by too much insulin, oral hypoglycemic agents activity, or lack of food. Clients who live alone need a realistic plan to obtain emergency help for severe hypoglycemia (ADA, 1997).

3. Ability to administer insulin independently	3. Devices such as the "Magni Guide" by Bectin and Dickinson allow visually impaired patients to measure their own insulin doses accurately. Because this device holds the vial of insulin and magnifies the numbers on the syringe, it is also valuable for older people with arthritis or decreased motor function.
4. Position sense, tactile sensation	4. Elevated glucose levels cause thickening of nutrient vessels to nerves, which results in decreased oxygen to nerves. Elevated glucose levels also cause demyelinization of the nerves with decreased conduction. This causes loss of feeling, touch, and position sense (Porth, 2002).
5. Visual acuity	5. Elevated glucose levels cause capillary basement thickening, which decreases microcirculation to the retina. Proliferation of new blood vessels in an attempt to increase circulation actually causes more problems. These vessels are prone to bleeding, which results in loss of vision (Porth, 2002).

(continues on page 196)

Interventions continued	Rationales continued
6. History of falls or injuries, or fear of falling	6. Visually handicapped clients differ as much as members of any group. The potential for injury may be nonexistent in one client and a major problem for another. An individualized assessment may identify the client's specific needs.

Goals

1. The client will monitor blood glucose.
2. The client will know how to treat episodes of decreased blood glucose.
3. The client will teach family/friends, coworkers how to assist in severe episodes of decreased BG.

Interventions	Rationales

1. Advise the client to
  a. Monitor blood glucose level frequently.
  b. Prevent decreased BG with scheduled meals.
  c. Carry glucose tablets to decrease BG.
  d. Wear diabetes identification.
	1. Monitoring BG level may detect low BG before it results in serious injury (Peragallo-Dittko, Godley & Meyer, 1993).

2. Teach client treatment options for mild and moderate decreased BG.	2. Commercial products like such as glucose tablets are convenient for decreased BG. Glucose gels such as glutose are valuable when clients are unable to swallow (Peragallo-Dittko et al., 1993).
3. Teach the client's significant other(s) to prepare and administer glucagon for severe episodes of decreased BG when client is unconscious.	3. Commercial glucagon is an injectable treatment for severe hypoglycemia. Glucagon acts by changing glycogen in the liver to a usable form of glucose. The stability of Glucagon is short; therefore, it must be mixed just before use. Because another person must administer it, the client's family or friends must be taught to prepare and administer it in an emergency (Guthrie & Guthrie, 1997).
4. Refer to the nursing diagnosis High Risk for Ineffective Therapeutic Regimen Management for additional teaching strategies.	

 Documentation

Discharge summary record
  Client teaching
  Status of outcome achievement

High Risk for Ineffective Sexuality Patterns (Male) Related to Erectile Problems Secondary to Peripheral Neuropathy or Psychological Stresses Associated With Diabetes

Focus Assessment Criteria	Clinical Significance
1. Sexual activity: a. Erectile problems 2. Relationship with partner 3. Cultural influences	1–3. Assessment of relationships enables the nurse to initiate discussions of possible sexual concerns (Davidson, 1998).
4. Conflicts (e.g., in values, body image, and self-esteem) 5. Emotional status (e.g., anxious, depressed, or irritable)	4,5. Psychogenic impotence is characterized by abrupt onset, nocturnal emissions, and the capacity for masturbation. The client's knowledge of the high incidence of impotence in diabetes may trigger psychogenic impotence (Davidson, 1998).
6. Use of prescribed medications, other drugs, and alcohol	6. Drugs such as antihypertensives, antidepressants, and phenothiazines may cause impotence. Alcohol may cause impotence by impairing neural reflexes.
7. Presence of peripheral neuropathy	7. Neuropathy may cause impotence.
8. Control of BG	

Goals

1. The client will relate an intent to share his feelings with his partner.
2. The client will identify treatment options.

Interventions	Rationales
1. Discuss the common effects of diabetes on male sexuality.	1. Sexual dysfunction is a complex problem that may result from physiological damage to the nervous systems.
2. A willingness to discuss the client's feelings and concerns projects an attitude of concern and empathy.	2. Open, honest dialogue may reduce the client's embarrassment and reluctance to share his fears and concerns.
3. If the client is physiologically unable to sustain an erection sufficient for intercourse, give information on alternative methods.	3. Penile implants provide the erections needed for intercourse without altering sensations or the ability to ejaculate (LeRoith, Taylor & Olefsky, 1996).

(continues on page 198)

Interventions continued	Rationales continued
4. Reaffirm the need for closeness and expressions of caring; involve the client's partner in touching and other means of sexual expression.	4. Sexual pleasure and gratification are not limited to intercourse. Other expressions of sexuality and caring may prove more meaningful and gratifying (LeRoith et al., 1996).
5. If indicated, refer the client to a specialist for evaluation and treatment of sexual problems.	5. The client may need specialized assessment and treatment.

 Documentation

Progress notes
  Assessment data
  Interactions
  Referrals

High Risk for Sexual Dysfunction (Female) Related to Genitourinary Infections and Physical and Psychological Stressors Associated with Diabetes

Focus Assessment Criteria	Clinical Significance

1. Sexual patterns
  a. Libido
  b. Satisfaction with sex role
  c. Frequency of activity
  d. Discomfort during intercourse
	1. Assessment of sexual patterns and relationships enables the nurse to initiate discussions of the client's sexual problems or concerns (Peragallo-Dittko et al., 1993).

2. Relationship with partner 3. Conflicts (e.g., in values, body image, and self-esteem) 4. Emotional status (e.g., anxious, depressed, or irritable) 5. Pregnancy and contraception history 6. Cultural influences	2–6. Diabetes, like any chronic disease, affects a client's life physically, emotionally, and financially and may negatively affect sexual function. Diabetes affects family planning decisions related to the genetics of the disease (Porte & Sherwin, 1997).
7. BG control	

Goals

1. The client will express feelings about her sexual concerns.
2. The client will relate an intent to share feelings with her partner.
3. The client will identify preventive treatments for genitourinary infections.

Interventions	Rationales
1. Discuss the effects of diabetes on female sexuality. Explain that poor control of blood glucose is a major contributing factor to decreased sexual satisfaction.	1. Helping the client understand the causes of sexual dysfunction may reduce her guilt and anxiety.

(continues on page 199)

Interventions continued	Rationales continued
2. Encourage the client to verbalize her concerns; listen attentively with a non-judgmental attitude.	2. This may help to reduce the client's embarrassment and reluctance to share concerns.
3. Explain the importance of planned pregnancies.	3. Family planning is essential for the woman with diabetes. Research has shown that tight control of BG before conception and throughout pregnancy helps to ensure a positive outcome (LeRoith et al., 1996).
4. Teach the client strategies to prevent perineal irritation, vaginitis, and urinary tract infection. a. Maintain good hygiene. b. Wear cotton underwear. c. Avoid tight jeans. d. Use a water-soluble vaginal lubricant. e. Maintain a high fluid intake.	4. Vaginitis and UTI occur more often in women with diabetes. Elevated BG levels enhance fungal and bacterial growth in the vagina and urinary tract (DeGrott et al., 1995).
5. Encourage regular physical exercise at least three times a week for 30 minutes.	5. Regular exercise may promote a sense of well-being and positively affect self-esteem; these changes may enhance the client's sense of sexuality (ADA, 1996).
6. If indicated, refer the client to a specialist for information, evaluation, or treatment of sexual problems.	6. The client may need specialized evaluation and treatment.

 Documentation

Progress notes
  Assessment data
  Interaction
  Referrals

Risk for Noncompliance Related to the Complexity and Chronicity of the Prescribed Regimen

Focus Assessment Criteria	Clinical Significance
1. Client's understanding of the disease process and chronic/acute complications related to diabetes 2. Client's perception of BG control 3. Perceived effects on life style	1–3. Assessing these factors provides information on the client's response to loss of control, perception of the loss, individual coping patterns, personal characteristics, and response to others.
4. Discuss the impact of BG control related to the chronic complications of diabetes.	4. The Diabetes Control and Complication Trial showed that intensive BG control delays the onset and progression of the chronic complications of diabetes (ADA, 1997).

Goal
The client will report a desire to increase adherence to achieve Hgb A, C <7.0.

Indicators
- State the risks and benefits of following the prescribed treatment regimen.
- Enter into a contract with the health care provider to set goals.

Interventions	Rationales

1. Explore with the patient the goals and treatment options.
2. Explore the client's perception of the effects of diabetes on the following:
  a. Occupation
  b. Role responsibilities
  c. Relationships
	1–2. Diabetes causes serious complications, requires a complex therapeutic regimen, and may trigger feelings of vulnerability and lack of control. It affects the client's life style, personality, and overall emotional well-being (Wysocki, 1997).

3. Determine the client's usual response to problems.	3. Discussions help to determine if the client usually seeks to change his own behaviors and to control problems.

 Documentation

Progress notes
  Participation in self-care and goal setting
  Emotional status
  Interactions

High Risk for Ineffective Therapeutic Regimen Management Related to Insufficient Knowledge of Diabetes, Monitoring of BG, Medications, Meal Planning, Treatment of Hypoglycemia, Weight Control, Sick Day Management, Exercise Routine, Foot Care, Risks of Complications

Focus Assessment Criteria	Clinical Significance

1. Knowledge of self management skills of diabetes (e.g., monitoring of BG)
2. Contributing factors:
  a. Anxiety
  b. Recent diagnosis of diabetes
  c. Lack of education
3. Community, family, and economic resources
4. Attitudes, feelings, and concerns related to diabetes
5. Readiness to learn
	1–5. These criteria identify factors that interfere with learning. A client who does not succeed in learning basic self-care requires a home care referral postdischarge. Comprehensive outpatient diabetes education is essential for everyone with diabetes (ADA, 1997).

6. Physical limitations	6. The management of diabetes mellitus requires dexterity and good vision for BG monitoring, insulin administration, and foot inspection. Clients with limitations may need assistance or devices to help overcome their limitations.

Interventions continued	Rationales continued
6. Recommend a meter for BG monitoring based on the client's motivation, physical ability, and financial resources.	6. BG meters vary in ease of use, maintenance, and optional features. Helping the client to choose a monitor that best fits her or his needs is an important role for the educator.
7. Assist client to obtain third-party reimbursement for BG monitoring.	7. Comparative shopping and third-party reimbursement may reduce the expense of BG monitoring. Medicare will pay for BG supplies for anyone who has diabetes (ADA, 1997).
8. Discuss with clients their specific BG goal, the frequency of BG monitoring, and the value of recording their results.	8. BG records help client and health care provider evaluate patterns of food intake, insulin administration, and exercise.
9. Teach the need for increased BG monitoring when meals are delayed, before exercise, and when sick.	9. These situations may change dietary or insulin requirements.
10. Assist client to identify the brand, type, dosage, action, and side effects of prescribed medications for controlling diabetes.	10. A client needs to know the dose, action, and side effects to make appropriate decisions for adjusting food and exercise (ADA, 1997).
11. Monitor for the effectiveness of insulin therapy.	11. BG monitoring identifies hypoglycemia and hyperglycemia.
12. Advise client about prescription drugs and over-the-counter remedies such as cough syrups, throat lozenges, and so on that affect BG levels.	12. Oral agents, insulin, glucagon, aspirin, and beta-adrenergic blockers decrease blood glucose; whereas corticosteroids, birth control pills, diuretics, and cold remedies containing decongestants increase BG.
13. Explain the need to adhere to the prescribed meal plan and exercise program.	13. These are essential for the treatment of diabetes.

14. Teach the client insulin administration, including
  a. Measuring an accurate dose
  b. Mixing insulin
  c. Injecting the insulin
  d. Rotating injection sites
	14. Return demonstration allows the nurse to evaluate the client's ability to administer insulin unassisted. Studies have found no evidence of infection when clients reuse syringes. Decreased cost has been the single most important motivation for

(continues on page 203)

Goals

The goals for this diagnosis represent those associated with discharge planning. Refer to the discharge criteria.

Interventions	Rationales
1. Instruct client and family on the etiology of diabetes treatment: meal planning, exercise, and medications.	1. Diabetes education prepares the client for self-management.
2. Explain the risk of complications of diabetes: a. Chronic: • Coronary artery disease • Peripheral vascular disease • Retinopathy • Neuropathy • Nephropathy b. Acute: • Hypoglycemia • DKA • Hyperglycemic, hyperosmolar, or HHNK	2. When teaching risk of complications, stress the importance of regular office visits including those with ophthalmologic and podiatric specialists (DeGrott et al., 1995).
3. Teach signs and symptoms of hyperglycemia: a. BG > 200 mg/dL b. Polyuria c. Polydipsia d. Polyphagia e. Fatigue f. Blurred vision g. Weight loss	3. Elevated BG causes dehydration from osmotic diuresis. Potassium is elevated because of hemoconcentration. Because carbohydrates are not metabolized, the client loses weight (LeRoith et al., 1996).
4. Teach the causes of hyperglycemia: a. Increased food intake b. Decreased insulin c. Decreased exercise d. Infection/illness e. Insulin resistance f. Dehydration	4. Increased food intake requires increased insulin or exercise; otherwise, hyperglycemia will ensue. Infections, illnesses, or both increase insulin requirements (LeRoith et al., 1996).
5. Discuss the rationale for BG monitoring:	5. BG monitoring assists clients to control diabetes by regulating food, exercise, and medications, and has become an essential component of diabetes management. BG monitoring has allowed flexible mealtimes, made strenuous exercise safe, and made successful pregnancy outcomes more likely.

(continues on page 202)

Interventions continued	**Rationales** continued
e. Reusing syringes f. Injecting insulin through clothing	clients to consider reusing syringes (Kahn, 1994). Clients have been injecting insulin through clothing for more than 50 years without medical advice. A 1997 study found this technique safe and convenient (Fleming, Jacober, Vandenberg, Fitzgerald & Grunberger, 1997).
15. Assist client to decrease fear of injections.	15. Using the same area repetitively may cause hypertrophy. Insulin is absorbed at different rates in the arms, abdomen, and thighs. It is recommended that rotation occur within the same anatomic area. For example, inject morning insulin into the abdomen and evening insulin into the thighs (ADA, 1997). Have client and family practice injections of normal saline solutions before beginning insulin therapy. Actively listen to concerns related to injections and correct any misconceptions.
16. Teach proper storage of insulin.	16. Insulin may be safely stored at room temperature. Spare vials are usually kept in the refrigerator. Insulin may not be frozen or kept at temperature extremes (ADA, 1997).
17. Strongly advise client to have an individualized meal plan developed by a registered dietitian (RD).	17. A nutrient balance helps to maintain normal blood glucose level. The ADA recommends an individualized meal plan based on assessment of the client. The exchange list, food pyramid, or gram counting methods are all acceptable (Powers, 1996).
18. Explain the goals of dietary therapy for the client after consultation with a RD.	18. Reinforcing the goals of dietary therapy may help improve success.
19. Help client to identify problems that interfere with following the meal plan.	19. This intervention may increase adherence to the recommendations.
20. Refer client to a dietitian to plan and implement meal plan: a. Provide a resource list of current publications on nutrition. b. Suggest a pocket guide of the meal plan for quick reference. c. Assist with planning a restaurant meal.	20. Individualized assessment and meal plan are required for success (Powers, 1996).

(continues on page 204)

Interventions continued	**Rationales** continued
d. Stress the importance of food preparation and portion sizes. e. Reinforce the need to limit saturated fat. f. Encourage increased dietary fiber.	
21. Encourage client to subscribe to journals such as the *Diabetes Forecast* or *Diabetes Self-Management.*	21. The journals provide up-to-date information on research, new products, recipes, meal plans, and exercise.
22. Assist client to make a list of favorite "legal foods."	22. Teaching foods that are permitted emphasizes positive rather than negative aspects.
23. Stress the *importance of consultations* with a nutritionist.	23. Periodic sessions with a nutritionist provides assessment evaluation of diet and support (Powers, 1996).
24. Teach s/s of hypoglycemia to client and family. a. Mild hypoglycemia: • Sudden plunges • Tingling in hands, lips, and tongue • Cold, clammy pale skin. • Tachycardia/palpitations b. Moderate hypoglycemia (<50 mg/dL) • Uncooperative • Irritable • Often requires assistance c. Severe hypoglycemia (central nervous-system): (< 40 mg/dL) • Incoherent speech • Lack of motor coordination • Mental confusion • Seizure or coma/convulsions	24. Early detection of hypoglycemia enables prompt intervention and may prevent serious complications (ADA 1997). Insulin reaction, insulin shock, and hypoglycemia are all synonymous with low blood glucose (<70 mg/dL). Hypoglycemia may result from too much insulin, too little food, or too vigorous activity. Low BG may occur just before meal times, during or after exercise, and/or when insulin is at its peak action.
25. Teach client to prevent hypoglycemia: a. Routine BG monitoring b. Scheduled meal plan c. BG monitoring before exercise or strenuous activity d. Guidelines for decreasing insulin or increasing food before exercise e. Awareness of changes in daily routines that may precipitate hypoglycemia f. Need to carry some form of glucose for emergencies g. Need to plan food intake carefully when drinking alcohol (drink 1 to 2 drinks only) h. Need to wear diabetes identification	25. Regular BG monitoring may help to minimize fluctuations in BG levels.

(continues on page 205)

Interventions continued	**Rationales** continued

26. Teach self-management of hypoglycemia:
  a. Treat BG ≤ 69 mg/dL with or without symptoms based on the following criteria:

Blood Glucose Level	*Treatment*
50–69 mg/dL	One fruit exchange
<50 mg/dL	Two fruit exchanges

  • Additional fruit exchanges should be taken every 15 minutes until blood glucose level is >69 mg/dL.
  • If hypoglycemia occurs at night or following significant exercise after BG level >69 mg/dL is established, eat ½ bread and ½ meat exchange to avoid repeated episodes.
  b. Teach client examples of appropriate treatment for hypoglycemia:
  • *Fruit exchange* (15 g CHO):
    ½ cup fruit juice
    ½ cup regular (not diet) soda
    ½ cup apple sauce
    6–7 Lifesavers
  • *Bread exchange* (15 g CHO)
    6 saltines
    1 slice bread
    ½ English muffin
  • *Meat exchange*
    1 oz cheese
    ¼ cup cottage cheese
  b. 1 tbsp peanut butter
  c. Discuss commercial products available for treating hypoglycemia:
  • Dextrosol tablets (Orange Medical)
  • Glucose tablets (B-D)
  • Monoject gel (Sherwood)
  • Glutose liquid (Paddock)
  • Glucagon injection (Eli Lilly)
  d. Teach family members and friends to prepare and administer Glucagon.

26.
  a,b. Quick-acting carbohydrates (CHO) are needed to increase BG quickly. Slowly digested CHO helps to maintain BG levels if the client is 2 hours from next meal (Guthrie & Guthrie, 1997).

  c. Commercial products may be more appropriate if client tends to overeat during decreased BG episodes. Glucose gels or liquids are treatments of choice for a semiconscious person.

  d. Commercial glucagon is an injectable treatment for severe hypoglycemia. It is available by prescription and recommended for clients who may be confused or unconscious and are unable to take food or drink by mouth. The stability of glucagon is short; therefore, it must be mixed just before use. Because glucagon must be administered by another person, the client's family or friends must be taught how to prepare and administer it in case of an emergency (ADA, 1996).

(continues on page 206)

Interventions continued	**Rationales** continued
27. Teach importance of achieving and maintaining normal weight. (Refer to the Obesity care plan for specific strategies.)	27. An obese client has fewer available insulin receptors. Weight loss restores the number of insulin receptors, making insulin more effective.
28. Explain how illness influences BG levels.	28. Anticipating the effects of illness on the BG level may alert the client to take precautions. Extra fluids help to prevent dehydration.
29. Teach the client to monitor BG and urine for ketones at least every 4 hours when ill.	29. Early detection of ketones in urine can enable prompt intervention to prevent ketoacidosis. Clients with type I diabetes are susceptible to ketosis.
30. Teach client to take insulin and maintain CHO intake when ill by substituting liquids or easily digested solids for regular food. Assist client to identify the total amount of grams of CHO in 24 hours. Instruct client to *always* consume CHO even when ill. Examples of CHO for sick days: a. *Bread exchange* = 15 g CHO 1 slice bread or toast ½ English muffin ½ bagel (2 oz) ½ cup cooked cereal 6 saltines 6 pretzels 20 oyster crackers b. *Fruit exchange* = 15 g CHO 1 cup Gatorade ½ twin bar popsicle ½ cup orange juice ½ cup apple cider ½ cup unsweetened applesauce ½ cup ginger ale or cola (not diet) c. CHO content other foods ½ cup regular Jello = 24 g 2 level tsp. sugar = 8 g 1 can chicken noodle soup = 15 g	30. Illness often causes loss of appetite. Liquids or semisoft foods may be substituted for the client's normal diet. A client on insulin therapy needs to maintain a consistent CHO intake that will supply glucose. When there is a lack of CHO, fats are used for energy. Ketones form from the metabolism of fat (DeGrott et al., 1995). Amount of CHO in standard meals plans: **Kcal** **CHO (g)** 1,000 134 1,200 150 1,500 214 1,800 259 2,000 295
31. Instruct the client to notify a health care professional if not eating, vomiting, or has diarrhea.	31. Immediate interventions are required to prevent dehydration and hypoglycemia.

(continues on page 207)

Interventions continued	**Rationales** continued
32. Explain the benefits of regular exercise: a. Improved fitness b. Psychological benefits such as enhanced ability to relax, increased self-confidence, improved self-image c. Reduction of body fat d. Weight control	32. Emphasizing the benefits of exercise may help client to succeed with the prescribed exercise regimen (ADA, 1996).
33. Explain the effects of exercise on glucose use. Teach the risks of exercise and diabetes.	33. Exercise is contraindicated when BG level exceeds 300 mg/dL, because it causes a rise in BG and an increase in ketone production as hepatic production of glucose becomes disproportionately greater than the body's use of insulin.
34. Instruct client to seek the advice of a health care provider before beginning an exercise program.	34. Exercise may be contraindicated with certain complications (e.g., severe nephropathy, proliferative retinopathy).
35. Teach client to avoid injecting insulin into a body part that is about to be exercised.	35. Insulin absorption increases in a body part that is exercised, which alters the insulin's absorption (ADA, 1996).
36. Encourage the client to exercise with others or where other informed persons are nearby and always to wear diabetes identification.	36. Exercising with others ensures that assistance is available should hypoglycemia occur.
37. Explain how to reduce serious hypoglycemic episodes related to exercise: a. Monitor BG before and after exercise. b. Exercise when BG level tends to be higher such as shortly after a meal. c. Carry a source of sugar for emergency. d. Identify a relative or friend who is willing and able to inject glucagon if necessary. e. Have glucagon available whenever strenuously exercising.	37. Proper timing of exercise, monitoring BG, and adjusting food or insulin decreases the risk of exercise-induced hypoglycemia. In the event of a severe reaction, a semiconscious or unconscious client may require glucagon (ADA, 1996).
38. Explain that people with diabetes are at high risk for foot problems and should watch for and promptly report any injuries or problems in the feet.	38. Foot lesions result from peripheral neuropathy, vascular disease, and superimposed infection. Feet that are deformed, insensitive, and ischemic are prime targets for lesions and susceptible to trauma (Davidson, 1998).

(continues on page 208)

Interventions continued	**Rationales** continued
39. Teach the importance of daily foot inspection.	39. Treatment may be delayed if the client is unaware of the injury until it has spread through the foot and possibly to bone. Infected tissue kills healthy tissue, causing gangrene. Decreased vascular circulation prevents healing and may lead to amputation; about 50% of amputations could be prevented.

40. Teach the client to prevent foot problems:
 	
  a. Maintain normal BG and cholesterol levels.
 	
  b. Remove shoes and socks at every office visit.
  c. Contact your health care provider at the first sign of a foot problem.
 	
  d. Trim toenails straight across or seek professional care regularly for corns, calluses, or ingrown/thickened toenails.
  e. Make foot inspection part of the daily routine.
  f. Avoid exposing the feet to temperature extremes.
  g. Wear warm, natural fiber socks and well-made, properly fitting shoes.
 	
  h. Nonsmoking status is essential.
	40. Diabetes makes the feet more prone to injury from decreased circulation.
	  a. This reduces conditions (i.e., hyperglycemia) that contribute to microorganism growth.
	  b. This reminds the provider to examine the client's feet.
	  c. Early detection and prompt treatment can prevent serious foot problems.
	  d. Proper toenail trimming can prevent injury. If unable to care for feet, the client needs to see a professional (ADA, 1996).
	  e. Daily inspection can detect early problems.
	  f. These precautions help to prevent burns and vasoconstriction.
	  g. Warm socks and well-fitted shoes absorb perspiration and help to prevent corns, calluses, and blisters.
	  h. The nicotine in tobacco causes blood vessels to contract and decreases blood flow to the already compromised feet.

41. Teach client and family to contact the health care provider with
  a. Unexplained fluctuations in BG
  b. Unexplained urinary ketones
 	
  c. A foot injury that does not show signs of healing in 24 hours
  d. Changes in vision
 	
  e. Vomiting/diarrhea for >24 hours
 	
  f. Signs of infection
	41.
	
	a,b. Severe BG fluctuations and DKA may be life-threatening and require careful investigation of the cause.
	  c. Early treatment may prevent serious infections.
	  d. Visual changes may indicate retinal hemorrhage.
	  e. Extra fluids may prevent dehydration.
	  f. Infection may necessitate medication adjustments.

(continues on page 209)

Interventions continued	**Rationales** continued
42. Provide informational materials and/or referrals that may assist the client to reach goals: 　a. Comprehensive Outpatient Diabetes 　b. Support groups 　c. *Diabetes Forecast, Diabetes Self-Management,* and *Clinical Diabetes* 　d. American Diabetes Association 　e. Books and/or videos on diabetes 　f. American Association Diabetes Educators (AADE)	42. A client who feels well supported can cope more effectively. A chronically ill person with multiple stressors needs to identify an effective support system. Knowing a friend or neighbor with diabetes, participating in a walk-a-thon for the ADA, and reading about people successfully coping with diabetes are some helpful examples (Wysocki, 1997).

 Documentation

Discharge summary record
　Client teaching
　Status of outcome achievement
　Referrals

HEPATITIS (VIRAL)

Hepatitis is an inflammation of the liver caused by one of five different viral agents (Table 1). Hepatitis ranges from mild and curable to chronic and fatal (Kucharski, 1993).

⊙⊙ DIAGNOSTIC CLUSTER	
Collaborative Problems	**Refer to**
△ PC: Fulminant Hepatitic Failure	
△ PC: Portal Systemic Encephalopathy	Cirrhosis
△ PC: Hypokalemia	Cirrhosis
△ PC: Hemorrhage	Cirrhosis
△ PC: Drug Toxicity	Cirrhosis
△ PC: Renal Insufficiency	Renal Calculi
Nursing Diagnoses	**Refer to**
▲ High Risk for Infection Transmission related to contagious nature of viral agents	
▲ Imbalanced Nutrition: Less Than Body Requirements related to anorexia, epigastric distress, and nausea	Cirrhosis
△ High Risk for Ineffective Therapeutic Regimen Management related to lack of knowledge of condition, rest requirements, precautions to prevent transmission, nutritional requirements, and activity restrictions.	
△ Impaired Comfort related to pruritus secondary to accumulation of bilirubin pigment and bile salts	Cirrhosis
△ Pain related to swelling of inflamed liver	Pancreatitis

▲ This diagnosis was reported to be monitored for or managed frequently (75%–100%).
△ This diagnosis was reported to be monitored for or managed often (50%–74%).

TABLE 1. Types of Viral Hepatitis

	Type A	Type B	Type C	Type D	Type E	Type G
Method of Transmission	Fecal–oral 98% Transfusion <2%	Parenteral Sexual Perinatal	Parenteral (IV drugs) 70% Sexual 6% Unknown 25–30%	Primary Parenteral Rare sexually Perinatal	Fecal–oral	Same as C
Severity, Chronicity	Never chronic but can relapse	90% Recover 5–10% Chronic	Subclinical infection Can take 10–30 years to develop chronic hepatitis		None	Probably no chronicity
Incubation	2–6 weeks	4 weeks to 6 months	15–150 days	4–6 Weeks	2–9 Weeks	?
Complications	Fulminant hepatitis <1%	Fulminant hepatitis <1% Hepatocellular carcinoma	Cirrhosis 15–20% Hepatocellular carcinoma 10–20% Chronic hepatitis 75%		Fulminant in pregnant women 20%	?
Prevention	Pre-exposure HAURIX Postexposure immuno-globulin	Postexposure HBIG+ Recombivax Preexposure Recombivax	None	Vaccine against B will protect against D	None	None

Discharge Criteria

Before discharge, the client or family will

1. Describe the modes of disease transmission.
2. State signs and symptoms that they must report to a health care professional.

Collaborative Problems

Potential Complication: Fulminant Hepatic Failure

Nursing Goal

The nurse will detect early signs/symptoms of fulminant hepatic failure and collaboratively intervene to stabilize the client.

Indicators
- Blood glucose <140 2 hours after eating
- Prothrombin time (PT) 11–12.5 seconds
- Partial prothrombin time (PTT) 60–70 seconds
- Aspartate aminotransferase (AST)
  - Male 7–21 u/L
  - Female 6–18 u/L
- Alanine aminotransferase (ALT) 5–35 u/L
- Alkaline phosphatase 30–150 u/L
- Blood urea nitrogen (BUN) 5–25 mg/dL
- Serum electrolytes (refer to laboratory values in institution)
- Prealbumin 20–50 mg/dL
- Alert, oriented
- Pulse 60–100 beats/min
- BP >90/60, <140/90
- Temperature 98–99.5°F
- Respiration 16–20 per min
- EEG normal

Interventions	Rationales

1. Monitor for fulminant hepatic failure.
  a. Coagulation defects
  b. Renal failure
  c. Electrolyte imbalance
  d. Infection
  e. Hypoglycemia
  f. Encephalopathy
  g. Cerebral edema
	1. Fulminant hepatic failure is the sudden onset of severely impaired liver function. Older adults with hepatitis are at serious risk for this problem.

2. Refer to index of collaborative problems for specific interventions for each physiologic complication above.	

◤ Related Physician-Prescribed Interventions

Medications. Hepatitis C antivirals (Acyclovir, Ribavirin); antiemetics; antidiarrheals; antacids; interferon alpha (Hep-C); vitamins

Intravenous Therapy. Total parenteral therapy, protein hydrolysates

Laboratory Studies. Bilirubin; alkaline phosphatase; prothrombin time; serum albumin; hepatitis C viral load, hepatitis C genotype; hepatitis panels; serum alanine aminotransferase (ALT)

Diagnostic Studies. Liver scan, aspartate aminotransferase (AST), liver biopsy

Therapies. Dietary restrictions depending on fat and protein tolerance, bed rest

Documentation

Flow records
   Intake and output
Progress notes
   Evaluation of signs and symptoms

Nursing Diagnoses

High Risk for Infection Transmission Related to Contagious Nature of Viral Agents

(This diagnosis is not currently on the NANDA list but has been included for clarity or usefulness.)

Focus Assessment Criteria	Clinical Significance

1. Mode of transmission:
  a. Feces and saliva
  b. Blood
  c. Semen and vaginal fluids
	1. Appropriate precautions depend on the mode of transmission.

Goal

The client will report precautions needed to release transmission.

Indicators
- Remain in isolation until noninfectious.
- Demonstrate meticulous handwashing during hospitalization.

Interventions	Rationales

1. Use appropriate universal body substance precautions for all body fluids:
  a. Wash hands before and after all client or specimen contact.
  b. Handle blood as potentially infectious.
  c. Wear gloves for potential contact with blood and body fluids.
  d. Place used syringes immediately in nearby impermeable container; do not recap or manipulate needle in any way.
  e. Use protective eye wear if splatter with blood or body fluids is possible (e.g., bronchoscopy, oral surgery).
  f. Wear gowns when splash with blood or body fluids is anticipated.
  g. Handle all linen soiled with blood or body secretions as potentially infectious.
  h. Process all laboratory specimens as potentially infectious.
	1. Refer to Table 1 for specific modes of transmission.

2. Use appropriate techniques for disposal of infectious waste, linen, and body fluids and for cleaning contaminated equipment and surfaces.	2. These techniques help to protect others from contact with infectious materials and prevent disease transmission.

(continues on page 214)

Interventions continued	Rationales continued
3. Refer the infection control practitioner for follow-up with the appropriate Health Department.	3. This referral is necessary to identify the source of exposure and other possibly infected persons.
4. Explain the importance of frequent hand-washing to client, family, other visitors, and health care personnel.	4. Handwashing removes the organism and breaks the chain of infection transmission.

Documentation

Flow records
    Isolation precautions required
Discharge summary record
    Client teaching

High Risk for Ineffective Therapeutic Regimen Management Related to Lack of Knowledge of Condition, Rest Requirements, Precautions to Prevent Transmission, Nutritional Requirements, and Contraindications

Focus Assessment Criteria	Clinical Significance
1. Client's or family's readiness and ability to learn and retain information	1. A client or family who does not achieve the goals for learning requires a referral for assistance postdischarge.

Goals

The goals for this diagnosis represent those associated with discharge planning. Refer to the discharge criteria.

Interventions	Rationales
1. Explain the mode of infection transmission to client and family. Refer to Table 1.	1. Understanding how infection can be transmitted is the first step in prevention.
2. If appropriate, explain to contacts such as family and peers that they should receive hepatitis B or A vaccines or immune globulin.	2. For their protection, family and associates should receive active or passive immunization for hepatitis B.
3. Explain the need to rest and to avoid strenuous activity.	3. As the liver repairs itself, excessive physical activity depletes the body of the energy needed for healing. Adequate rest prevents relapse. It may take 3 to 6 months for energy levels to return to normal.

(continues on page 215)

Interventions continued	Rationales continued
4. Explain the need for a diet high in protein and calories. (Refer to the nursing diagnosis Imbalanced Nutrition in the Cirrhosis care plan.)	4. Protein and caloric requirements increase during periods of tissue healing.
5. Explain the hazards of certain medications: oral contraceptives, narcotics, sedatives, tranquilizers, and acetaminophen.	5. Certain drugs are hepatotoxic. Moreover, in hepatitis, impaired liver function slows drug metabolism; this causes drug levels to accumulate in the body.

6. Teach client and family to watch for and report signs and symptoms of complications:
 	
  a. Unusual bleeding (e.g., gums, stools)
 	
  b. Hypokalemia (manifested by muscle cramps, nausea, vomiting)
 	
  c. Confusion, altered speech patterns
 	
  d. Increasing severity of symptoms
 	
  e. Rapid weight loss or gain
	6. Early recognition and reporting enable prompt intervention to prevent serious complications.
	  a. Bleeding indicates decreased prothrombin time and clotting factors.
	  b. Overproduction of aldosterone causes sodium and water retention and potassium excretion.
	  c. Neurologic impairment results from cerebral hypoxia owing to high serum ammonia levels caused by the liver's impaired ability to convert ammonia to urea (Porth, 2002).
	  d. Worsening symptoms indicate progressive liver damage.
	  e. Rapid weight loss points to negative nitrogen balance; weight gain, to fluid retention.

7. Explain the importance of avoiding alcohol.	7. Alcohol increases hepatic irritation and may interfere with recovery. With Hepatitis C, alcohol leads to rapid progression of cirrhosis (Vail, 1997).
8. Stress the importance of follow-up care and laboratory studies.	8. Follow-up care enables evaluation of liver function and detection of relapse or recurrence. New therapies are available for severe liver disease (Kowdley, 1996).

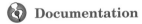 **Documentation**

Discharge summary record
  Client teaching
  Outcome achievement
  Referrals when indicated

HYPOTHYROIDISM

In hypothyroidism, thyroid gland dysfunction results in a deficiency of thyroid hormones thyroxine (T_4) and triiodothyronine (T_3). These hormones are responsible for maintaining body metabolism. Factors that contribute to hypothyroidism are hypothalamic dysfunction, thyroid-releasing hormone or thyroid-stimulating hormone deficiency, iatrogenic (e.g., surgery), iodide medications (e.g., lithium), pituitary disorders, thyroid deficiencies, or destruction (Porth, 2002).

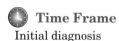 **Time Frame**
Initial diagnosis

⊗ DIAGNOSTIC CLUSTER*

Collaborative Problems

PC: Metabolic
PC: Myxedema Coma
PC: Atherosclerotic Heart Disease
PC: Hematologic
PC: Acute Organic Psychosis

Nursing Diagnoses	Refer to
Impaired Comfort related to cold intolerance secondary to decreased metabolic rate	
High Risk for Ineffective Therapeutic Regimen Management related to insufficient knowledge of condition, treatment regimen, signs and symptoms of complications, dietary management, pharmacological therapy, and activity restrictions.	
Imbalanced Nutrition: Less Than Body Requirements related to intake greater than metabolic needs secondary to slowed metabolic rate	Corticosteroid Therapy
Constipation related to decreased peristaltic action secondary to decreased metabolic rate and decreased physical activity	General Surgery

* This medical condition was not included in the validation study.

Discharge Criteria

Before discharge, the client or family will

1. Describe dietary restrictions.
2. Relate the importance of adhering to the medication schedule.
3. Describe risk factors.
4. Relate signs and symptoms that must be reported to a health care professional.
5. Identify community resources available for assistance.

Collaborative Problems

Potential Complication: Metabolic

Potential Complication: Myxedema Coma

Potential Complication: Atherosclerotic Heart Disease

Potential Complication: Hematologic

Potential Complication: Acute Organic Psychosis

Nursing Goal

The nurse will detect early signs and symptoms of (a) metabolic dysfunction, (b) atherosclerotic heart disease, (c) hematologic dysfunction, and (d) acute psychosis and collaboratively intervene to stabilize the client.

Indicators

- Temperature 98–99.5°F (a)
- Heart rhythm regular (a, b, c)
- Heart rate 60–100 beats/min (a, b, c)
- BP >90/60, <140/90 mm Hg
- Respiratory 16–20 breaths/min (a, c)
- Intact peripheral sensation (a)
- Alert, orient, and calm (a, b, c, d)
- Intact memory (b, d)
- Clear speech (b, d)
- Intact muscle strength (b, d)
- Regular menses (a)
- No jaundice (a)
- Urine, stool, emesis—negative for blood (c)
- No signs of bleeding, bruises (c)
- Thyroid-stimulating hormone 2–10 U/ml (a)
- Triiodothyronine (T_3) 0.2–0.6 µg/dL (a)
- Thyroxine (T_4) 5–12 µg/dL (a)
- Serum glucose 70–115 mg/dL (a)

Interventions	Rationales
1. Monitor metabolic function:	1. Deficiencies in circulating hormones reduce metabolism, thus affecting all body systems. Severity of signs and symptoms depends on the duration and degree of thyroid hormone deficiency (Porth, 2002).

(continues on page 218)

Interventions continued	**Rationales** continued

a. Cardiac:
  • Decreased cardiac output
  • Low blood pressure or decreased pulse
  • Low blood pressure or decreased pulse pressures
  • Decreased or normal heart rate
	a. Cardiac tissue changes, decreased stroke volume, and heart rate reduce cardiac output. Impaired peripheral circulation accounts for changes in cardiac performance.

b. Respiratory	b. Hypoventilation occurs partly because of mucopolysaccharide deposits in respiratory system with subsequent decreased vital capacity. Hypercarbia also further decreases respiratory rate.

c. Neurologic:
  • Paresthesias of fingers and toes
  • Changes in affect, mentation, short-term memory, delusions
  • Slowed, slurred speech
  • Seizures
	c. Hyponatremia may be responsible for some neurologic symptoms. Paresthesias result from direct metabolic changes on nerves and interstitial edema of surrounding tissues. Changes in affect, mentation, short-term memory, and delusions are caused by cerebral edema resulting from changes in adrenal gland affecting water retention and by cerebral hypoxia, resulting from decreased cerebral blood flow. Speech problems result from edema in the cerebellar region of the brain. Seizures may occur in up to 25% of people with long-standing hypothyroidism.

d. Musculoskeletal:
  • Muscle weakness
  • Pathologic fractures
	d. Mucoprotein edema separating muscle fibers causes muscle weakness and stiffness. Pathologic fractures result from impaired calcium transport and use caused by decreased calcitonin levels (produced by thyroid gland).

e. Gastrointestinal:
  • Constipation
  • Impaired digestion
	e. GI tract motility is decreased because of mucoproteins in the interstitial spaces. Poor food digestion occurs throughout the GI tract because of mucosal atrophy and decreased production of hydrochloric acid.

f. Hormonal:
  • Hypoglycemia
  • Increased thyroid-stimulating hormone (TSH)
  • Decreased T_3 or T_4
  • Menorrhagia or amenorrhea, decreased libido
	f. Hypoglycemia results from changes in the adrenal cortex. Increased TSH usually confirms the diagnosis of primary hypothyroidism, which accounts for approximately 90% of cases of hypothyroidism. TSH levels tend to increase with age. Levothyroxine (T_4) and triiodothyronine (T_3) are produced and distributed by the thyroid gland; T_4 is responsible for maintaining a steady metabolic rate. Altered levels of sexual hormones in early hypothyroidism result in prolonged heavy menstrual periods and changes in libido. Prolonged hypothyroidism leads to amenorrhea, anovulation, and infertility resulting from effects of myxedema on luteinizing hormone.

(continues on page 219)

Interventions continued	**Rationales** continued

g. Integumentary:
  • Thickened, dry skin
  • Yellowish skin color in absence of jaundiced sclera
  • Thin, brittle nails with transverse grooves
  • Coarse, dry hair with beginning hair loss (e.g., medial third of eyebrows)
	g. Hyperkeratosis, an overgrowth of the horny layer of the epidermis, occurs with subsequent decrease in activity of sweat glands and resulting skin dryness. Monopolysaccharide accumulation in subcutaneous tissue results in thickened skin. Low-density lipoprotein, the primary plasma carrier of carotene, increases with low levels of thyroid hormone resulting in yellowed skin. Dry skin, hair loss, and nail changes result in altered cell replication resulting from decreased thyroid hormones.

2. Monitor for myxedema coma:
  • Comatose
  • Hypothermia
  • Bradycardia
  • Hypoventilation
  • Hypotension
  • Hyponatremia
  • Hypoglycemia
	2. Myxedema coma, although rare, may result from untreated progressive myxedema. It occurs more frequently in older women. Many of the cases occur when the individual with long-standing hypothyroidism is hospitalized for another condition. It carries a 50% mortality rate. Precipitating events for myxedema coma include infections, surgery, trauma, hypothermia, and effects of various drugs such as sedatives or hypnotics (McMorrow, 1996).

3. Monitor a myxedematous client for signs and symptoms of myocardial ischemia and infarction after initiating thyroid hormone replacement:
  a. Abnormal rate or rhythm
  b. Palpitations
  c. Syncope
  d. Cardiac emergencies (e.g., arrest or ventricular fibrillation)
	3. As oxygen requirements increase with increased metabolism, angina may result if the client has atherosclerosis or coronary artery disease caused by reduced lipid metabolism with monopolysaccharide deposits in the myocardium (Porth, 2002).

4. Monitor for signs and symptoms of atherosclerotic heart disease:
  a. Elevated blood pressure
  b. Vertigo
  c. Chest pain
	4. Atherosclerosis can occur rapidly in a client with hypothyroidism because the protein-bound iodine and T_4 levels are low and blood cholesterol levels are high. Sometimes a decrease in atherosclerosis occurs after thyroid hormone replacement is initiated. However, excessive doses of thyroid hormone replacement initially may result in vascular occlusion due to atherosclerosis.

(continues on page 220)

Interventions continued	Rationales continued
5. Monitor for signs and symptoms of acute organic psychosis: a. Agitation b. Acute anxiety c. Paranoia d. Delusions e. Hallucinations	5. Often a client with severe behavioral symptoms has an underlying psychiatric disorder that may not improve and actually may be exacerbated by thyroid hormone therapy.
6. Monitor for signs and symptoms of anemia: a. Fatigue b. Hypoxia c. Easy bruising d. Confusion	6. Normochromic, normocytic anemia results from a decrease in erythrocyte mass as a compensatory response to decreased oxygen demand.
7. Monitor for signs of abnormal bleeding: a. Petechiae b. Bleeding gums c. Ecchymotic areas d. Blood in urine, stool, or emesis	7. Thyroid hormone deficiencies cause increased capillary fragility, prolonged clotting time, and decreased platelet adhesiveness (Braverman, Dworkin & MacIndoe, 1997).
8. Avoid administering sedatives and narcotics or reduce dosage to one-half or one-third the regular dose.	8. Slowed breakdown of these medications prolongs high circulating levels, resulting in heightened responses and possibly respiratory depression.

 Related Physician-Prescribed Interventions

Medications. Levothyroxine, liothyronine

Intravenous Therapy. Not indicated

Laboratory Studies. Serum T_4, T_3; serum cholesterol; serum sodium; resin T_3 uptake; alkaline phosphate; thyroid-stimulating hormone assay; triglyceride levels

Diagnostic Studies. Radioactive iodine uptake, electrocardiogram, thyroid scan, MRI—head

Therapies. Weight loss diet

 Documentation

Flow records
   Vital signs
   Intake and output
   Rhythm strips
Progress notes
   Unusual events

Nursing Diagnoses

Impaired Comfort Related to Cold Intolerance Secondary to Decreased Metabolic Rate

(This diagnosis is currently not on the NANDA list and has been added for clarity and usefulness.)

Focus Assessment Criteria	Clinical Significance

1. Presence of discomfort:
  a. Description
  b. Site
  c. Onset
  d. Precipitating factors
2. Body temperatures
3. Skin color and temperature
	1–3. A baseline assessment aids the nurse in planning interventions and client teaching.

Goals

1. The client will report episodes of cold intolerance.
2. The client will report improved tolerance to cold after body heat retention measures are employed.

Interventions	Rationales

1. Monitor for signs of hypothermia:
  a. Rectal temperature <96°F
  b. Decreased pulse and respiration rate
  c. Cool skin
  d. Blanching, redness, or pallor
  e. Shivering
	1. Decreased circulating thyroid hormones reduce the metabolic rate; the resulting vasoconstriction increases the risk of hypothermia.

2. Explain measures to prevent chilling:
  a. Increase temperature in the living environment.
  b. Eliminate drafts.
  c. Use several blankets at night.
  d. Protect from cold exposure (e.g., wear several layers of clothing and wool hats, socks, and gloves.)
	2. Chilling increases the metabolic rate and puts increased stress on the heart.

3. Explain the needs for gradual rewarming after cold exposure and avoiding application of external heat to rewarm rapidly.	3. Vascular collapse can result from a rapid increase in metabolic rate by heating and subsequent strain on the heart from increased myocardial oxygen requirements.
4. Encourage the client to avoid smoking cigarettes.	4. Smoking further increases the vasoconstriction caused by a decreased metabolic rate, increasing susceptibility to cold in peripheral areas.

 Documentation

Flow records
  Vital signs including rectal temperature
Discharge summary record
  Client teaching
  Outcome achievements

High Risk for Ineffective Therapeutic Regimen Management Related to Insufficient Knowledge of Condition, Treatment Regimen, Signs and Symptoms of Complications, Dietary Management, Pharmacological Therapy, and Contraindication

Focus Assessment Criteria	Clinical Significance
1. Client's or family's readiness and ability to learn and retain information 2. Concerns regarding the effects of the condition on the client's life style	1,2. Depressed mentation and short attention span can prevent retention of learning. A client or family that does not achieve goals for learning requires a referral for assistance postdischarge.

Goal

The goals for this diagnosis represent those associated with discharge planning. Refer to the discharge criteria.

Interventions	Rationales
1. Explain the pathophysiology of hypothyroidism by using teaching aids appropriate to client's or family's educational level (e.g., pictures, slide-tapes, models).	1. Presenting relevant and useful information in an easily understandable format greatly decreases learning frustration and may help to increase compliance.
2. Explain risk factors that can be eliminated or modified: a. Exposure to cold b. Tobacco use c. Regular alcohol intake d. High-fat diet e. Stressors (e.g., emotional stress, infections)	2. The client's understanding that certain risk factors can be controlled may help to improve compliance with the therapeutic regimen. a–c. Exposure to cold as well as tobacco and alcohol use increases vasoconstriction. a–d. Decreased thyroid hormone levels increase blood lipids. a–e. Stress produces an increase in metabolic rate in hypothyroidism.
3. Instruct client and family to observe for and report signs and symptoms of disease complications: a. Progression of disease signs and symptoms b. Behavioral changes (e.g., agitation, confusion, delusions, paranoia, hallucinations) c. Angina d. Extreme fatigue e. Seizure activity f. Edema in the feet and ankles	3. Early detection and reporting complications enables prompt treatment.
4. Reinforce explanations for therapeutic diet. Consult dietitian when indicated.	4. Understanding the reasons for the therapeutic diet may encourage the client to comply with it.

(continues on page 223)

Interventions continued	**Rationales** continued
a. Low-calorie diet	a. A low-calorie diet compensates for a decreased metabolic rate.
b. Small portions of nutritious foods	b. Small portions compensate for impaired digestion secondary to decreased production of hydrochloric acid.
c. Avoid excessive fluid intake	c. Limited fluid intake may help to reduce fluid retention secondary to increased capillary permeability.
d. Fiber	d. Increased fiber intake can help to increase gastrointestinal motility.
e. Avoid soybeans, white turnips, cabbage, and peanuts	e. These foods interfere with thyroid hormone production.

5. Explain why precautions are required when taking certain medications:
  a. Antihyperlipidemics, phenothiazines, sedatives, narcotics, anesthetics: Chemical reactions are slowed, causing delayed breakdown of medications and prolonged high circulating levels; this results in increased somnolence.
  b. Insulin: Thyroid hormones may increase blood glucose levels.
  c. Digitalis, indomethacin, anticoagulants: Delayed metabolism can potentiate their effects.
  d. Phenytoin (Dilantin), lovastatin (Mevacor), and carbamazepine (Tegretol) lower circulating T_4 levels by increasing rate of clearance.
  e. Lithium inhibits secretion of thyroid hormones from the thyroid gland.
	5. Understanding that the delayed metabolism of medications can cause sustained elevated levels may encourage the client to adhere to the dosage schedule (Eisenhaurer, Nichols, Spencer, & Bergan, 1997).

6. Explain that side effects of thyroid hormone therapy can produce signs and symptoms similar to those of hyperthyroidism:
  a. Tachycardia
  b. Increased respiratory rate
  c. Restlessness or irritability
  d. Heat intolerance
  e. Increased perspiration
  f. Diarrhea
  g. Osteopenia or reduction in bone density
	6. Excessive dosage can cause hyperthyroidism and a too-rapid metabolic rate. These signs and symptoms tend to be less exaggerated in an elderly client than in a younger one. Studies have shown 9% to 13% decrease in bone density with use of thyroxine >5 years (Franklyn & Sheppard, 1990).

7. Teach the client to observe for symptoms of a too-rapid change in metabolic rate:
  a. Headaches
  b. Palpitations
  c. Angina
	7. The client must begin the medication regimen slowly so as to not significantly increase cardiac workload, causing dysrhythmias and angina.

(continues on page 224)

Interventions continued	Rationales continued
8. Explain the importance of continuing daily medication and periodic laboratory testing throughout the rest of the client's life. Explain the following: a. The client should take thyroid hormone at the same time each day. b. T_3 and T_4 testing should be done periodically to check thyroid hormone blood levels. c. The brand of thyroid replacement therapy should not be changed.	8. a–b. Fluctuations in drug blood levels produce signs and symptoms of hypothyroidism. c. Different brands of the drug are *not* bioequivalent (Eisenhaurer et al., 1997).
9. Reinforce the need for follow-up care; note that it may take several months to achieve control.	9. Follow-up enables evaluation for signs of hypothyroidism or hyperthyroidism and laboratory tests to determine if medication adjustments are needed.

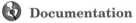 **Documentation**

Discharge summary record
   Discharge instructions
   Follow-up instructions
   Status at discharge
   Achievement of goals (family or individual)

OBESITY

More than 97 million Americans are overweight or obese. BMI (body mass index) describes relative weight for height and is significantly correlated with total body fat content. A BMI of 25–29.9 kg/m² is defined as overweight. A BMI above 30 kg/m2 defines obesity (Blackwell, Miller & Chun, 2002). Obesity is a complex problem involving social, psychological, and metabolic issues. Most commonly, obesity is caused by overeating and insufficient exercise. Behavioral characteristics common to obese persons include the following:

- Response to external cues rather than internal cues as to when to eat or stop eating
- Eating in response to feelings of depression, elation, loneliness, sadness, or boredom
- Excessive eating in a short time span followed by feelings of remorse
- Inactivity or underactivity (Dudek, 2001)

 DIAGNOSTIC CLUSTER*

Nursing Diagnoses

- Ineffective Health Maintenance related to imbalance between caloric intake and energy expenditure
- Ineffective Coping related to increased food consumption secondary to response to external stressors

---

* This medical condition was not included in the validation study.

Discharge Criteria

Before discharge, the client or family will

1. Relate caloric, nutritional, and exercise requirements.
2. State condition of home behavioral management of food consumption and energy expenditure.
3. Relate community resources or professionals to contact after discharge.

Nursing Diagnoses

Ineffective Health Maintenance Related to Imbalance Between Caloric Intake and Energy Expenditure

Focus Assessment Criteria	Clinical Significance
1. Height, weight, and vital signs	1–8. To help ensure success when planning a weight reduction program, all factors contributing to the client's obesity should be identified. Baseline data is needed to evaluate progress.
2. Medical problems; presence of risk factors	

(continues on page 226)

Focus Assessment Criteria continued	Clinical Significance continued
3. Food intake and exercise history	
4. Dieting and body weight history including recent gains or losses	
5. Factors contributing to excessive caloric intake: a. Knowledge deficit related to balanced nutritional intake b. Inappropriate response to external cues (e.g., urge rather than hunger, boredom, stress, anger, or guilt) c. Lack of initiative or motivation d. Imbalance in nutritive composition of diet (e.g., excessive fat or simple carbohydrate intake) e. Cultural or familial factors f. Poor eating habit (e.g., eating fast foods, eating on the run, or skipping meals)	
6. Factors contributing to inadequate energy expenditure: a. Knowledge deficit of the importance of exercise in weight reduction and maintenance b. Inadequate exercise program c. Sedentary life style or occupation d. Fatigue e. Lack of initiative or motivation f. Activity intolerance g. Poor time management, prioritization, or planning	
7. Support or sabotage from family and friends in weight reduction efforts	
8. Client's current desire and readiness (physiological and psychological) to comply with a controlled caloric intake and exercise program	
9. Rule out an eating disorder such as anorexia nervosa or bulimia or other conditions requiring treatment by other health care professionals.	9. Certain conditions or weight loss modes may require specific therapies beyond the scope of nursing (e.g., bulimia, conditions requiring special diets, conditions requiring carefully planned exercise, and weight loss through a protein-sparing modified fast requiring careful laboratory monitoring).

Goals

The client will commit to a weight loss program:

1. Identify present eating and exercise patterns.
2. Describe the relationship between metabolism, intake, and exercise.

Relate a plan to lose weight.

Interventions	Rationales
1. Increase the client's awareness of how body weight is affected by the balance between food intake and activity. Explain that successful weight reduction and maintenance hinge on achieving a balance between reduced caloric intake and increased caloric expenditure through regular exercise. To determine the number of calories the client should consume daily to reach and maintain his or her ideal weight, multiply the client's ideal weight in pounds by 11, if female, or 12, if male. One pound of fat roughly equals 3,500 calories. Thus, to lose 2 lb/week, the client must cut 7000 calories from his or her current weekly intake. Exercise caloric expenditure charts may be used to determine the calories burned during various activities.	1. Weight loss goals may be achieved through a combination of reduced caloric intake and increased caloric expenditure through exercise. Any increase in physical activity increases energy output and caloric deficits in a person following a reduced-calorie dietary regimen (Blackburn et al., 1997).
2. Help the client to develop a safe, realistic weight-loss program that considers these factors: a. Amount of loss desired b. Duration of program c. Cost d. Nutritional soundness e. Compatibility with life style	2. Realistic goals increase the likelihood of success. Successes give the client an incentive to continue the program.
3. Help the client to identify environmental factors that contribute to poor eating patterns by discussing the following (Dudek, 2001): a. Friends, family, coworkers: What are their habits? Would they be supportive? b. What types of foods are found in the home? At parties? At work? In the lunch room? c. In what type of leisure or recreational activities does the client engage? Is the client sedentary? d. What route(s) does the client take to and from work? Does the client pass by fast food restaurants?	3. Helping the client to identify external factors that may increase his internal motivation to overcome them (Dudek, 2001).

(continues on page 228)

Interventions continued	**Rationales** continued
e. Who does the housework? Gardening and yard work? Errands? f. How much television does the client watch? g. Has the client responded to any advertisements for rapid weight loss programs or devices?	
4. Instruct the client to keep a diary for 1 week that includes these things: a. Food intake and exercise b. Location and times of meals c. Emotions during mealtimes d. Person(s) with whom the client ate e. Any skipped meals f. Snacks	4. Such a diary helps the client to become aware of his food intake patterns.
5. Discuss the hazards of the following activities: a. Eating while doing another activity, such as watching TV or reading b. Eating while standing up which can give the illusion of not eating a meal c. Eating out of boredom, stress, or another psychological reason d. Eating because everyone else is eating	5. Certain situations may be identified as cues that trigger inappropriate eating.
6. Teach the client the basics of balanced nutritional intake including supportive measures: a. Choose a diet plan that encourages high intake of complex carbohydrates and limited fat intake. Recommended U.S. dietary goals are 30% of total calories from fat, 12% from protein, 48% from complex carbohydrates, and 10% from simple carbohydrates. b. Be aware that method of preparation also affects total calorie and fat content. For example, a chicken-fried steak is a protein with a high fat content owing to its method of preparation (frying). c. Try to obtain as many calories as possible from fruits and vegetables instead of from meat and dairy products. d. Eat more chicken and fish, which contain less fat and total calories per ounce than red meat. e. Limit high-fat salad dressings, especially dressing containing mayonnaise (216–308 calories per 2-oz serving).	6. Successful weight loss and long-term maintenance can be achieved through a diet low in fat and high in complex carbohydrates (Dudek, 2001).

(continues on page 229)

Interventions continued   **Rationales** continued

f. Avoid fast foods that have a high fat and total calorie content.

g. When dining in a restaurant, make special requests (e.g., serve salad dressing on the side; omit sauce from entree).

h. Plan meals in advance.

i. If attending a party or dining out, plan your eating ahead of time and stick to it.

j. When food shopping, prepare a shopping list and adhere to it.

k. Involve the family in meal planning for better nutrition.

l. Buy the highest quality ground beef to limit fat content. (Ground round has about 10% fat; regular hamburger, 25% fat.)

m. Choose a wide variety of appropriate foods to reduce feelings of deprivation.

n. Avoid eating at family-style buffets that increase the chance of overeating.

o. Drink 8 to 10 glasses (8 oz) of water daily to help excrete the by-products of weight loss.

p. Measure foods and count calories; keep records.

q. Read food labels and note ingredients, composition, and total calories per serving. Choose low-fat or no-fat products when possible. Be aware that many prepared foods have hidden ingredients such as salt and saturated fats and that some so-called "natural" foods, such as granola, are high in fat and sugar.

r. Eat slowly and chew food thoroughly.

s. Experiment with spices, fat substitutes, and low-calorie recipes.

t. Chew gum while preparing meals to deter eating while cooking.

7. Discuss the benefits of exercise:
   a. Reduces caloric absorption
   b. Acts as an appetite suppressant
   c. Increases metabolic rate and caloric expenditure
   d. Preserves lean muscle mass
   e. Increases oxygen uptake
   f. Improves self-esteem and decreases depression, anxiety, and stress
   g. Aids restful sleep
   h. Improves body posture
   i. Provides fun, recreation, and diversion
   j. Increases resistance to degenerative diseases of middle and later years, e.g., cardiovascular disorders

7. A significant amount of lean mass (muscle), up to 30%, can be lost on a calorie-restricted diet. Exercise minimizes this loss. Exercise also contributes to an overall feeling of well-being, which can positively influence self-esteem during dieting.

(continues on page 230)

Interventions continued	Rationales continued

8. Help the client to develop a safe, realistic exercise program by considering the following factors (Williamson et al., 1992):
  a. Personality and life style
  b. Time availability
  c. Occupation: sedentary or active
  d. Safety (e.g., sports injuries, environmental hazards)
  e. Cost of club membership or equipment
  f. Age, physical size, and physical condition
	8,9. The client is more likely to comply with a regular exercise program that is convenient and enjoyable. A gradually progressing exercise program minimizes discomfort and injury and encourages compliance.

9. Discuss beginning an exercise program. If indicated, instruct the client to consult with a physician before starting. Advise the client as follows:
  a. Start slow and easy.
  b. Choose activities that exercise many parts of the body.
  c. Choose activities that are vigorous enough to cause "healthful fatigue."
  d. Do reading, consult with experts, and talk with friends and coworkers who exercise.
  e. Develop a regular exercise program and chart progress.
  f. Add supplemental activities, e.g., park far away and walk, work on garden, walk up stairs, spend weekends at leisure activities that require walking, such as festivals or art fairs.
  g. Eliminate time- and energy-saving devices when practicable.
  h. Work up to ½ to 1 hour of exercise per day at least 4 days per week.
  i. To maintain optimum conditioning, avoid lapses of more than 2 days between exercise sessions.	

10. Teach the client about the risks of obesity:
  a. Metabolic abnormalities
  b. Arteriosclerosis
  c. Hypertension
  d. Left ventricular hypertrophy
  e. Diabetes mellitus
  f. Gallbladder disease
  g. Increased risk of complications of surgery
  h. Respiratory disease
	10. The client must understand that obesity is a multiple-system health hazard. A diet high in fat and simple cholesterol contributes to atherosclerosis, diabetes, gallbladder disease, breast cancer, and colon cancer. A sedentary life style decreases muscle tone and strength; compromised mobility and balance increase the risk of falls and injury. Fatty tissue is less vascular and more susceptible to infection. Increased peripheral resistance causes

(continues on page 231)

Interventions continued	Rationales continued
i. Increased risk of cancer (e.g., breast, colon) j. Increased risk of accident and injury	increased cardiac workload, which raises blood pressure. Excessive abdominal fatty tissue compromises diaphragmatic movement, which can lead to hypoventilation (Skelton, 1992).
11. Discuss the value of weekly goals versus the larger weight loss goal (e.g., will walk 20 minutes 3–5 days weekly).	11. Weekly goals enable achievement and foster compliance. Unsatisfactory habits can be targeted (e.g., the client doubles eating time by actively slowing consumption) and healthy habits can be promoted (e.g., the client eats plain popcorn as an evening snack). Because weight loss may vary from week to week, a primary focus on pounds lost may be discouraging.

Documentation

Progress notes
   Client teaching
Planning:
   Weight loss goal
   Exercise (type, frequency)
   Weekly goals

Ineffective Coping Related to Increased Food Consumption Secondary to Response to External Stressors

Focus Assessment Criteria	Clinical Significance
1. Personal stressors 2. Stressors contributing to the eating behavior 3. Effective and ineffective response to stressors	1–3. Often, inappropriate responses to external cues, particularly stressors, facilitate or aggravate obesity. They trigger an ineffective coping pattern in which the client eats in response to stress cues rather than to physiological hunger.
4. Coping strengths 5. Cultural or familial patterns that enhance or impair positive outcomes 6. Insight into eating in response to external rather than internal cues 7. Motivation to alter destructive patterns 8. Ability to distinguish "urges" from physiologic hunger	4–8. The client's insight into his or her eating problem is a certain factor in predicting the success of treatment.

Goal

The client will identify alternative responses to stressors besides eating.

Indicators

- Identify stressors contributing to overeating.
- Verbalize strengths.

Interventions	Rationales

1. Assist the client to do the following:
  a. Alter ways of thinking (e.g., think of "cheating" as "off-target behavior)" "eating" as "energy intake;" "exercise" as "energy consumption."
  b. Reduce fears of loss of control (e.g., learn to take a taste without fear of a binge).
  c. Take risks and reward successes.
  d. Identify potential problem areas and have a definite plan for getting back "on target."
  e. Understand that weight management simply involves balancing energy intake and energy consumption.
  f. Observe role models and understand that persons who maintain their weight are not "just lucky."
  g. Examine personal meanings for eating and food other than as a means to meet physiologic needs and sustain life.
	1. Our society places a high priority on thinness and typically labels obese persons as undesirable and undisciplined. These measures attempt to alter the client's attitude toward obesity, weight reduction, and exercise.

2. Encourage and assist the client to do the following:
  a. Contract reduction and exercise programs with realistic goals.
  b. Keep intake and exercise records.
  c. Hang an admired photograph on the refrigerator.
  d. Increase knowledge about weight loss and exercise by talking with health-conscious friends, relatives, and associates.
  e. Make new friends who are health-conscious and active.
  f. Get a friend to join the program or to serve as a support person.
  g. Reward himself or herself for progress.
  h. Keep in mind that self-image and behavior are learned and can be unlearned.
  i. Build a support system of people who value growth and appreciate him or her as an individual.
  j. Be aware of rationalization (e.g., a lack of time may actually be poor prioritization).
  k. Keep a list of positive outcomes.
	2. Significant weight loss takes many months. These activities help to increase the client's interest and maintain motivation throughout the long program.

(continues on page 233)

Interventions continued	**Rationales** continued
3. If possible, involve the client's family in the weight-reduction project. Determine if support is present.	3. Family support is important. If support is not present, open discussions are needed to elicit family support.
4. Instruct the client to limit body measurements and weighing to once per week.	4. Fluctuations in body weight are common, especially in females, owing to water retention. Daily weights are misleading and often disheartening; body measurements provide a better indicator of losses. Moreover, consistent exercising results in lean muscle mass gain. Because muscle weighs more than fat, this may be reflected as a weight gain on the scale.
5. Encourage the client to avoid persons who may sabotage weight loss attempts if possible.	5. Certain persons and relationships may be threatened by the client's weight loss.
6. Teach the client to do the following: 　a. Distinguish between an urge and actual hunger. 　b. Use distraction, relaxation, and guided imagery. 　c. Make a list of external cues or situations that lead to off-target behavior. 　d. List constructive actions to substitute for off-target behavior, e.g., take a walk. 　e. Post the list of alternative behaviors on the refrigerator. 　f. Adhere to the list and reward himself or herself when appropriate. 　g. Every 1 or 2 weeks reevaluate if the plan is realistic.	6. Identification and reduction of inappropriate or destructive responses to stressors can be the critical factors for successful weight loss and maintenance.

 Documentation

Progress Notes
Interactions

PANCREATITIS

Pancreatitis is an inflammatory response and potential necrosis of pancreatic endocrine and exocrine cells resulting from activation of pancreatic enzymes. The most common causes are alcohol abuse and biliary tract obstruction related to gallstones (Munoz & Katerndahl, 2000). Mechanical causes are those that obstruct or damage the pancreatic duct system such as cancer, cholelithiasis, abdominal trauma, radiation therapy, parasitic diseases, and duodenal disease. Metabolic causes are those that alter the secretory processes of the acinar cells such as alcoholism, certain medications, genetic disorders, and diabetic ketoacidosis. Miscellaneous etiologic factors include infections, ischemic injury, embolism, and hypovolemia. The substrates released cause local inflammation and pathology in and around the pancreas as well as trigger systemic complications. The mortality rate for acute pancreatitis is 2% to 9% and is 20% to 50% if hemorrhage is present (Munoz & Katerndahl, 2000).

 Time Frame

Initial diagnosis
Recurrent acute episode

 DIAGNOSTIC CLUSTER

Collaborative Problems

▲ PC: Hyperglycemia
▲ PC: Hypovolemia/Shock
▲ PC: Hypercalcemia
▲ PC: Delirium Tremens (refer to Alcohol Withdrawal)
* PC: Acute Respiratory Distress Syndrome
* PC: Sepsis
* PC: Hematologic
* PC: Acute Renal Failure

Nursing Diagnoses

▲ Acute Pain related to nasogastric suction, distention of pancreatic capsule, and local peritonitis
▲ Imbalanced Nutrition: Less Than Body Requirements related to vomiting, anorexia, impaired digestion secondary to decreased pancreatic enzymes
▲ Ineffective Denial related to acknowledgment of alcohol abuse or dependency
▲ High Risk for Ineffective Therapeutic Regimen Management related to lack of knowledge of disease process, treatments, contraindications, dietary management, and follow-up care

---

▲ This diagnosis was reported to be monitored for or managed frequently (75%–100%).
△ This diagnosis was reported to be monitored for or managed often (50%–74%).
* This diagnosis was not included in the validation study.

Discharge Criteria

The client or family will

1. Explain the causes of symptoms.
2. Describe signs and symptoms that must be reported to a health care professional.
3. Relate the importance of adhering to dietary restrictions and avoiding alcohol.
4. If alcohol abuse is present, admit to the problem.
5. Relate community resources available for alcoholism.

Collaborative Problems

Potential Complication: Hyperglycemia

Potential Complication: Hypovolemia/Shock

Potential Complication: Hypercalcemia

Potential Complication: Acute Respiratory Distress Syndrome

Potential Complication: Sepsis

Potential Complication: Hematologic

Potential Complication: Acute Renal Failure

Nursing Goals

The nurse will detect early signs and symptoms of (a) cardiovascular complications, (b) respiratory complications, (c) metabolic complications, (d) alcohol withdrawal, (e) sepsis, (f) renal insufficiency, and (g) hematologic complications and collaboratively intervene to stabilize the client.

Indicators

- Cardiac: rhythm regular, rate 60 to 100 beats/min (a)
- B/P >90/60, <140/90 mm Hg (a, b)
- Respiratory rate 16 to 20 breaths/min (a, b)
- Urinary output >30 ml/hr (a)
- Capillary refill <3 seconds (a)
- Calm, alerted (a, b)
- Dry skin (a, b)
- No nausea or vomiting (c, e)
- Temperature 98–99.5°F (c, e)
- White blood cells 4300–10,800 mm^3 56–190 IV/L (c, e)
- Serum amylase alkaline phosphatase 30–85/mU/ml (e)
- Fasting serum glucose 70–115 mg/dL (c)
- Aspartate aminotransferase (AST) (c)
  - Male: 7–21 u/L
  - Female: 6–18 u/L
- Alanine aminotransferase 5–35 U/L (c)
- Lactic dehydrogenase (LDH) 100–225 u/L (c)
- Hematocrit (g)
  - Male: 42%–52%
  - Female: 37%–47%
- Serum calcium 8.5–10.5 mg/dL (f)
- Oxygen saturation (pulse oximeter) >96% (a, b)
- pH 7.35–7.45 (a, b, c)
- Stool occult blood negative (g)
- Urine specific gravity 1.005–1.030 (f)
- Blood urea nitrogen (BUN) 10–20 mg/dL (e)
- Serum potassium 3.8–5 mEq/L (e)

Interventions	Rationales

1. Monitor for signs and symptoms of hypovolemia and shock:
  a. Increasing pulse rate, normal or slightly decreased blood pressure
  b. Urine output <30 mL/hr
	1. The release of vasoactive compounds during autodigestion of the pancreas results in increased capillary permeability, causing a plasma shift from the circulatory system to the peritoneal cavity. Hypo-

(continues on page 236)

Interventions continued	**Rationales** continued
c. Restlessness, agitation, change in mentation d. Increasing respiratory rate e. Diminished peripheral pulses f. Cool, pale, or cyanotic skin g. Thirst	volemic shock can result. The compensatory response to decreased circulatory volume is to increase blood oxygen by increasing heart and respiratory rates and to decrease circulation to the extremities, causing decreased pulse and cool skin. Diminished oxygen to the brain causes changes in mentation.
2. Monitor cardiovascular response and fluid volume carefully: • Blood pressure • Peripheral pulses • Capillary refill • Intake • Output	2. The degree of inflammation will influence the amount of fluid sequestered and resulting hypovolemia (Banks, 1997).
3. Monitor for respiratory complications: a. Hypoxemia b. Atelectasis c. Pleural effusion	3. Sixty percent of deaths in acute pancreatitis occur in the first 7 days from respiratory complications. The cause is believed to be enzyme-induced inflammation of the diaphragm or pulmonary microvasculature (Munoz & Katerndahl, 2000).
4. Monitor for sepsis: a. Persistent abdominal pain or tenderness b. Prolonged fever c. Abdominal distention d. Palpable abdominal mass e. Vomiting, nausea f. Increased WBC count, increased C-reactive protein g. Persistent elevation of serum amylase h. Hyperbilirubinemia i. Elevated alkaline phosphatase j. Positive culture and Gram's stain k. Jaundice	4. Septic complications from pancreatic abscess, infected pancreatic necrosis, and infected pseudocyst have a high mortality rate (Munoz & Katerndahl, 2000). Twenty to thirty percent of people with acute pancreatitis will develop complications of necrosis.
5. Monitor for signs and symptoms of hypocalcemia: a. Change in mental status b. Cardiac dysrhythmias c. Numbness, tingling of fingers, toes d. Muscle cramps e. Seizures f. Positive Chvostek's sign (spasm of face after tapping) g. Positive Trousseau's sign (contracture of fingers and hands after B/P cuff is inflated above systolic BP for 3 minutes)	5. Several causes of hypocalcemia have been proposed. Calcium may bind with free fats that are excreted owing to the lack of lipase and phospholipase needed for digestion. Low serum calcium levels produce increased neural excitability, resulting in muscle spasms (cardiac, facial, extremities) and central nervous system irritability (seizures). Hypomagnesemia also may cause hypocalcemia because it inhibits parathyroid hormone secretion (Bullock & Henze, 2000).

(continues on page 237)

Interventions continued	**Rationales** continued
6. Monitor glucose levels in blood and urine.	6. Injury to pancreatic beta cells decreases insulin production; injury to pancreatic alpha cells increases glucagon production.

7. Monitor for signs and symptoms of hyperglycemia:
  a. Early signs:
    • Polyuria
    • Polydipsia
  b. Later manifestations (ketoacidosis):
    • Polyphagia
    • Fruity breath odor
    • Weakness
    • Warm, flushed, dry skin
    • Hypotension
    • Blood glucose >300 mg/dL
	7. Without insulin, cells cannot use glucose. Protein and fats are then metabolized, producing ketones. Ketoacidosis results with the lungs and kidneys attempting to return the pH to normal. Increased urine excretion causes losses of water, sodium, potassium, magnesium, calcium, and phosphate. Respiration increases to reduce CO_2 levels.

8. Evaluate whether or not client abuses alcohol.	8. Alcoholism contributes to pancreatitis by lowering gastric pH, which triggers release of pancreatic enzymes. Alcohol also triggers excess production of hydrochloric acid, which causes spasms and partial obstruction of ampulla of Vater. Alcohol also directly irritates the pancreas, causing protein precipitates that obstruct the acinar ductules (Banks, 1997).

9. Monitor for signs and symptoms of alcohol withdrawal:
  a. Tremors
  b. Diaphoresis
  c. Anorexia, nausea, vomiting
  d. Increased heart rate and respiratory rate
  e. Agitation
  f. Hallucinations (visual or auditory)
  g. Delirium tremens (grand mal seizures, disorientation to time and place, panic level anxiety, visual hallucinations)
	9. Because chronic alcohol abuse can cause pancreatitis, the nurse must be alert for the signs even when the client denies alcoholism. Signs of alcohol withdrawal begin 24 hours after the last drink and can continue for 1 to 2 weeks. Refer to Alcohol Withdrawal care plan.

10. Consult with a physician for sedation in appropriate dosage to control symptoms.	10. Alcohol withdrawal often requires large doses of sedatives to prevent seizures.

11. Identify high-risk clients:
  a. At diagnosis:
    • Age >55 years
    • WBC count >16,000/mm³
    • Blood glucose >200 mg/dL
    • Serum lactic dehydrogenase >350 IU/L
	11. Ransen's prognostic signs have a 96% accuracy rate. People with fewer than three signs have a 1% mortality rate; three to four signs, 16% rate; five to six signs, 40% rate; and more than six signs, 100% rate (Munoz & Katerndahl, 2000).

(continues on page 238)

Interventions continued	**Rationales** continued

• Serum glutamic oxaloacetic transaminase >250 IU/L
• Aspartate aminotransferase
b. During initial 48 hours:
  • Hematocrit decrease >10 percentage points
  • Serum calcium level <8 mg/dL
  • Arterial PO_2 <60 mm Hg
  • BUN rise >5 mg/dL
  • Base deficit >4 mEq/L
  • Estimated fluid sequestration >6,000 mL	

12. Monitor for hematologic complications:
  a. Thrombosis
  b. Disseminated intravascular coagulation
	12. Elevated levels of fibrinogen and factor VIII contribute to a hypercoagulable state (Munoz & Katerndahl, 2000).

13. Monitor:
  a. Coagulation profiles
  b. Hemoglobin and hematocrit
  c. Stool, urine, and GI drainage for occult blood
  d. For ecchymosis (blackened bruises)
	13. Early detection of signs of bleeding or DIC can reduce morbidity.

14. Refer to collaborative problem index under thrombosis and disseminated intravascular coagulation for specific monitoring criteria.	

15. Monitor for renal insufficiency:
  a. Oliguria
  b. Elevated urinary sodium
  c. Elevated specific gravity
  d. Elevated BUN
	15. Hypovolemia and hypotension activate the renin-angiotensin system; this results in increased renal vasculature resistance, which decreases renal plasma flow and glomerular filtration rate (Bullock & Henze, 2000).

16. Monitor for hypokalemia:
  a. Muscle weakness
  b. Polyuria
  c. Hypotension
  d. Electrocardiogram changes
	16. Pancreatic enzymes are high in potassium; losses into the peritoneal cavity may result in a potassium deficiency (Krumberger, 1993).

17. Monitor for:
  a. Hiccups
	17.
	  a. Hiccups may be related to phrenic nerve irritation resulting from subdiaphragmatic collection of purulent debris.

(continues on page 239)

Interventions continued	Rationales continued
b. Cardiac rate, rhythms, and pattern c. Temperature	b. Electrolyte imbalance can cause cardiac dysrhythmias. c. Fever in pancreatitis may indicate cholangitis, cholecystitis, peritonitis, intra-abdominal abscesses, or fistula.
18. Maintain strict nothing-by-mouth (NPO) status. Explain to client that even ice chips are not allowed.	18. NPO reduces or ceases secretion of pancreatic enzymes, which reduces the inflammatory process (Krumberger, 1993).
19. Explain use of nasogastric tube and suctioning.	19. Nasogastric suctioning is used to remove gastric juices, which, if present, will stimulate the release of secretions in the duodenum. Secretions stimulate the pancreas to secrete enzymes (Krumberger, 1993).
20. If total parenteral nutrition (TPN) is used, refer to TPN care plan.	20. Oral intake should not be resumed until abdominal pain subsides and serum amylase levels are normal (Krumberger, 1993).

Related Physician-Prescribed Interventions

Medications. Antibiotic therapy, replacement pancreatic enzymes, vitamins, analgesics, insulin, antacids, anticholinergics, tranquilizers/sedatives, histamine H_2 receptor blockers, glucagon, somatostatin, calcitonin

Intravenous Therapy. Fluid/electrolyte replacement, TPN

Laboratory Studies. Fresh frozen plasma; CBC with differential; partial thromboplastin time (PTT); serum amylase; prothrombin time (PT); serum, trypsin/elastase C-reactive protein; creatine protein transaminase; coagulation studies; urine amylase; serum magnesium; serum lipase and bilirubin; serum ionized calcium; serum albumin, protein; serum isoamylase P_4; serum glucose; WBC; serum calcium and potassium; liver enzymes; triglycerides; arterial blood gases; LDH; AST

Diagnostic Studies. Computed tomographic (CT) scan, ultrasonography, endoscopy, endoscopic retrograde cholangiopancreatography, upper GI series

Therapies. NPO; peritoneal lavage; nasogastric suction; low-fat, high-protein, and moderate CHO diet

 Documentation

Flow records
  Vital signs
  Intake and output
Progress notes
  Behavior, orientation
  Changes in physiologic status
  Actions taken
Response

Acute Pain Related to Nasogastric Suction, Distention of Pancreatic Capsule, and Local Peritonitis

Focus Assessment Criteria	Clinical Significance

1. Source of pain:
  a. Epigastric area
  b. Back, chest
  c. Abdomen
  d. Nasogastric tube
	1. Determining the source and nature of the pain helps to guide interventions.

2. Severity of pain based on a scale of 0 to 10 (0 = no pain; 10 = worst pain), rated:
  a. At its best
  b. At its worst
  c. After each pain relief measure
	2. The degree of pain correlates with the extent of pancreatic damage.

Goal
The client will relate satisfactory relief after pain-relief interventions.

Indicators
- Relate factors that increase pain.
- Relate effective interventions.
- Rate pain level lower after measures.

Interventions	Rationales
1. Collaborate with client to determine what methods could be used to reduce the pain's intensity.	1. Pain related to pancreatitis produces extreme discomfort in addition to increasing metabolic activity, with a corresponding increase in pancreatic secretory activity (Krumberger, 1993).

2. Relate to client your acceptance of his or her response to pain:
  a. Acknowledge the pain.
  b. Listen attentively to descriptions of the pain.
  c. Convey that you are assessing pain because you want to understand it better.
  d. Ask client to rate pain (0–10) at its highest and to rate pain level that is satisfactory after relief measures.
	2. A client who must try to convince health care providers that he or she has pain experiences increased anxiety that may increase the pain.
	
	  d. Subjective assessment of pain can be quantified with 0–10 scale.

3. Provide accurate information and correct any misconceptions the client may have:
  a. Explain the cause of the pain.
  b. Relate how long the pain should last, if known.
	3. Movement of inflammatory exudates and enzymes into the retroperitoneum produces a chemical burn to tissue, resulting in the pain of pancreatitis. The pain is severe and knife-like, twisting, or band-like (Brown,

(continues on page 241)

Interventions continued	**Rationales** continued
	1991). A client who is prepared for a painful experience through an explanation of the actual sensations tends to experience less stress than a client who receives vague or no explanation.

4. Provide nasogastric tube care if indicated:
  a. Explain that the tube is used to reduce gastric contents, which reduces pancreatic secretions.
  b. Apply a water-soluble lubricant around nares to prevent irritation.
  c. Monitor nares for pressure points and signs of necrosis. Frequently retape tube when soiled or nonadherent or to reposition.
  d. Provide frequent oral care with gargling; avoid alcohol-based mouthwashes that dry mucosa.
	4. These interventions can reduce some discomfort associated with nasogastric tube use.

5. Explain the need for bed rest.	5. Rest decreases metabolism, reduces gastric secretions, and allows available energy to be used for healing.
6. Position sitting upright in bed with knees and spine flexed.	6. This position relieves tension on the abdominal muscles (Brown, 1991).
7. When client is NPO, avoid all exposure to food (e.g., sight and smell).	7. The sight and smell of food can cause pancreatic stimulation (Brown, 1991).
8. Discuss with physician the use of analgesics such as meperidine, barbiturates, and fentanyl. Avoid the PRN approach and morphine.	8. These analgesics do not cause spasm of the sphincter of Oddi (Munoz & Katerndahl, 2000). A regular time schedule maintains a steady drug blood level (Agency for Health Care Policy and Research, 1992).

9. Explain the need for the following:
  a. To reduce pancreatic activity, advance diet slowly, and avoid large meals.
  b. Take antacids to neutralize gastric acid.
  c. Restrict dietary fats (e.g., fried foods, ice cream, whole milk, nuts, gravies, meat fat, bacon) that require pancreatic enzymes for digestion.
	9. Decreasing pancreatic enzyme release through modifications in eating habits may reduce the pain of pancreatitis.

 Documentation

Medication administration record
   Type, route, and dosage of all medications

Progress notes
   Status of pain
   Degree of relief from pain-relief measures

Imbalanced Nutrition: Less Than Body Requirements Related to Vomiting, Anorexia, Impaired Digestion Secondary to Decreased Pancreatic Enzymes

Focus Assessment Criteria	Clinical Significance
1. Weight and intake	1. During acute pancreatitis, NPO status is maintained to reduce production of pancreatic enzymes and TPN is used. As the client improves, oral feedings are slowly initiated. Weight can serve as an indicator of nitrogen balance. The diet's adequacy in meeting nutritional requirements also must be evaluated.
2. Stools (amount, characteristics)	2. Steatorrhea indicates impaired digestion.
3. Complaints of nausea, vomiting, stomatitis, gastritis, and flatus	3. These symptoms can adversely affect eating patterns.
4. Laboratory values: BUN; serum albumin, protein, and cholesterol; hematocrit; and hemoglobin	

Goal

The client will ingest daily nutritional requirements in accordance with activity level and metabolic needs.

Indicators
• Describe reasons for dietary restrictions.
• Weigh within norm for height and age.

Interventions	Rationales
1. Promote foods that stimulate eating and increase calorie consumption.	1. Nausea and fear of pain associated with eating negatively influence appetite.
2. Maintain good oral hygiene before and after meals.	2. This decreases microorganisms that can cause foul taste and odor that inhibit appetite.
3. Offer small, frequent feedings.	3. Small, frequent feedings can reduce malabsorption and distention by decreasing protein metabolized at one time.

(continues on page 243)

Interventions continued	Rationales continued
4. Determine what time of the day the client's appetite is greatest and plan the most nutritious meal for this time.	4. This can help to ensure intake of nutrients needed for cell growth and repair.
5. Explain the need for a high-carbohydrate, low-protein, low-fat diet.	5. A diet low in protein and fat reduces secretion of secretin and cholecystokinin, thus decreasing autodigestion and destruction of pancreatic cells (Dudek, 2001).
6. Explain the need to avoid alcohol, caffeine, and gas-forming and spicy foods.	6. Alcohol produces hypersecretion of protein in pancreatic secretions that causes protein plugs and obstructs pancreatic ducts. Caffeine and spicy foods increase gastric and pancreatic secretions. Gas-forming foods increase gastric distention (Dudek, 2001).

Documentation

Flow records
    Intake (amount, type, time)
    Weight
    Output (urine, stool, vomitus)

Ineffective Denial Related to Acknowledgment of Alcohol Abuse or Dependency

Focus Assessment Criteria	Clinical Significance
1. Alcohol use (reported by client or family)	1–4. Denial in alcoholism may include denial of loss of control, family pain, or the alcoholic's part in the family problem (Smith-DiJulio, 2002).
2. Occupational functioning	
3. Family and social functioning	
4. Previous rehabilitation attempts	

Goal

The client will acknowledge an alcohol/drug abuse problem.

Indicators

- Explain the psychological and physiologic effects of alcohol or drug use.
- Abstain from alcohol/drug use.

Interventions	Rationales
1. Approach client nonjudgmentally. Be aware of your own feelings regarding alcoholism.	1. The client probably has been reprimanded by many and is distrustful. The nurse's personal experiences with alcohol may increase or decrease empathy for the client.
2. Help client to understand that alcoholism is an illness, not a moral problem.	2. Historically alcoholics have been viewed as immoral and degenerate. Acknowledgment of alcoholism as a disease can increase the client's sense of trust.
3. Assist client to examine how drinking has affected relationships, work, and so on. Ask how he or she feels when not drinking.	3. During acute pancreatitis, the client may be more likely to acknowledge his or her drinking problem.
4. Encourage significant others to discuss with the client how alcohol has affected their lives.	4. Confrontation with family and peers may help to break down the client's denial.
5. Focus on how the client can avoid alcohol and recover, not on reasons for drinking.	5. The client may try to focus on the reasons for using alcohol in an attempt to minimize the problem's significance.
6. Explain that inpatient treatment programs or self-help groups are critical for assistance in recovering. Specific treatment programs include lectures, psychotherapy, peer assistance, recreational therapy, and support groups.	6. Participation in a structured treatment program greatly increases the chance of successful recovery from alcoholism.
7. If sanctioned, schedule interactions with recovering alcoholics.	7. Recovering alcoholics provide honest, direct confrontation with the realities of alcoholism.
8. If sanctioned, schedule a visit with an expert from a detoxification program for ongoing treatment.	8. Affording the client direct contact with an expert who can help can promote a sense of hope.
9. Refer the family to Al-Anon and Al-Ateen as appropriate.	9. The client's family needs assistance to identify enabling behavior and strategies for dealing with a recovering or existing alcoholic (Smith-DiJulio, 2002).
10. Refer to care plan on Alcohol Withdrawal.	

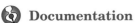 **Documentation**

Progress notes
  Dialogues
Discharge summary record
Client teaching
  Outcome achievement
  Referrals

High Risk for Ineffective Therapeutic Regimen Management Related to Lack of Knowledge of Disease Process, Treatments, Contraindications, Dietary Management, and Follow-up Care

Focus Assessment Criteria	Clinical Significance
1. Client's readiness to learn and retain information	1. A client who does not achieve the goals for learning requires a referral for assistance postdischarge.

Goals

The goals for this diagnosis represent those associated with discharge planning. Refer to discharge criteria.

Interventions	Rationales
1. Explain causes of acute and chronic pancreatitis.	1. Inaccurate perceptions of health status usually involve misunderstanding the nature and seriousness of the illness, susceptibility to complications, and need for restrictions to control illness.

2. Teach client to report these symptoms:
  a. Steatorrhea
  b. Severe back or epigastric pain
  c. Persistent gastritis, nausea, or vomiting
  d. Weight loss
  e. Elevated temperature
	2. They can indicate worsening of inflammation and increased malabsorption. Elevated temperature could indicate infection or abscess formation.

3. Explain the relationship of hyperglycemia to pancreatitis; teach client to observe for and report signs and symptoms.	3. Early detection and reporting enables prompt intervention to prevent serious complications.

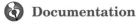 **Documentation**

Discharge summary record
  Client teaching
  Outcome achievement
  Referrals, when indicated

Gastrointestinal Disorders

GASTROENTEROCOLITIS/ENTEROCOLITIS

An infectious agent (bacterial or viral) can cause inflammation of the small bowel (enterocolitis) or both the small and large colons (gastroenterocolitis). Enterocolitis causes cramps and diarrhea, whereas gastroenterocolitis produces nausea, vomiting, diarrhea, and cramps. Hospitalization is indicated with severe fluid and electrolyte imbalances or for high-risk clients (older adults, people with diabetes, people with compromised immune systems) (Cheskin & Lacy, 2003).

 Time Frame
Acute episode

⊙⊙ DIAGNOSTIC CLUSTER*

Collaborative Problems

PC: Fluid/Electrolyte Imbalance

Nursing Diagnoses

- High Risk for Deficient Fluid Volume related to losses secondary to vomiting and diarrhea
- Acute Pain related to abdominal cramping, diarrhea, and vomiting secondary to vascular dilatation and hyperperistalsis
- High Risk for Ineffective Therapeutic Regimen Management related to lack of knowledge of condition, dietary restrictions, and signs and symptoms of complications

---

*This medical condition was not included in the validation study.

Discharge Criteria

Before discharge, the client or family will

1. Describe the causes of gastroenteritis and its transmission.
2. Identify dietary restrictions that promote comfort and healing.
3. State signs and symptoms of dehydration.
4. State signs and symptoms that must be reported to a health care professional.

Collaborative Problems

Potential Complication: Fluid/Electrolyte Imbalance

Nursing Goals

The nurse will detect early signs and symptoms of dehydration and electrolyte imbalances and collaboratively intervene to stabilize client.

Indicators
- Urine output >30ml/hr
- Urine specific gravity 1.005–1.030
- Moist skin/mucous membranes
- Serum sodium 135–145 mEq/L
- Serum potassium 3.8–5 mEq/L
- Serum chloride 95–105 mEq/L

Interventions	Rationales

1. Monitor for signs and symptoms of dehydration:
  a. Dry skin and mucous membrane
  b. Elevated urine specific gravity
  c. Thirst
	1. Rapid propulsion of feces through the intestines decreases water absorption. Low circulatory volume causes dry mucous membranes and thirst. Concentrated urine has an elevated specific gravity.

2. Carefully monitor intake and output.	2. Intake and output records help to detect early signs of fluid imbalance.

3. Monitor for electrolyte imbalances:
  a. Sodium
  b. Chloride
  c. Potassium
	3. Rapid propulsion of feces through the intestines decreases electrolyte absorption. Vomiting also causes electrolyte loss.

Related Physician-Prescribed Interventions

Medications. Antidiarrheals, antiemetics, antibiotics (if bacterial)

Intravenous Therapy. Fluid/electrolyte replacement

Laboratory Studies. CBC with differential; stool examination/cultures for amoeba, bacteria, parasites, leukocytes; electrolytes

Diagnostic Studies. Endoscopy (if severe)

Therapies. Diet as tolerated (e.g., clear fluids, full fluids, bland, soft); oral electrolyte preparations

Documentation
Flow records
  Intake and output
  Stools (amount, consistency)

Nursing Diagnoses

High Risk for Deficient Fluid Volume Related to Losses Secondary to Vomiting and Diarrhea

(If client is NPO, this is then a collaborative problem: refer to index: PC: Hypovolemia.)

Focus Assessment Criteria	Clinical Significance
1. Vital signs: blood pressure, temperature, pulse, respirations	1–4. These assessments provide baseline data for comparison with subsequent assessment findings.
2. Skin turgor, mucous membranes, urine output	
3. Consistency and frequency of stools	
4. Laboratory studies: electrolytes, urine specific gravity, blood urea nitrogen (BUN)	

Goal

The client will have a urine specific gravity between 1.005 and 1.030.

Indicators

- Intake is 1.5 ml of fluids every 24 hours.
- Urinate at least every 2 hours.

Interventions	Rationales

1. Monitor for early signs and symptoms of fluid volume deficit:
  a. Dry mucous membranes (lips, gums)
  b. Amber urine
  c. Specific gravity >1.025
	1. Decreased circulating volume causes drying of tissues and concentrated urine. Early detection enables prompt fluid replacement therapy to correct deficits.

2. Monitor parenteral fluid infusion and administer parenteral antiemetic medications as ordered.	2. Antiemetics prevent vomiting by inhibiting stimuli to the vomiting center.

3. Provide fluids often and in small amounts so that the urge to urinate occurs every 2 hours:
  a. Broths
  b. Noncarbonated soft drinks
  c. Electrolyte-supplemented drinks
  d. Apple juice
	3. Carbonated beverages replace sodium and potassium lost in diarrhea and vomiting.

4. Instruct to
  a. Avoid products (drinks, gum) with sorbitol.
  b. Put a small amount (¼ teaspoon) of sugar in carbonated beverages.
	a. Sorbitol can cause or aggravate diarrhea.
	  b. Sugar will disperse bubbles to reduce gastric distention.

5. Monitor intake and output, making sure that intake compensates for output.	5. Output may exceed intake that already may be inadequate to compensate for insensible losses. Dehydration may decrease glomerular filtration rate, making output inadequate to clear wastes properly and leading to elevated BUN and electrolyte levels.
6. Weigh the client daily.	6. Accurate daily weights can detect fluid loss.

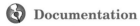 **Documentation**

Flow records
  Vital signs
  Intake and output
  Daily weights
  Medications
  Vomiting episodes

Acute Pain Related to Abdominal Cramping, Diarrhea, and Vomiting Secondary to Vascular Dilatation and Hyperperistalsis

Focus Assessment Criteria	Clinical Significance
1. Complaints of abdominal cramps, diarrhea, vomiting 2. Factors that may precipitate symptoms	1,2. This assessment helps to evaluate the client's status and identify possible sources of irritation.

Goal

The client will report less painful symptoms.

Indicators

- Report reduced abdominal cramping.
- List foods and fluids to avoid.

Interventions	Rationales
1. Encourage the client to rest in the supine position with a warm heating pad on the abdomen.	1. These measures promote GI muscular relaxation and reduce cramping.
2. Encourage frequent intake of small amounts of cool clear liquids (e.g., dilute tea, flat ginger ale, jello, water): 30 to 60 mL every ½ to 1 hour.	2. Small amounts of fluids do not distend the gastric area and thus do not aggravate symptoms.
3. Eliminate unpleasant sights and odors from the client's environment.	3. Unpleasant sights or odors can stimulate the vomiting center.

4. Instruct the client to avoid these items:
  a. Hot or cold liquids
  b. Foods containing fat or fiber (e.g., milk, fruits)
  c. Caffeine
	4. Cold liquids can induce cramping; hot liquids can stimulate peristalsis. Fats also increase peristalsis, and caffeine increases intestinal motility.

5. Protect the perianal area from irritation.	5. Frequent stools of increased acidity can irritate perianal skin.

⊗ Documentation

Flow records
   Intake and output
   Tolerance of intake
   Stools (frequency, characteristics, consistency)
   Bowel sounds

High Risk for Ineffective Therapeutic Regimen Management Related to Lack of Knowledge of Condition, Dietary Restrictions, and Signs and Symptoms of Complications

Focus Assessment Criteria	Clinical Significance
1. Knowledge of causative agents of gastroenteritis a. Food eaten b. Similar illness in others c. Onset of symptoms after eating (immediate, 1–2 days, longer) d. Recent uses of antimicrobials e. Neurologic symptoms f. Risk factors for HIV infection	1. A thorough history of onset of symptoms and other factors can assist in identifying etiologic agents.
2. Readiness for learning and possible barriers that might interfere	
3. Support person(s) who will assist the client	

Goal

The goals for this diagnosis represent those associated with discharge planning. Refer to the discharge criteria.

Interventions	Rationales
1. Discuss the disease process in understandable terms; explain the following: a. Causative agents b. Reason for enteric precautions c. Preventive measures d. Importance of scrupulous handwashing	1. The client's understanding may increase compliance with dietary restrictions and hygiene practices.
2. Explain dietary restrictions: a. High-fiber foods (e.g., bran, fresh fruit) b. High-fat foods (e.g., whole milk, fried foods) c. Very hot or cold fluids d. Caffeine e. High carbohydrate foods	2. These foods can stimulate or irritate the intestinal tract.
3. Instruct on dietary options: a. Rice b. Toast, crackers c. Bananas d. Tea e. Apple juice/sauce	3. Foods with complex carbohydrates facilitate fluid absorption into the intestinal mucosa (Cheskin & Lacy, 2003).

(continues on page 254)

Interventions continued	**Rationales** continued

4. Teach the client and family to report these symptoms:
  a. Inability to retain fluids
  b. Dark amber urine persisting for more than 12 hours
  c. Bloody stools
	4. Early detection and reporting of the signs of dehydration enable prompt interventions to prevent serious fluid or electrolyte imbalances.

5. Explain the benefits of rest and encourage adequate rest.	5. Inactivity reduces peristalsis and allows the GI tract to rest.

6. Explain preventive measures:
  a. Proper food storage/refrigeration
  b. Proper cleaning of kitchen utensils especially wooden cutting boards
  c. Handwashing before and after handling food
	6. The most common cause of gastroenteritis is ingestion of bacteria-contaminated food.

7. Instruct to wash hands and:
  a. Disinfect surface areas with disinfectants that contain high proportion of alcohol.
  b. Suspend eating utensils and thermometers in alcohol solution or use dishwasher for eating utensils and dishes.
  c. Do not permit sharing of objects used by ill person (toys, games).
	7. The spread of virus can be controlled by disinfecting surface areas (bathrooms) and eating utensils. Disinfectants with low proportions of alcohol are ineffective against some viruses.

8. If stool culture is needed, instruct to refrigerate stool in container until transported to lab. Advise only to send watery stool for culture.	8. Most bacteria that cause diarrhea die quickly at room temperature.
9. Explain the risks of ill persons working in food service, institutions, elementary school, and day care.	9. The risk for transmission is high, especially in such groups as children and the elderly.

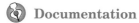 **Documentation**

Discharge summary record
  Discharge instructions
  Progress toward goal attainment
  Status at discharge

INFLAMMATORY BOWEL DISEASE

Inflammatory bowel disease (IBD) is a generic term comprising both Crohn's disease and ulcerative colitis. Both are inflammatory conditions of the GI tract and have similar clinical presentations. The causes of IBD are unknown. Crohn's disease has transmural lesions that can involve the entire intestinal tract. Ulcerative colitis consists of mucosal inflammation limited to the colon involving the rectal mucosal 95% of the time (Arcangelo & Peterson, 2001; Cheskin & Lacy, 2003). Crohn's disease can involve the entire intestinal tract from the mouth to the anus with discontinuous focal ulceration, fistula formation, and perianal involvement. Small bowel or upper GI involvement, fistulas, fissures, and abscesses are absent. The causes of IBD are not known.

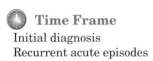 **Time Frame**

Initial diagnosis
Recurrent acute episodes

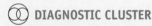 **DIAGNOSTIC CLUSTER**

Collaborative Problems

▲ PC: Fluid/Electrolyte Imbalances
▲ PC: Intestinal Obstruction
▲ PC: GI Bleeding
▲ PC: Anemia
△ PC: Fistula/Fissure/Abscess
△ PC: Renal Calculi
▲ PC: Growth Retardation

Nursing Diagnoses

▲ Chronic Pain related to intestinal inflammatory process
▲ Imbalanced Nutrition: Less Than Body Requirements related to dietary restrictions, nausea, diarrhea, and abdominal cramping associated with eating or painful ulcers of the oral mucous membrane
▲ Diarrhea related to intestinal inflammatory process
△ High Risk for Ineffective Coping related to chronicity of condition and lack of definitive treatment
△ High Risk for Ineffective Therapeutic Regimen Management related to lack of knowledge of condition, diagnostic tests, prognosis, treatment, and signs and symptoms of complications

Related Care Plan

Corticosteroid Therapy

▲ This diagnosis was reported to be monitored for or managed frequently (75%–100%).
△ This diagnosis was reported to be monitored for or managed often (50%–74%).

Discharge Criteria

Before discharge, the client or family will

1. Discuss management of activities of daily living.
2. State signs and symptoms that must be reported to a health care professional.
3. Verbalize an intent to share feelings and concerns related to IBD with significant others.
4. Identify available community resources or self-help groups.

Collaborative Problems

Potential Complication: Fluid/Electrolyte Imbalances

Potential Complication: Intestinal Obstruction

Potential Complication: GI Bleeding

Potential Complication: Anemia

Potential Complication: Fistula/Fissure/Abscess

Potential Complication: Renal Calculi

Potential Complication: Growth Retardation

Nursing Goal

The nurse will detect early signs/symptoms of (a) fluid/electrolyte imbalances, (b) intestinal obstruction, (c) abscess, (d) GI bleeding, (e) anemia, and (f) renal calculi.

Indicators

- Temperature 98–99.5°F (c, f)
- Respiratory rate 16–20 breaths/min (a, d)
- Normal breath sounds, no adventitious sounds (a, d)
- Normal relaxed, quiet, even breathing (a, d)
- Peripheral pulses full, bounding (a)
- Pulse 60–100 beats/min (a)
- Blood pressure >90/60, <140/90 mm Hg
- Serum pH 7.35–7.45
- Warm, dry skin (a)
- Pinkish, ruddy brownish, or olive skin tones
- Calm, oriented (d)
- No nausea or vomiting (b)
- Urine output >30 ml/hour (a, f)
- Urine specific gravity 1.005–1.030 (a, f)
- Blood urea nitrogen 5–25 mg/dL (f)
- Serum pre-albumin 20–50 mg/dL (f)
- Red blood cells (e)
  - ○ Male 4.6–5.9 million/mm^3
  - ○ Female 4.2–5.4 million/mm^3
- White blood count 4,300–10,800 mm^3 (c)
- Serum potassium 3.5–5.0 mEq/L (a)
- Creatinine clearance (a)
  - ○ Male 95–135 ml/mm
  - ○ Female 85–125 ml/mm
- Serum sodium 135–145 mEq/L (a)
- Capillary refill <3 seconds
- Bowel sounds present in all quadrants (b)
- Stool occult blood-negative
- Usual weight (a)
- No abdominal pain (b)
- B$_{12}$ 130–785 pg/ml (e)
- Folate 2.5–20 ng/ml (e)
- Hemoglobin (d, e)
  - ○ Males 13.18 gm/dL
  - ○ Females 12.16 gm/dL
- No abdominal pain (c)
- No rectal pain or discharge (c)

Interventions	Rationales

1. Monitor laboratory values for electrolyte imbalances:
  a. Potassium
  b. Sodium
  c. Calcium
  d. Phosphorus
  e. Magnesium
  f. Zinc
	1. Chronic diarrhea and inadequate oral intake can deplete electrolytes. Small intestine inflammation impairs absorption of fluid and electrolytes (Bullock & Henze, 2000).

2. Monitor for signs and symptoms of dehydration:
  a. Tachycardia
  b. Dry skin/mucous membrane
  c. Elevated urine specific gravity
  d. Thirst
	2. When circulating volume decreases, heart rate increases in an attempt to supply tissues with oxygen. Low circulatory volume causes dry mucous membranes and thirst. Concentrated urine has an elevated specific gravity.

3. Monitor intake and output.	3. Intake and output monitoring provides early detection of fluid imbalance.
4. Collect 24-hour urine samples weekly for evaluation of electrolytes, calcium, phosphates, urea, and nitrogen.	4. This enables evaluation of electrolyte status and renal function.

5. Monitor for signs and symptoms of intestinal obstruction:
  a. Wavelike abdominal pain
  b. Vomiting (gastric juices, bile, progressing to fecal material)
  c. Abdominal distention
  d. Change in bowel sounds (initially hyperactive progressing to none)
	5. Inflammation and edema cause the obstruction. Intestinal contents are then propelled toward the mouth instead of the rectum.

6. If you suspect intestinal obstruction, withhold all food and fluids and notify the physician.	6. Avoidance of foods and fluids prevents further distention and prepares the GI tract for surgery.

7. Monitor for signs and symptoms of fistula, fissures, or abscesses:
  a. Purulent drainage
  b. Fecal drainage from vagina
  c. Increased abdominal pain
  d. Burning rectal pain following defecation
  e. Perianal induration, swelling, redness, and cyanotic tags
  f. Signs of sepsis (e.g., fever, increased WBC count)
	7. The inflammation and ulceration of Crohn's disease can penetrate the intestinal wall and form an abscess or fistula to other parts of the intestine or skin. Abscesses and fistulas may cause cramping, pain, and fever and may interfere with digestion. Sepsis may arise from seeding of the bloodstream from fistula tracts or abscess cavities (Botoman, Bonner & Botoman, 1998).

(continues on page 258)

Interventions continued	Rationales continued

8. Monitor for signs and symptoms of GI bleeding:
  a. Decreased hemoglobin and hematocrit
  b. Fatigue
  c. Irritability
  d. Pallor
  e. Tachycardia
  f. Dyspnea
  g. Anorexia
	8. Chronic inflammation can cause erosion of vessels and bleeding.

9. Monitor for signs of anemia:
  a. Decreased hemoglobin
  b. Decreased red blood cells
  c. B_{12} deficiency
  d. Folate deficiency
	9. Anemia may result from GI bleeding, bone marrow depression (associated with chronic inflammatory diseases), and inadequate intake or impaired absorption of vitamin B_{12}, folic acid, and iron. Sulfasalazine therapy can cause hemolysis, which contributes to anemia (Bullock & Henze, 2000).

10. Monitor for signs and symptoms of urolithiasis (refer to the renal calculi [urolithiasis] care plan if they occur):
  a. Flank pain
  b. Fever, chills
	10. Severe diarrhea can lead to a decreased volume of concentrated urine. This, combined with intestinal bicarbonate loss and lowered pH, leads to the development of urate stones. With ileal resection or severe IBD, the calcium normally available to bind with oxalate binds instead with fatty acids, freeing dietary oxalate for absorption. Decreased urine volume enhances the precipitation of calcium oxalate in the kidney, pre-disposing to stone formation (Bullock & Henze, 2000).

11. Monitor an adolescent client for signs of growth retardation:
  a. Delayed bone growth
  b. Weight loss
  c. Delayed development of secondary sex characteristics
	11. Possible causes include decreased nutritional intake, loss of protein and nutrients by rapid passage through the GI tract, increased metabolic requirements secondary to bowel inflammation, and corticosteroid therapy (Cheskin & Lacy, 2003).

Related Physician-Prescribed Interventions

Medications. Aminosalicylates, immunosuppressants, antibiotics, corticosteroids, IgG (infliximab), (oral, enemas), vitamins/minerals, erythropoietin, tumor necrosis factor inhibitors, opioids

Intravenous Therapy. Fluid/electrolyte replacement, 5-aminosalicylic acid

Laboratory Studies. Stool specimens (bacteria), ova, parasites; CBC; serum protein electrophoresis; serum electrolytes; sedimentation rate; blood urea nitrogen; alkaline phosphatase; creatinine; prothrombin time

Diagnostic Studies. Endoscopy, biopsy (rectal), GI x-ray film, D-xylose test, proctosigmoidoscopy, barium enema, abdominal MRI, abdominal CT scan

Therapies. Low-residue, high-protein diet; surgery; total parenteral nutrition

⚘ Documentation

Flow records
    Abnormal laboratory values
    Vital signs
    Intake and output
    Bowel sounds
    Diarrhea episodes
    Vomiting episodes
    Drainage (wound, rectal, vaginal)
    Urine specific gravity

Nursing Diagnoses

Chronic Pain Related to Inflammatory Intestinal Process

Focus Assessment Criteria	Clinical Significance
1. Client's pain experience: intensity and tolerance	1. Pain tolerance differs among clients and may vary in the same client in different circumstances.
2. Factors that increase or decrease pain (e.g., eating, passing stool, flatus)	2. Increased pain without relief from usual interventions may indicate complications such as intestinal obstruction or peritonitis.
3. Effects of pain on client's life style and ability to perform ADLs 4. Knowledge of pain management techniques	3,4. This assessment may indicate the need for alternative pain management strategies.

Goal

The client will relate improvement of pain and an increase in ability to perform activities of daily living (ADLs).

Indicators

- Relate that others acknowledge and validate the pain.
- Practice noninvasive pain relief measures to manage pain.

Interventions	Rationales
1. Acknowledge the presence of the client's pain.	1. Acknowledging and validating a client's pain may help reduce his or her anxiety, which can decrease pain.
2. Have the client rate pain intensity on a scale of 1 to 10 (1 = no pain; 10 = greatest pain possible), and level of pain tolerance (1 = can tolerate; 10 = cannot tolerate at all).	2. Such a rating scale provides a good method of evaluating the subjective experience of pain.

(continues on page 260)

Interventions continued	Rationales continued
3. Determine the relationship between eating and drinking and abdominal pain.	3. The client may link eating or drinking to onset of abdominal pain and may limit intake to avoid pain.
4. Determine the relationship between passage of stool or flatus and pain relief.	4. Pain not relieved by passage of feces or flatus may be a sign of intestinal obstruction or peritonitis.
5. Determine the effects of chronic pain on the client's life style.	5. Chronic pain can cause withdrawal, depression, anger, and dependency.
6. Determine if pain occurs during the night.	6. Abdominal cramps or a feeling of urgency to defecate may awaken the client at night. This usually occurs less often in Crohn's disease than in ulcerative colitis.

7. Provide for pain relief:
   a. Assist with position changes.
 	
   b. Apply a warm heating pad to the abdomen, *except* during an acute flare-up of IBD.
   c. Encourage relaxation exercises.
 	
   d. Encourage diversional activities such as family visits, telephone calls, and involvement in self-care.
	7.
	   a. Repositioning may help to move air through the bowel and relieve cramps.
	   b. Warmth relaxes abdominal muscles.
	
	   c. Relaxation may enhance the therapeutic effects of pain medication.
	   d. Diversion may help to distract the client from pain.

8. Evaluate the effectiveness of the pain management plan.	8. Frequent evaluation of pain relief enables regimen adjustment for maximum effectiveness. Failure to manage chronic pain may lead to depression.

 Documentation

Medication administration record
  Type, dosage, and route of all medications
Progress notes
  Pain descriptions
  Unsatisfactory relief from pain relief measures

Imbalanced Nutrition: Less Than Body Requirements Related to Dietary Restrictions, Nausea, Diarrhea, and Abdominal Cramping Associated with Eating or Painful Ulcers of the Oral Mucous Membrane

Focus Assessment Criteria	Clinical Significance
1. Appetite and energy level	1. A client with IBD typically suffers from malnourishment because of the malabsorption of nutrients in the bowel wall. In addition, the client tends to eat less because he associates nausea and abdominal cramping with food intake.

(continues on page 261)

Focus Assessment Criteria continued	Clinical Significance continued
2. Current body weight and history of recent weight loss	2. Weight loss is reported in 65% to 70% of clients with IBD. Weight loss may exceed 10 lb a month.
3. Food intolerance, if any	3. A client with IBD may have food intolerance to milk, fried or spicy foods, and foods high in fiber. In Crohn's disease, structural changes in the intestinal villi result in decreased absorption area and loss of the intestinal enzyme lactase.
4. Condition of oral mucosa	4. A client with Crohn's disease is susceptible to painful ulcers of the mouth.
5. Anthropometric measurements: mid-arm circumference, triceps pain	5. Anthropometric measurements help to evaluate nutritional status. Midarm circumference measures somatic muscle mass; triceps skin fold estimates subcutaneous fat stored.
6. Relationship of eating to onset of nausea, diarrhea, or abdominal pain	6. This assessment helps to determine patterns and differentiate complications (intestinal obstruction and peritonitis).

7. Laboratory data:
  a. Serum albumin
 	
  b. Serum transferrin and iron
 	
  c. Hemoglobin and hematocrit
  d. Total lymphocyte count
  e. Zinc, trace minerals
	7.
	  a. Serum albumin levels reflect the body's protein status. Serum albumen takes about 3 weeks for protein repletion to be reflected. Clients with acute IBD have been shown to lose from two to 60 times the amount of albumin lost by healthy persons.
	  b. Transferrin is the major transport protein for iron. Serum transferrin reflects protein repletion in 1 week.
	  c,d. Protein malnutrition results in decreased WBC count and anemia.
	  e. A client with IBD often has chronic zinc deficiency manifested by anxiety, depression, alopecia, acrodermatitis, and diarrhea. Daily intravenous replacement improves these symptoms dramatically. Within hours mental depression and anxiety are relieved, diarrhea responds to treatment, and the dermatitis begins resolving. Alopecia reverses within 2 weeks (Cheskin & Lacy, 2003).

Goal

The client will be in positive nitrogen balance as evidenced by weight gain of 2–3 lb/wk.

Indicators

- Verbalize understanding of nutritional requirements.
- List foods to avoid.

Interventions	Rationales
1. Administer total parenteral nutrition (TPN) therapy as ordered and intervene as follows: a. Teach long-term venous access catheter care. (Refer to the Long-Term Venous Access Devices care plan for more information.)	1. a. TPN is the treatment of choice when weight loss, nutritional depletion, and symptoms of IBD are severe. In TPN, the client requires 45 to 50 kcal and about 2 g of protein/kg of body weight/day to remain in positive nitrogen balance. This allows weight gain of about 8 oz/day. Clients with ulcerative colitis do not benefit from TPN therapy as greatly as do those with Crohn's disease. (Galica, 1997)
b. Maintain nothing-by-mouth (NPO) status.	b. NPO status decreases the mechanical, physical, and chemical activities of the bowel.
c. Provide psychosocial support and reassurance during bowel rest and TPN.	c. Prolonged NPO status is disturbing both socially and psychologically.
d. Assist the client to ambulate with an intravenous pole.	d. Ambulation enhances the client's sense of well-being and helps to maintain or improve physical conditioning.
2. Wean the client from TPN feedings when ordered (Dudek, 2001): a. Use a relaxed, confident, consistent approach to TPN catheter care. b. Provide emotional support during the weaning process.	2. a,b. A client receiving TPN typically views the TPN catheter as his or her "lifeline." He or she may feel protective of it and question the expertise of the professional staff caring for it.
c. Reassure client that weight loss during the first week off TPN is due to fluid loss.	a,c. Client generally loses 4 to 5 lb of fluid during the first week off TPN.
d. Help client to set realistic expectations for gaining weight after discontinuation of TPN.	a,d. Client may expect to gain weight on oral feeding at the same rate as when on TPN, however, this is not a realistic expectation.
e. Encourage use of high-protein drinks with meals.	a,e. Dietary supplements may be needed to meet nutritional requirements.
f. Arrange for a dietitian to spend time with the client.	a,f. Consultation may be needed to plan an adequate dietary regimen.
3. Assist client in resuming oral food intake:	3. Client may need encouragement to resume oral intake because he or she may resist for fear of pain.
a. Encourage liquids with caloric value rather than coffee, tea, water, or diet soda.	a. Calorie-rich liquids can help to prevent malnutrition.
b. Assess client's acceptance of and response to oral fluid intake.	b. The ability to absorb nutrients must be evaluated daily.
c. Start formula feedings in dilute form and progress to full strength as tolerated.	c. If the client cannot tolerate a regular diet, elemental feedings may be ordered. They are better tolerated because they are residue-free, low in fat, nutritionally balanced, and digested mainly in the upper jejunum. They do not stimulate pancreatic, biliary, and intestinal secretions as does regular food.

(continues on page 263)

Interventions continued	Rationales continued
d. Offer a variety of flavors of elemental feedings and keep them chilled.	d. Elemental diets have an unpleasant odor and taste because of the amino acids present. Adding flavor and keeping them chilled increase their palatability.
e. Assist with progression to soft, bland, and low-residue solids and encourage small frequent feedings high in calories, protein, vitamins, and carbohydrates.	e. Gradual introduction of solid foods is needed to reduce pain and increase tolerance.
f. Teach the client to avoid raw fruits, vegetables, condiments, whole-grain cereals, gas-forming and fried foods, alcohol, and iced drinks.	f. These foods and liquids can irritate the GI tract.
g. As ordered, supplement the client's diet with folic acid, ascorbic acid, iron, calcium, copper, zinc, vitamin D, and vitamin B_{12}.	g. Nutrient deficiencies result from decreased oral intake, malabsorption, or both.

 Documentation

Flow records
  Acceptance of food
  Tolerance of food
  Type and amount of food taken orally
  Daily weight
Progress notes
  Energy level

Diarrhea Related to Intestinal Inflammatory Process

Focus Assessment Criteria	Clinical Significance

1. Frequency, consistency, odor, and amount of stools
2. Onset of diarrhea in relationship to any of the following:
  a. Pain
  b. Eating
  c. Activity
  d. Stress
3. Urgency to expel stool
4. Flatus
	1–4. In IBD, an inflamed colon fails to reabsorb water and electrolytes, the rectum loses its capacity to retain a fluid load, and the small intestine may fail to absorb water, bile, salts, and lactose. All these factors contribute to diarrhea. The severity of the diarrhea relates directly to the extent of bowel involvement.

5. Steatorrhea	5. Steatorrhea results from high unabsorbed fat content.
6. Blood, mucus, or pus in stools	6. Blood, mucus, or pus in stools may indicate bleeding or abscess.
7. Serum albumin level	7. Hypoalbuminemia may be associated with severe diarrhea.

Goal

The client will report less diarrhea.

Indicators

- Describe factors that cause diarrhea.
- Explain the rationales for interventions.
- Have fewer episodes of diarrhea.
- Verbalize signs and symptoms of dehydration and electrolyte imbalances.

Interventions	Rationales

1. Assess for the following:
  a. Decreased number of stools
  b. Increased consistency of stools
  c. Decreased urgency to expel stool
	1. Stool assessment helps to evaluate the effectiveness of antidiarrheal agents and dietary restrictions.

2. Maintain an odor-free patient environment:
  a. Empty the bedpan or commode immediately.
  b. Change soiled linens.
  c. Provide a room deodorizer.
	2. Fecal odor can cause embarrassment and self-consciousness and can increase the stress of living with IBD.

3. Provide good perianal care.	3. Perianal irritation from frequent liquid stool should be prevented.
4. Decrease physical activity during acute episodes of diarrhea.	4. Decreased physical activity decreases bowel peristalsis.
5. Determine the relationship between diarrheal episodes and ingestion of specific foods	5. Identification of irritating foods can reduce diarrheal episodes.

6. Observe for signs and symptoms of electrolyte imbalance:
  a. Decreased serum potassium
 	
  b. Decreased serum sodium
	6.
	
	  a. In osmotic diarrhea, impaired fluid absorption by the intestines is caused by ingested solutes that cannot be digested or by a decrease in intestinal absorption. Water and electrolytes are drawn into the intestine in greater quantities than can be absorbed, and the diarrheal fluid is high in potassium (Bullock & Henze, 2000).
	  b. Secretory diarrhea occurs when the gut wall is inflamed or engorged or when it is stimulated by bile salts. The resulting diarrheal stool is high in sodium.

(continues on page 265)

Interventions continued	Rationales continued

7. Replace fluid and electrolytes with oral fluid containing appropriate electrolytes:
  a. Gatorade, a commercial preparation of glucose-electrolyte solution
  b. Apple juice, which is high in potassium but low in sodium
  c. Colas, root beer, and ginger ale that contain sodium but negligible potassium content.
	7. The type of fluid replacement depends on the electrolyte(s) needed.

Documentation

Flow records
  Intake and output
  Number of stools
  Consistency of stools
Medication administration record
  Frequency of as-needed anti-diarrheal medication

High Risk for Ineffective Coping Related to Chronicity of Condition and Lack of Definitive Treatment

Focus Assessment Criteria	Clinical Significance

1. Emotional status and defense mechanisms:
  a. Independence or dependence
  b. Anger, denial of IBD
  c. Self-control, perfectionism, internal demands
  d. Self-confidence
  e. Perceived stressors and changes in health status
  f. Perceived coping status
	1. IBD is a life-disrupting illness that can dominate the lives of those it affects. The client may have heard that IBD is a "psychosomatic" disease and may misinterpret this to mean that it is all in the mind. One study with a one-year follow-up found that 40–60% of clients with IBD described their quality of life as fair to poor (Irvine et al., 1994).

2. Sleep disturbances:
  a. Changes in sleep patterns
  b. Cramping or diarrheal episodes during sleep hours
  c. Energy levels in evening and morning
	2. Some clients with IBD report inability to sleep because of being "wound up" and full of energy at bedtime. This may be related to use of corticosteroids in the treatment of IBD. Lack of sleep may contribute to a lack of ability to cope effectively with a chronic condition.

3. Family and social interactions:
  a. Social participation
  b. Availability of and satisfaction with support systems
  c. Demands of others on client
  d. Demands of clients on others
	3. The ever-present risk of uncontrollable diarrhea can isolate the client and restrict the activities of all family members.

Goal

The client will make appropriate decisions to cope with condition.

Indicators
• Verbalize factors that contribute to anxiety and stress.
• Verbalize methods to improve the ability to cope with the chronic condition.

Interventions	Rationales
1. Clear up misconceptions about IBD. Stress that psychological symptoms are a reaction to, not the cause of, IBD.	1. Correcting misconceptions may help to reduce the guilt associated with this belief.
2. Identify and minimize factors that contribute to anxiety: a. Explain all diagnostic tests and support the client during each procedure. b. Do not label the client as "demanding" or a "big baby."	2. Understanding procedures can reduce anxiety. Labels lead to overt or subtle rejection by others and further exaggerate the client's feelings of helplessness and isolation.
3. Allow the client to have some control over care. Demonstrate acceptance and concern when caring for the client.	3. A client with IBD typically feels as if he or she has lost control over other aspects of life.
4. Set appropriate limits if the client demands constant attention. Explain that frequent checks will be made at specified intervals to ensure that needs are met.	4. Demanding behavior is a sign of fear and dependency. If the client feels sure that the caregiver will return, he or she will feel more secure and be less demanding of time.
5. Set aside 15 to 30 minutes a day to allow the client time to verbalize fears and frustrations.	5. The nurse can use this time to help the client develop new, more effective coping strategies.
6. Reinforce effective coping strategies.	6. Reinforcement may promote continued use of effective coping strategies.
7. Involve family members or significant others in care, if possible.	7. Family members and others play a very important role in supporting clients and helping them to cope with and accept their disease.
8. Refer the client and family to the National Foundation for Ileitis and Colitis. (Each state has a chapter that offers self-help support groups for clients and families and annual conferences on coping with inflammatory bowel disease.)	8. Discussing IBD with others with the same problem can reduce feelings of isolation and anxiety. Sharing experiences in a group led by professionals gives the client the benefit of others' experiences with IBD and the interpretation of those experiences by health professionals.
9. Refer to the nursing diagnosis Ineffective Individual Coping in the Ostomy care plan for role-playing strategies to increase coping abilities.	

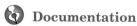 **Documentation**

Progress notes
    Participation in self-care
    Emotional status
    Interactions with staff and significant others

High Risk for Ineffective Therapeutic Regimen Management Related to Lack of Knowledge of Condition, Diagnostic Tests, Prognosis, Treatment, and Signs and Symptoms of Complications

Focus Assessment Criteria	Clinical Significance
1. Knowledge of intestinal signs and symptoms of IBD 2. Knowledge of extraintestinal signs and symptoms of IBD 3. Knowledge of diagnostic tests 4. Family history of IBD 5. Knowledge of etiology, prognosis, and treatment measures 6. Knowledge of potential complications	1–6. Assessing the client's and family's learning needs prior to teaching allows the nurse to determine the appropriate content and teaching methods and evaluate their readiness and ability to learn.

Goal

The goals for this diagnosis represent those associated with discharge planning. Refer to the discharge criteria.

Interventions	Rationales

1. Explain the diagnostic tests:
 	
  a. Colonoscopy is done to explore the large intestine with a long, flexible tube. A clear liquid diet is maintained for 24 to 48 hours before the procedure, and a cleansing enema may be given before the examination. Medication is given to promote relaxation and aid insertion of the lubricated tube into the anus. The procedure takes about 1 hour. The client may feel pressure and cramping; breathing slowly and deeply may help relieve discomfort.
  b. GI X-ray films: The role of the barium enema is to determine the extent of the disease early in its progression. It also helps the endoscopist to determine the configuration of the colon and indicates suspicious areas that should be observed directly by endoscopy.
	1. Explanations of what to expect can reduce the client's anxiety associated with the unknown.
	  a. Colonoscopy may be used to diagnose the medical problem. Polyps can be removed and tissue collected for further study. The procedure may reduce the need for surgery.
	
	  b. Contrast studies of the colon using barium have been used historically as a surveillance technique. The repetition of barium enema every 6 to 12 months raises the question of the effect of long-term radiation on intestinal mucosa that is already at risk.

(continues on page 268)

Interventions continued	**Rationales** continued
c. Biopsy to differentiate ulcerative colitis and Crohn's disease and to detect dysplasia.	c. If dysplasia is found in multiple areas of the colon, the patient is in a high-risk group for developing carcinoma of the colon.
d. Blood tests: • CBC • Serum electrolytes • BUN • Creatinine • Serum protein electrophoresis • Sedimentation rate • Alkaline phosphatase	d. Bone marrow depression of blood cells may be present with fulminating types of colitis. The white blood count may be elevated and the sedimentation rate increased. Electrolyte imbalance is common with severe acute IBD. A decreased serum albumin and negative-nitrogen balance may result from decreased protein intake and increased metabolic needs. Anemia may be caused by iron deficiency or by chronic inflammation.
2. Explain the familial aspects of IBD. Although the cause of IBD is unknown, 15% to 35% of clients with IBD have a relative with the disorder; thus it is considered a familial disorder.	2,3. A client with IBD may have been led to believe that anxiety or psychological problems caused the disorder. Dispelling this belief can help the client to accept the disorder and encourage compliance with treatment.
3. Explain the possible etiology of IBD; theories center on the body's immune system and include the following: a. Hypersensitivity reaction in the gut b. Autoimmune antibody–mediated damage to the epithelial cells c. Tissue deposition of antigen–antibody complexes d. Lymphocyte-mediated cytotoxicity e. Impaired cellular immune mechanisms Emotional and psychological factors have not been identified or implicated in the etiology of IBD. However, stress seems to provoke hyperreactivity of the colon in susceptible persons.	
4. Discuss the prognosis of IBD. IBD typically is a chronic illness with remissions and relapses. In Crohn's disease, the client is much more likely to develop fistulas and abscesses. In ulcerative colitis, the client is more likely to develop toxic megacolon and carcinoma of the colon. In ulcerative colitis, total colectomy and ileostomy is considered a cure because ulcerative colitis involves only the colon. Crohn's disease can affect any portion of the intestinal tract and tends to recur in the proximal bowel even after colectomy.	4. A client usually can deal with a frank and realistic discussion of the prognosis better than with a lack of information about the prognosis.

(continues on page 269)

Interventions continued	**Rationales** continued

5. Discuss the treatment of IBD:
 	
a. Medical
  • Medications (Botoman et al., 1998)
    A. 5-aminosalicylic acid components (sulfasalazine, Dipentum Pentasa, Asacol Rowasa)
 	
    B. Metronidazole (Flagyl)
 	
    C. Corticosteroids (systemic, topical)
 	
    D. Immunosuppressants (6-mercapto purine, azathioprine, methotrexate, cyclosporine)
  • Diet (Refer to the nursing diagnosis Altered Nutrition: Less Than Body Requirements in this care plan.)
  • TPN and bowel rest (Refer to the nursing diagnosis Altered Nutrition: Less Than Body Requirements in this care plan.)
b. Surgical (ulcerative colitis)
  • Bowel resection
    A. Total colectomy and ileostomy (Refer to the Ileostomy care plan.)
    B. Partial colectomy and colostomy (Refer to the Colostomy care plan.)
  • Incision, drainage, or resection of perianal fistulas and abscesses
	5. Treatment of IBD is symptomatic (Botoman et al., 1998).
	
	A. It is thought that the 5-ASA component is therapeutic through its local anti-inflammatory effect on the intestinal mucosa. The agents are available in tablets, suppositories, and enema forms.
	B. Bacterial flora are thought to play an important role in the pathogenesis of IBD.
	C. Corticosteroids are used to treat a moderate to severe exacerbation of IBD. Once a remission is achieved, the goal is to taper and discontinue steroids as quickly as possible.
	D. These agents may be used in clients who fail to respond to sulfasalazine and corticosteroid therapy. The combination of agents increases the immuno-suppressive effects.
	
	b. Surgical treatment is indicated only when medical treatment fails and the client becomes disabled. Surgery for Crohn's disease is not curative because of recurrence in remaining intestines.

6. Explain the potential complications of IBD. (refer to the Collaborative Problems in this care plan for specific signs and symptoms): a. Fissures, fistulas, and perianal abscesses b. Anemia c. Toxic megacolon marked by a sharp increase in number of stools and flatus, bloody diarrhea, increasing abdominal pain and distention, and hypoactive or absent bowel sounds	6. The client's understanding of IBD complications can help to ensure early detection and enable prompt treatment. b. Anemia may result from either malabsorption of iron (vitamin B_{12}) or folate deficiency.

(continues on page 270)

Interventions continued	**Rationales** continued
d. Intestinal obstruction or perforation	
e. Erythema nodosum or pyoderma gangrenosum: A condition exhibiting red, raised, and tender nodules, erythema nodosum occurs in 5% to 15% of clients with IBD.	
f. Arthritis, migratory polyarthritis, or ankylosing spondylitis	f. The National Cooperative Crohn's Disease Study reported that 14% of clients studied had arthritis or arthralgia at the time of diagnosis.
g. Ocular lesions	g. Conjunctivitis, iritis, uveitis, or episcleritis occurs in 3% to 10% of clients with IBD.
h. Nephrolithiasis	h. Severe diarrhea can lead to decreased volume of concentrated urine. This combined with intestinal bicarbonate loss and decreased pH leads to the development of urate stones. With ileal resection or extensive IBD, the calcium normally available to bind with oxylate instead binds with fatty acids, freeing dietary oxylate for absorption. Decreased urine volume leads to increased precipitation of calcium oxylate in the kidneys.
i. Cholelithiasis	i. Gallstones occur in 30% to 35% of clients with Crohn's disease of the terminal ileum. The ileal dysfunction causes bile acid malabsorption and a decrease in the concentration of bile salts. The decrease in bile salt to cholesterol ratio predisposes the client to the precipitation of cholesterol stones.
j. Colon cancer	j. The incidence of colon cancer is 10 to 20 times greater in clients with ulcerative colitis than in the general population. The etiology of cancer in IBD is unknown. Close surveillance is needed because cancer may mimic the signs and symptoms of IBD.
k. Growth retardation	k. Growth is impaired in 30% to 50% of young clients with IBD occurring before puberty. Possible causes include decreased nutritional intake, loss of protein and nutrients by rapid passage through the GI tract, increased metabolic requirements secondary to inflammatory bowel, and corticosteroid therapy.
7. Teach the importance of maintaining optimal hydration.	7. Optimal hydration prevents dehydration and reduces the risk of renal calculi formation.

(continues on page 271)

Interventions continued	Rationales continued
8. Avoid oral contraceptives and tobacco use.	8. These two agents have been found to exacerbate Crohn's disease but not ulcerative colitis (Arcangelo & Peterson, 2001).
9. Teach measures to preserve perianal skin integrity: a. Use soft toilet tissue. b. Cleanse area with mild soap after bowel movements. c. Apply a protective ointment (e.g., A&D, Desitin, Sween Cream).	9. These measures can help to prevent skin erosion from diarrheal irritation.
10. Teach the client to report the following signs and symptoms: a. Increasing abdominal pain or distention b. Persistent vomiting c. Unusual rectal or vaginal drainage or rectal pain d. Change in vision e. Continued amber urine f. Flank pain or ache g. Heart palpitations	10. Early reporting enables prompt intervention to reduce the severity of complications. a. Increasing abdominal pain or distention may indicate obstruction or peritonitis. b. Persistent vomiting may point to obstruction. c. Unusual drainage or rectal pain may indicate abscesses or fistulas. d. Vision changes may indicate ocular lesions. e. Amber urine indicates dehydration. f. Flank pain may indicate renal calculi. g. Palpitations may point to potassium imbalance.
11. Provide information on available community resources (e.g., self-help groups, counseling) and patient education material on how to live with IBD.	11. Communicating with others with IBD may help the client to cope better with the disorder's effect on his life style.

 Documentation

Discharge summary record
    Client teaching
    Outcome achievement or status
    Referrals, if indicated

PEPTIC ULCER DISEASE

Peptic ulcer disease involves erosion in the mucosal wall of the stomach, pylorus, duodenum, or esophagus. The eroded areas are circumscribed and occur only in the areas of the gastrointestinal tract exposed to hydrochloric acid and pepsin. Duodenal ulcers are usually caused by hypersecretion of gastric acid. Peptic ulcers are primarily caused by Helicobacter pylori bacterium and long-term use of non-steroidal anti-inflammatory drugs (NSAIDS). Other causes are cancer and hypersecretory disorders such as Zollinger-Ellison syndrome. With gastric ulcers, gastric acid secretion may be normal or even subnormal. Stress ulcers are ulcers usually in the fundus of the stomach. A major physiologic stress causes an imbalance of aggressive factors that promote ulceration (e.g., acid, bile, urea) and defense factors that protect against ulceration: mucosal barrier, mucosal blood flow, mucus secretion, epithelial regeneration, and prostaglandins. The incidence of stress ulcers in critically ill clients is nearly 100%. *Helicobacter pylori* is an organism found in gastric epithelium. Eradication of *H. pylori* accelerates duodenal ulcer healing (Damianos & McGarrity, 1997; National Institutes of Health [NIH], 1994).

 Time Frame

Initial diagnosis
Recurrent acute episodes

 DIAGNOSTIC CLUSTER

Collaborative Problems

▲ PC: Hemorrhage
▲ PC: Stress Ulcer
△ PC: Pyloric Obstruction

Nursing Diagnoses

▲ Acute/Chronic Pain related to lesions secondary to increased gastric secretions
△ High Risk for Ineffective Therapeutic Regimen Management related to lack of knowledge of disease process, contraindications, signs and symptoms of complications, and treatment regimen

---

▲ This diagnosis was reported to be monitored for or managed frequently (75%–100%).
△ This diagnosis was reported to be monitored for or managed often (50%–74%).

Discharge Criteria

Before discharge, the client or family will

1. Identify the causes of disease symptoms.
2. Identify behaviors, substances, or foods that may alter gastric activity.
3. Identify necessary adjustments to prevent ulcer formation.
4. State signs and symptoms that must be reported to a health care professional.
5. Relate community resources that can provide assistance with life style modifications.

Collaborative Problems

Potential Complication: Hemorrhage

Potential Complication: Stress Ulcer

Potential Complication: Pyloric Obstruction

Nursing Goal

The nurse will detect early signs and symptoms of (a) hemorrhage, (b) stress ulcer, and (c) pyloric obstruction and collaboratively intervene to stabilize client.

Indicators

- Heart rate 60–100 beats/min (a)
- Cardiac rhythm regular (b)
- Respiratory rate 16–20 breaths/min (c)
- B/P >90/60, <40/90 mm Hg (d)
- Urinary output >30 ml/hr
- No abdominal pain (b, c)
- Alert, oriented, calm (a, b, c)
- Dry, warm skin
- Capillary refill <3 seconds (a, b, c)
- Gastric pH 3.5–5.0 (b)
- Gastric aspirates negative for occult blood (b)

Interventions	Rationales

1. Identify clients at high risk for stress ulcers (Prevost, 1993).
   a. Shock, hypotension
   b. Prolonged mechanical ventilation
   c. Multiple trauma
   d. Major surgery (>3 hours)
   e. Sepsis
   f. Head injury
   g. Acute renal, hepatic failure
   h. Respiratory insufficiency
   i. Cardiovascular disease
   j. Severe vascular disease
   k. Burns (>35% of body)
	1. Decreased blood supply to mucosa limits the production of bicarbonate, which results in an inability to control hydrogen ions. These ions damage mucosal cells and capillaries, which leads to the formation of mucosal lesions. Ischemia with a hyper-secretion of gastric acid and pepsinogen also interferes with blood flow to the mucosa. Normally this limited diffusion and bicarbonate neutralization maintain a slightly acid mucosa. Epithelial cells of the stomach are sensitive to even slight decreases in blood supply, which results in necrosis (Porth, 2002).

2. Monitor for occult blood in gastric aspirates and bowel movements.	2. Frequent and careful assessment can help diagnose bleeding before the client's status is severely compromised (Prevost, 1993).

3. Monitor gastric pH every 2 to 4 hours (Prevost, 1993).
 	
   a. Use pH paper with a range from 0 to 7.5.
   b. Use good light to interpret the color on the pH paper.
   c. Position client on left side, lying down.
 	
   d. Use two syringes (>30 mL) to obtain the aspirate. Aspirate a gastric sample and discard. Use aspirate in second syringe for testing.
	3. Maintenance of gastric pH below 5 has decreased bleeding complications by 89% (Eisenberg, 1990).
	   a,b. The user error in pH testing is considerable (Prevost, 1993).
	
	   c. The left-side-down position allows the tip of the nasogastric or gastrostomy tube to move into the greater curvature of the stomach and usually below the level of gastric fluid.
	   d. The first aspirate will clear the tube of antacids and other substances that can alter the pH of the sample (Prevost, 1993).

(continues on page 274)

Interventions continued	Rationales continued

4. Evaluate for other factors that will affect the pH readings.
  a. Medications (e.g., Cimetidine)
  b. Tube feeding
  c. Irrigations
	4. False positives and negatives can result when aspirate contains certain substances.

5. Consult with the physician for the specific prescription for titration ranges of pH and antacid administration.	5. Most investigators recommend a pH range of 3.5 to 5.0 (Eisenberg, 1990).

6. Monitor for signs and symptoms of hemorrhage and report promptly:
  a. Hematemesis
  b. Dizziness
  c. Generalized weakness
  d. Melena
  e. Increasing pulse rate with normal or slightly decreased blood pressure
  f. Urine output <30 mL/hr
  g. Restlessness, agitation, change in mentation
  h. Increasing respiratory rate
  i. Diminished peripheral pulses
  j. Cool, pale, or cyanotic skin
  k. Thirst
	6. Hemorrhage is the most common complication of peptic ulcer disease and occurs in 15% to 20% of clients. Signs and symptoms of hemorrhage may be insidious and present gradually or be quite demonstrative and massive. The compensatory response to decreased circulatory volume increases blood oxygen by increasing heart and respiratory rates and decreases circulation to extremities; this is marked by changes such as decreased pulse and cool skin. Diminished oxygen to the brain causes changes in mentation.

7. If saline lavage is ordered, use tepid saline.	7. Ice saline lavages have been shown to damage stomach mucosa and promote bleeding (Prevost, 1993).

▼ Related Physician-Prescribed Interventions

Medications. Bismuth subsalicylate, sedatives, tetracycline, misoprostal, histamine-2 (H₂) receptor antagonists, anticholinergics, antacids, sucralfate, triple therapy for *H. pylori* (clarithromycin, metronidazole, amoxicillin), proton pump inhibitors, prostaglandins

Intravenous Therapy. Variable depending on severity of illness

Laboratory Studies. Serum gastrin, guaiac testing, CBC, stool antigen test, electrolytes, immunoglobin A anti-h (detects *H. pylori* antibodies)

Diagnostic Studies. Fasting gastric levels, barium study, endoscopy with biopsy, arteriography, C urea breath test

Therapies. NPO or diet as tolerated, nasogastric intubation/gastrostomy

Documentation

Flow records
  Vital signs
  Intake and output
  Weight
  Gastric pH
  Stool characteristics
  Bowel sounds
Progress notes
  Unusual events

Acute/Chronic Pain Related to Lesions Secondary to Increased Gastric Secretions

Focus Assessment Criteria	Clinical Significance
1. Pain characteristics: onset, duration, location, quality, quantity, and aggravating and alleviating factors 2. Pattern of discomfort in relation to food ingestion 3. Intake of substances that damage or irritate the mucosal barrier (e.g., alcohol, caffeine, tobacco, and certain foods and medications)	1–3. Contact of hydrochloric acid with exposed ulcer nerve endings presumably causes pain. Duodenal ulcer pain characteristically begins as an epigastric gnawing that occurs ½ to 3 hours after eating and frequently awakens the client during the night. Food or antacids commonly relieve the pain. The pain of gastric ulcers occurs immediately after eating (Porth, 2002).

Goal

The client will report improvement of pain and an increase in daily activities.

Indicators

- Report symptoms of discomfort promptly.
- Verbalize increased comfort in response to treatment plan.
- Identify changes in life style to reduce recurrence.

Interventions	Rationales
1. Explain the relationship between hydrochloric acid secretion and onset of pain.	1. Hydrochloric acid (HCl) presumably is an important variable in the appearance of peptic ulcer disease. Because of this relationship, control of HCl secretion is considered an essential aim of treatment (Porth, 2002).
2. Explain the risks of nonsteroidal anti-inflammatory drugs (NSAIDs) (e.g., Motrin, Aleve, Relafen).	2. NSAIDS cause superficial irritation of the gastric mucosa and inhibit the production of prostaglandins that protect gastric mucosa (Arcangelo & Peterson, 2001)
3. Administer antacids, anticholinergics, sucralfate, and H_2 blockers as directed	3. HCl secretion can be regulated by neutralizing it with various drug therapies.
4. Encourage activities that promote rest and relaxation.	4. Relaxation of muscles decreases peristalsis and decreases gastric pain
5. Help the client to identify irritating substances (e.g., fried foods, spicy foods, coffee).	5. Avoidance of irritating substances can help to prevent the pain response.

(continues on page 276)

Interventions continued	Rationales continued
6. Teach diversional techniques for stress reduction and pain relief.	6. The relationship between stress and peptic ulcer disease is based on the higher incidence of peptic ulcers in those with chronic anxiety.
7. Advise the client to eat regularly and to avoid bedtime snacks.	7. Contrary to popular belief, certain dietary restrictions do not reduce hyperacidity. Individual intolerances first must be identified and used as a basis for restrictions. Avoidance of eating prior to bedtime may reduce nocturnal acid levels by eliminating the postprandial stimulus to acid secretion. During the day, regular amounts of food particles in the stomach help to neutralize the acidity of gastric secretions.
8. Encourage the client to avoid smoking and alcohol use.	8. Smoking decreases pancreatic secretion of bicarbonate; this increases duodenal acidity. Tobacco delays the healing of gastric duodenal ulcers and increases their frequency (Katz, 2003).
9. Encourage the client to reduce intake of caffeine-containing and alcoholic beverages, if indicated.	9. Gastric acid secretion may be stimulated by caffeine ingestion. Alcohol can cause gastritis.
10. Teach the client the importance of continuing treatment even in the absence of pain.	10. Dietary restrictions and medications must be continued for the prescribed duration. Pain may be relieved long before healing is complete.

 Documentation

Progress record
    Complaints of pain
    Response to treatment plan

High Risk for Ineffective Management of Therapeutic Regimen Related to Lack of Knowledge of Disease Process, Contraindications, Signs and Symptoms of Complications, and Treatment Regimen

Focus Assessment Criteria	Clinical Significance
1. Knowledge level of therapeutic indications and requirements	1. Determining the client's or family's knowledge level helps to guide teaching.
2. Readiness to learn and barriers that might impede teaching	2. A client or family that does not achieve goals for learning requires a referral for assistance postdischarge.

Goals

The goals for this diagnosis represent those associated with discharge planning. Refer to discharge criteria.

Interventions	Rationales
1. Explain the pathophysiology of peptic ulcer disease using terminology and media appropriate to the client's and family's levels of understanding.	1. Understanding helps to reinforce the need to comply with restrictions and may improve compliance.
2. To reduce the risk of recurrence, explain behaviors that can be modified or eliminated: a. Tobacco use b. Excessive alcohol intake c. Intake of caffeine-containing beverages and foods d. Large quantities of dairy products	2. Alcohol on an empty stomach causes gastritis. Smoking decreases pancreatic secretion of bicarbonate; this increases duodenal acidity. Excessive calcium and protein cause more gastric acid production (Katz, 2003).
3. If the client is being discharged on antacid therapy, teach the following (Arcangelo & Peterson, 2001): a. Chew tablets well and follow with a glass of water to enhance absorption. b. Lie down for ½ hour after meals to delay gastric emptying. c. Take antacids 1 hour after meals to counteract the gastric acid stimulated by eating. d. Avoid antacids high in sodium (e.g., Gelusil, Amphojel, Mylanta II); excessive sodium intake contributes to fluid retention and elevated blood pressure.	3. Proper self-administration of antacids can enhance their effects and minimize side effects.
4. If the client is being discharged on therapy for *H. pylori,* explain • The relationship of *H. pylori* and gastric ulcers, including its occurrence and reoccurrence • The need to be on therapy for 14 days • The need to take all three types of medication.	4. Triple therapy for 2 weeks eradicates *H. pylori* at a 90% rate. Eradication of *H. pylori* promotes healing of the ulcer and prevents reoccurrence for at least 7 years. *H. pylori* is also present in 90% of persons with cancer of the stomach (Damianos & McGarrity, 1997).
5. Discuss the importance of continued treatment, even in the absence of overt symptoms.	5. Continued therapy is necessary to prevent recurrence or development of another ulcer.
6. Instruct the client and family to watch for and report these symptoms: a. Red or black stools b. Bloody or brown vomitus	6. These signs and symptoms may point to complications such as peritonitis, perforation, or GI bleeding. Early detection enables prompt intervention.

(continues on page 278)

Interventions continued	Rationales continued
c. Persistent epigastric pain d. Sudden, severe abdominal pain e. Constipation (not resolved) f. Unexplained temperature elevation g. Persistent nausea or vomiting h. Unexplained weight loss	
7. Explain the risks of aspirin and anti-inflammatory drugs (NSAIDs).	7. Aspirin disrupts the gastric mucosa and causes ulcer formation. Enteric-coated and buffered aspirin are also ulcerogenic. NSAIDs can also cause ulcers, especially in persons older than 60 years (Katz, 2003).
8. Refer to community resources if indicated (e.g., smoking cessation program, stress management class).	8. The client may need assistance with life style changes after discharge.

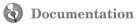 Documentation

Discharge summary record
   Client teaching
   Status of goal achievements
   Referrals

For a care map on peptic ulcer disease, visit http://connection.lww.com

Renal and Urinary Tract Disorders

ACUTE KIDNEY FAILURE

Acute kidney failure involves the sudden loss of renal function as a result of reduced renal blood flow or glomerular or tubular dysfunction. Hypotension, hypovolemia, or shock can reduce renal blood flow. Calculi or tumors also can obstruct renal blood flow, leading to tubular dysfunction. Reduced glomerular filtration or tubular damage can result from toxic precipitates (e.g., proteins and hemoglobin released from injured muscles in burns or infection) that become concentrated in renal tubules. Some nonsteroidal anti-inflammatory medications impair renal blood flow, especially in older adults. Certain antibiotics (e.g., streptomycin) and heavy metals (e.g., mercury) also are nephrotoxic.

The stages of acute kidney failure are initiating oliguric, diuretic, and recovery. Acute kidney failure can be reversed if identified and treated promptly before the kidneys are permanently damaged. The prognosis is good for 50% to 60% of clients. Of the remaining 40% to 50%, 25% to 30% of clients ultimately will develop chronic kidney disease, of which 15% to 20% will die (Baer & Lancaster, 1992).

 Time Frame
Initial diagnosis (postintensive care)
Recurrent acute episodes

⊘ DIAGNOSTIC CLUSTER	
Collaborative Problems	**Refer to**
▲ PC: Fluid Overload	
▲ PC: Metabolic Acidosis	
▲ PC: Electrolyte Imbalances	
* PC: Acute Albuminemia	
Nursing Diagnoses	**Refer to**
▲ High Risk for Infection related to invasive procedure	
△ Imbalanced Nutrition: Less Than Body Requirements related to anorexia, nausea, vomiting, loss of taste, loss of smell, stomatitis, and unpalatable diet	Chronic Kidney Disease
* High Risk for Injury related to stress, retention of metabolic wastes and end products, altered capillary permeability, and platelet dysfunction	Chronic Kidney Disease
Related Care Plans	
Hemodialysis or Peritoneal Dialysis	
Chronic Kidney Disease	

▲ This diagnosis was reported to be monitored for or managed frequently (75%–100%).
△ This diagnosis was reported to be monitored for or managed often (50%–74%).
* This diagnosis was not included in the validation study.

Discharge Criteria

Before discharge, the client or family will

1. Relate the intent to comply with agreed-on restrictions and follow-up.
2. State signs and symptoms that must be reported to a health care professional.
3. Identify how to reduce the risk of infection.

Collaborative Problems

Potential Complication: Fluid Overload

Potential Complication: Metabolic Acidosis

Potential Complication: Electrolyte Imbalances

Nursing Goal

The nurse will detect early signs and symptoms of (a) fluid overload, (b) metabolic acidosis, and (c) electrolyte imbalances and will intervene collaboratively to stabilize the client.

Indicators

- Alert, calm, oriented (a, c)
- BP > 90/160, < 140/90 mm Hg (a)
- Respirations relaxed and rhythmic (a)
- Pulse 60–100 beats/min (a)
- Respirations 16–20 breaths/min (a)
- EKG normal sinus rhythm (b, c)
- Flat neck veins (a)
- No edema (pedal, sacral, periorbital) (a)
- No seizure activity (b, c)
- No complaints of numbness/tingling in fingers or toes (b, c)
- No muscle cramps (b, c)
- Intact strength (b, c)
- Skin warm, dry, usual color (a)
- Serum albumin 3.5–5 g/dL (b, c)
- Serum prealbumin 1–3 g/dL (b, c)
- Serum sodium 135–145 mEq/L (b, c)
- Serum potassium 3.8–5 mEq/L (b, c)
- Serum calcium 8.5–10.5 mg/dL (b, c)
- Serum phosphates 125–300 mg/dL (b, c)
- Blood urea nitrogen 10–20 mg/dL (b)
- Creatinine 0.2–0.8 mg/dL (b)
- Alkaline phosphate 30–150 IU/mL (b)
- Creatinine clearance 100–150 mL/min (a, b)
- Oxygen saturation (SaO_2) > 94% (a)
- Carbon dioxide ($PaCO_2$) 35–45 mm Hg (a)
- Urine output > 30 mL/hr (a)
- Urine specific gravity 1.005–1.030 (a)
- Usual or desired weight (a)
- Bowel sounds all quadrants (c)

Interventions	Rationales

1. Monitor for signs of fluid overload:
  a. Weight gain
  b. Increased blood pressure and pulse rate, neck vein distention
	1. The oliguric phase of acute kidney failure usually lasts from 5 to 15 days and often is associated with excess fluid volume. Functionally the changes result in decreased

(continues on page 283)

Interventions continued	Rationales continued
c. Dependent edema (periorbital, pedal, pretibial, sacral) d. Adventitious breath sounds (e.g., wheezes, crackles) e. Urine specific gravity < 1.010	glomerular filtration, tubular transport of substances, urine formation, and renal clearance (Baer & Lancaster, 1992).
2. Weigh client daily or more often if indicated. Ensure accuracy by weighing at the same time every day on the same scale and with client wearing the same amount of clothing.	2. Daily weights can help to determine fluid balance and appropriate fluid intake.
3. Maintain strict intake and output records; determine net fluid balance and compare with daily weight loss or gain for correlation.	3. A 1-kg weight gain should correlate with excess intake of 1 L (1 L of fluid weighs 1 kg, or 2.2 lb).
4. Inform client about fluid management goals.	4. Client's understanding can help gain his or her cooperation.
5. Adjust client's fluid intake so it approximates fluid loss plus 300 to 500 mL/day. Consider all sensible and insensible losses when calculating replacement fluids.	5. Careful replacement can prevent fluid overload.
6. Distribute fluid intake fairly evenly throughout the entire day and night.	6. Toxins can accumulate with decreased fluid and cause nausea and sensorium changes. It may be necessary to match fluid intake with loss every 8 hours or even every hour if client is critically imbalanced.
7. Encourage client to express feelings and frustrations; give positive feedback.	7. Fluid and diet restrictions can be extremely frustrating.
8. Consult with dietitian regarding fluid plan and overall diet.	8. Fluid content of nonliquid food, amount and type of liquids, liquid preferences, and sodium content all are important in fluid management.
9. Administer oral medications with meals whenever possible. If medications must be administered between meals, give with the smallest amount of fluid necessary.	9. This prevents the fluid allowance from being used up unnecessarily.
10. Avoid continuous IV fluid infusion whenever possible. Dilute all necessary IV drugs in the smallest amount of fluid safe for IV administration.	10. A small IV bag, Buretrol, or an infusion pump is preferred to avoid accidental infusion of a large volume of fluid.

(continues on page 284)

Interventions continued	**Rationales** continued

11. Monitor for signs and symptoms of metabolic acidosis:
   a. Rapid, shallow respirations
   b. Headache
   c. Nausea and vomiting
   d. Low plasma bicarbonate
   e. Low pH of arterial blood (< 7.35)
   f. Behavior changes, drowsiness, and lethargy
	11. Acidosis results from the kidney's inability to excrete hydrogen ions, phosphates, sulfates, and ketone bodies. Bicarbonates are lost when the kidney reduces its reabsorption. Hyperkalemia, hyperphosphatemia, and decreased bicarbonate levels aggravate metabolic acidosis. Excessive ketone bodies cause headaches, nausea, vomiting, and abdominal pain. Respiratory rate and depth increase to increase CO_2 excretion and to reduce acidosis. Acidosis affects the central nervous system (CNS) and can increase neuromuscular irritability because of the cellular exchange of hydrogen and potassium (Baer & Lancaster, 1992).

12. Limit fat and protein intake. Ensure caloric intake (consult dietitian for appropriate diet).	12. Fats and protein are not used as main energy sources, so acidic end products do not accumulate.
13. Assess for signs and symptoms of hypocalcemia, hypokalemia, and alkalosis as acidosis is corrected.	13. Rapid correction of acidosis may cause rapid excretion of calcium and potassium and rebound alkalosis.

14. Consult with physician to initiate bicarbonate/acetate dialysis if above measures do not correct metabolic acidosis.
   a. Bicarbonate dialysis for severe acidosis: Dialysate—$NaHCO_3 = 100$ mEq/L
   b. Bicarbonate dialysis for moderate acidosis: Dialysate—$NaHCO_3 = 60$ mEq/L
	14. The acetate anion that the liver converts to bicarbonate is used in dialysate to combat metabolic acidosis. Use of bicarbonate dialysis is indicated for clients with liver impairment, lactic acidosis, or severe acid-base imbalance.

15. Monitor for signs and symptoms of hypernatremia with fluid overload:
   a. Thirst
   b. CNS effects ranging from agitation to convulsions
   c. Edema, weight gain
   d. Hypertension
   e. Tachycardia
   f. Dyspnea
   g. Rales
	15. Hypernatremia results from excessive sodium intake or increased aldosterone output. Water is pulled from the cells, which causes cellular dehydration and produces CNS symptoms. Thirst is a compensatory response to dilute sodium (Baer & Lancaster, 1992).

16. Maintain sodium restriction.	16. Hypernatremia must be corrected slowly to minimize CNS deterioration.

(continues on page 285)

Interventions continued	**Rationales** continued

17. Monitor for signs and symptoms of hyponatremia:
   a. CNS effects ranging from lethargy to coma
   b. Weakness
   c. Abdominal pain
   d. Muscle twitching or convulsions
   e. Nausea, vomiting, and diarrhea
	17. Hyponatremia results from sodium loss through vomiting, diarrhea, or diuretic therapy; excessive fluid intake; or insufficient dietary sodium. Cellular edema, caused by osmosis, produces cerebral edema, weakness, and muscle cramps.

18. Monitor for signs and symptoms of hyperkalemia:
   a. Weakness to paralysis
   b. Muscle irritability
   c. Paresthesias
   d. Nausea, abdominal cramping, or diarrhea
   e. Irregular pulse
   f. Electrocardiogram (ECG) changes: tall tented T-waves, ST segment depression, prolonged PR interval (>0.2 second), first-degree heart block, bradycardia, broadening the ORS complex, eventual ventricular fibrillation, and cardiac standstill
	18. Hyperkalemia results from the kidney's decreased ability to excrete potassium or from excess intake of potassium. Acidosis increases release of potassium from cells. Fluctuations in potassium affect neuromuscular transmission; this produces cardiac dysrhythmias, reduces action of GI smooth muscle, and impairs electrical conduction (Baer & Lancaster, 1992).

19. Intervene for hyperkalemia:
   a. Restrict potassium-rich foods and fluids. Do not allow salt substitute that contains potassium as the cation.
   b. Hemodialysis on a potassium-free bath removes K+ rapidly and efficiently from the plasma.
   c. Administer blood transfusions during hemodialysis so hemodialysis treatment can remove excess K+.
	19. High potassium levels necessitate a reduced potassium intake. Prolonged dwell time during dialysis increases potassium excretion.

20. Monitor for signs and symptoms of hypokalemia:
   a. Weakness or paralysis
   b. Decreased or no deep tendon reflexes
   c. Hypoventilation
   d. Polyuria
   e. Hypotension
   f. Paralytic ileus
   g. ECG changes: U wave, flat T wave, dysrhythmias, and prolonged Q-T interval
   h. Increased risk of digitalis toxicity
   i. Nausea, vomiting, and anorexia
	20. Hypokalemia results from losses associated with vomiting, diarrhea, or diuretic therapy or from insufficient potassium intake. Hypokalemia impairs neuromuscular transmission and reduces efficiency of respiratory muscles. Kidneys are less sensitive to antidiuretic hormone (ADH) and thus excrete large quantities of dilute urine. Gastrointestinal smooth muscle action also is reduced. Abnormally low potassium levels also impair electrical conduction of the heart (Baer & Lancaster, 1992).

21. Intervene for hypokalemia. Encourage increased intake of potassium-rich foods.	21. Increased dietary potassium intake helps to ensure potassium replacement.

(continues on page 286)

Interventions continued	Rationales continued

22. Monitor for signs and symptoms of hypocalcemia:
   a. Altered mental status
   b. Numbness or tingling in fingers and toes
   c. Muscle cramps
   d. Seizures
   e. ECG changes: prolonged Q-T interval, prolonged ST segment, and dysrhythmias
	22. Hypocalcemia results from the kidneys' inability to metabolize vitamin D (needed for calcium absorption); retention of phosphorus causes a reciprocal drop in serum calcium level. Low serum calcium level produces increased neural excitability resulting in muscle spasms (cardiac, facial, extremities) and CNS irritability (seizures). It also causes cardiac muscle hyperactivity as evidenced by ECG changes (Porth, 2002).

23. Intervene for hypocalcemia. Administer a high-calcium, low-phosphorus diet.	23. Elevated phosphate levels lower serum calcium level, necessitating dietary replacement.

24. Monitor for signs and symptoms of hypermagnesemia:
   a. Weakness
   b. Hypoventilation
   c. Hypotension
   d. Flushing
   e. Behavioral changes
	24. Hypermagnesemia results from the kidneys' decreased ability to excrete magnesium. Its effects include CNS depression, respiratory depression, and peripheral vasodilation (Porth, 2002).

25. Monitor for signs and symptoms of hyperphosphatemia:
   a. Tetany
   b. Numbness or tingling in fingers and toes
	25. Hyperphosphatemia results from the kidneys' decreased ability to excrete phosphorus. Elevated phosphorus itself does not cause symptoms but contributes to tetany and other short-term neuromuscular symptoms (Porth, 2002).

26. For a client with hyperphosphatemia, administer phosphorus-binding antacids, calcium supplements, or vitamin D, and restrict phosphorus-rich foods.	26. The client needs supplements to overcome vitamin D deficiency and to compensate for a calcium-poor diet. High phosphate decreases calcium, which increases parathyroid hormone (PTH). PTH is ineffective in removing phosphates (as a result of kidney failure) but causes calcium reabsorption from bone and decreases tubular reabsorption of phosphate.

▼ Related Physician-Prescribed Interventions

Medications. Diuretics; antihypertensives; electrolyte inhibitors or replacements (e.g., calcium gluconate, aluminum hydroxide gels)

Intravenous Therapy. Fluid and electrolyte replacement

Laboratory Studies. Urine pH, osmolality, creatinine clearance, specific gravity, sodium, HCO_3, casts, protein, RBCs, hemoglobin, albumin, serum pH, prealbumin, blood urea nitrogen, creatinine

Diagnostic Studies. ECG; x-ray film (kidney-ureter-bladder [KUB]); retrograde pyelogram

Therapies. Dialysis, pulse oximetry, indwelling catheter, fluid restrictions

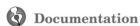 **Documentation**

Flow records
  Vital signs
  Respiratory assessment
  Weight
  Edema (sites, amount)
  Specific gravity
  Intake and output
  Complaints of nausea, vomiting, or muscle cramps
  Treatments
Progress notes
  Changes in behavior and sensorium
  ECG changes

Nursing Diagnoses

High Risk for Infection Related to Invasive Procedure

Focus Assessment Criteria	Clinical Significance
1. IV lines (peripheral and subclavian), arterial catheters, central venous lines, venipuncture sites, and dialysis accesses for signs of infection	1,2. Prompt recognition of signs of infection and immediate institution of appropriate treatment can help to prevent systemic infection.
2. Cloudy or odorous urine, dysuria	

Goal

The client will continue to be infection free.

Indicators
• Describe the reasons for increased susceptibility.
• Relate precautions to prevent infection.

Interventions	Rationales
1. Instruct the client about his or her increased susceptibility to infection and responsibility in prevention.	1. Infections are a leading cause of death in acute kidney failure; urinary tract infection is a major type. A client with acute kidney failure has altered immunity and nutritional status, disruptive biochemical status, poor healing potential, edema, and decreased activity—all of which predispose him or her to infection. Therefore implementation of preventive measures is mandated (Baer & Lancaster, 1992).
2. Use an indwelling bladder catheter only when necessary, for the shortest time possible, and with diligent care.	2,3. Avoiding catheters and invasive procedures helps to prevent introducing microorganisms into the body (Baer & Lancaster, 1992).

(continues on page 288)

Interventions continued	**Rationales** continued

3. Avoid other invasive procedures as much as possible:
  a. Repeated venous punctures
  b. IV lines
  c. Central venous lines
  d. Arterial catheters	

4. Whenever possible, avoid placing client with a roommate who has an indwelling catheter, urinary tract infection, or upper respiratory infection.	4. Selected isolation can decrease risk of cross-contamination and possible spread of infection.
5. Use aseptic technique with all invasive procedures and when caring for lines, catheters, dressing changes, suctioning, and dialysis accesses. Do not use access catheters for blood sampling.	5. Each disruption of invasive lines introduces microorganisms. Aseptic technique reduces the quantity of microorganisms introduced.

6. Assess for and report signs of infection at invasive sites.
  a. Redness
  b. Swelling
  c. Drainage
  d. Warmth
	6. Traumatized tissue predisposes to inflammation and infection. Uremic toxins decrease neutrophil phagocytosis and chemotaxis that increase susceptibility to infection (Baer & Lancaster, 1992).

7. Never cannulate an inflamed area of an arteriovenous fistula.	7. Cannulation will increase the risk of introducing microorganisms.
8. Teach client to avoid contacting people with any infection especially an upper respiratory tract infection.	8. Selected isolation can help to protect client against contacting an infection.
9. Use written signs to alert visitors to wash hands before and after contact with client.	9. Handwashing reduces risk of cross-contamination.

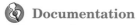 Documentation

Flow records
  Urine color and other characteristics
Progress notes
  Redness, swelling, drainage, or warmth at sites

CHRONIC KIDNEY DISEASE

Chronic kidney disease involves the progressive loss of glomerular filtration, a process that can be slowed but is irreversible and eventually results in end-stage kidney disease. The kidney cannot maintain metabolic, fluid, and electrolyte balance; this results in uremia. Causes of chronic kidney disease are hypertension, diabetes, and glomerular disease as well as congenital and hereditary factors. Table 1 outlines the stages of chronic kidney disease. As the condition progresses, dialysis or transplantation is considered.

 Time Frame
Acute exacerbations

⊗ DIAGNOSTIC CLUSTER

Collaborative Problems	Refer to
△ PC: Fluid Imbalance	
▲ PC: Anemia	
PC: Hyperparathyroidism	
PC: Pathological Fractures	
△ PC: Polyneuropathy	
△ PC: Hypoalbuminemia	
△ PC: Congestive Heart Failure	
△ PC: Metabolic Acidosis	
△ PC: Pleural Effusion	
PC: Pericarditis, Cardiac Tamponade	Acute Kidney Failure
▲ PC: Fluid/Electrolyte Imbalance	Acute Kidney Failure
▲ PC: Fluid Overload	Hemodialysis
* PC: Hypertension	

Nursing Diagnoses	Refer to
△ Imbalanced Nutrition: Less Than Body Requirements related to anorexia, nausea, vomiting, loss of taste or smell, stomatitis, and unpalatable diet	
Ineffective Sexuality Patterns related to decreased libido, erectile dysfunction, amenorrhea, or sterility	
△ Powerlessness related to feeling of loss of control and life style restrictions	
▲ High Risk for Ineffective Therapeutic Regimen Management related to insufficient	

(continues on page 290)

Nursing Diagnoses continued	
knowledge of condition, dietary restrictions, daily recording, pharmacological therapy, and signs and symptoms of complications, and insufficient resources (e.g., financial, caregiver), follow-up visits, and community resources	
▲ High Risk for Infection related to invasive procedures	Acute Kidney Failure
△ Impaired Comfort related to calcium phosphate or urate crystals on skin	Cirrhosis
Related Care Plan Hemodialysis	

▲ This diagnosis was reported to be monitored for or managed frequently (75%–100%).
△ This diagnosis was reported to be monitored for or managed often (50%–74%).
*This diagnosis was not included in the validation study.

Discharge Criteria

Before discharge, the client or family will

1. Describe dietary restrictions, medications, and treatment plan.
2. Maintain contact and follow-up with health care providers.
3. Keep complete daily records as instructed.
4. Verbalize community resources available.
5. Relate the intent to comply with agreed-on restrictions and follow-up.
6. State the signs and symptoms that must be reported to a health care professional.
7. Relate the importance of an outlet for feelings and concerns.

Collaborative Problems

Potential Complication: Fluid Imbalance

TABLE 1   Stages of Chronic Kidney Disease: A Clinical Action Plan

Stage	Description	GFR (mL/min/1.732)	Action*
1	Kidney damage with normal or increase GFR	>90	Diagnosis and treatment; treatment of comorbid conditions; slowed progression; CVD risk reduction
2	Kidney damage with mild decrease GFR	60–89	Estimating progression
3	Moderate decrease GFR	30–59	Evaluating and treating complications
4	Severe decrease GFR	15–29	Preparation for kidney replacement therapy
5	Kidney failure	<15 (or dialysis)	Replacement (if uremia present)

Chronic kidney disease is defined as either kidney damage or GFR, 60 mL/min/1.73 m² for ≥ 3 months. Kidney damage is defined as pathologic abnormalities or markers of damage including abnormalities in blood or urine tests or imaging studies.

*Includes actions form preceding stages

Potential Complication: Anemia

Potential Complication: Hyperparathyroidism

Potential Complication: Pathological Fractures

Potential Complication: Polyneuropathy

Potential Complication: Hypoalbuminemia

Potential Complication: Congestive Heart Failure

Potential Complication: Metabolic Acidosis

Potential Complication: Pleural Effusion

Potential Complication: Pericarditis, Cardiac Tamponade

Nursing Goal

The nurse will monitor for early signs and symptoms of (a) fluid imbalance, (b) anemia, (c) hyperparathyroidism, (d) pathological fractures, (e) polyneuropathy, (f) hypoalbuminemia, (g) congestive heart failure, (h) metabolic acidosis, (i) pleural effusion, and (j) pericarditis/cardiac tamponade and will intervene collaboratively to stabilize the client.

Indicators

- Alert, calm, oriented (a, g)
- Respirations 16–20 breaths/min (g, h, i)
- Respirations relaxed and rhythmic (g, h, i)
- Breath sounds present all lobes (g, i)
- Pulse 60–100 beats/min (a, g, h)
- EKG normal sinus rhythm (c, d, e, f, g)
- BP > 90/60, < 140/90 mm Hg (g, h, j)
- Temperature 98.5–99°F (j)
- No seizure activity (c)
- Flat neck veins (g, j)
- Full range of motion (c)
- No c/o numbness of toes/fingers (e)
- No c/o of palpitations (g)
- Sensation intact (e)
- Strength intact (c, e)
- No foot drop (e)
- Intact reflexes (e)
- No or minimal edema (a, f)
- Ideal or desired weight (a, f)
- Urine output > 30 mL/hr (a, f)
- No substernal pain (a, i)
- Red blood cells 4,000,000–6,200,000 cu mm (b)
- White blood cells 48,000–100,000 cu mm (j)
- Hematocrit (b)
  - Male 42%–50%
  - Female 40%–48%
- Hemoglobin (b)
  - Male 13–18 g/dL
  - Female 12–16 g/dL
- Serum albumin 3.5–5 g/dL (f)
- Serum prealbumin 1–3 g/dL (f)
- Total cholesterol < 200 mg/dL (f)
- Transferrin saturation 230–320 mg/dL (b)
- Serum ferritin (b)
  - Males 29–438 ng/mL
  - Females 9–219 ng/mL

- Serum potassium 3.8–5 mEq/L (b)
- Serum sodium 135–145 mEq/L (a)
- Serum calcium 8.5–10.5 mg/dL (c)
- Folic acid 2.5–20 ng/mL (b)
- Vitamin B_{12} 13–785 pg/mL (b)
- Serum phosphate 125–300 mg/dL (c, d)
- Blood urea nitrogen 10–20 mg/dL (h)
- Creatinine 0.2–0.8 ng/ml (h)
- Negative DEXA scan (c, d)
- Alkaline phosphatase 30–150 m/Uml (c)
- Urine sodium 130–200 mEq/24h (a)
- Creatinine clearance 100–150 mL per min (f)
- Oxygen saturation (SaO_2) > 94% (a, h)
- Carbon dioxide ($PaCO_2$) 35–45 mm Hg (a, h)

Interventions	Rationales
1. Monitor for fluid imbalances: a. Weight changes b. B/P changes c. Increased pulse d. Increased respirations e. Neck vein distention f. Dependent, peripheral edema g. Increased fluid intake h. Increased sodium intake i. Orthostatic hypotension (decreased fluid volume)	1. Fluid imbalance, usually hypervolemia, results from failure of kidney to regulate extracellular fluids by decreased sodium and water elimination.
2. Consult with nephrology staff if fluid volume changes. 3. Refer to dialysis care plans for specific fluid management strategies.	2,3. Adjustments to the dialysis treatment may be needed.
4. Frequently monitor vital signs particularly blood pressure and pulse.	4. Circulating volume must be monitored with chronic kidney disease to prevent severe hypervolemia.
5. Monitor hematocrit each treatment.	5. A decline is directly proportional to the frequency and volume of blood loss associated with phlebotomy-related blood drawing and blood loss during dialysis (Robbins, Serger, Kerhailas, & Fishbane, 1997).
6. Administer bulk-forming laxatives or stool softeners if client is constipated. Avoid magnesium-containing laxatives.	6. Certain laxatives elevate serum magnesium levels. Clients with kidney disease already have difficulty excreting usual intake of magnesium in foods.

(continues on page 293)

Interventions continued	Rationales continued
10. Prepare for and administer total parenteral nutrition (TPN) as ordered. (Refer to the TPN Care Plan for more information.)	10. For a client who cannot maintain nutritional status through the GI route, TPN can provide amino acids necessary for healing, especially renal tissue, and for preventing a catabolic state.
11. Prepare for dialysis as indicated and monitor for potential complications. (Refer to the Hemodialysis and Peritoneal Dialysis Care Plans for more information.)	11. Dialysis is indicated for rising BUN that dietary management cannot control. It also may be necessary to remove excess fluid administered with TPN.
12. Work with client to develop a plan to incorporate diet prescription successfully into his or her daily life.	12. Collaboration provides opportunities for client to exert control; this tends to increase compliance.

Documentation

Flow records
Nursing
 Daily weights
 Intake (specify food types and amounts)
 Output
 Mouth assessment
Discharge summary records
 Client teaching
  Referrals

Ineffective Sexuality Patterns Related to Decreased Libido, Erectile Dysfunction, Amenorrhea, or Sterility

Focus Assessment Criteria	Clinical Significance
1. Knowledge of condition's effect on sexual function 2. Sexual function: a. Pattern b. Satisfaction c. Libido d. Erectile problems	1,2. As the disorder progresses, client experiences a narrowing of existence; mobility decreases and pain, discomfort, and fatigue commonly increase. These all contribute to decreased libido. In men, erectile dysfunction may result from neuropathy, vascular insufficiency, hormonal changes, and possibly antihypertensive medications. More than 50% of men with ESRD suffer from sexual or reproductive problems (Zarifian, 1992).
3. Relationship and communication between client and partner	3. The interaction between partners critically affects sexuality.
4. Menstrual pattern	4. Amenorrhea may result from malnourishment, anemia, or chronic debilitation.

Goal

The client will discuss own feelings and partner's concerns regarding sexual functioning.

Indicators

- Relate the causes of decreased libido and impaired sexual functioning.
- Verbalize an intention to discuss concerns with partner.

Interventions	Rationales
1. Explore client's patterns of sexual functioning; encourage him or her to share concerns. Assume that all clients have had some sexual experience and convey a willingness to discuss feelings and concerns.	1. Many clients are reluctant to discuss sexuality. The proper approach can encourage them to share feelings and concerns.
2. Explain the possible effects of chronic kidney disease on sexual functioning and sexuality.	2. Explaining that impaired sexual functioning has a physiologic basis can reduce feelings of inadequacy and decreased self-esteem; this actually may help improve sexual function.
3. Reaffirm the need for frank discussion between sexual partners.	3. Both partners probably have concerns about sexual activity. Repressing these feelings negatively influences the relationship.
4. Explain how client and partner can use role-playing to discuss sexual concerns.	4. Role-playing helps a person to gain insight by placing himself or herself in another's position and allows more spontaneous sharing of fears and concerns.
5. Reaffirm the need for closeness and expressions of caring through touching, massage, and other means.	5. Sexual pleasure and gratification is not limited to intercourse. Other expressions of caring may prove more meaningful.
6. Suggest that sexual activity need not always culminate in intercourse but that the partner can reach orgasm through non-coital manual or oral stimulation.	6. Sexual gratification is an individual matter. It is not limited to intercourse but includes closeness, touching, and giving pleasure to others.
7. Explain the function of a penile prosthesis: point out that both semirigid and inflatable penile prostheses have a high rate of success.	7. Explaining penile prostheses can give client hope for renewed sexual function.
8. Refer client to a certified sex or mental health professional if desired.	8. Certain sexual problems require continuing therapy and the advanced knowledge of specialists.

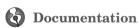 **Documentation**

Progress notes
   Dialogues
   Client teaching

Powerlessness Related to Progressive Disabling Nature of Illness

Focus Assessment Criteria	Clinical Significance
1. Understanding disease process 2. Perception of control 3. Effects on life style and dietary management 4. Previous health care experience 5. Previous/current lifestyle 6. Family role expectations 7. Effects of illness	1–7. A client's response to loss of control depends on the meaning of the loss, individual patterns of coping, personal characteristics, and responses of others.

Goal

The client will participate in decision making for plan of care.

Indicators
- Identify personal strengths.
- Identify factors that he or she can control.

Interventions	Rationales

1. Explore the condition's effects on the following:
  a. Occupation
  b. Leisure and recreational activities
  c. Role responsibilities
  d. Relationships
  e. Finances
	1. Illness can negatively affect client's self-concept and ability to achieve goals. Specifically in chronic kidney disease, fatigue can interfere with client's abilities to work and play.

2. Determine client's usual response to problems.	2. To plan effective interventions, nurse must determine if client usually seeks to change his or her own behaviors to control problems or if he or she expects others or external factors to control problems.
3. Encourage client to verbalize concerns about potential changes in body image, life style, close relationships, role expectations, and life goals.	3. Clients with chronic kidney disease experience the formal loss of self. Former self-image changes negatively because of a restricted life style, social isolation, unmet expectations, and dependence on others (Ferrans & Powers, 1993).

(continues on page 304)

Interventions continued	Rationales continued
4. Help client to identify personal strengths and assets.	4. Clients with chronic illness need assistance to not see themselves as helpless victims. People with a sense of hope, self-control, direction, purpose, and identity can better meet the challenges of their disease (Molzann, Northcott, & Dosseto, 1997).
5. Assist client to identify energy patterns and to schedule activities around these patterns.	5. A review of client's daily schedule can help nurse and client to plan activities that promote feelings of self-worth and dignity and to schedule appropriate rest periods to prevent exhaustion.
6. Discuss the need to accept help from others and to delegate some tasks.	6. Client may need assistance to prevent exhaustion and hypoxia.
7. Help client seek support from other sources (e.g., self-help groups, support groups).	7. Client may benefit from opportunities to share similar experiences and problem solving with others in the same situation.
8. Encourage client to make decisions that might increase ability to cope.	8. Self-concept can be enhanced when clients actively engage in decisions regarding health and life style.
9. Develop a plan of care with client that reinforces positive coping mechanisms, uses personal strengths, and acknowledges limitations.	9. Research has shown that clients who adjust their aspiration levels to fit their new circumstances have a higher quality of life (Ferrans & Powers, 1993).
10. Provide adequate information about the multiple facets of illness and therapy options.	10. This will help to increase active participation in care.
11. Provide anticipatory guidance and counseling.	11. Therapy can address major stressors to be encountered.
12. Provide opportunity for client to meet others who have had similar experiences.	12. Sharing experiences can help a person to identify options previously unknown.

Documentation

Progress notes
Interactions with the client

High Risk for Ineffective Therapeutic Regimen Management Related to Insufficient Knowledge of Condition, Dietary Restrictions, Daily Recording, Pharmacological Therapy, Signs/Symptoms of Complications, Follow-up Visits, and Community Resources

Focus Assessment Criteria	Clinical Significance
1. Knowledge of disease, therapeutic regimen, and future treatment alternatives 2. Ability and readiness to learn considering level of literacy 3. Barriers to learning (e.g., pain, fatigue, stress) 4. Past experiences influencing current health status 5. Nature of concerns and fears	1–5. Effective client teaching involves guided interaction between nurse and client that results in a change in client behavior. A warm, accepting environment helps ensure learning success. The timing and content of teaching are crucial to client's understanding, acceptance, and compliance with the plan of care.

Goals

The goals for this diagnosis represent those associated with discharge planning. Refer to the discharge criteria.

Interventions	Rationales
1. Develop and implement a teaching plan using techniques and tools appropriate to client's understanding. Plan several teaching sessions.	1. Presenting relevant and useful information in an understandable format greatly reduces learning frustration and enhances teaching efforts. Some factors specific to a client with chronic kidney disease influence the teaching—learning process (Lancaster, 1995): • Depressed mentation that necessitates repeating information • Short attention span that may limit teaching sessions to 10 to 15 minutes • Altered perceptions that necessitate frequent clarification and reassurance • Sensory alterations cause a better response to ideas presented using varied audio-visual formats.

2. Implement teaching that includes but is not limited to (Burrows-Hudson, 1999) renal function
  a. Normal function
  b. Altered function
    • Disease process
    • Causes
    • Physiologic and emotional response to uremia
	2. Amount and depth of teaching will depend on client's present readiness to learn. Several sessions will be needed; include written materials to take home.

(continues on page 306)

Interventions continued	**Rationales** continued

Treatment modalities
a. Conservative management
b. Hemodialysis
- Home staff-assisted, self-care, daily dialysis
- In-center (staff-assisted, self-care)
c. Peritoneal dialysis
- Continuous ambulatory peritoneal dialysis (CAPD)
- Continuous cycling peritoneal dialysis (CCPD)
- Intermittent peritoneal dialysis (IPD)
d. Transplantation:
- Living related/unrelated donor
- Cadaveric donor
- Multiple organ transplantation
e. No treatment

Renal replacement therapies
a. Definitions
b. Process/procedures
c. Vascular/peritoneal access
d. Availability
e. Benefits/risks
f. Life style adaptation
g. Nutritional considerations
h. Mobility/activity/rehabilitation
i. Financial considerations

Laboratory, x-rays, routine tests
a. Purpose of each
b. Expected ranges
c. Monitoring frequency

Nutrition
a. Incorporation of prescribed diet into life style
b. Shopping, preparation, dining out
c. Nutritional requirements
- Energy
- Protein
- Sodium and water
- Potassium
- Vitamins
- Calcium and phosphorus

Medication therapy
a. Identification/name
b. Purpose
c. Dosage
d. Route
e. Side effects
f. Instructions for missed dose
g. Drug interactions
h. Relationship to diet
i. Avoidance of over-the-counter medications
j. Use of complementary and/or alternative medicine/treatments

(continues on page 307)

Interventions continued	**Rationales** continued

Psychosocial issues
a. Emotional aspects: coping, self-concept
b. Sexual function
c. Rehabilitation
d. Energy/activity level
e. Body image
 	
Financial aspects
a. Medicare/Medicaid/other payor-sources
b. Disability
 	
Client involvement
a. Client's rights
b. Client's responsibilities
c. Advanced directives
d. Long-term care program
e. Short-term care plan
f. Medical record
  • Access for client review
  • Confidentiality	

3. Encourage client to verbalize anxiety, fears, and questions.	3. Recognition of client's fear of failure to learn is vital to successful teaching.
4. Identify factors that may help to predict noncompliance: a. Lack of knowledge b. Noncompliance in the hospital c. Failure to perceive disorder's seriousness or chronicity d. Belief that condition will "go away" on its own e. Belief that condition is hopeless	4. Openly addressing barriers to compliance may help to minimize or eliminate these barriers.
5. Include significant others in teaching sessions. Encourage them to provide support without acting as "police."	5. Significant others must be aware of the treatment plan so they can support client. "Policing" client can disrupt positive relationships.
6. Emphasize to client that ultimately it is his or her choice and responsibility to comply with therapeutic regimen.	6. Client must understand that he or she has control over choices and that his or her choices can improve or impair health.
7. If cost of medications is a financial burden for client, consult with social services.	7. A referral for financial support can prevent discontinuation because of financial reasons.
8. Assist client to identify his or her ideal or desired weight.	8. Establishing an achievable goal may help to improve compliance.

(continues on page 308)

Interventions continued	Rationales continued
9. Teach client to record weight and urinary output daily.	9. Daily weight and urine output measurements allow client to monitor his or her own fluid status and limit fluid intake accordingly.
10. Explain signs and symptoms of electrolyte imbalances and the need to watch for and report them. (See Collaborative Problems in this entry for more information.)	10. Early detection of electrolyte imbalance enables prompt intervention to prevent serious complications.
11. Teach client measures to reduce risk of urinary tract infection: a. Perform proper hygiene after toileting, to prevent fecal contamination of urinary tract. b. To prevent urinary stasis, drink maximum fluids allowed.	11. Repetitive infections can cause further renal damage.
12. Reinforce the need to comply with diet and fluid restrictions and follow-up care. Consult with dietitian regarding fluid plan and overall diet.	12. Compliance reduces the risk of complications.
13. Teach client who has fluid restrictions to relieve thirst by other means: a. Sucking on a lemon wedge, a piece of hard candy, a frozen juice pop, or an ice cube b. Spacing fluid allotment over 24 hours	13. Strategies to reduce thirst without significant fluid intake reduce risk of fluid overload.
14. Encourage client to express feelings and frustrations; give positive feedback for adherence to fluid restrictions.	14. Fluid and diet restrictions can be extremely frustrating; positive feedback and reassurance can contribute to continued compliance.
15. Explain importance of Epoetin alfa therapy and iron supplements to achieve an Hct of 33% to 36%.	15. When Hct is maintained between 33% and 36%, there are incremental improvements in survival, left ventricle hypertrophy, exercise capacity, cognitive function, sleep dysfunction, and overall quality of life (Cutler, 1997).
16. Teach client to take oral medications with meals whenever possible. If medications must be administered between meals, give with the smallest amount of fluid possible.	16. Planning can reduce unnecessary fluid intake and conserve fluid allowance.

(continues on page 309)

Interventions continued	Rationales continued
17. Encourage client to maintain his or her usual level of activity and continue activities of daily living to the extent possible.	17. Regular activity helps to maintain strength and endurance and promotes overall well-being.
18. Teach client and family to watch for and report the following: a. Weight gain greater than 2 lb or weight loss b. Shortness of breath c. Increasing fatigue or weakness d. Confusion, change in mentation e. Palpitations f. Excessive bruising; excessive menses; excessive bleeding from gums, nose, or cut; or blood in urine, stool, or vomitus g. Increasing oral pain or oral lesions	18. Early reporting of complications enables prompt intervention (Lancaster, 1995). a. Weight gain greater than 2 lb may indicate fluid retention; weight loss may point to insufficient intake. b. Shortness of breath may be an early sign of pulmonary edema. c. Increasing fatigue or weakness may indicate increasing uremia. d. Confusion or other changes in mentation may point to acidosis or fluid and electrolyte imbalances. e. Palpitations may indicate electrolyte imbalances (K, Ca). f. Excessive bruising, excessive menses, and abnormal bleeding may indicate reduced prothrombin, clotting factors III and VIII, and platelets. g. Oral pain or lesions can result as excessive salivary urea is converted to ammonia in the mouth, which is irritating to the oral mucosa.
19. Discuss with client and family any anticipated disease-related stressors: a. Financial difficulties b. Reversal of role responsibilities c. Dependency	19. Discussing the nonphysiologic effects of chronic kidney disease in family dynamics can help client and family to identify effective coping strategies (Flaherty & O'Brien, 1992).
20. Provide information about or initiate referrals to community resources (e.g., American Kidney Association, counseling, self-help groups, peer counseling, Internet information sites, publications).	20. Assistance with home management and dealing with the potential destructive effects on client and family may be needed.

 Documentation

Discharge summary record
   Client teaching
   Outcome achievement or status
   Referrals if indicated

Neurologic Disorders

CEREBROVASCULAR ACCIDENT (STROKE)

Cerebrovascular accident, or stroke, involves a sudden onset of neurological deficits ND-2 because of insufficient blood supply to a part of the brain. Insufficient blood supply is caused by a thrombus (80%) usually secondary to atherosclerosis, an embolism originating elsewhere in the body, or a hemorrhage (20%) from a ruptured artery (aneurysm).

Preventable and costly, stroke, or brain attack, is the third leading cause of death and the leading cause of long-term disability in the United States. A recent estimate from the American Heart Association is that at least 600,000 new or recurrent strokes occur each year (Pajeau, 2002). Preventing first and recurrent strokes requires prompt identification of vulnerable clients. Some risk factors can be modified (Pajeau, 2002) including hypertension, cigarette smoking, unhealthy eating habits, sedentary lifestyle, lipid imbalance, poor glycemic control, and immoderate alcohol intake. Nonmodifiable risk factors include age, gender, genetic predisposition, and history of previous stroke, transient ischemic attacks (TIAs), or other cardiac conditions (Pajeau, 2002).

Time Frame
Initial diagnosis
Recurrent episodes

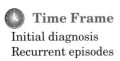 **DIAGNOSTIC CLUSTER**

Collaborative Problems

- ▲ PC: Increased Intracranial Pressure
- * PC: Pneumonia, Atelectasis
- ▲ PC: Adult Respiratory Distress Syndrome
- * PC: Seizures
- * PC: Gastrointestinal (GI) Bleeding
- • PC: Hypothalamic Syndromes

Nursing Diagnoses	Refer to
▲ Impaired Communication related to the effects of hemisphere (left or right) damage on language or speech.	
▲ High Risk for Injury related to visual field, motor, or perception deficits	
▲ Impaired Physical Mobility related to decreased motor function of (specify) secondary to damage to upper motor neurons	

(continues on page 314)

Nursing Diagnoses continued	Refer to continued
▲ Functional Incontinence related to inability and difficulty in reaching toilet secondary to decreased mobility or motivation	
▲ Impaired Swallowing related to muscle paralysis or paresis secondary to damage to upper motor neurons	
▲ Self-Care Deficit related to impaired physical mobility or confusion	Immobility or Unconsciousness
△ Unilateral Neglect related to (specify site) secondary to right hemispheric brain damage	
△ High Risk for Ineffective Therapeutic Regimen Management related to altered ability to maintain self at home secondary to sensory/motor/cognitive deficits and lack of knowledge of caregivers of home care, reality orientation, bowel/bladder program, skin care, signs and symptoms of complications, and community resources	
△ Total Incontinence related to loss of bladder tone, loss of sphincter control, or inability to perceive bladder cues	Neurogenic Bladder
△ High Risk for Disturbed Self-Concept related to effects of prolonged debilitating condition on achieving developmental tasks and life style	Multiple Sclerosis
* Disuse Syndrome	Immobility or Unconsciousness
Related Care Plan • Immobility or Unconsciousness	

▲ This diagnosis was reported to be monitored for or managed frequently (75%–100%).
△ This diagnosis was reported to be monitored for or managed often (50%–74%).
* This diagnosis was not included in the validation study.

Discharge Criteria

Before discharge, the client or family will

1. Describe measures for reducing or eliminating selected risk factors.
2. Relate intent to discuss fears and concerns with family members after discharge.

3. Identify methods for management (e.g., of dysphagia, of incontinence).
4. Demonstrate or relate techniques to increase mobility.
5. State signs and symptoms that must be reported to a health care professional.
6. Relate community resources that can provide assistance with management at home.

Collaborative Problems

Potential Complication: Increased Intracranial Pressure (ICP)

Potential Complication: Pneumonia, Atelectasis

Potential Complication: Adult Respiratory Distress Syndrome

Potential Complication: Seizures

Potential Complication: GI Bleeding

Potential Complication: Hypothalamic Syndromes

Nursing Goal

The nurse will detect early signs/symptoms of increased ICP, hypoxia, pneumonia, seizures, GI bleeding, and hypothalamic dysfunction and collaboratively intervene to stabilize the client.

Indicators

- Alert, oriented
- Pulse 60–100 per min
- B/P >90/60, <140/90 mm Hg
- Respirations 16–20 per min
- Pupils equal, reactive to light
- Temperature 98–99.5°F
- Breath sounds-equal, no adventitious sounds
- Oxygen saturation (pulse oximetry) (SaO_2) >95
- Stool-negative for occult blood
- Urine specific gravity 1.005–1.030
- Serum sodium 135–145 mEq/L

Interventions	Rationales
1. Monitor for signs and symptoms of increased ICP.	1. Cerebral tissue is compromised by deficiencies of cerebral blood supply caused by hemorrhage, hematoma, cerebral edema, thrombus, or emboli. Monitoring ICP is an indicator of cerebral perfusion.
a. Assess the following: • Best eye opening response: spontaneously to auditory stimuli or to painful stimuli, or no response • Best motor response: obeys verbal commands, localizes pain, flexion-withdrawal, flexion-decorticate, extension-decerebrate, or no response • Best verbal response: oriented to person, place, and time; confused conversation, inappropriate speech, incomprehensible sounds, or no response	a. The Glasgow Coma Scale evaluates the client's ability to integrate commands with conscious and involuntary movements. Cortical function can be assessed by evaluating eye opening and motor response. No response may indicate damage to the midbrain.

(continues on page 316)

Interventions continued	**Rationales** continued
b. Assess for changes in vital signs: • Pulse changes: slowing rate to 60 or below or increasing rate to 100 or above • Respiratory irregularities: slowing of rate with lengthening periods of apnea • Rising blood pressure or widening pulse pressure c. Assess pupillary responses: • Inspect the pupils with a flashlight to evaluate size, configuration, and reaction to light. Compare both eyes for similarities and differences. • Evaluate gaze to determine whether it is conjugate (paired, working together) or if eye movements are abnormal. • Evaluate eyes' ability to adduct and abduct. d. Note the presence of the following: • Vomiting • Headache (constant, increasing in intensity, or aggravated by movement or straining) • Subtle changes (e.g., lethargy, restlessness, forced breathing, purposeless movements, and changes in mentation)	b. These vital sign changes may reflect increasing ICP. • Changes in pulse may indicate brainstem pressure by being slowed at first, then increasing to compensate for hypoxia. • Respiratory patterns vary with impairments at various sites. Cheyne-Stokes breathing (a gradual increase followed by a gradual decrease then a period of apnea) points to damage in both cerebral hemispheres, midbrain, and upper pons. Ataxic breathing (irregular with random sequence of deep and shallow breaths) indicates medullar dysfunction. • Blood pressure and pulse pressure changes are late signs indicating severe hypoxia. c. Pupillary changes indicate pressure on oculomotor or optic nerves. • Pupil reactions are regulated by the oculomotor nerve (cranial nerve III) in the brain stem. • Conjugate eye movements are regulated from parts of the cortex and brain stem. • Cranial nerve VI, or the abducent nerve, regulates abduction and adduction of the eyes. Cranial nerve IV, or the trochlear nerve, also regulates eye movement. d. • Vomiting results from pressure on the medulla that stimulates the brain's vomiting center. • Compression of neural tissue movement increases ICP and increases pain. • These changes may be early indicators of ICP changes.
2. Elevate the head of the bed 15 to 30 degrees unless contraindicated. Avoid changing position rapidly.	2. Slight head elevation can aid venous drainage to reduce cerebrovascular congestion.

(continues on page 317)

Interventions continued	**Rationales** continued
3. Avoid the following:	3. These situations or maneuvers can increase ICP.
a. Carotid massage	a. Carotid massage slows heart rate and reduces systemic circulation; this is followed by a sudden increase in circulation.
b. Neck flexion or rotation >45 degrees	b. Neck flexion or extreme rotation disrupts cerebrospinal fluid and venous drainage from intracranial cavity.

c. Digital anal stimulation
    d. Breath holding, straining
    e. Extreme flexion of hips and knees
	c.–e. These activities initiate Valsalva's maneuver, which impairs venous return by constricting the jugular veins and increases ICP.

4. Consult with the physician for stool softeners if needed.	4. Stool softeners prevent constipation and straining that initiate Valsalva's maneuver.
5. Maintain a quiet, calm, softly lit environment. Plan activities to minimize ICP.	5. These measures promote rest and decrease stimulation, helping decrease ICP. Suctioning, position changes, and neck flexion in succession will markedly increase cranial pressure.
6. Monitor for signs and symptoms of pneumonia:	6. Pneumonia is a common complication of many major illnesses. Swallowing, respiratory therapy, and deep breathing exercises help to decrease the risk of pneumonia (American Stroke Association, 2001).
a. Increased respiratory rate	a. Increased respiratory rate is a compensatory mechanism for hypoxia.
b. Fever, chills (sudden or insidious)	b. Bacteria can act as pyrogen by raising the hypothalamic thermostat through the production of endogenous pyrogen that may mediate through prostaglandins. Chills can occur when the temperature setpoint of the hypothalamus rapidly changes.
c. Productive cough	c. Productive cough indicates increased mucus production in response to irritant (bacteria).
d. Diminished or absent breath sounds	d. Airflow through the tracheobronchial tree is affected or obstructed by the presence of fluid or mucus.
e. Pleuritic pain	e. Pleuritic pain results from the rubbing together of inflamed pleural surfaces during respiration.

(continues on page 318)

Interventions continued	**Rationales** continued

7. Monitor for signs and symptoms of atelectasis:
    a. Pleuritic pain
 	
    b. Diminished or absent breath sounds
    c. Dull percussion sounds over area
 	
    d. Tachycardia
    e. Increased respiratory rate
    f. Elevated temperature
 	
    g. Marked dyspnea
    h. Cyanosis
	7. Inactivity can cause retained secretions, leading to obstruction or infection.
	    a. Pleuritic pain results from the rubbing together of inflamed pleural surfaces during respiration.
	    b,c. Changes in breath and percussion sounds represent increased density of lung tissue secondary to fluid accumulation.
	    d,e. Tachycardia and tachypnea are compensatory mechanisms for hypoxia.
	    f. Bacteria can act as pyrogen by raising the hypothalamic thermostat through the production of endogenous pyrogen, which may mediate through prostaglandins.
	    g. Dyspnea indicates hypoxia.
	    h. Cyanosis indicates vasoconstriction in response to hypoxia.

8. Monitor high-risk clients closely for changes in respiratory status. Report changes immediately.	8. CVA clients who have pneumonia, sepsis, ICP, or gastric aspirations are at high risk for adult respiratory distress syndrome (ARDS). Mortality rate for ARDS is 50% to 60%.

9. Monitor for signs and symptoms of ARDS:
    a. Respiratory discomfort
    b. Noisy tachypnea
    c. Tachycardia
    d. Diffuse rales and rhonchi
	9. Damaged type II cells release inflammatory mediators that increase alveolocapillary membrane permeability, causing pulmonary edema. Decreased surfactant production decreases alveolar compliance. Respiratory muscles must greatly increase inspiratory pressures to inflate lungs.

10. Monitor hydration status by evaluating the following:
    a. Oral intake
    b. Parenteral therapy
    c. Intake and output
    d. Urine specific gravity
	10. A balance must be maintained to ensure hydration to liquefy secretions while simultaneously preventing hypervolemia, which increases ICP.

11. Monitor the effectiveness of airway clearance by evaluating:
    a. Effectiveness of cough effort
    b. Need for tracheobronchial suctioning
	11. Lower cranial deficits can affect swallowing ability. The prevalence of aspiration post-CVA is reported to be 25% to 30%.

(continues on page 319)

Interventions continued	Rationales continued
12. Monitor for seizures.	12. Ischemic areas may serve as epileptogenic foci or metabolic disturbances can lower seizure threshold (American Stroke Association, 2001).
13. Refer to care plan on Seizure Disorders if indicated.	
14. Monitor stools for blood.	14. Hypersecretion of gastric juices occurs during periods of stress.
15. Monitor for: a. Low serum sodium b. Elevated urine sodium c. Elevated urine specific gravity	15. Damage to the hypothalamic region may result in increased secretion of ADH.
16. Monitor for diabetes insipidus: a. Excess urine output b. Extreme thirst c. Elevated serum sodium d. Low specific gravity	16. Compression of posterior pituitary gland or its neuronal connections can cause a decrease of antidiuretic hormone (ADH).
17. Monitor body temperature.	17. Hypothalamic pituitary compression can compromise the temperature-regulating mechanism.

Related Physician-Prescribed Interventions

Medications. Anticonvulsants, antihypertensives, stool softeners, peripheral vasodilators, corticosteroids, anticoagulants, antiplatelets (aspirin, ticlopidine), analgesics

Intravenous Therapy. Fluid/electrolyte replacements

Laboratory Studies. Complete blood count, urinalysis, chemistry profile, sedimentation rate, prothrombin time, RPR serology, single-photon tomography

Diagnostic Studies. Computed tomography (CT) scan of head, lumbar puncture, cerebral angiography, magnetic resonance imaging (MRI), positron emission, tomography scan, brain scan, Doppler ultrasonography, electroencephalography (EEG), skull X-ray film

Therapies. Swallowing studies, antiembolism stockings, speech therapy, physical therapy, occupational therapy, craniotomy endarterectomy

Documentation

Flow records
  Neurologic assessment
  Vital signs
Complaints of vomiting or headache
Changes in status
Respiratory assessment

Nursing Diagnoses

Impaired Communication Related to the Effects of Hemisphere (Left or Right) Damage on Language or Speech

Focus Assessment Criteria	Clinical Significance
1. Ability to comprehend simple commands and complete ideas	1. Damage to a language center located on the dominant side of the brain (known as Broca's area) causes expressive aphasia. Damage to a language center located on a rear position of the brain (called Wernicke's area) results in receptive aphasia (National Institute of Neurological Disorder and Stroke, 2000).

2. Ability to speak:
  a. Clear
  b. Slurred
  c. Stuttering
  d. Appropriate use of words
	2. Damaged cells in the frontal lobe near the motor cortex and cranial nerves control the movement of lips, jaw, tongue, soft palate, and vocal cords (National Institute of Neurological Disorders and Stroke, 2000).

3. Ability to read and write	3. Injury to Wernicke's area also disrupts the ability to read and write (National Institute of Neurological Disorders and Stroke, 2000).
4. Ability to hear and the functioning of hearing aids, if applicable 5. Ability to see and the correctness of glasses, if applicable	4,5. Hearing or vision impairment calls for specific interventions (National Institute of Neurological Disorders and Stroke, 2000).

Goal

The client will report improved satisfaction with ability to communicate.

Indicators
- Demonstrate improved ability to express self and understand others.
- Report decreased frustration during communication efforts.

Interventions	Rationales
1. Differentiate between language disturbances (dysphagia/aphasia) and speech disturbances (dyspraxia/apraxia).	1. Language involves comprehension and transmission of ideas and feelings. Speech is the mechanics and articulations of verbal expression.

(continues on page 321)

Interventions continued	**Rationales** continued
2. Collaborate with the speech therapist to evaluate client and create a plan.	2. A detailed assessment is required to diagnose a language dysfunction. Most clients have more than one type of dysfunction (National Institute of Neurological Disorders and Stroke, 2000).
3. Provide frequent, short therapy and practice sessions. Try to incorporate topics of interest to client.	3. These sessions are more beneficial than lengthy, infrequent ones (National Institute of Neurological Disorders and Stroke, 2000).
4. Provide an atmosphere of acceptance and privacy: a. Do not rush. b. Speak slowly and in a normal tone. c. Decrease external noise and distractions. d. Encourage client to share frustrations; validate client's nonverbal expressions. e. Provide client with opportunities to make decisions about his care when appropriate. f. Do not force client to communicate. g. If client laughs or cries uncontrollably, change subject or activity.	4. Communication is the core of all human relations. Impaired ability to communicate spontaneously is frustrating and embarrassing. Nursing actions should focus on decreasing the tension and conveying an understanding of how difficult the situation must be for the client.
5. Make every effort to understand client's communication efforts: a. Listen attentively. b. Repeat client's message back to him or her to ensure understanding. c. Ignore inappropriate word usage; do not correct mistakes. d. Do not pretend you understand; if you do not, ask client to repeat. e. Try to anticipate some needs (e.g., Do you need something to drink?).	5. Nurse should make every attempt to understand the client. Each success, regardless of how minor, decreases frustration and increases motivation.
6. Teach the client techniques to improve speech: a. Instruct client to speak slowly and in short phrases. b. Initially ask questions that client can answer with a "yes" or "no." c. With improvement, allow person to complete some phrases, e.g. ("This is a _____."). d. As the client is able, encourage her or him to share feelings and concerns.	6. Deliberate actions can be taken to improve speech. As the client's speech improves, her or his confidence will increase and she or he will make more attempts at speaking.

(continues on page 322)

Interventions continued	Rationales continued

7. Use strategies to improve the client's comprehension:
  a. Gain the client's attention before speaking; call client by name.
  b. Practice consistent speech patterns:
    • Speak slowly.
    • Use common words and use the same words consistently for a task.
    • Repeat or rephrase when indicated.
  c. Use touch and behavior to communicate calmness.
  d. Add other nonverbal methods of communication:
    • Point or use flash cards for basic needs.
    • Use pantomime.
    • Use paper/pen or spelling board.
    • Display the most effective methods at the client's bedside.
	7. Improving the client's comprehension can help to decrease frustration and increase trust. Clients with aphasia can correctly interpret tone of voice.

8. Refer to the Parkinson's disease care plan for further strategies to manage dysarthria.	

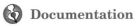 **Documentation**

Progress notes
  Dialogues
  Method to use (care plan)

High Risk for Injury Related to Visual Field, Motor, or Perception Deficits

Focus Assessment Criteria	Clinical Significance

1. Acuity:
  a. Vision
  b. Hearing
  c. Thermal and tactile perception
	1. Determining what specific risks are present will determine specific interventions.

2. Mental status	2. This assessment helps to determine if the client can detect environmental hazards and request help.
3. Mobility for ambulation and for self-care activities	3. This assessment determines if the client needs assistance or assistive devices.
4. Gait	4. A client with unstable gait needs assistance with ambulation.

Goal
The client will relate no injuries.

Indicators
- Identify factors that increase the risk for injury.
- Demonstrate safety measures to prevent injury.
- Request assistance when needed.

Interventions	Rationales

1. Take steps to reduce environmental hazards:
  a. Orient the client to his surroundings.
  b. Instruct client to use a call bell to summon assistance. Post high-risk status at bedside.
  c. Keep the bed in a low position with all side rails up.
  d. Keep paths to the bathroom obstacle-free.
  e. Provide adequate lighting in all areas.
  f. Provide a night light.
  g. Ensure that a light switch is accessible next to the bed.
	1. Emphasizing safety can help to reduce injuries.

2. If decreased tactile sensitivity is a problem, teach the client to do the following:
  a. Carefully assess temperature of bath water and heating pads prior to use; measure with a thermometer if possible.
  b. Assess extremities daily for undetected injuries.
  c. Keep feet warm and dry and skin softened with emollient lotion (e.g., lanolin or mineral oil).
	2. Post-CVA sensory impairment can interfere with the client's perception of temperature and injuries.

3. Take steps to reduce risks associated with assistive devices:
  a. Assess for proper use of devices.
  b. Assess devices for fit and condition.
  c. Consult with a physical therapist for gait training.
  d. Instruct client to wear shoes with non-skid soles.
	3. Improper use or fit of assistive devices can cause straining or falls.

4. Teach client and family to maximize safety at home: a. Eliminate throw rugs, clutter and litter, and highly polished floors.	4. A client with mobility problems needs such safety devices installed and hazards eliminated to aid in activities of daily living.

(continues on page 324)

Interventions continued	Rationales continued
b. Provide nonslip surfaces in bathtub or shower by applying traction tapes. c. Provide hand grips in the bathroom. d. Provide railings in hallways and on stairs. e. Remove protruding objects (e.g., coat hooks, shelves, and light fixtures) from stairway walls.	

Documentation
Discharge summary record
   Client teaching

Impaired Physical Mobility Related to Decreased Motor Function of (Specify) Secondary to Damage to Upper Motor Neurons

Focus Assessment Criteria	Clinical Significance
1. Dominant hand	1. If the client's dominant hand is impaired, he or she requires more assistance.
2. Motor function; range of motion; and strength in hands, arms, and legs 3. Mobility: ability to turn, sit, stand, transfer, and ambulate	2,3. These assessments provide baseline data to determine the assistance needed and to evaluate progress.

Goal
The client will report an increase in strength and endurance of limbs.

Indicators
* Demonstrate the use of adaptive devices to increase mobility.
* Use safety measures to minimize potential for injury.
* Describe rationale for interventions.
* Demonstrate measures to increase mobility.

Interventions	Rationales
1. Teach the client to perform active range-of-motion (ROM) exercises on unaffected limbs at least four times a day if possible.	1. Active ROM increases muscle mass, tone, and strength and improves cardiac and respiratory functioning.
2. Perform passive ROM on affected limbs three to four times daily. Do the exercises	2. A voluntary muscle will lose tone and strength and become shortened from

(continues on page 325)

Interventions continued	Rationales continued
slowly to allow the muscles time to relax, and support the extremity above and below the joint to prevent strain on joints and tissues. Stop at the point when pain or resistance is met.	reduced range of motion or lack of exercise (American Stroke Association, 2001).
3. When the client is in bed, take steps to maintain alignment: a. Use a footboard. b. Avoid prolonged periods of sitting or lying in the same position. c. Change position of shoulder joints every 2 to 4 hours. d. Use a small pillow or no pillow when in Fowler's position. e. Support hand and wrist in natural alignment. f. If client is supine or prone, place a rolled towel or small pillow under the lumbar curvature or the end of the rib cage. g. Place a trochanter roll or sand bags alongside hips and upper thighs. h. If client is in the lateral position, place pillow(s) to support the leg from groin to foot and a pillow to flex the shoulder and elbow slightly; if needed, support the lower foot in dorsal flexion with a sandbag. i. Use hand–wrist splints.	3. Prolonged immobility and impaired neurosensory function can cause permanent contractures (American Stroke Association, 2001). a. This measure helps prevent foot drop. b. This measure prevents hip flexion contractures. c. This measure prevents shoulder contractures. d. This measure prevents flexion contracture of the neck. e. This measure prevents dependent edema and flexion contracture of the wrist. f. This measure prevents flexion or hyperflexion of lumbar curvature. g. This measure prevents external rotation of femurs and hip. h. These measures prevent internal rotation and adduction of the femurs and hip, internal rotation and adduction of the shoulder, and foot drop. i. These splints prevent flexion or extension contractures of fingers and abduction of the thumb.
4. Provide progressive mobilization: a. Maintain head of bed at least at 30-degree angle unless contraindicated. b. Assist the client slowly from the lying to the sitting position and allow the client to dangle legs over the side of the bed for a few minutes before standing up. c. Initially limit the time out of bed to 15 minutes three times a day. d. Increase time out of bed by 15-minute increments as tolerated. e. Progress to ambulation with or without assistive devices. f. If the client cannot walk, assist her or him out of bed to a wheelchair or chair. g. Encourage short, frequent walks (at least three times daily) with assistance if unsteady. h. Increase the length of walks each day.	4. Prolonged bed rest or decreased blood volume can cause a sudden drop in blood pressure (orthostatic hypotension) as blood returns to peripheral circulation. Gradual progression to increased activity reduces fatigue and increases endurance (Michael, 2002).

(continues on page 326)

Interventions continued	Rationales continued
5. Gradually help client progress from active ROM to functional activities as indicated.	5. Incorporating ROM exercises into the client's daily routine encourages their regular performance.

Documentation

Flow records
 Intake and output
 Incontinent episodes

Functional Incontinence Related to Inability or Difficulty in Reaching Toilet Secondary to Decreased Mobility or Motivation

Focus Assessment Criteria	Clinical Significance
1. Mobility and desire to be continent	1. Specific assessments are needed to evaluate self-care ability.
2. Ability to delay urination after urge	2. A small bladder capacity interferes with retraining.
3. Interpretation of need to void	3. The client's ability to interpret and act on urge bladder cues is necessary to enable participation in bladder retraining.
4. Incontinence episodes	4. A baseline assessment provides a means for evaluating progress.

Goal

The client will report no or fewer episodes of incontinence.

Indicators

- Remove or minimize environmental barriers at home.
- Use proper adaptive equipment to assist with voiding, transfers, and dressing.
- Describe causative factors for incontinence.

Interventions	Rationales
1. Assess environment for barriers to the client's access to the bathroom.	1. Barriers can delay access to the toilet and cause incontinence if client cannot delay urination.
2. Provide grab rails and a raised toilet seat if necessary.	2. These devices can promote independence and reduce toileting difficulties.

(continues on page 327)

Interventions continued	Rationales continued
3. If client requires assistance, provide ready access to a call bell and respond promptly when summoned.	3. A few seconds' delay in reaching the bathroom can make the difference between continence and incontinence.
4. Encourage client to wear pajamas or ordinary clothes.	4. Wearing normal clothing or nightwear helps to simulate the home environment where incontinence may not occur. A hospital gown may reinforce incontinence.
5. For a client with cognitive deficits, do the following: a. Offer toileting reminders every 2 hours after meals and before bedtime. b. Provide verbal instruction for toileting activities. c. Praise success and good attempts.	5. A client with a cognitive deficit needs constant verbal cues and reminders to establish a routine and reduce incontinence (American Stroke Association, 2001).
6. Maintain optimal hydration (2,000 to 2,500 mL/day unless contraindicated). Space fluids every 2 hours.	6. Dehydration can prevent the sensation of a full bladder and can contribute to loss of bladder tone. Spacing fluids helps to promote regular bladder filling and emptying.
7. Minimize intake of coffee, tea, colas, and grapefruit juice.	7. These beverages act as diuretics, which can cause urgency.

 Documentation

Flow records
  Range of motion exercises
  Progress in activities and ambulation

Impaired Swallowing Related to Muscle Paralysis or Paresis Secondary to Damage to Upper Motor Neurons

Focus Assessment Criteria	Clinical Significance
1. Ability to swallow food and liquid	1. Post-CVA paresis or paralysis can interfere with the ability to chew and swallow.
2. Gag and swallowing reflexes	2. Impaired reflexes increase the risk of aspiration.

Goal

The client will report improved ability to swallow.

Indicators

• Describe causative factors when known.
• Describe rationale and procedures for treatment.

Interventions	Rationales
1. Consult with speech pathologist for evaluation and a specific plan.	1. The speech pathologist has the expertise needed to perform the dysphagia evaluation.
2. Establish a visual method to communicate at bedside to staff that client is dysphagic.	2. The risk of aspiration can be reduced if all staff are alerted.
3. Plan meals when client is well rested; ensure that reliable suction equipment is on hand during meals. Discontinue feeding if client is tired.	3. Fatigue can increase the risk of aspiration.
4. If indicated, use modified supraglottic swallow technique: a. Position the head of the bed in semi- or high Fowler's position with the client's neck flexed forward slightly and chin tilted down. b. Use cutout cup (remove and round out ⅓ of side of foam cup). c. Take bolus of food and hold in strongest side of mouth for 1 to 2 seconds, then immediately flex the neck with chin tucked against chest. d. Without breathing, swallow as many times as needed. e. When client's mouth is emptied, raise chin and clear throat. f. Avoid straws.	4. a. This position uses the force of gravity to aid downward motion of food and decreases risk of aspiration. b. This prevents neck extension, which will open airway and risk aspiration. c–e. This maneuver triggers the protective mechanisms of epiglottis movement, laryngeal elevation, and vocal cord adduction (closure). f. Straws hasten transit time and increase the risk of aspiration (National Institute of Neurological Disorders and Stroke, 2000).
5. Offer high viscous foods first at meal (e.g., mashed bananas, mashed potatoes, gelatin, gravy).	5. Post-CVA clients may have slowed peristalsis. Viscous foods increase peristaltic pump action.
6. Offer thick liquids (e.g., milk shakes, slushes, nectars, or cream soups).	6. Thicker fluids have a slower transit time and allow more time to trigger the swallow reflex (National Institute of Neurological Disorders and Stroke, 2000).
7. Establish a goal for fluid intake.	7. These clients are at risk for dehydration because of self-imposed fluid restrictions related to fear of choking.

(continues on page 329)

Interventions continued	Rationales continued

8. If drooling is present, use a quick-stretch stimulation just before each meal and toward the end of the meal.
  a. Digitally apply short, rapid, downward strokes to edge of bottom lip mostly on affected side.
  b. Use a cold washcloth over finger for added stimulation.
	8. This maneuver stimulates the orbicularis oris muscle to facilitate labial adduction. Damage to VII cranial nerves causes this motor impairment.

9. If a bolus of food is pocketed in the affected side, teach client how to use tongue to transfer food or apply external digital pressure to cheek to help remove the trapped bolus.	9. Poor tongue control with impaired oral sensation allows food into affected side.

10. For a client with cognitive deficits, do the following:
  a. Divide eating tasks into the smallest steps possible.
  b. Describe and point out food.
  c. Provide a verbal command for each step.
  d. Progress slowly. Limit conversation.
  e. Continue verbal assistance at each meal as needed.
  f. Provide several small meals to accommodate short attention span.
  g. Provide a written checklist for other staff.
	10. A confused client needs repetitive, simple instructions.

 Documentation

Flow records
  Intake of foods and fluids
Progress notes
  Swallowing difficulties

Unilateral Neglect Related to (Specify Site) Secondary to Right Hemispheric Brain Damage

Focus Assessment Criteria	Clinical Significance
1. Cuts in visual acuity and visual field	1. Loss of vision may occur on the side contralateral to the brain injury.
2. Sensory losses	2. Perceptual deficits result from right hemispheric brain damage.
3. Presence of neglect in one side of the body or face or in one limb	3. This assessment identifies what areas are neglected.

Goal

The client will demonstrate an ability to scan the visual field to compensate for loss of function or sensation in affected limb(s).

Indicators
- Describe the deficit and the rationale for treatments.
- Identify safety hazards in the environment.

Interventions	Rationales

1. Initially adapt the client's environment:
  a. Place the call light, telephone, and bedside stand on the unaffected side.
  b. Always approach client from the center or midline.
	1. This will minimize sensory deprivation initially; however, attempts should be made to have the person attend to both sides (American Stroke Association, 2001).

2. Orient the client to the environment and teach client to recognize the forgotten field (e.g., place the telephone out of client's visual field).	2. These reminders can help the client to adapt to the environment.

3. Provide a simplified, uncluttered environment:
  a. Provide a moment between activities.
  b. Provide concrete cues such as "You are on your side facing the wall."
	3.
	  a. Rapid movements can precipitate anxiety.
	  b. Cues can help with adjustment to position changes.

4. Reassure person that the problem is the result of CVA.	4. Clients know that something is wrong but may attribute it to being "disturbed."

5. Teach client to:
  a. Stroke the affected side.
  b. Watch the body part as she or he strokes.
  c. Vary tactile stimulation (e.g., warm, cold, rough, soft).
	5. Tactile stimulation of the affected parts promotes their integration into the whole body.

6. Teach client to scan the entire environment, turning the head to compensate for visual field cuts. Remind client to scan when ambulating.	6. Scanning can help to prevent injury and increase awareness of entire space.

7. Teach client to:
  a. Wear an arm sling when upright.
  b. Position the arm on a lapboard.
  c. Use a Plexiglas lapboard to view the affected leg.
  d. Recognize the danger of sources of cold and heat and moving machinery to the affected limb(s).
	7. Decreased sensation or motor function increases vulnerability to injury.

(continues on page 331)

Interventions continued	Rationales continued

8. For self-care, instruct the client to
  a. Attend to the affected side first.
  b. Use adaptive equipment as needed.
  c. Always check the affected limb(s) during activities of daily living (ADLs).
	8. The client may need specific reminders to prevent her or him from ignoring non-functioning body parts.

Documentation

Progress notes
  Presence of neglect
Discharge summary record
  Client teaching
  Response to teaching

High Risk for Ineffective Therapeutic Regimen Management Related to Altered Ability to Maintain Self at Home Secondary to Sensory/Motor/Cognitive Deficits and Lack of Knowledge of Caregivers of Home Care, Reality Orientation, Bowel/Bladder Program, Skin Care, and Signs and Symptoms of Complications, and Community Resources

Focus Assessment Criteria	Clinical Significance
1. Readiness and ability to learn and retain information	1. A client or family who does not achieve goals for learning requires a referral for assistance postdischarge.

Goals

The goals for this diagnosis represent those associated with discharge planning.

Interventions	Rationales
1. Teach about the condition, its cause, and treatments.	1. Understanding can reinforce the need to comply with the treatment regimen.

2. Identify risk factors that can be controlled:
 	
  a. Hypertension
 	
  b. Smoking
 	
  c. Obesity
  d. High-fat diet
	2. Focusing on factors that can be controlled can improve compliance, increase self-esteem, and reduce feelings of helplessness.
	  a. Hypertension with increased peripheral resistance damages the intima of blood vessels, contributing to arteriosclerosis.
	  b. Smoking produces tachycardia, raises blood pressure, and constricts blood vessels.
	  c. Obesity increases cardiac workload.
	  d. A high-fat diet may increase arteriosclerosis and plaque formation.

(continues on page 332)

Interventions continued	**Rationales** continued
e. High-sodium diet	e. Sodium controls water distribution throughout the body. A gain in sodium causes a gain in water, thus increasing the circulating volume.
3. Explain signs and symptoms of complications, and stress the need for prompt reporting: a. Development of or increase in weakness, lethargy, dysphagia, aphasia, vision problems, confusion b. Seizures	3. These signs and symptoms may indicate increasing ICP or cerebral tissue hypoxia.
4. Discuss with family the anticipated stressors associated with CVA and its treatment: a. Financial b. Changes in role responsibilities c. Dependency (Refer to Chapter 3, the Ill Adult: Issues and Responses, for information regarding the effects of chronic illness on families.) d. Caregiver responsibilities (Refer to Caregiver Role Strain in index for specific interventions.) • Assess for signs and symptoms of depression and treat accordingly.	4. Serious illness of a family member can cause disruption of family functioning. • Post-stroke depression affects two-thirds of clients (Eslinger, 2002). Post-stroke depression has negative effects on functional recovery; pharmacological treatment of depression can counterbalance this effect (Gainotti, 2001).
5. Provide information about or initiate referrals to community resources, e.g., counselors, home health agencies, and American Heart Association.	5. Such resources can provide needed assistance with home management and help to minimize the potentially destructive effects on the client and family.

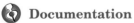 **Documentation**

Discharge summary record
   Client teaching
   Outcome achievement or status
   Referrals if indicated

For a care map on cerebrovascular accident (stroke), visit http://connection.lww.com

GUILLAIN-BARRÉ SYNDROME

Guillain Barró syndrome (GBS) is a complicated degenerative disorder that can be chronic or acute. Its etiology is unclear, but it is believed to be an autoimmune response to a viral infection. The syndrome affects all age groups, races, and both sexes; has presented in all countries; and is considered a non-seasonal syndrome. Statistics show that 5% of clients will die of respiratory–cardiovascular complications, 20% will suffer irreversible distal paresthesia (glove and stocking anesthesia), and 75% will "recover with little or no" residual deficits. The pathophysiologic findings are multiple and varied, including inflammation, demyelinization of the peripheral nerves, loss of granular bodies, and degeneration of the basement membrane of the Schwann cell resulting in an ascending symmetric flaccid paralysis and loss of cranial nerve functions (Hickey, 2001). The four different variants of GBS reflect the degree of peripheral nerve involvement: ascending GBS, descending GBS, Miller-Fisher variant, and pure motor GBS (Hickey, 2001, p. 690). Another term for GBS is chronic idiopathic demyelinating polyneuropathy (CIDP).

Time Frame
Initial diagnosis: 1 year

DIAGNOSTIC CLUSTER*

Collaborative Problems

PC: Acute Respiratory Failure (ARF)
PC: Autonomic Nervous System Failure
PC: Peripheral Nervous System Failure

Nursing Diagnoses	Refer to
High Risk for Ineffective Airway Clearance related to impaired ability to cough	Thoracic Surgery
High Risk for Impaired Skin Integrity related to immobility, incontinence, sensory-motor deficits	Immobility
Impaired Swallowing related to swallowing/chewing problems secondary to cranial nerve impairment	Cerebrovascular Accident [Stroke]
Activity Intolerance related to fatigue and difficulties in performing activities of daily living	Chronic Obstructive Pulmonary Disease

(continues on page 334)

Nursing Diagnoses continued	Refer to continued
Powerlessness related to the unpredictable nature of the condition	Chronic Obstructive Pulmonary Disease
High Risk for Self-Care Deficits related to flaccid paralysis, paresis, and fatigue	Immobility
High Risk for Deficient Diversional Activity related to inability to perform usual job-related/recreational-related activities	
High Risk for Interrupted Family Process related to nature of disorder, role disturbances, and uncertain future	
High Risk for Ineffective Therapeutic Regimen Management related to lack of knowledge of condition, treatments required, stress management, signs and symptoms of complications, and availability of community resources	

* This medical condition was not included in the validation study.

Discharge Criteria

Before discharge the client or family will

1. Relate intent to discuss fears and concerns with family/trusted friends after discharge.
2. Relate necessity of continuation of therapeutic programs.
3. Identify strategies to increase independence.
4. Relate safety precautions to prevent falls/injury.
5. Identify signs and symptoms that must be reported to a health care professional.

Collaborative Problems

Potential Complication: Acute Respiratory Failure (ARF)

Potential Complication: Autonomic Nervous System Failure

Potential Complication: Peripheral Nervous System Failure

Nursing Goal

The nurse will detect early signs/symptoms of (a) acute respiratory failure, (b) autonomic nervous system dysfunction, and (c) cranial nerve dysfunction and collaboratively intervene to stabilize the client.

Indicators
- Respirations 16–20 breaths/min (a)
- Oxygen saturation (pulse oximeter) >95% (a)
- Serum pH 7.35–7.45 (a)

- Serum PCO_2 35–45 mm Hg (a)
- Cardiac normal sinus rhythm (a)
- Bowels sounds present (b)
- Alert, oriented (a)
- Cranial nerves II–XXII intact (c)
- Urine output >30ml/hour (a)
- Dry, warm skin (b)

Interventions	Rationales
1. Monitor for signs and symptoms of acute respiratory failure (ARF) position to assist with breathing.	1. Ventilation may become necessary as acute Guillain-Barré progresses, due to increased damage to the phrenic and intercostal nerves.
a. Auscultate breath sounds.	a. Auscultating breath sounds assesses adequacy of air flow and detects the presence of adventitious sounds. (See Mechanical Ventilation for more information.)
b. Assess for secretions: • Encourage client to deep breathe and cough. • Position client side to side to assist movement of secretions. • Suction if client is unable to manage secretions. • Reassure client by maintaining a calm environment.	b. When the respiratory muscles fatigue, cough becomes ineffective leading to the accumulation of mucus and formation of mucous plugs in the airway. This accumulation of secretions causes alveolar collapse leading to acute respiratory failure.
c. Assess O_2 saturation via pulse oximetry.	c. Pulse oximetry provides ongoing data on O_2 saturation.
d. Assess blood gases: • Monitor for signs of decreased respiratory functions, pH, $PaCO_2$, O_2 saturation, and HCO_3.	d. An increase in the $PaCO_2$ levels indicates hypoventilation and that the client requires intubation to avoid acute respiratory failure.
e. Explain the necessity to intubation to the client and family.	e. Intubation is initiated to relieve shortness of breath to avoid acute respiratory failure, aspiration, and pneumonia.
f. Provide assurance and encouragement for the client.	f. This will reduce fear of disease process. Most Guillain-Barré clients have been healthy active individuals and suddenly are victims of dependency.
g. Report to physician condition status changes regarding: • Respiratory status and reduced vital capacity and arterial blood gases • Neurologic status • GI status	g. Early recognition enables prompt intervention to prevent further complications.
2. Monitor signs and symptoms of autonomic nervous system dysfunction: a. Blood pressure variations and cardiac dysrhythmias	2. a. The vagal nerve involvement causes hypertension, postural hypotension, bradycardia, sinus tachycardia, and diaphoresis.

(continues on page 336)

Interventions continued	Rationales continued
b. Cardiac monitor to evaluate cardiac status	b. Client may experience chest discomfort.
c. Urinary retention	c. Urinary retention is associated with autonomic nervous system dysfunction.
3. Monitor signs and symptoms of cranial nerve dysfunction: a. Assess the following: • Cranial nerve VII • Cranial nerve XI • Cranial nerve V • Cranial nerves III, IV, and VI • Cranial nerves IX, X, and XII	3. Demyelination of the efferent fibers of the spinal and cranial nerve creates a delay in conduction, resulting in motor weakness or loss of conduction, producing paralysis (Hickey, 2001). • Involvement of this cranial nerve will decrease the client's ability to wrinkle forehead and close eyes; client will present a flat affect (Hickey, 2001). • With involvement of this cranial nerve, client will lack the ability to turn head and have dropping of shoulders (Hickey, 2001). • Involvement of this cranial nerve will cause client to have loss of sensation in the face, forehead, and temples and to have problems with chewing (Hickey, 2001). • Involvement of these cranial nerves will cause client to have visual problems: pilosis, diplopia, deviations in upward, and outward movement of the eyeball (Hickey, 2001). • Involvement of these cranial nerves will cause client to have problems with coughing, swallowing, and the gag mechanism (Hickey, 2001).

 Related Physician-Prescribed Interventions

Medications. Steroids, antidysrhythmics (beta blocker, atropine)

Diagnostic Studies. Electrophysiologic studies (EMG), spinal tap

Therapies. EKG monitoring, plasmapheresis, mechanical ventilation

 Documentation

Flow records
    Vital signs
    Intake and output
    Neurologic assessment findings
Progress notes
    Changes in respiratory status
    Response to interventions
    Neurologic changes

Nursing Diagnoses

High Risk for Deficient Diversional Activity Related to the Inability to Perform Usual Job-Related/Recreational Activities

Focus Assessment Criteria	Clinical Significance
1. Fears	1–4. Previous history of the client's activity levels will influence the response to reduced activity levels.
2. Previous activity levels	
3. Vocational skills	
4. Interest and hobbies	

Goal

The client will report more satisfaction with activity level.

Indicators
- Report participation in activity each day.
- Relate methods of coping with feelings caused by boredom.

Interventions	Rationales

1. Identify the client's fears:
  a. Provide an environment conducive for verbalization of fears.
  b. Be a good listener.
  c. Provide accurate information to questions.
	1. The rapid onset of GBS causes the disease to equally affect mind and spirit. There are feelings of dependency and a constant fear of permanent paralysis or disability.

2. Identify client's vocation:
  a. Student
  b. Clerical
  c. Laborer
  d. Professional
  e. Retired
	2. Using client's previous work environment as a source of stimulation in performing self-care activities promotes an attitude of wellness and reduces anxiety of dependency.

3. Encourage visitors.	3. Visitors provide socialization. Have a select former GBS client visit with client for emotional support.
4. Discuss interests and hobbies.	4. Discussion will assist to identify recreational activities.

(continues on page 338)

Interventions continued	Rationales continued
5. Use variations in the physical environment and daily routines to increase mental stimulation: a. Select a room with a view for the client. b. Provide a variety of reading material. c. Provide reading stand if necessary. d. Obtain talking books. e. Encourage participation in board games with visitors. f. Use video tapes and games. g. Encourage family and friends to bring in pictures and small prized items. Allow client the choice of the arrangement of items. h. Change hygiene routines two or three times a week. i. Allow and encourage client to dress in street clothes. j. Allow trips to the hospital cafeteria with family and friends. Allow trips on hospital grounds with family, friends, and volunteers when condition is considered safe for the above activities. k. Encourage family and friends to bring the client's favorite foods. l. When the client is able to perform any vocational skills, encourage use of lap-top computers and preparation of reports. Continue studies of the client's physical tolerance and mental needs.	5. Change reduces boredom.
6. Encourage client to participate in open discussions with nursing staff and visitors concerning experiences, activities, and events of interest.	6. Discussions will give clients opportunities to involve themselves with various topics beyond self-concerns.

 Documentation

Progress notes
Participation in self-care activities

High Risk for Interrupted Family Process Related to Nature of Disorder, Role Disturbances, and Uncertain Future

Focus Assessment Criteria	Clinical Significance
1. Understanding of condition	1–4. The family unit is a system based on interdependent members and patterns that provide structure and support. Hospitalization can disrupt these patterns and possibly lead to excessive stressors for the family.
2. Usual family coping skills	
3. Current responses to condition	
4. Available community resources	

Goal

Family members will maintain functional system of mutual support for one another.

Indicators

- Frequently verbalize feelings to professional nurse and one another.
- Identify appropriate external resources available.

Interventions	Rationales
1. Provide family members with accurate, simply stated information regarding the condition.	1. Anxiety and stressful states produced by hospitalization impair the client's ability to process information effectively. Simple, brief explanations can relay valuable information effectively.
2. Identify the family's perception of the client's condition.	2. Evaluate each family member's learning level and provide teaching at this level of understanding.
3. Observe the dynamics of client–family interactions: a. Need to visit b. Effects of visit on client c. Family interactions d. Physical contact	3. These observations provide vital information regarding family roles, interrelationships, and the quality and amount of support family members are able to provide each other. Family members may need nursing permission to have physical contact with the client because of fear that they may "hurt" the client.
4. Observe and determine the family's coping skills: a. Assist the family with rethinking role responsibilities at home, redistributing tasks, and setting priorities.	4. The illness' rapid onset may create the necessity of role changes that place a family in a high-stress situation.
5. Assess emotional responses to stressors of hospitalization: a. Explain procedures. b. Explain therapies.	5. An understanding of the multiple procedures and therapies involved with diagnosis of condition will relieve the family's fears and enhance cooperation.
6. Encourage family members to reorganize their schedules to meet their own physical and psychological needs: a. Encourage calls to the nursing unit or client for condition reports. b. Encourage select friends to visit. c. Adjust visiting hours to accommodate family's schedules. d. Provide information on living accommodations near the hospital.	6. Family members who ignore their own health requirements are prone to becoming ill, which may reduce their effectiveness as support persons. A family member who falls ill may cause the client to have feelings of guilt.

(continues on page 340)

Interventions continued	Rationales continued

7. Observe and promote family strengths:
  a. Gradually involve family members in physical care of the client.
  b. Show your appreciation of the family involvement.
	7. Allowing involvement of family members with care will maintain a supportive family structure and strengthen the family unit.

8. Address the client's financial concerns and responsibilities:
  a. Provide an environment for client to verbalize concerns.
  b. Initiate a referral to Social Services for assistance.
	8. The sudden lack of income can be overwhelming, causing excessive mental anguish and slowing progress with goal setting.

High Risk for Ineffective Therapeutic Regimen Management Related to Lack of Knowledge of Condition, Treatments Required, Stress Management, Signs and Symptoms of Complications, and Availability of Community Resources

Focus Assessment Criteria	Clinical Significance
1. Readiness to learn and apply information	1. The client and family will require reinforcement of hospital learning from home health assistance on discharge.

Goals
Refer to discharge criteria.

Interventions	Rationales
1. Teach client and family the basic pathology of condition.	1. Understanding can improve compliance and reduce the family unit's frustrations.
2. Assist client with identification of realistic short-term goals.	2. Preparation of the client to set realistic goals for recovery will reduce feelings of depression if goals are not attainable.
3. Teach the client the value of continued strengthening–stretching exercise programs. Consult Physical Therapy.	3. Exercise will recondition all muscle groups.

4. Teach the client energy conservation techniques:
  a. Schedule planned rest periods.
  b. Exercise consistent with tolerance levels.
	4. Energy conservation can reduce fatigue (Penrose, 1993).

(continues on page 341)

Interventions continued	**Rationales** continued

5. Teach care of alterations in body functions:
  a. Bowel and bladder functions: Encourage an intake of fluids to 2,000 mL every day unless contraindicated.
  b. Nutritional requirements: Provide a diet high in calories and protein.
  c. Self-care deficits if necessary: Areas of concern:
    • Dressing
    • Grooming
    • Safe ambulation
	5.
	  a. These are required to prevent constipation resulting from reduced peristalsis and activity.
	  b. Protein and calories are required to rebuild muscle mass.
	  c. Encourage maximum client self-care with ADL activities for purpose of strengthening muscles and increasing independence.

6. Initiate a referral to rehabilitation services.	6. Client will require outpatient or home care for therapies postdischarge.

7. Explanation of signs and symptoms that must be reported to a health care professional:
  a. Productive cough
  b. Difficulty with urination or odor to urine
  c. Prolonged constipation
  d. Increased weakness or fatigue
  e. Weight loss
	7. Early interventions will minimize complications of the condition.

8. Provide information and literature to assist the client and family to manage at home. Refer to following resources:
  a. Guillain-Barré Syndrome Foundation provides emotional and educational support to client and family.
  b. Home health agency
  c. Case manager referral
	8. When client and family receive community support, they are able to cope more effectively with home management.
	  a. The mainstay of treatment is supportive care. Guillain Barré Syndrome Foundation, P.O. Box 262, Wynnewood, PA 19096

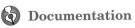 **Documentation**

Discharge summary record
  Client teaching
  Outcome achievement or status
  Referrals if indicated

MULTIPLE SCLEROSIS

Multiple sclerosis (MS) is an inflammatory demyelinating disease of the central nervous system (CNS) and can be characterized by acute exacerbations or gradual worsening of neurological function and disability (Ben-Zacharia, 2001). MS affects some 300,000 Americans, 75% of whom are female. The disease typically strikes during young adulthood with peak incidence between 20 and 40 years of age. MRI studies have shown clear evidence that central to the disease process is the gradual destruction of the myelin sheath surrounding nerve cells; this stripping of nerve fibers interferes with nerve conduction, which leads to various degrees of paralysis and the other symptoms of the disease (Glaser, 2000). MS can profoundly affect the client's quality of life. With its disability and chronic and unforeseeable features, MS brings about a series of changes in the client's life (Landoni, 2000). In people with MS, the range of main symptoms includes the loss of mobility and spasticity, pain tremors, abnormal eye movements, paroxysmal symptoms, bladder and bowel dysfunction, sexual disturbances, fatigue, and depression (Clanet, 2000).

 Time Frame

Initial diagnosis
Recurrent acute exacerbations

DIAGNOSTIC CLUSTER*

Collaborative Problems

Potential Complications:

Urinary Tract Infection
Renal Insufficiency
Pneumonia

Refer to:

Cerebrovascular Accident [Stroke]

Nursing Diagnoses

- High Risk for Disturbed Self-Concept related to the effects of prolonged debilitating condition on life style and on achieving developmental tasks and uncertain prognosis

- Impaired Comfort related to demyelinated areas of the sensory tract

- High Risk for Injury related to visual disturbances, vertigo, and altered gait

- Interrupted Family Processes related to nature of disorder, role disturbances, and uncertain future

---

(continues on page 343)

Nursing Diagnoses continued

- High Risk for Ineffective Therapeutic Regimen Management related to lack of knowledge of condition, treatments, prevention of infection, stress management, aggravating factors, signs and symptoms of complications, and community resources

• Impaired Swallowing related to cerebellar lesions	• Cerebrovascular Accident [Stroke]
• Impaired Verbal Communication related to dysarthria secondary to ataxia of muscles of speech	• Parkinson's Disease
• Fatigue related to extremity weakness, spasticity, fear of injury, and stressors	• Inflammatory Joint Disease
• Urinary Retention related to sensorimotor deficits	• Neurogenic Bladder
• Incontinence (specify) related to poor sphincter control and spastic bladder	• Neurogenic Bladder
• Powerlessness related to the unpredictable nature of condition (remission/exacerbation)	• Chronic Obstructive Pulmonary Disease

Related Care Plans

Immobility or Unconsciousness
Corticosteroid Therapy

* This medical condition was not included in the validation study.

Discharge Criteria

Before discharge, the client and family will

1. Relate an intent to share concerns with other family members or trusted friend(s).
2. Identify one strategy to increase independence.
3. Describe actions that can reduce the risk of exacerbation.
4. Identify signs and symptoms that must be reported to a health care professional.

Collaborative Problems

Potential Complication: Urinary Tract Infections

Potential Complication: Renal Insufficiency

Nursing Goal

The nurse will detect early signs/symptoms of (a) urinary tract infections and (b) renal insufficiency, and collaboratively intervene to stabilize the client.

Indicators

- Temperature 98–99.5°F (a)
- Urine specific gravity 0.005–0.030 (b)
- Urine output >30mg/hr (b)
- Clear urine (a, b)
- Blood urea nitrogen 5–25 mg/hr (b)
- Creatinine (b)
  - Male: 0.6–1.5 mg/dL
  - Female 0.6–1.1 mg/dL
- Potassium 3.5–5.0 mEq/L (b)
- Phosphate 1.8–2% mEq/L (b)
- Urine creatinine clearance (b)
  - Male 95–135 ml/min
  - Female 85–125 ml/min

Interventions	Rationales
1. Monitor for signs and symptoms of urinary tract infection:	1. MS exacerbation can be precipitated by any infection. MS can cause urinary retention owing to lesions of afferent pathways from the bladder. Resulting urine stasis contributes to microorganism growth. Also, corticosteroid therapy reduces the effectiveness of WBCs against infection.
a. Chills, fever	a. Bacteria can act as a pyrogen by raising the hypothalamic thermostat through the production of endogenous pyrogen that may mediate through prostaglandins. Chills can occur when the temperature setpoint of the hypothalamus changes rapidly.
b. Costovertebral angle (CVA) pain (a dull, constant backache below the 12th rib)	b. CVA pain results from distention of the renal capsule.
c. Leukocytosis	c. Leukocytosis reflects an increase in WBCs to fight infection through phagocytosis.
d. Foul odor or pus in urine	d. Bacteria change the odor and pH of urine.
e. Dysuria, frequency	e. Bacteria irritate bladder tissue, causing spasms and frequency.
2. Monitor for early signs and symptoms of renal insufficiency:	2. Repeated infections can alter renal function.
a. Sustained elevated urine specific gravity	a,b. Decreased ability of the renal tubules to reabsorb electrolytes causes increased urine sodium levels and increased specific gravity.
b. Elevated urine sodium levels	
c. Sustained insufficient urine output (30 mL/hr)	c,d. Decreased glomerular filtration rate eventually causes sustained insufficient urine output (<30 ml/m) and stimulates renin production that raises blood pressure in an attempt to increase blood flow to the kidneys.
d. Elevated blood pressure	

(continues on page 345)

Interventions continued	Rationales continued
e. Increasing blood urea nitrogen (BUN) and pressure serum creatinine, phosphate, and potassium, and decreased creatinine clearance	e. Decreased excretion of urea potassium and creatinine in the urine results in elevated BUN potassium and creatinine levels. The kidneys' inability to excrete hydrogen ions, phosphates, sulfates, and ketone bodies causes increased levels of acidosis.

3. Instruct client to:
  a. Drink a minimum of six to eight glasses of fluids per day.
  b. Empty bladder completely using Credé technique or self-cathing (see Credé and Clean Intermittent Self-Catheterization techniques in Neurogenic Bladder).
  c. Wipe from front to back especially after a bowel movement.
  d. Avoid undergarments made of synthetic materials.
  e. Empty bladder before and after intercourse.
  f. Change wet or soiled undergarments frequently in situations of dribbling or incontinence.
  g. Identify and notify the physician of urinary tract infection (UTI) signs and symptoms:
    • Foul-smelling urine
    • Increased frequency and urge to urinate
    • Change in color—dark yellow
    • Change in consistency—cloudy, sediment, or flecks of blood
	3.
	  a. Dilute urine reduces incidence of bacterial growth leading to infection
	  b. Reduces incidence of urinary stasis.
	
	  c. Reduces introduction of inappropriate bacterial exposure to the urinary tract.
	
	e,f. Reduces incidence of urinary stasis.

◤ Related Physician-Prescribed Treatments

Medications. Muscle relaxants, vitamin B, tricyclic antidepressants, corticosteroids, immunosuppressives, bulk-forming laxative, antibiotics, Beta Seron, beta blockers, Vitamin C: 1,000 mg four times/day (Shapiro, 1987), Avonex, glatiramer, spasmolytic (Urispas or Ditropan), urinary tract antiseptics (Macrodantin or Hyprex)

Intravenous Therapy. Adrenocorticotropic hormone (ACTH)

Laboratory Studies. Electrophoresis gammaglobulin level, white blood count, gamma globulin levels

Diagnostic Studies. EEG, MRI, CT scan of the brain, lumbar puncture, urinary retention study, evoked potential studies, electrophoresis, cerebrospinal fluid analysis

Therapies. Dependent on deficits (e.g., urinary and motor); dependent on bladder emptying problems (Credé technique, clean intermittent self-catheterization [CISC], indwelling Foley catheter, and suprapubic)

 Documentation

Flow records
Intake and output
Urine specific gravity

Nursing Diagnoses

High Risk for Disturbed Self-Concept Related to the Effects of Prolonged Debilitating Condition on Life Style and on Achieving Developmental Tasks, and Uncertain Prognosis

Focus Assessment Criteria	Clinical Significance
1. Previous exposure to persons with MS 2. Ability to express feelings about condition 3. Ability to share feelings with family members or significant others 4. Evidence of or others' reports of negative self-concept	1–4. This information helps the nurse to detect patterns of response due to adaptation. It may be helpful to note how the client's support persons view the client's self-concept; they can provide insight into factors that may have had a negative impact on self-concept and tend to be sensitive to subtle changes.
5. Participation in self-care 6. Evidence of adapting life style to disabilities	5,6. Participation in self-care and adapting goals to the disability indicate attempts to cope with the changes.

Goal

The client will report an improved sense of well-being and increased satisfaction with relationships, life style, and with himself or herself.

Indicators

- Acknowledge changes in body structure and function.
- Communicate feelings about disability.
- Participate in self-care.

Interventions	Rationales
1. Contact client frequently and treat her or him with warm, positive regard.	1. Frequent contact by the caregiver indicates acceptance and may facilitate trust. The client may be hesitant to approach the staff because of negative self-concept.

2. Encourage client to express feelings and thoughts about the following:
  a. Condition
  b. Progress
  c. Prognosis
  d. Effects on lifestyle
  e. Support system
  f. Treatments
	2. Encouraging client to share feelings can provide a safe outlet for fears and frustrations and can increase self-awareness.

3. Provide reliable information and clarify any misconceptions.	3. Misconceptions can needlessly increase anxiety and damage self-concept.

(continues on page 347)

Interventions continued	**Rationales** continued
4. Help client to identify positive attributes, hopefulness, and possible new opportunities. Explore new techniques to increase hopefulness such as relaxation techniques, exercise programs, religious and social activities (Glaser, 2000).	4. Client may tend to focus only on the change in self-image and not on the positive characteristics that contribute to the whole concept of self. The nurse must reinforce these positive aspects and encourage the client to reincorporate them into his new self-concept.
5. Assist with hygiene and grooming as needed.	5. Participation in self-care and planning can aid positive coping.
6. Encourage visitors.	6. Frequent visits by support persons can help the client feel that she or he is still a worthwhile, acceptable person; this should promote a positive self-concept.
7. Help the client to identify strategies to increase independence and maintain role responsibilities such as the following: a. Prioritizing activities b. Getting assistance with less valued or most fatiguing activities (e.g., shopping and housekeeping) c. Using energy conservation techniques (Refer to the nursing diagnosis Fatigue in the Inflammatory Joint Disease care plan for specific strategies.) Refer the MS client to an occupational therapist. d. Using mobility aids and assistive devices as needed	7. Occupational Therapy helps people with disabilities remain as independent as possible. Clients are taught to use special equipment and adapt to their home, workplace, or vehicle for greater safety and comfort (National Multiple Sclerosis Society, 2002).
8. Discuss ways that the client can provide support to support persons: a. Actively listening to their problems b. Attempting to decrease the focus on disabilities (Refer to Chapter 3, the Ill Adult: Issues and Responses, for more information.)	8. The nurse can help the client learn how to balance relationships and preserve the family system.
9. Allow client's support persons to share their feelings regarding the diagnoses and actual or anticipated effects.	9. Multiple sclerosis can have a big impact on families. They may have to share the financial burden, tackle additional chores, and help the person with MS deal with illness emotionally (National Multiple Sclerosis Society, 2002).

(continues on page 348)

Interventions continued	Rationales continued

10. Assess for signs of negative response to changes in appearance:
  a. Refusal to discuss loss
  b. Denial of changes
  c. Decreased self-care ability
  d. Social isolation
  e. Refusal to discuss the future
	10. These signs may indicate that the client is at high risk for unsuccessful adjustment.

11. Refer an at-risk client for professional counseling	11. Follow-up therapy may be indicated to assist with adjustment.

 Documentation

Progress notes
Present emotional status
Interventions
Response to interventions

Impaired Comfort Related to Demyelinated Areas of the Sensory Tract

Focus Assessment Criteria	Clinical Significance

1. Complaints of pain:
  a. Location
  b. Description
  c. Intensity
  d. Duration
 	
2. Effects of pain relief interventions
	1,2. The client is the best source of information about her or his pain and the degree of relief obtained from interventions.

Goals

- The client will relate improvement of pain and an increase in daily activities as evidenced by (specify).
- The client's family and significant others will support the management plan.

Indicators

- Participate in developing, carrying out, and evaluating the pain management plan.
- Report an improved sense of well-being and increased satisfaction with relationships, life style, and with himself or herself.

Interventions	Rationales
1. Acknowledge the existence of pain.	1. This establishes a trusting relationship (Glaser, 2000).
2. Identify location, nature, intensity, and duration of pain.	2,3. Pain has such a pervasive impact on role, mood, capacity to work and rest, and interpersonal relationships. Optimal therapy

(continues on page 349)

Interventions continued	Rationales continued
3. Assist client to identify the pain patterns (situations and factors that precipitate or intensify the pain).	treatment involves a commitment to the goal of controlled pain and improved quality of life (National Multiple Sclerosis Society, 2000).
4. Collaborate with pain management specialists to develop appropriate cutaneous, affective, and cognitive treatment modalities. 5. Collaborate with other care providers to establish management plan.	4,5. Team collaboration will establish an individualized and comprehensive pain management plan.
6. Review pain management options with client. 7. Teach the individual, family, and significant others about the nature of the pain. 8. Provide guidance regarding anticipated life-style changes. 9. Provide opportunities for the client to verbalize feelings related to the chronicity of pain.	6–9. Understanding the pain management plan and options will empower the client to make his or her own choices, which allows for greater acceptance.

 Documentation

Progress notes
Present description of client's pattern of pain
Interventions
Client's response to interventions
Discharge summary record
Client/family teaching
Outcome achievement or status
Referrals if indicated

High Risk for Injury Related to Visual Disturbances, Vertigo, and Altered Gait

Focus Assessment Criteria	Clinical Significance
1. Understanding/acceptance of potential visual problems 2. Client/family coping patterns 3. Current responses 4. Available resources	1–4. A clients' inability to understand and accept the visual disturbances related to MS will require a referral for assistance postdischarge depending on the severity of the visual disturbances.

Goal

The client will relate fewer injuries.

Indicators

- Relate the intent to use safety measures to prevent injury.
- Relate the intent to practice selected prevention measures.

Interventions	Rationales
1. Identify the type of visual disturbance the client is experiencing (diplopia, nystagmus, optic neuritis, or blurred vision).	1–4. Identifying the types of visual disturbances and options available will allow the client to take the necessary precautions. Optic neuritis is a common presenting symptom of MS; it often lasts for days to weeks but eventually will remit (Glaser, 1999).
2. Explain the options available (i.e., eye patch for diplopia, rest for fatigue-related disturbances, or environmental precautions for the visually impaired.)	
3. Reassure client that blindness seldom occurs, and many of these disturbances frequently remit (Glaser, 1999).	
4. Refer the client to the Association for the Blind.	

 Documentation

Progress notes
Present visual disturbances
Interventions
Client's response to interventions
Discharge summary record
Client teaching
Outcome achievement or status
Referrals if indicated

Interrupted Family Processes Related to Nature of Disorder, Role Disturbances, and Uncertain Future

Focus Assessment Criteria	Clinical Significance
1. Understanding of condition	1–4. The family unit is a system based on interdependency between members and patterns that provides structure and support. Chronic illness in one family member disrupts these relationships and patterns.
2. Family coping patterns	
3. Current response	
4. Available resources	

Goal
Family members will maintain functional system of mutual support for each other.

Indicators
- Frequently verbalize feelings to professional nurse and each other.
- Identify appropriate external resources available.

Interventions	Rationales
1. Convey an understanding of the situation and its impact on the family.	1. Communicating understanding and a sense of caring and concern facilitates trust and strengthens the nurse's relationships with the client and family.
2. Explore family members' perceptions of the situation. Encourage verbalization of feelings such as guilt, anger, and blame.	2. Verbalization can provide opportunities for clarification and validation of feelings and concerns; this contributes to family unity.
3. Determine if present coping mechanisms are effective.	3. Illness of a family member may cause great changes, putting the family at high risk for maladaptation. Multiple Sclerosis also involves the family: relatives must revise certain plans and projects made before the illness (Landoni, 2000).
4. Take steps to promote family strengths: a. Acknowledge the assistance of family members. b. Involve the family in the client's care. c. To prevent burnout, encourage family members to take time away from caregiving. d. Encourage humor. (Refer to Chapter 3, The Ill Adult: Issues and Responses, for more information.)	4. This can help to maintain the existing family structure and its function as a supportive unit.
5. Assist the family to reorganize roles at home, set new priorities, and redistribute responsibilities.	5. Planning and prioritizing can help to maintain family integrity and reduce stress.
6. Prepare the family for signs of depression, anxiety, anger, and dependency in the client and other family members.	6. Anticipatory guidance can alert members to potential problems before they occur; this enables prompt intervention at early signs.

(continues on page 352)

Interventions continued	Rationales continued
7. Encourage the family to call on its social network (e.g., friends, relatives, church members) for emotional and other support. Refer the family to receive psychological support.	7. Outside assistance may help to reduce the perception that the family must "go it alone." Psychological support could help relatives with the emotions associated with care giving. Support will also give them a listening space for their distresses and fears (Landoni, 2000).
8. Identify dysfunctional coping mechanisms: a. Substance abuse b. Continued denial c. Exploitation of one or more family members d. Separation or avoidance (Glaser, 2000) Refer for counseling as necessary.	8. A family with a history of unsuccessful coping may need additional resources. A family with unresolved conflicts prior to diagnosis is at high risk.
9. Direct to community agencies and other sources of assistance (e.g., financial, housekeeping, or direct care) as needed.	9. The family may need assistance to help with management at home.

 Documentation

Progress notes
Present family functioning
Interventions
Family's response to interventions
Discharge summary record
Referrals if indicated

High Risk for Ineffective Therapeutic Regimen Management Related to Lack of Knowledge of Condition, Treatments, Prevention of Infection, Stress Management, Aggravating Factors, Signs and Symptoms of Complications, and Community Resources

Focus Assessment Criteria	Clinical Significance
1. Readiness and ability to learn and retain information	1. A client or family that does not achieve goals for learning requires a referral for assistance postdischarge.

Goals

The goals for this diagnosis represent those associated with discharge planning. Refer to the discharge criteria.

Interventions	Rationales
1. Assist in formulating and accepting realistic short- and long-term goals.	1. Mutual goal setting reinforces the client's role in improving his or her quality of life.

(continues on page 353)

Interventions continued	Rationales continued
2. Teach about the diagnosis and management techniques including alternative methods.	2. Understanding can help to improve compliance and reduce exacerbations (MS Exchange, 1997a).
3. Discuss the importance of strengthening and stretching exercises for the arms, legs, and facial and respiratory muscles. Consult with a physical therapist (Glaser, 2000).	3. Exercise can prevent underused muscles from becoming weak. Facial and respiratory muscle exercises can improve speech deficits. Disability and loss of function can improve with physical therapy (Glaser, 2000).
4. Discuss the factors known to trigger exacerbation (Glaser, 1999): a. Undue fatigue or excessive exertion b. Overheating or excessive chilling or cold exposure c. Infections d. Hot environments e. Fever f. Emotional stress g. Pregnancy h. Cigarette smoking i. Alcohol use	4. This information gives the client insight into aspects of the condition that can be controlled; this may promote a sense of control and encourage compliance. As body temperature rises above the normal range, it blocks conduction across demyelinated regions in the brain and can worsen MS (Glaser, 1999).
5. Teach energy conservation techniques. (Refer to the nursing diagnosis Fatigue in the Inflammatory Joint Disease care plan for more information.)	5. Energy conservation can prevent fatigue.
6. Instruct a pregnant client or one contemplating pregnancy to consult a physician about the problems associated with pregnancy.	6. Pregnancy is associated with onset and exacerbations of MS.
7. Explain the hazards of infection and ways to reduce the risk: a. Avoid contact with infected persons. b. Receive immunization against influenza and streptococcal pneumonia if advised. c. Cleanse all equipment and utensils well. d. Eat a well-balanced diet and get sufficient rest. e. Drink 2000 mL of fluids daily unless contraindicated by renal insufficiency.	7. Minor infections can cause serious problems in a client with MS. a. This precaution reduces the risk of cross-infection. b. Immunization confers protection against these infections. c. Proper cleansing removes microorganisms and secretions that are media for microorganism growth. d. Adequate nutrition and rest promote overall good health and increase resistance to infection. e. Adequate hydration prevents concentrated urine with high levels of bacteria.

(continues on page 354)

Interventions continued	**Rationales** continued

8. Teach the importance of constructive stress management and reduction; explain measures such as the following:
  a. Progressive relaxation techniques
  b. Self-coaching
  c. Thought-stopping
  d. Assertiveness techniques
  e. Guided imagery
If possible, refer to community resources for specific courses or assistance.
	8. Managing stress helps the multiple sclerosis client to cope and adapt to changes caused by MS. Approaches to stress management include massage therapy, exercise programs, and involvement in religious and social activities (Glaser, 2000).

9. Teach the effects of MS on bowel function and the techniques to prevent constipation or incontinence. (Refer to appropriate nursing diagnoses in the Immobility or Unconsciousness care plan for specific interventions.)	9. Clients rate constipation and fecal incontinence as having a major impact on their lives (Wiesel, 2000). Preparing the client for these bowel symptoms helps him or her to handle them. Constipation results from decreased paralysis because of immobility and decreased fluid and fiber intake. Bowel incontinence is caused by lesions of the efferent pathways of the corticospinal tract, resulting in loss of sphincter control.

10. Explore with the client and partner, current and previous sexual patterns and partner problems that may interfere with sexual activity:
  a. Low self-esteem
  b. Fatigue
  c. Ejaculatory disorders
  d. Thigh muscle spasms
  e. Fear of bowel or bladder incontinence
	10. Libido is negatively influenced by stress, fatigue, and low self-esteem. Ejaculatory disorders result from lesions in the pyramidal tracts of the spinal cord.
	
	  Many people with multiple sclerosis are able to enjoy a completely normal sex life. Others may have some problems. Communicating openly and being flexible about sexual expression are often the keys to enjoyment (National Multiple Sclerosis Society, 2002).

11. Discuss options available for sexual enjoyment:
  a. Medication management
 	
  b. Phospho diesterase Type 5 inhibitor (Viagra), Prostaglandins; or penile prosthetics
  c. Positioning
	11.
	
	  a. Client may be taking medications that interfere with the normal sexual response (i.e., some antihypertensives, antidepressants or tranquilizers) or may need the appropriate medication relating to the specific MS problem (i.e., spasticity or leg spasms can be reduced by timing antispastic medications to maximize effectiveness during sexual activity).
	  b. Client may be experiencing insufficient erections secondary to MS lesions.
	
	  c. Proper positions may reduce spasticity problems.

(continues on page 355)

Interventions continued	Rationales continued
12. Refer to appropriate health care professional (neurologist, urologist, or counselor).	12. The client may need follow-up therapy.
13. Refer to a counselor for continued therapy.	
14. Explain the signs and symptoms that must be reported to a health care professional: a. Worsening of symptoms (e.g., weakness, spasticity, visual disturbances) b. Temperature elevation c. Change in urination patterns or cloudy, foul-smelling urine d. Productive cough with cloudy greenish sputum e. Cessation of menses	14. Early detection enables prompt intervention to minimize complications. a. Worsening symptoms may herald an exacerbation. b–d. These symptoms may indicate infection (urinary tract or pulmonary). e. Cessation of menses may indicate pregnancy, which can exacerbate MS.
15. Provide information and materials to assist the client and family to maintain goals and manage at home from sources such as the following: a. Multiple Sclerosis Society b. Home health agencies c. American Red Cross d. Individual/family counselors e. Jimmie Heuga Center	15. A client who feels well supported can cope more effectively with the multiple stressors associated with chronic debilitating disease.

Documentation

Discharge summary record
Client teaching
Outcome achievement or status
Referrals if indicated

Refer to website http://connection.lww.com for critical paths for this condition.

MYASTHENIA GRAVIS

Myasthenia gravis (MG) is a chronic, unpredictable autoimmune disease that is characterized by the destruction of acetylcholine receptors at the neuromuscular junctions, producing muscle weakness and excessive fatigue. The disease affects voluntary skeletal muscles in single or multiple groups with involvement of the external ocular muscle only to generalized muscle groups affecting respirations, speech, chewing, and swallowing (Hickey, 2001).

A thymectomy is beneficial in 60% to 70% of patients with MG by providing relief of symptoms. The role of the thymus gland is unclear but may be a source of immunologic stimulus. Exacerbations of MG may be triggered by infection, stress, ultraviolet light, and pregnancy (Kernich & Kaminski, 1995).

The age of onset of MG is 20 to 30 years for women and 40 to 60 years for men; after 60 years of age, the incidence is similar for both sexes (Kernich & Kaminski, 1995). The onset of MG is usually gradual, although rapid onset has been reported in association with respiratory infections or emotional upsets. The course of the illness is extremely variable (Hickey, 2001).

 Time Frame

Initial diagnosis
Acute exacerbations
Remissions

⟨⟩ DIAGNOSTIC CLUSTER*

Collaborative Problems

PC: Respiratory Insufficiency
PC: Myasthenia/Cholinergic Crisis

Nursing Diagnoses	**Refer to**
• High Risk for Ineffective Airway Clearance related to impaired ability to cough	• Chronic Obstructive Pulmonary Disease
• High Risk for Impaired Swallowing related to cerebellar dysfunction	• Cerebrovascular Accident [Stroke]
• High Risk for Injury related to visual disturbances, unsteady gait, weakness	• Cerebrovascular Accident [Stroke]
• High Risk for Impaired Verbal Communications related to involvement of muscles for speech	• Parkinson's

---

(continues on page 357)

Nursing Diagnoses continued	Refer to continued
• High Risk for Impaired Skin Integrity related to immobility	• Immobility
• High Risk for Activity Intolerance related to fatigue and difficulty in performing activities of daily living	• Pressure Sores
• High Risk for Powerlessness related to the unpredictable nature of the condition (remissions/exacerbations)	• Cerebrovascular Accident [Stroke]
• High Risk for Ineffective Therapeutic Regimen Management related to insufficient knowledge of condition, treatments, prevention of infections, stress management, aggravating factors, signs and symptoms of complications, and community resources	• Chronic Obstructive Pulmonary Disease

*This medical condition was not included in the validation study.

Discharge Criteria

1. Relate intent to share concerns with other family members or a trusted friend.
2. Relate side effects of medications.
3. Identify strategies to reduce stress.
4. Identify signs and symptoms that must be reported to a health care professional.
5. Describe long-term management of the disease.
6. State the value of wearing a Med-Alert bracelet.
7. Receive information/referral to the local chapter of the Myasthenia Gravis Foundation.

Collaborative Problems

Potential Complication: Respiratory Distress

Potential Complication: Myasthenic/Cholinergic Crisis

Nursing Goal

The nurse will detect early signs/symptoms of (a) respiratory insufficiency and (b) myasthenia/cholinergic crisis and collaboratively intervene to stabilize client.

Indicators
• Respirations 16–20 breaths/min (a)
• Clear breath sounds with no adventitious sounds (a)
• Vital capacity 4600 ml (a)
• Expiratory reserve volume 1100 ml (a)
• Total long capacity 5800 ml (a)
• Intact cough-gag reflexes (b)
• Heart rate 60–100 beats/min (a, b)
• Intact muscle strength (b)
• Dry, warm skin (a, b)

- B/P >90/60, <140–90 mm Hg (a, b)
- No nausea/vomiting (b)
- No muscle twitching/cramping (b)

Interventions	Rationales
1. Monitor for signs and symptoms of respiratory distress: a. Monitor for changes in respiratory status: • Respiratory rate increase • Change in respiratory pattern • Change in breath sounds • Serial vital capacity measurements b. Monitor for increased pulse rate. c. Elevate head of bed 30 to 40 degrees.	1. The most dangerous aspect of MG is weakened muscle contraction and resultant ineffective inspiration. The client's first complaint may be dyspnea at rest. a. Antibodies to acetylcholine receptors at muscle sites block nerve transmission to the striated muscles, specifically the intercostal muscles and diaphragm, that control respiratory functions (Porth, 2001). b. This sign indicates difficulty with air exchange. c. Elevation will enhance diaphragmatic movement.
2. Assess ability to clear airway: a. Cough-gag reflexes b. Suction secretions as necessary every ½ to 1 hour. c. Postural drainage d. Position client side to side.	2. a. The absence or presence of reflexes denotes weakness of muscle group innervated by the 10 cranial nerves originating in the brain stem. These are the muscles necessary for chewing, swallowing, eye movements, neck movements, and facial expressions (Hickey, 2001). b. If the person cannot manage secretions, this can lead to intubation for secretion control or ventilation support. c. To mobilize secretions d. To reduce pooling of secretions and prevent aspiration and pneumonia
3. Assess communication ability: a. Anxiety and panic: • Provide a calm, reassuring environment. • Provide explanations for treatment. b. Increased muscle weakness involving speech: • Listen to client and repeat requests for accuracy. • Ask questions that require yes or no answers. • Ask client to move fingers or toes, or give yes or no answer.	3. Weakness in facial muscles can affect facial expression, phonation, and articulation. A normal smile may look like a snarl, and speech may become slurred (Hickey, 2001). a. To reduce anxiety and promote easier respirations b. Establish a method of communication to reduce anxiety, panic.

(continues on page 359)

Interventions continued	**Rationales** continued
4. Monitor response of patient to Tensilon test (edrophonium chloride).	4. This medication is administered intravenously, providing a differentiated diagnosis of myasthenia gravis/cholinergic crisis. A positive Tensilon test equals an increase in muscle strength in 30 to 90 seconds after administration, suggesting the diagnosis of a myasthenia gravis (O'Donnell, 1996).
5. Report to physician status changes in respiratory status, increased difficulty with swallowing and speech.	5. To adjust treatment
6. Monitor for signs and symptoms of myasthenic/cholinergic crisis: a. Monitor for • Restlessness, anxiety • Dyspnea • Generalized muscle weakness • Increased bronchial selections/sweating • Difficulty swallowing/speaking • Bradycardia/tachycardia • Hypotension/hypertension	6. Myasthenic crises result from inadequate amounts of acetylcholine (ACh) due to disease progression or undermedication. Cholinergic crises can result from excessive amounts of ACh from overmedication with anticholinesterase drugs. These are often difficult to distinguish clinically. a. Refer to rationale above.
7. Monitor for: a. Nausea and vomiting b. Diarrhea and abdominal cramping c. Sweating d. Increased salivation/bronchial secretions e. Tachycardia/bradycardia/hypotension f. Increased muscle weakness g. Increased fatigue h. Bronchial relaxation (collapse) i. Muscle twitching/cramping	7. These symptoms are adverse effects of cholinergic drugs. The anticholinesterase medication that helps to improve acetylcholine effects at neuromuscular junctions and helps to control symptoms also has an effect on the autonomic nervous system. Acetylcholine activates muscarinic receptors that have an effect on smooth muscle cardiac muscles and granular tissue. Acetylcholine activates nicotinic receptors; this involves function of skeletal muscle and the ganglion cells (O'Donnell, 1996).
8. Assess for diplopia (double vision): a. Alternate patching of eyes for short periods.	8. An eye patch will relieve double vision and provide comfort and ability to do self-care.
9. Assess for ptosis: a. Tape eyes open for short intervals. b. Use artificial tears to prevent corneal damage. c. Use sunglasses to reduce photophobia.	9. To provide comfort and avoid eye injuries (Hickey, 2001)

Related Physician-Prescribed Interventions

Medications. Mestinon (pyridostigmine bromide), Prostigmin (neostigmine bromide), Mytelase (ambenonium chloride), corticosteroids, immunosuppressants (azathioprine, cyclophosphamide, intravenous immunoglobulin [IVIG])

Diagnostic Studies. Electrophysiologic studies (electromyogram), nerve conduction studies, Tensilon (edrophonium chloride), chest x-ray, swallowing video

Therapies. Plasmapheresis, tracheotomy, thymectomy, mechanical ventilation

Documentation
Vital signs
Neurologic
Progress notes
   Change in status
   Response to interventions

Nursing Diagnoses

High Risk for Ineffective Therapeutic Regimen Management Related to Insufficient Knowledge of Condition, Treatments, Prevention of Infections, Stress Management, Aggravating Factors, Signs and Symptoms of Complications, and Community Resources

Focus Assessment Criteria	Clinical Significance
1. Readiness to learn and apply information	1. The client–family may need home health assistance for management on discharge.

Goals
The goals for this diagnosis represent those associated with discharge planning. Refer to the discharge criteria.

Interventions	Rationales
1. Teach regarding diagnosis and long-term management of disease and determine client-family level of learning.	1. The client–family must have a good understanding of this chronic disease process to enable them to recognize symptoms leading to complications.

2. Teach client the signs and symptoms of myasthenic crisis versus cholinergic crisis:
  a. Myasthenic crisis:
    • Increased blood pressure
    • Tachycardia
    • Restlessness
    • Apprehension
    • Increased bronchial secretions, lacrimation, and sweating
    • Generalized muscle weakness
    • Absent cough reflex
	2. A myasthenic crisis results from an insufficiency of acetylcholine, usually induced by a change or withdrawal of medications. Client needs to know the symptoms of overdose and underdose of his or her medications.
	   Cholinergic crises result from excessive amounts of acetylcholine, usually from overmedication with anticholinesterase medication.

(continues on page 361)

Interventions continued | **Rationales** continued

- Dyspnea
- Difficulty swallowing
- Difficulty speaking
  b. Cholinergic crisis:
  - Decreased blood pressure
  - Bradycardia
  - Restlessness
  - Apprehension
  - Increased bronchial secretions, lacrimation, and sweating
  - Generalized muscle weakness
  - Fasciculations
  - Dyspnea
  - Difficulty swallowing
  - Difficulty speaking
  - Blurred vision
  - Nausea and vomiting
  - Abdominal cramps and diarrhea

---

3. Teach incompatibility of medications:
   a. Quinine—also found in tonics.
   b. Alcohol—speeds drugs' absorption and should be consumed 1 hour after taking anticholinesterase medications.
   c. Aminoglycoside antibiotics are to be used with caution.
   d. Other medications known to aggravate MG are morphine, diuretics, procainamide, and beta blockers (O'Donnell, 1996).

3. The client–family need to know that these medications will aggravate the disease. Other medical professionals may unknowingly order these medications.

---

4. Teach administration of medications:
   a. Correct time—1 hour before meals
   b. Accurate dosage
   c. Advise client to keep a medication diary to determine peak function of medications.

4. The exact time of an accurate medication dosage coincides with increases in energy demands. Taking medications before meals is essential to provide muscle strength for chewing food.

---

5. Teach how to manage diplopia and ptosis:
   a. Use eye patch; alternate eye every 2 to 4 hours.

   b. Use lubricating eye drops.

5.
   a. Eye patch will relieve double vision and provide the patient with comfort and ability to do self-care (Hickey, 2001).
   b. Eye drops will prevent corneal abrasions (Hickey, 2001).

---

6. Teach energy conservation.

6. Rest periods should be scheduled when medication peaks are low. Client should learn to space tasks. Teach family the importance of vital rest periods and planning activities.

(continues on page 362)

Interventions continued	**Rationales** continued
7. Teach strategies of stress management: a. Use of relaxation tapes b. Guided imagery c. Referral to community resource for stress management course	7. Uncontrolled stress factors can lead to an acute exacerbation of the disease.
8. Inform client of factors that are known to trigger exacerbations: a. Excessive weakness b. Increased stressors c. Upper respiratory infection d. Exposure to ultraviolet light e. Surgery f. Pregnancy g. Hot and cold temperatures	8. This information can provide client with insight of disease and promote a sense of personal control. If client is pregnant or considering a pregnancy, she should consult with physician as the course of pregnancy with MG is unpredictable and she will require close observation.
9. Explain signs and symptoms that must be reported to a health care professional: a. Increased muscle weakness b. Progressive symptoms of visual disturbance. Difficulty with breathing, chewing and swallowing, and sweating c. Productive cough	9. Early intervention can minimize pending complications. These symptoms can be warnings of a crisis.
10. Teach chewing and swallowing techniques: a. Sit in an upright position with head slightly forward when eating. b. Wear a soft cervical collar for neck support while eating. c. Limit hot food intake. d. Refer to Impaired Swallowing—CVA Care Plan for specific teaching to prevent aspiration.	10. a. This position will create a gravity force for the downward motion of food. b. A collar will help to support the neck and head and reduce fatigue. c. Hot foods tend to increase muscle weakness.
11. Provide information and literature to assist client—family to manage long-term goals at home. Resources as follows: a. Myasthenia Gravis Foundation b. Home health agency c. Case manager referral	11. The client—family who receives community support will cope more effectively with this progressive chronic disease.

 Documentation
Discharge summary record
   Client teaching
   Outcome achievement or status
   Referrals if indicated

NEUROGENIC BLADDER

A neurogenic bladder is defined as any bladder disturbance attributable to motor or sensory pathways in the central or peripheral nervous systems that have input to the bladder (Hickey, 2001). Lapides and Diokno (1976) classified neurogenic bladders into five groups to help pinpoint the underlying pathologic process: reflex, autonomous, uninhibited, sensory paralytic, and motor paralytic neurogenic bladders.

- *Autonomous* neurogenic bladder results from destruction of the *bladder center in the sacral spinal cord.* The client feels no conscious sensation to void and has no micturition reflex; the bladder empties irregularly.
- A *reflex* neurogenic bladder occurs with damage between the sacral spinal cord and the cerebral cortex. The client has no sensation to void and cannot void volitionally. The uninhibited detrusor contractions may be poorly sustained with inefficient bladder emptying. If the micturition reflex arc is intact, reflex voiding can occur. If there is detrusor-sphincter dyssynergy (DSD), there will be increased bladder pressure and high residual urine.
- *Motor paralytic* neurogenic bladder occurs when there is damage in the anterior horn cells of S2–S4 ventral roots and the motor side of the micturition reflex arc is damaged. The client has intact sensation but experiences partial or complete motor loss of function. Bladder capacity may increase and have a large residual urine. There may be overflow incontinence.
- *Sensory paralytic* or neurogenic bladder occurs when the dorsal roots of S2–S4 are damaged. The client loses sensation but can void volitionally. Bladder capacity may increase, with subsequent overflow incontinence.
- In *uninhibited* neurogenic bladder resulting from damage to the *bladder center in the cerebral cortex,* the client has limited sensation of bladder distention but no ability to inhibit urination. Urgency results from the short time between limited sensation to void and the uninhibited bladder contraction. The bladder usually empties completely.

Time Frame
Secondary diagnosis (hospitalization not usual for neurogenic bladder)

⦾ DIAGNOSTIC CLUSTER*

Collaborative Problems

PC: Renal Calculi
PC: Vesicoureteral Reflux
PC: Urinary Tract Infection
PC: Renal Failure/Hydronephrosis/Multiple Sclerosis

Nursing Diagnoses	Refer to
Urinary Retention related to chronically overfilled bladder with loss of sensation of bladder distention	
Urinary Retention related to detrusor–sphincter dyssynergy (DSD)	

(continues on page 364)

Nursing Diagnoses continued	Refer to continued
Reflex Incontinence related to absence of sensation to void and loss of ability to inhibit bladder contraction	
High Risk for Infection related to retention of urine or introduction of urinary catheter	
Urge Incontinence related to inability to inhibit urination after urge is perceived	
High Risk for Loneliness related to embarrassment of incontinence in front of others and fear of odor from urine	
High Risk for Ineffective Therapeutic Regimen Management related to insufficient knowledge of etiology of incontinence, management, bladder retraining programs, signs and symptoms of complications, and community resources	
High Risk for Dysreflexia related reflex stimulation of sympathetic nervous system secondary to loss of autonomic control	Spinal Cord Injury
High Risk for Impaired Skin Integrity related to constant irritation from urine	Pressure Ulcers

* This medical condition was not included in the validation study.

Discharge Criteria

Before discharge, the client or family will

1. Identify measures to reduce incontinence.
2. Relate the intent to discuss fears and concerns with family after discharge.
3. Relate signs and symptoms that must be reported to a health care professional.
4. Demonstrate correct self-catheterization technique.
5. Relate the intent to continue exercises and fluid intake program at home.

Collaborative Problems

Potential Complication: Renal Calculi

Potential Complication: Urinary Tract Infection

Nursing Goal

- The nurse will detect early signs/symptoms of (a) renal calculi and (b) urinary tract infections and collaboratively intervene to stabilize the client.

Indicators

- Temperature 98–99.5°F (a, b)
- Urine specific gravity 0.005–0.030 (a, b)
- Urine output >30 ml/min (a, b)
- Clear urine (a, b)
- Prealbumin 20–50 mg/dL (a, b)
- No flank pain (a, b)

Interventions	Rationales

1. Monitor for signs and symptoms of renal calculi:
 	
  a. Acute flank pain
  b. CVA (costovertebral angle) pain (a dull, constant backache below the 12th rib)
 	
  c. Hematuria
 	
  d. Nausea and vomiting
	1. Urinary stasis and infection increase the risk of renal calculi because of increased precipitants in the urine.
	a,b. Stones can cause severe pain owing to obstruction and ureter spasms or CVA pain due to distention of the renal capsule.
	c. The abrasive action of the stone can sever small blood vessels.
	d. Afferent stimuli in the renal capsule may cause pylorospasm of the smooth muscle of the GI tract.

2. Monitor for signs of urinary tract infection:
  a. Change in urine color, odor, volume
  b. Fever
  c. Increased urgency, frequency, or incontinence
	2. UTIs, especially if frequent or chronic, will place a person at risk for upper tract disease as well as sclerosis of ureters, causing increased renal pressure.

3. Monitor for urinary retention by paying attention to output amounts vs. intake amounts.	3. Urine retention, especially associated with high pressure, can cause reflux at the vesicoureteral junction with potential hydronephrosis.

◤ Related Physician-Prescribed Interventions

Medications. Antimuscarinics, terazosin, alpha-adrenergic stimulators, phenoxybenzamine, pseudophedrine, dicyclomine, flavoxate, imipramine, propantheline, methantheline

Diagnostic Studies. Voiding cystourethrogram

Therapies. Corrective surgery

 Documentation

Flow records
  Urine output and characteristics
  Intake and output
Progress notes
  Complaints of pain, nausea, vomiting
  Urination pattern
  Complaints of change in urinary status

Nursing Diagnoses

Urinary Retention Related to Chronically Overfilled Bladder with Loss of Sensation of Bladder Distention

Focus Assessment Criteria	Clinical Significance
1. Perception of need to void	1–5. The client may perceive bladder fullness but cannot volitionally empty the bladder, or may have no sensation of fullness or volitional control to empty. When sufficient urine collects in the bladder to stretch the detrusor muscle, bladder pressure exceeds urethral pressure resulting in overflow incontinence or dribbling.
2. Complaints of incontinence or dribbling	
3. Reports of relief after voiding	
4. Urine characteristics	
5. Bladder distention and capacity	

Goal

The client will achieve a state of dryness that is personally satisfactory.

Indicators
- Empty the bladder using Credé's or Valsalva maneuver with a residual urine of less than 50 mL, if indicated.
- Void voluntarily.

Interventions	Rationales

1. Teach the client methods to empty the bladder.
  a. Credé's maneuver:
    • Place the hands (either flat or in fists) just below the umbilical area, one hand on top of the other.
    • Firmly press down and in toward the pelvic arch.
    • Repeat six or seven times until no more urine is expelled.
    • Wait several minutes, then repeat again to ensure complete emptying.
  b. Valsalva's maneuver (bearing down):
    • Lean forward on thighs.
    • Contract abdominal muscles, if possible, and strain or bear down while holding the breath.
    • Hold until urine flow stops; wait 1 minute, then repeat.
    • Continue until no more urine is expelled.
  c. Clean intermittent self-catheterization (CISC) used alone or in combination with the above methods. (Refer to the nursing diagnosis High Risk for Ineffec-
	1.
	
	a. In many clients, Credé's maneuver can help to empty the bladder. This maneuver is inappropriate, however, if the urinary sphincters are chronically contracted. In this case, pressing the bladder can force urine up the ureters as well as through the urethra. Reflux of urine into the renal pelvis may result in renal infection.
	
	b. Valsalva's maneuver contracts the abdominal muscles which manually compresses the bladder.
	
	c. CISC prevents overdistention, helps to maintain detrusor muscle tone, and ensures complete bladder emptying. CISC may be used initially to determine

(continues on page 367)

Interventions continued	Rationales continued
tive Therapeutic Regimen Management in this care plan for specific teaching points.)	residual urine following Credé's maneuver or tapping. As residual urine decreases, catheterization may be tapered. CISC may recondition the voiding reflex in some clients.
d. A baseline cystometrogram (CMG) may be warranted.	d. Discuss diagnostic testing CMD to progress a bladder program.

🐾 Documentation

Flow records
   Fluid intake
   Voiding patterns (amount, time, method used)
Discharge summary record
   Client teaching
   Outcome achievement or status

Urinary Retention Related to Detrusor–Sphincter Dyssynergy (DSD)

Focus Assessment Criteria	Clinical Significance
1. Level of cord injury	1–8. Urinary retention related to DSD occurs with a reflex bladder. Sensation may be present and the client may perceive urgency. Inability of the distal sphincter to relax in coordination with detrusor contraction results in increased bladder pressure with emptying and large amounts of residual urine. Urine may be released in small amounts with premature closure of the sphincter, causing urine to be retained. Clients may report frequency of urination because the bladder never empties.
2. Perception of need to void	
3. Voiding pattern	
4. Relief after voiding	
5. Reflexes (anal, bulbocavernosus)	
6. Bladder distention, residual urine (amount)	
7. Fluid intake pattern	
8. Urine characteristics	

Goal

Refer to Goals for Urinary Retention p 366.

Interventions	Rationales
1. Cutaneous triggering by suprapubic tapping (see under Reflex Incontinence)	
2. The anal stretch maneuver (see under Reflex Incontinence)	

(continues on page 368)

Interventions continued	Rationales continued
3. Intermittent catheterization (see under Urinary Retention related to chronically overfilled bladder)	

🕊 Documentation

Flow records
    Fluid intake
    Urine output
    Amount from IC immediately after voiding
Discharge summary record
    Client teaching
    Outcome achievement or status

Reflex Incontinence Related to Absence of Sensation to Void and Loss of Ability to Inhibit Bladder Contraction

Focus Assessment Criteria	Clinical Significance
1. Level of cord injury	1–9. Reflex incontinence entails partial or complete loss of the sensation of bladder distention resulting in repeated involuntary reflexes that produce spontaneous voiding. Data collection is indicated to determine the extent of bladder control and identify appropriate interventions.
2. Perception of need to void	
3. Relief after voiding	
4. Voiding pattern	
5. Reflexes (anal, bulbocavernosus)	
6. Bladder distention, residual urine (amount)	
7. Fluid intake pattern	
8. Urine characteristics	
9. Use of external stimuli (triggering)	

Goal

The client will report a state of dryness that is personally satisfactory.

Indicators
• Have a residual urine volume of less that 50 mL.
• Use triggering mechanisms to initiate reflex voiding.

Interventions	Rationales
1. Ensure adequate fluid intake (at least 2,000 mL/day unless contraindicated).	1. Adequate fluid intake prevents concentrated urine that can irritate the bladder and cause increased bladder instability.

(continues on page 369)

Interventions continued	Rationales continued
2. Consult with the physician about prescribing medication to relax the bladder (e.g., anticholinergics).	2. Anticholinergic medications can eliminate hyperirritable and uninhibited bladder contractions and allow successful bladder retraining.

3. Teach techniques to trigger reflex voiding.
  a. Place client in half-sitting position.
  b. Tap on bladder wall at a rate of 7 to 8 times in 5 seconds for ½ minute.
 	
  c. Tell client to contract abdominal muscles.
	3.
	  a,b. Stimulating the reflex arc relaxes the internal sphincter of the bladder and allows urination. Stimulating the bladder wall or cutaneous sites (e.g., suprapubic, pubic) can trigger the reflex arc.
	  c. Contraction of abdominal muscles compresses the bladder to empty it.

4. Cutaneous triggering by suprapubic tapping:
  • Assume a half-sitting position.
  • Using the fingers of one hand, aim tapping directly at the bladder wall; tap at a rate of 7 or 8 times every 5 seconds for a total of 50 taps.
  • Shift the site of tapping over the bladder to find the most effective site.
  • Continue stimulation until a good stream starts.
  • Wait about 1 minute, then repeat stimulation until bladder is empty. (One or two series of stimulations without urination indicates bladder emptying.)
  • If tapping is ineffective, perform each of the following for 2 to 3 minutes each:
 	
    Stroke the glans penis.
    Lightly punch the abdomen above the inguinal ligaments.
    Stroke the inner thigh.
	4. External cutaneous stimulation can stimulate the voiding reflex.

5. The anal stretch maneuver:
  • Sit on the commode or toilet, leaning forward on the thighs.
  • Insert one or two lubricated fingers into the anus to the anal sphincter.
  • Spread fingers apart or pull in the posterior direction to stretch the anal sphincter.
  • Bear down and void while performing the Valsalva maneuver.
  • Relax then repeat the procedure until the bladder is empty.
	5. Anal sphincter stimulation can stimulate the voiding reflex.

6. Teach measures to help reduce detrusor activity: a. Resist voiding for as long as possible.	6. To increase comfort associated with voiding, the client must condition the voiding reflex by ingesting adequate fluids and

(continues on page 370)

Interventions continued	Rationales continued
b. Drink sufficient fluid to distend the bladder. c. Time fluid intake so that detrusor activity is restricted to waking hours.	inhibiting bladder contractions. Frequent toileting causes chronic low-volume voiding and increases detrusor activity. Resisting the urge to void may increase voiding intervals and reduce detrusor muscle activity.
7. Encourage the client to void or trigger at least every 3 hours.	7. A regular voiding pattern can prevent incontinent episodes.
8. Manage incontinence with CISC and incontinence products, whichever are most appropriate for the client and caregiver. External urine collection devices may be used if urodynamic studies show complete bladder emptying. Protect skin.	8. Loss of both the sensation to void and the ability to inhibit contractions makes bladder retraining impossible. CISC, often in conjunction with medications, is then the procedure of choice for managing incontinence. Incontinence is a factor in skin breakouts.

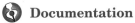 **Documentation**

Flow records
    Fluid intake
    Voiding patterns (amount, time, method used)
Discharge summary record
    Client teaching
    Outcome achievement or status

High Risk for Infection Related to Retention of Urine or Introduction of Urinary Catheter

Focus Assessment Criteria	Clinical Significance
1. Urine color, odor, volume 2. Temperature 3. Urethral orifice condition	1–3. The catheter, as a foreign body in the urethra, irritates mucosa and can introduce bacteria into the urinary tract, which increases the risk of infection.
4. Presence of urinary retention	4. Stagnant urine provides a good medium for bacterial growth.

Goal

The client will be free of bladder infection.

Indicators

• Urine is clear.
• Temperature is between 98–99.5°F.
• Demonstrate techniques to prevent infection.

Interventions	Rationales
1. Ensure adequate fluid intake (at least 2,000 mL/day unless contraindicated).	1. Dilute urine helps to prevent infection and bladder irritation.
2. Eliminate residual urine by aiding urine outflow through methods such as these: a. Credé maneuver b. Suprapubic tapping c. Multiple voiding d. Valsalva's maneuver, Credé maneuver e. Intermittent catheterization	2. Bacteria multiply rapidly in stagnant urine retained in the bladder. Moreover, overdistention hinders blood flow to the bladder wall, increasing the susceptibility to infection from bacterial growth. Regular, complete bladder emptying greatly reduces the risk of infection.
3. Consult with the physician for medication to relieve detrusor/sphincter dyssynergia (DSD).	3. DSD is associated with large amounts of residual urine.
4. As ordered, administer vitamin C and cranberry tablets.	4. Acidic urine deters the growth of most bacteria implicated in cystitis.
5. Monitor residual urine (should be no more than 50 mL).	5. Careful monitoring detects problems early, enabling prompt intervention to prevent urine stasis.
6. Test an uncontaminated urine sample for bacteria.	6. A bacteria count over 10^5/mL of urine suggests infection when pyuria is present. Some physicians may not want to treat until client has symptoms.
7. Maintain sterile technique for intermittent catheterization while the client is hospitalized.	7. The most common cause of infection is bacteria introduced by a caregiver who did not wash hands adequately between clients.
8. Avoid using an indwelling catheter unless it is indicated by a client's individual situation: Mobility inability to perform CISC.	8. Indwelling catheters are associated with urinary tract infection related to the catheter sliding in and out of the urethra, which introduces pathogens.

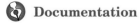 **Documentation**

Flow records
    Urine characteristics
    Temperature
    Elimination pattern (amount, time)
    Urine retention > 50 mL

Urge Incontinence Related to Disruption of the Inhibitory Efferent Impulses Secondary to Brain or Spinal Cord Dysfunction

Focus Assessment Criteria	Clinical Significance
1. Incontinence history (onset; pattern, complaints of frequency or urgency)	1. Descriptions of the incontinence can help to distinguish urge incontinence from other types.
2. History of cerebrovascular accident, brain tumor, spinal cord injury or tumor, or demyelinating disease (e.g., multiple sclerosis)	2. Defects in corticoregulatory pathways (cerebral, spinal cord) can cause urgency, frequency, and decreased bladder capacity.
3. Bladder sensation, bulbocavernosus reflex	3. If bladder sensation and bulbocavernosus reflex remain intact, stimulated voiding is possible.

Goals

The client will report no or fewer episodes of incontinence (specify).

Indicators
- Explain causes of incontinence.
- Describe bladder irritants.

Interventions	Rationales
1. Reduce any impediments to voiding routine by providing the following, if necessary: a. Velcro straps on clothes b. Handrails or mobility aids to bathroom c. Bedside commode d. Urinal	1. These measures ensure the client's ability to self-toilet before incontinence occurs. Often, little time exists between onset of the sensation to void and the bladder contraction.
2. Assess voiding patterns and develop a schedule of frequent timed voiding.	2. Frequent timed voiding can reduce urgency from bladder overdistention.
3. If incontinence occurs, decrease the time between planned voidings.	3. Bladder capacity may be insufficient to accommodate the urine volume, necessitating more frequent voiding.
4. If indicated, restrict fluid intake during the evening.	4. Evening fluid restrictions may help to prevent enuresis.

(continues on page 373)

Interventions continued	**Rationales** continued
5. If needed, teach trigger voiding, external manual compression, or abdominal straining. Refer to nursing diagnosis, Reflex Bladder.	5. A client with an intact reflex arc may be taught parasympathetic stimulation of the detrusor muscle, which will initiate and sustain bladder contractions to aid bladder emptying.
6. Teach pelvic floor exercises (Kegel exercises) to help restore bladder control if the client is a candidate (Newman & Smith, 1992): a. Obtain an audio cassette tape and exercise booklet from National Association For Continence (AAFC), P.O. Box 8310, Spartanburg, SC 29305, 1-800-Bladder. b. Help client to identify the muscles that start and stop urination. c. Instruct client to try the exercises for 3 to 4 months to strengthen periurethral tissue.	6. Useful for some clients with stress incontinence, Kegel exercises strengthen the pelvic floor muscles, which in turn may increase urinary sphincter competence.
7. Reinforce the need for optimal hydration (at least 2,000 mL/day unless contraindicated).	7. Optimal hydration is needed to prevent urinary tract infection and renal calculi.
8. Teach biofeedback if the client is a candidate. (Client must be alert and have a good memory.) Client may be able to learn to control the sphincter and prevent uninhibited bladder contractions by watching information on a screen as the bladder fills during cystometry or by hearing movement of the sphincter muscles in action.	8. Effective for some clients with urge incontinence, biofeedback uses behavior modification to habituate the client to recognize and control unwanted bladder spasms.
9. If other measures fail, plan for managing incontinence: a. Incontinent males can manage fairly easily by using an external condom drainage system and leg bag or pubic pressure urinal. b. Incontinent females have a more difficult problem. Incontinence pads are frequently used; new external collection devices are being marketed but are not yet perfected.	9. If bladder emptying techniques are unsuccessful, other methods of managing incontinence are necessary.

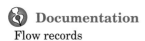 **Documentation**

Flow records
   Intake
   Voidings (amount, time)

Method used
    Incontinent episodes
Discharge summary record
    Client teaching

High Risk for Loneliness Related to Embarrassment of Incontinence in Front of Others and Fear of Odor From Urine

Focus Assessment Criteria	Clinical Significance
1. Socialization history 2. Anticipated or actual decrease in social contacts	1,2. Feelings of embarrassment, rejection, and low self esteem may contribute to isolation. An at-risk client must be assessed carefully because the suffering associated with social isolation is not always readily apparent.

Goals

The client will report decreased feelings of loneliness.

Indicators
• Identify the reasons for feelings of isolation.
• Discuss ways of increasing meaningful relationships.

Interventions	Rationales
1. Acknowledge the client's frustration with incontinence.	1. To the client, incontinence may seem like a reversion to an infantile state in which he or she has no control over body functions and feels ostracized by others. Acknowledging the difficulty of the situation can help to reduce feelings of frustration.
2. Determine the client's eligibility for bladder training, CISC, or other methods to manage incontinence.	2. These measures can increase control and reduce fear of accidents. CISC has a low incidence of UTI compared with Foley indwelling catheters (Webb, Lawson, & Neal, 1990).
3. Teach the client ways to control wetness and odor. Many products make wetting manageable by providing reliable leakage protection and masking odors.	3. Helping the client to manage incontinence encourages socialization.
4. Encourage the client to initially venture out socially for short periods, then to increase the length of social contacts as success at managing incontinence increases.	4. Short trips help the client to gradually gain confidence and reduce fears.

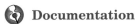 **Documentation**
Progress notes
  Significant dialogue
  Discharge summary record
Client teaching

High Risk for Ineffective Therapeutic Regimen Management Related to Insufficient Knowledge of Etiology of Incontinence, Management, Bladder Retraining Programs, Signs and Symptoms of Complications, and Community Resources

Focus Assessment Criteria	Clinical Significance
1. Readiness and ability to learn and retain information	1. A client or family failing to achieve learning goals requires a referral for assistance postdischarge.

Goals

The goals for this diagnosis represent those associated with discharge planning. Refer to the discharge criteria.

Interventions	Rationales
1. Teach about the condition, its cause, and management.	1. Understanding can encourage compliance with and participation in the treatment regimen.

2. If the client has voluntary control, institute a bladder training program.
  a. Document fluid intake, incontinence episodes, periods of continence, and client behavior on a voiding chart; this provides reinforcement for the client.
  b. Have client void "by the clock" rather than from an urge.
  c. Ensure that the client assumes an anatomically correct position for voiding attempts.
  d. Ensure privacy.
  e. Encourage use of the toilet 30 minutes before any usual incontinent episodes.
  f. Increase the scheduled time between voidings as the client remains continent for longer periods.
	2. Bladder training, an acceptable treatment for urge incontinence, can help to increase bladder volume and extend the length of time between voidings.

3. Encourage an obese client to lose weight.	3. Obesity places excessive intra-abdominal pressure on the bladder, which can aggravate incontinence.

(continues on page 376)

Interventions continued	**Rationales** continued

4. Teach client about any drugs prescribed for managing incontinence:
  a. Anticholinergics decrease uninhibited bladder contractions.
  b. Smooth muscle relaxants increase bladder capacity.
  c. Alpha-adrenergic agents stimulate the urethral sphincter.
  d. Alpha-blocking agents decrease neural sphincter resistance and help to reduce overflow incontinence.
	4. Understanding the medications' actions may encourage the client's compliance with the therapeutic regimen.

5. Explain possible surgical options as appropriate:
  a. Artificial urinary sphincters are increasing in popularity for clients with a malfunctioning sphincter or those who have undergone prostatectomy.
  b. Prostate resection often can eliminate overflow incontinence.
  c. Subarachnoid block, sacral rhizotomy, sacral nerve dissection, sphincterectomy, and urinary diversions may benefit spinal cord-injured clients with severe spasticity. The client must have a complete neurological and urodynamic evaluation to identify the appropriate surgical or medical treatment.
	5. The client may be a candidate for surgery to control or cure incontinence.

6. If indicated, teach CISC to the client or caregiver.
  a. In women, follow this procedure:
  • Wash hands thoroughly.
  • Hold the catheter $1\frac{1}{2}$ inches from the tip. With the other hand, separate the labia, using the second and fourth fingers, and locate the urethral meatus with the middle finger. Use this finger as a guide for insertion.
  • Gently insert the catheter into the urethral meatus by slipping the catheter tip just under the middle finger. Advance the catheter in an upward direction.
  • Guide the catheter into the bladder, about 1 inch past the point at which urine begins to flow.
  • Drain the bladder of urine. When urine stops flowing, slowly begin removing the catheter. If urine flow begins again during removal, hold the catheter in position and wait until flow stops.
	6. Intermittent self-catheterization is appropriate for children and adults who are motivated and physically able to perform the procedure. Often a caregiver may be taught to catheterize the client. CISC stimulates normal voiding, prevents infection, and maintains integrity of the uretero-vesical junction. In the hospital, aseptic technique is used because of increased microorganisms in the hospital environment. At home, clean technique is used. CISC entails fewer complications than an indwelling catheter and is the procedure of choice for clients who are unable to empty the bladder completely.

(continues on page 377)

Interventions continued	**Rationales** continued
• After removal, cleanse the outer surface of the catheter with water and the same soap used to wash hands, then rinse the inside and outside with clear water. Let catheter dry before storing it in its container. Remember to discard a catheter that becomes too stiff or soft. b. In men, use the following procedure: • Wash hands and prepare the catheter. Generously apply water-soluble lubricant to the catheter tip. • Hold the catheter about $1\frac{1}{2}$ inches from the tip. With the other hand, hold the penis straight out from the body. • Insert the catheter into the urinary meatus until slight resistance is felt. Then, using gentle but firm pressure, advance the catheter to the bladder, 1 inch past the point at which urine begins to flow. • Drain the bladder of urine. When urine stops flowing, slowly begin removing the catheter. If urine flow begins again during removal, hold the catheter in position and wait until flow stops. • After removal, cleanse the outer surface of the catheter with water and the same soap used to wash hands, then rinse the inside and outside with clear water. • Dry and store catheter in its container. Remember to discard a catheter that becomes too stiff or soft.	
7. Teach the client to keep a record of catheterization times, amount of fluid intake and urine output, and any incontinent periods.	7. Accurate record-keeping aids in evaluating status. Teach client about the dehydrating effects of alcohol.
8. Teach the client to notify the physician of the following: a. Bleeding from urethral opening b. Reactions from medications c. Difficulty inserting catheter d. Dark, bloody, cloudy, or strong-smelling urine	8. Early reporting enables prompt treatment to prevent serious problems. a. Bleeding may indicate trauma or renal calculi. b. Drug reactions may indicate overdose. c. Difficult catheter insertion may indicate a stricture. d. These urine changes may point to infection.

(continues on page 378)

Interventions continued	Rationales continued
e. Pain in the abdomen or back f. Elevated temperature	e. Pain may indicate renal calculi. f. Fever may be the first sign of urinary tract infection.
9. Explain available community resources (e.g., National Association for Continence [AAFC]; 1-800-BLADDER.)	9. The client and family may need assistance or more information for home care.
10. Provide AHCPR booklet *Urinary Incontinence in Adults: A Patient's Guide.*	

 Documentation

Discharge summary record
   Client teaching
   Outcome achievement or status

PARKINSON'S DISEASE

Parkinson's disease is a chronic degenerative disorder of the basal ganglia and includes striatum, globus pallidum, subthalamic nucleus, substantia nigra, and red nucleus. Dopamine is a neurotransmitter that is produced and stored in the substantia nigra and is depleted when substantia nigra cells are damaged. A decrease in dopamine disrupts the inhibitory effects of dopamine and causes an increase in the excitatory effect of acetylcholine. The dominant features of Parkinson's disease (PD) include resting tremors, bradykinesia, limb rigidity, postural instability, and dystonia (Dewey, Kelley, & Shulman, 2002). Initial symptoms typically develop after age 50. Onset is insidious, and a diagnosis may not be made for years.

 Time Frame

Secondary diagnosis (hospitalization not usual)

 DIAGNOSTIC CLUSTER*

Collaborative Problems

PC: Long-Term Levodopa Treatment Syndrome

Nursing Diagnoses

- Impaired Verbal Communication related to dysarthria secondary to ataxia of muscles of speech
- Impaired Physical Mobility related to effects of muscle rigidity, tremors, and slowness of movement on activities of daily living

Related Care Plans

- Immobility or Unconsciousness
- Multiple Sclerosis

---

*This medical condition was not included in the validation study.

Discharge Criteria

Before discharge, the client and family will

1. Relate the intent to share concerns with another family member or a trusted friend.
2. Identify one strategy to increase independence.
3. Describe measures that can reduce the risk of exacerbation.
4. Identify signs and symptoms that must be reported to a health care professional.

Collaborative Problems

Potential Complication: Long-Term Levodopa Treatment Syndrome

Nursing Goal

The nurse will detect early signs/symptoms of long-term levodopa treatment syndrome.

Indicator

- Less or no fluctuations between involuntary movements (tics, tremors, rigidity, and repetitive, bizarre movements) and bradykinesia (slowed movements)

Interventions	Rationales
1. Explain long-term levodopa treatment syndrome to client and family.	1. This syndrome occurs 2 to 6 years after beginning treatment and is characterized by a deterioration of the efficacy of levodopa (Dewey, Kelly, & Shulman, 2002).
2. Explain symptoms of syndrome (on-off syndrome): a. Fluctuates between being symptom free and severe Parkinson's symptoms. b. Symptoms may last minutes or hours.	2. This syndrome is believed to be caused by altered sensitivity of dopamine receptors or to serum level changes in levodopa (Dewey, Kelly, & Shulman, 2002).
3. Encourage client to discuss with physician the possibility of "drug holiday."	3. Some physicians advocate from 1 to 2 days to 10 to 14 days of a drug holiday in a hospital setting to permit resensitization of dopamine receptors.
4. Evaluate knowledge of dietary precautions: a. The need to avoid foods high in pyridoxine (e.g., B$_6$ vitamins, pork, beef, liver, bananas, ham, and egg yolks) b. Advise client to divide daily protein intake in equal amounts over the entire day. c. Wait 45 minutes before eating after taking levodopa. If nausea develops, client may take dosage with food. d. The need to have a diet high in fiber and fluid (unless contraindicated)	4. a. Pyridoxine accelerates the breakdown of levodopa to dopamine before it reaches the brain. b,c. Protein competes with levodopa for transport to the brain. Levodopa is best absorbed on an empty stomach. However, it may cause nausea so then should be taken with food. d. Constipation and nausea are side effects of levodopa (Dewey, Kelly, & Shulman, 2002).
5. Observe for psychiatric disturbances: a. Visual hallucinations b. Sleep disturbances c. Depression d. Confusion	5. Drug-related psychiatric disturbances can occur in 30% of treated clients; disturbances include hallucinations; confused, delusional, abnormal dreams; and sleep disturbances. b. Sleep disorders may be treated medically after sleep apnea is ruled out. c. Depression in Parkinson's is associated with advancing disease severity, recent disease deterioration, and occurrence of falls (Schrag, 2001). d. Confusion, although less common, is also a side effect of levodopa (Dewey, Kelly, & Shulman, 2002).
6. Prevent complications of exacerbation of symptoms. Refer to index under following subjects:	6.

(continues on page 381)

Interventions continued	Rationales continued
a. High risk for aspiration	a. Swallowing disorders are common in Parkinson's disease and may cause dehydration, weight loss, aspiration pneumonia, and airway obstruction.
b. Impaired swallowing	b. A barium swallow study is useful for identifying the swallowing disorder (Palmer, 2000).
c. Disuse syndrome	
d. Thrombophlebitis	
e. Avoid alcohol	e. Alcohol may antagonize the effects of levodopa.

 Related Physician-Prescribed Interventions

Medications. Dopaminergic agonists, dopaminergics, catechol-o-methyltransferase inhibitors

Intravenous Therapy. None

Laboratory Studies. Stereotaxic neurosurgery urine dopamine levels

Diagnostic Studies. Autologous tissue transplantation, CT scan or MRI (to rule out other disorders)

Therapies. Fetal tissue transplantation, physical therapy

 Documentation

Progress notes
Changes in symptoms

Nursing Diagnoses

Impaired Verbal Communication Related to Dysarthria Secondary to Ataxia of Muscles of Speech

Focus Assessment Criteria	Clinical Significance

1. Speech:
  a. Volume
  b. Intonation (monotone)
  c. Quality (breathy, hoarse)
  d. Rate
  e. Rhythm (hesitation)
2. Articulation
	1,2. Speech is a motor activity involving complex coordination of intrinsic and extrinsic larynx muscles with those of the pharynx, soft palate, lips, and tongue. Impairments of articulation, respiration, and phonation are common symptoms of Parkinson's disease and may result in reduced communication (Stelzig, 1999).

3. Hearing	3. Communication problems are complicated by hearing impairments.

Goal

The client will demonstrate improved ability to express self.

Indicator

Demonstrate techniques and exercises to improve speech and strengthen muscles.

Interventions	Rationales
1. Explain the disorder's effects on speech.	1. Understanding may promote compliance with speech improvement exercises.
2. Explain the benefits of daily speech improvement exercises.	2. Daily exercises help to improve the efficiency of speech musculature and increase rate, volume, and articulation.
3. Refer client to a speech pathologist to design an individualized speech program as recommended by the American Parkinson's Disease Association. Reinforce with client to: a. Practice in front of a mirror. b. Do exercises to improve voice loudness. c. Do exercises to improve voice variation: "I will" (softly) "I will" (a little louder) "I will" (much louder) • Say a sentence several times and stress a word. Change the word each time. For example, use the following sentence: *I* don't want that blue hat. I *don't* want that blue hat. I don't *want* that blue hat. I don't want *that* blue hat. I don't want that *blue* hat. I don't want that blue *hat.* • Practice asking questions and giving answers. Raise the voice after a question, lower it with an answer. d. Practice tongue exercises several times: • Stick tongue out as far as you can, hold, relax. • Stick tongue out and move slowly from corner to corner. • Stretch tongue to chin and then to nose. • Stick tongue out and put it back as fast as you can. • Move tongue in a circle as quickly as you can around lips. e. Practice lip and jaw exercises; repeat several times: • Open and close mouth slowly; close lips completely. Do another set but as fast as you can. • Close lips and press together tightly for a few seconds.	3. These exercises improve muscle tone and control and speech clarity. a. Practicing in front of a mirror allows the client to see and evaluate lip and tongue movements. b. These exercises increase air intake and improve control over air intake and exhalation during speech. c. These exercises enhance speech intelligibility. d. These exercises strengthen the tongue and increase its range of motion for to improved articulation. e. These exercises strengthen and increase the range of lip movements for the formation of speech sounds.

(continues on page 383)

Interventions continued	Rationales continued

• Stretch lips into a wide smile—hold—relax.
   • Pucker lips—hold—relax.
   • Pucker—hold—smile—hold.
   • Say "ma-ma-ma-ma" as fast as you can.
  f. Do exercises to slow the rate of speaking:
   • Say words in syllables:
    pos-si-bil-i-ty
    pa-ci-fic
    hor-ri-ble
   • Say phrases in syllables:
    when-ev-er pos-si-ble
    fam-i-ly bus-i-ness
  g. Practice varying facial expression: Using a mirror, make faces (e.g., smile, frown, laugh, grin, whistle, puff out cheeks).
  h. Read the newspaper out loud. Determine how many words you can speak in one breath before the volume decreases.
	f. These exercises help to improve deliberate word-by-word pronunciation.
	
	  g. Parkinson's disease causes limited movement of facial muscles, which produces a masklike facies; these exercises help to overcome this effect.
	  h. This helps the client learn to maintain volume for each syllable and final consonant sounds.

4. Refer the client to American Parkinson's Disease Association 1250 Hylan Blvd. Staten Island, NY 10305 1-800-223-2732	4. The client requires additional instruction.

 Documentation

Discharge summary record
Assessment of speech
Exercises taught
Outcome achievement or status
Referrals if indicated

Impaired Physical Mobility Related to Effects of Muscle Rigidity, Tremors, and Slowness of Movement on Activities of Daily Living

Focus Assessment Criteria	Clinical Significance
1. Gait, balance 2. Range of motion 3. Presence of tremors, akinesia (no movement), or bradykinesia (slowed movements)	1–3. Parkinson's disease disrupts the extrapyramidal motor system, which is responsible for control of posture and semicoordination of movements.
4. Muscle rigidity (trunk, facial, or intercostal)	4. Affected muscles include two-joint flexor muscles (e.g., trunk) and striated muscles (e.g., face and intercostal).

Goal

The client will describe measures to increase mobility.

Indicators
- Demonstrate exercises to improve mobility.
- Demonstrate a wide base gait with arm swinging.
- Identify one strategy to increase independence.
- Relate an intent to exercise at home.

Interventions	Rationales
1. Explain the cause of symptoms.	1. The client's understanding may help to promote compliance with an exercise program at home.
2. Teach the client to walk erect while looking at the horizon, with feet separated and arms swinging normally.	2. Conscious efforts to simulate a normal gait and position can improve mobility and reduce loss of balance.
3. Instruct the client to exercise three to five times a week.	3. Exercise has been proven to delay disability, ameliorate diseases, and fortify strength, balance, flexibility, and endurance, even in older clients who are frail or have a medical condition (Edelberg, 2002). Specific benefits include the following: a. Increased muscle strength b. Improved coordination and dexterity c. Reduced rigidity d. Help preventing contractures e. Improved flexibility f. Enhanced peristalsis g. Improved cardiovascular endurance h. Increased ability to tolerate stress i. A sense of control, which reduces feelings of powerlessness j. Slows osteoporosis k. Reduces LDL cholesterol l. Reduces systolic BP, raises HDL cholesterol
4. Consult with a primary care provider for a specific exercise program. Teach that an exercise program should include the following: a. Warm-up for 10 minutes. b. Exercise for 15 to 40 minutes. c. Cool down for 10 minutes.	4. An exercise program of range of motion and aerobic exercise (tailored to the person's ability) can help to preserve muscle strength and coordination (Arcangelo & Peterson, 2001). a. Warm-up stretches muscles to help prevent injury. b. The workout conditions the heart and tones other muscles. Walking, dancing, swimming, and riding a stationary bike are examples. c. Cool down promotes excretion of body wastes from exercise and reduces heart rate slowly.

(continues on page 385)

Interventions continued	**Rationales** continued
d. Lower body, torso, upper body, and head exercises	d. A range of exercises ensures that all affected muscle areas are exercised.
e. Relaxation exercises	e. Relaxation exercises provide some control over the anxiety associated with fear of "freezing" or falling.
f. Explain that short bouts of physical activity are also beneficial.	f. Exercise programs should begin with low intensity activities, and gradually intensify (Edelberg, 2002).
5. Stress to the client that compliance with the exercise program is ultimately his or her choice.	5. Promoting the client's feelings of control and self-determination may improve compliance with the exercise program.
6. Include family members or significant others in teaching sessions; stress that they are not to "police" the client's compliance.	6. Support from family members or significant others can encourage the client to comply with the exercise program (Hayes, 2002).
7. Refer to a physical therapist or reference material for specific exercise guidelines.	7. Physical or occupational therapy as well as some alternative therapies may help clients deal with disability, provide palliation, or reduce stress (Viliani, 1999).
8. Discuss strategies to maintain as much independence as possible. 9. Discuss the importance of accomplishing tasks and planning events to look forward to.	8,9. Parkinson's disease seems to advance more slowly in people who remain involved in their pre-Parkinson's activities or who find new activities to amuse them and engage their interests (Parkinson's Disease Foundation, 2002).
10. Refer to nursing diagnosis Fatigue in index for additional interventions.	

 Documentation

Discharge summary record
Assessment of mobility
Exercises taught
Outcome achievement or status
Referrals if indicated

Refer to website http://connection.lww.com for critical paths for this condition.

SEIGURE DISORDERS

Seizure disorders constitute a chronic syndrome in which a neurologic dysfunction in cerebral tissue produces recurrent paroxysmal episodes (seizures): disturbances of behavior, mood, sensation, perception, movement, and/or muscle tone. The disorder is thought to be an electrical disturbance in cerebral nerve cells that causes them to produce abnormal, repetitive electrical charges. Seizures are diagnosed as epileptic or reactive. Epilepsy is a chronic neurologic condition producing recurrent seizures. Reactive seizures are single or multiple seizures resulting from a transient systemic problem (fever, infection, alcohol withdrawal, tumors, stroke, toxic or metabolic disturbances). The International League Against Epilepsy has established a system of classification for seizures: partial (focal) (local) seizures or generalized (convulsive) (nonconvulsive) seizures. Partial seizures can be classified as either simple or complex (Walsh-D'Espiro, 1999).

 Time Frame

Initial diagnosis
Recurrent acute episodes

 DIAGNOSTIC CLUSTER

Collaborative Problems

* PC: Status Epilepticus

Nursing Diagnoses

▲ High Risk for Ineffective Airway Clearance related to relaxation of tongue and gag reflexes
   secondary to disruption in muscle innervation
Anxiety related to fear of embarrassment secondary to having a seizure in public
△ High Risk for Ineffective Therapeutic Regimen Management related to insufficient
   knowledge of condition, medication, care during seizures, environmental hazards, and
   community resources

▲ This diagnosis was reported to be monitored for or managed frequently (75%–100%).
△ This diagnosis was reported to be monitored for or managed often (50%–74%).
* This diagnosis was not included in the validation study.

Discharge Criteria

Before discharge, the client or family will

1. State the intent to wear medical identification.
2. Relate activities to be avoided.
3. Relate the importance of complying with the prescribed medication regimen.
4. Relate the side effects of prescribed medications.
5. State situations that increase the possibility of a seizure.
6. State signs and symptoms that must be reported to a health care professional.

Collaborative Problems

Potential Complication: Status Epilepticus

Nursing Goal

The nurse will detect early signs/symptoms of status epilepticus and collaboratively intervene to stabilize the client.

Indicators

- Respirations 16–20 breaths/min
- Heart rate 60–100 beats/min
- B/P >90/60, <140/90 mm Hg
- No seizure activity
- Serum ph 7.35–7.45
- Serum PCO_2 35–45 mmHg
- Pulse oximetry (SaO_2) >95

Interventions	Rationales

1. If person continues to have generalized convulsions, notify physician and initiate protocol:
   a. Establish airway.
   b. Do not attempt to open mouth to insert something.
   c. Do not try to restrain the person.
   d. Suction as needed.
   e. Administer oxygen via nasal catheter.
   f. Initiate an intravenous line.
	1. Status epilepticus is a medical emergency that requires prompt and appropriate intervention. Maintenance of adequate vital function with attention to airway, breathing, and circulation; prevention of systemic complications; and rapid termination of seizures must be coupled with investigating and treating any underlying cause (Hanhan, 2001).

2. Initiate pulse oximetry.	2. It provides an accurate measurement of oxygen saturation.
3. Provide medications as prescribed. Refer to pharmacological reference for specific information.	

4. Monitor for signs/symptoms of underlying cause:
   • Abrupt cessation of antiepileptic medication
   • Increased intracranial pressure
   • Metabolic disorders
   • Infectious process
	4. The underlying cause must be diagnosed and corrected for the seizures to be controlled (Hanhan, 2001).

 Related Physician-Prescribed Interventions

Medications. Antiseizure

Intravenous Therapy. Diazepam, lorazepam, glucose solution (IV) or fosphenytoin (IV)

Laboratory Studies. Drug levels (Tegretol, Dilantin); complete blood cell count; electrolytes; blood urea nitrogen; calcium; magnesium; fasting blood glucose; urinalysis

Diagnostic Studies. EEG; ECG; CT scan; cerebrospinal fluid examination; pulse oximetry; MRI

 Documentation

Progress notes
   Abnormal findings
   Interventions
   Response

Nursing Diagnoses

High Risk for Ineffective Airway Clearance Related to Relaxation of Tongue and Gag Reflexes Secondary to Disruption in Muscle Innervation

Focus Assessment Criteria	Clinical Significance
1. History of seizure activity 2. Respiratory status during seizure activity	1,2. The tonic/clonic movement during a seizure can cause the tongue to drop backward and obstruct the airway.

Goal

The client will demonstrate continued airway patency.

Indicator

The family will describe interventions to maintain a patent airway during seizures.

Interventions	Rationales

1. During a seizure, do the following:
    a. Provide privacy if possible.
    b. Ease the client to the floor if possible.
    c. Roll the person on his or her side.
    d. Remove anything that may cause injury.
    e. Loosen any restraining clothing.
    f. Allow person to proceed with seizure; do not restrain person as this could cause injury.
    g. Clear the airway (nose and mouth) so breathing is not obstructed.
    h. Never put anything in the person's mouth.
    i. If the seizure lasts more than 5 minutes, call 911 (Epilepsy Foundation, 2002).
	1. These measures can help to reduce injury and embarrassment (Epilepsy Foundation, 2002).

2. Observe the seizure and document its characteristics:
    a. Onset and duration
    b. Preseizure events (e.g., visual, auditory, olfactory, or tactile stimuli)
    c. Part of body where the seizure started, initial movement
    d. Eyes: open or closed, pupil size
    e. Body parts involved, type of movements
    f. Involuntary motor activities (e.g., lip smacking or repeated swallowing)
    g. Incontinence (fecal or urinary)
    h. Loss of consciousness
    i. Postseizure: ability to speak, sleeping, confusion, weakness, paralysis
	2. This information gives clues to the location of the epileptogenic focus in the brain and is useful in guiding treatment (Epilepsy Foundation, 2002).

(continues on page 389)

Interventions continued	Rationales continued
3. If the client reports an aura, have him or her lie down.	3. A recumbent position can prevent injuries from a fall.
4. Teach family members or significant others how to respond to the client during a seizure.	4. Others can be taught measures to prevent airway obstruction and injury.

 Documentation

Progress notes
  Description of seizures
Discharge summary record
  Client teaching

Anxiety Related to Fear of Embarrassment Secondary to Having a Seizure in Public

Focus Assessment Criteria	Clinical Significance

1. Usual socialization patterns:
  a. Hobbies
  b. Other interests
  c. Church
  d. Work
  e. Neighborhood
  f. School
	1. An at-risk client must be assessed carefully because the suffering associated with anxiety is not always readily apparent.

2. Concerns regarding socialization	2. Feelings of rejection and embarrassment are common.

Goal

The client will relate an increased in psychological and physiologic comfort.

Indicators
- Use effective copping mechanisms.
- Describe his or her anxiety and perceptions.

Interventions	Rationales
1. Allow opportunities to share concerns regarding seizures in public.	1. Stigma associated with epilepsy is a huge concern for people living with epilepsy. A client with epilepsy may tend to separate himself or herself from family, friends, and society (Blair, 2001).
2. Provide support and validate that client's concerns are normal.	2. Possible losses related to epilepsy are loss of control, independence, employment, self-

(continues on page 390)

Interventions continued	Rationales continued
	confidence, transportation, family, and friends. When a person feels listened to and understood, his or her loss is validated and normalized (Blair, 2001).
3. Assist the client in identifying activities that are pleasurable and nonhazardous.	3. Fear of injury may contribute to isolation.
4. Stress the importance of adhering to the treatment plan.	4. Adherence to the medication regimen can help to prevent or reduce seizure episodes.
5. Discuss sharing the diagnosis with family members, friends, coworkers, and social contacts.	5. Open dialogue with others forewarns them of possible seizures; this can reduce the shock of witnessing a seizure and possibly enable assistive action.
6. Discuss situations through which the client can meet others in a similar situation: a. Support groups b. Epilepsy Foundation of America	6. Sharing with others in a similar situation may give the client a more realistic view of seizure disorder and societal perception of it.

 Documentation

Progress notes
  Client's concerns
  Interaction with client

High Risk for Ineffective Therapeutic Regimen Management Related to Insufficient Knowledge of Condition, Medications, Care During Seizures, Environmental Hazards, and Community Resources

Focus Assessment Criteria	Clinical Significance

1. Current knowledge of seizures and their management
2. Contributing factors including the following:
  a. Anxiety
  b. New diagnosis
  c. Lack of previous instruction
3. Resources (e.g., family, financial, and community)
4. Attitudes, feelings, and concerns related to seizure disorders
5. Readiness and ability to learn
	1–5. Assessment helps to identify any factors that may interfere with learning. A client or family who does not achieve goals for learning requires a referral for assistance postdischarge.

Goals

The goals for this diagnosis represent those associated with discharge planning. Refer to the discharge criteria.

Interventions	Rationales
1. Teach about seizure disorders and treatment; correct misconceptions.	1. The client's and family's understanding of seizure disorders and the prescribed treatment regimen strongly influences compliance with the regimen.

2. If the client is on medication therapy, teach the following information:
  a. Never to discontinue a drug abruptly
 	
  b. Side effects and signs of toxicity
 	
  c. The need to have drug blood levels monitored
  d. The need for periodic complete blood counts if indicated
 	
  e. The effects of diphenylhydantoin (Dilantin), if ordered, on gingival tissue and the need for regular dental examinations
	2. Certain precautions must be emphasized to ensure safe, effective drug therapy:
	  a. Abrupt discontinuation can precipitate status epilepticus.
	  b. Early identification of problems enables prompt intervention to prevent serious complications.
	  c. Drug blood levels provide a guide for adjusting drug dosage.
	  d. Long-term use of some anticonvulsive drugs, such as hydantoins (e.g., phenytoin [Dilantin]), can cause blood dyscrasias.
	  e. Long-term phenytoin therapy can cause gingival hyperplasia.

3. Provide information regarding situations that increase the risk of seizure (Goroll & Mulley, 2000):
  a. Alcohol ingestion
  b. Excessive caffeine intake
  c. Excessive fatigue or stress
  d. Febrile illness
  e. Poorly adjusted television screen
  f. Sedentary activity level
  g. Lack of sleep
  h. Hypoglycemia
  i. Constipation
  j. Diarrhea
	3. Certain situations have been identified as increasing seizure episodes, although the actual mechanisms behind them are unknown (Goroll & Mulley, 2000).

4. Discuss why certain activities are hazardous and should be avoided:
  a. Swimming alone
  b. Driving (unless seizure free for 1 to 3 years, depending on state)
  c. Operating potentially hazardous machinery
  d. Mountain climbing
  e. Occupations in which the client could be injured or cause injury to others
	4. Generally a client prone to seizures should avoid any activity that could place him, her, or others in danger should a seizure occur. Teach the client how to recognize the warning signals of a seizure and what to do to minimize injury (Goroll & Mulley, 2000).

5. Provide opportunities for the client and significant others to express their feelings alone and with each other.	5. Witnessing a seizure is terrifying for others and embarrassing for the client prone to them. This shame and humiliation

(continues on page 392)

Interventions continued	Rationales continued
	contribute to anxiety, depression, hostility, and secrecy. Family members also may experience these feelings. Frank discussions may reduce feelings of shame and isolation.
6. Refer the client and family to community resources and reference material for assistance with management (e.g., Epilepsy Foundation of America, counseling, occupational rehabilitation).	6. Such resources may provide additional information and support.

 Documentation

Discharge summary record
   Client teaching
   Outcome achievement or status
   Referrals if indicated

Refer to website http://connection.lww.com for critical paths for this condition.

SPINAL CORD INJURY

Spinal cord injuries can be caused by four major mechanisms: acceleration/deceleration, deformation, vertical loading, and penetration wounds. Acceleration/deceleration-caused injuries (e.g., rear-end collisions) produce hyperextension and hyperflexion. Deformation-caused injuries involve tissues and other structures that support the spinal cord. In vertical loading-caused injuries (e.g., diving accidents), damage results from compression of the spinal column. Penetration wounds commonly result from knives or other sharp objects. The consequences of spinal cord injury depend on the location and extent of cord injury. The severity of cord injury is classified according to the American Spinal Injury (ASIA) Association Scale.

Time Frame
Initial acute episode (post-intensive care, pre-rehabilitation)
Secondary diagnosis

DIAGNOSTIC CLUSTER

Collaborative Problems	Refer to
△ PC: Fracture Dislocation	
▲ PC: Hypoxemia	
△ PC: Paralytic Ileus	
△ PC: Urinary Retention	
Pyelonephritis	
△ PC: Renal Insufficiency	
△ PC: Gastrointestinal (GI) Bleeding	
△ PC: Electrolyte Imbalance	Acute Renal Failure
▲ PC: Thrombophlebitis	Fractures

Nursing Diagnoses	Refer to
▲ Anxiety related to perceived effects of injury on life style and unknown future	
▲ Grieving related to loss of body function and its effects on life style	
△ High Risk for Disturbed Self-Concept related to effects of disability on achieving developmental tasks and life style	
△ Bowel Incontinence: Reflexic related to lack of voluntary sphincter control	

(continues on page 394)

Nursing Diagnoses continued	Refer to continued
secondary to spinal cord injury above the eleventh thoracic vertebra (T11)	
△ Bowel Incontinence: Areflexic related to lack of voluntary sphincter control secondary to spinal cord injury involving sacral reflex arc (S2–S4)	
△ High Risk for Dysreflexia related to reflex stimulation of sympathetic nervous system secondary to loss of autonomic control	
△ Interrupted Family Processes related to adjustment requirements, role disturbances, and uncertain future	
△ High Risk for Ineffective Sexuality Pattern related to physiologic, sensory, and psychological effects of disability on sexuality or function	
△ High Risk for Ineffective Therapeutic Regimen Management related to insufficient knowledge of the effects of altered skin, bowel, bladder, respiratory, thermoregulation, and sexual function and their management; signs and symptoms of complications; follow-up care; and community resources	
▲ Self-Care Deficit related to sensorimotor deficits secondary to level of spinal cord injury	Immobility or Unconsciousness
Related Care Plans Immobility or Unconsciousness Pressure Ulcer Neurogenic Bladder Tracheostomy	

▲ This diagnosis was reported to be monitored for or managed frequently (75%–100%).
△ This diagnosis was reported to be monitored for or managed often (50%–74%).

Discharge Planning

Before discharge, the client or family will

1. Describe the effects of injury on functioning and methods of home management.
2. Express feelings regarding the effects of injury on life style.
3. Relate an intent to share feelings with significant others after discharge.
4. State signs and symptoms that must be reported to a health care professional.

5. Identify a plan for rehabilitation and follow-up care.
6. Identify available community resources.

Collaborative Problems

Potential Complication: Fracture Dislocation

Potential Complication: Hypoxemia

Potential Complication: Electrolyte Imbalance

Potential Complication: Paralytic Ileus

Potential Complication: Urinary Retention

Potential Complication: Pyelonephritis

Potential Complication: Renal Insufficiency

Potential Complication: Gastrointestinal (GI) Bleeding

Nursing Goal

The nurse will monitor for early signs/symptoms of (a) fracture dislocation, (b) cardiovascular, (c) respiratory, (d) metabolic, (e) renal and (f) gastrointestinal dysfunction, and collaboratively intervene to stabilize client.

Indicators

- Correct alignment of cord (a)
- Heart rate 60–100 beats/min (b, c)
- B/P <140/90, >90/60 mm Hg (b, c)
- Lung sounds clear, no adventitious sounds (b)
- Temperature 98–99.5°F (c)
- Serum pH 7.35–7.45 (b, c)
- Serum PCO_2 35–45 mm Hg (b, c)
- Oxygen saturation (pulse oximeter) >95% (b, c)
- Alert, oriented (b, c, d)
- Urine output >30 ml/hr (b, c, e)
- Prealbumin 16–40 m/µ/ml (e)
- Urine specific gravity 1.005–1.030 (b, e)
- Urine sodium 130–200 mEq/24h (e)
- Blood urea nitrogen 5–25 mg/dL (e)
- Serum electrolytes (refer to laboratory range of normal) (e)
- 24-hour creatinine clearance (e)
    - Male: 95–135 ml/mm
    - Female: 85–125 ml/min
- Negative stool for occult blood (f)
- Hemoglobin (b)
    - Male: 14–18 g/dL
    - Female: 12–16 g/dL

Interventions	Rationales
1. Maintain immobilization with skeletal traction (e.g., tongs, calipers, collar or halo vest); ensure that ropes and weights hang freely. Check the orthopedic frame and traction daily (e.g., secure nuts/bolts).	1. Skeletal traction stabilizes the vertebral column to prevent further spinal cord injury and to allow reduction and immobilization of the vertebral column into correct alignment by constant traction force. Once traction is in place, pain is diminished by separating and aligning the injured vertebrae and reducing spasms (Hickey, 2001).

(continues on page 396)

Interventions continued	**Rationales** continued
2. Turn client every 2 hours around the clock while on bed rest with skeletal traction. Use the triple log-rolling technique with a fourth person to stabilize weights during turning (Hickey, 2001).	2. A change of position helps to maintain skin integrity, decrease lower extremity spasms, and mobilize secretions. Log-rolling helps to maintain spinal alignment during turning.
3. If traction disconnects or fails, stabilize the head, neck, and shoulders with a cervical collar, hands, or sand bags.	3. Stabilization of the injured area is vital to prevent misalignment and further damage.

4. Monitor for spinal shock
  a. Decreased blood pressure
  b. Decreased heart rate
  c. Absent reflexes below injury
  d. Decreased cardiac output
  e. Decreased PO_2 (if injury at cervical or thoracic level)
  f. Increased PCO_2 (if injury at cervical or thoracic level)
	4. Sudden depression of reflex activity in spinal cord caused complete paralysis of muscle innervated by that part of the cord (Hickey, 2001).

5. Monitor for complications of neuro-vascular injury:
  a. Bradycardia
 	
  b. Hypotension, orthostatic hypotension
 	
  c. Hypothermia/Hyperthermia
 	
  d. Hypoglycemia
	5.
	
	  a. Cardiac function is altered because of the vagal stimulation, which has no sympathetic control (unopposed parasympathetic response).
	  b. Sympathetic blockage causes vaso-dilatation with resulting decreased venous return. With time and conditioning the person can tolerate low BP with no symptoms (Teasell, Malcolm, & Delaney, 1996).
	  c. Temperature regulation is highly dependent on an intact sympathetic nervous system. High level SCI clients are unable to adapt to environmental temperature changes because of their inability to shiver or vasoconstrict cutaneous blood vessels. Hyperthermia can occur with increased environmental temperatures or in response to infection. There is a loss of the ability to sweat (Teasell, Malcolm, & Delaney, 1996). This phenomenon is called poikilothermia.
	  d. In quadriplegics, insulin-induced hypoglycemia does not raise levels of plasma adrenaline or noradrenaline that would cause clinical manifestations of anxiety, tremulousness, hunger, sweating, tachycardia, and a rise in systolic blood pressure. There-

(continues on page 397)

Interventions continued	Rationales continued
	fore, in these patients, sedation and a drop in systolic blood pressure are the only symptoms (Teasell, Malcolm & Delaney, 1996).
e. Deep vein thrombosis (DVT) (swelling, warmth, redness of lower extremities) (filters are not standard of care for SCI with DUT)	e. Pooling of blood coupled with immobility greatly increases the risk of vascular stasis. DVT may result in pulmonary embolus. Sequential compression boots and prophylactic heparin usually are indicated (Hickey, 2001).
6. Monitor for signs of hypoxemia:	6. Spinal cord injuries can impair the muscles of respiration depending on the level of injury (e.g., diaphragm [C3–C5], intercostals [T1–T7], accessory muscles [C2–C7], and abdominal muscles [T6–T12] [Nelson, Zejdlik & Love, 2002]).
a. Abnormal arterial blood gases (ABGs) (pH <7.35 and PCO_2 >46 mmHg)	a. ABG analysis helps to evaluate gas exchange in the lungs.
b. Increased and irregular heart rate c. Increased respiratory rate followed by decreased rate	b,c. Respiratory acidosis results from excessive CO_2 retention. A client with respiratory acidosis initially exhibits increased heart rate and respirations in an attempt to correct decreased circulating oxygen, then client begins to breathe more slowly and with prolonged expiration.
d. Changes in mentation	d. Altered mentation may indicate cerebral tissue hypoxia.
e. Decreased urine output (<30 mL/hr) f. Cool, pale, or cyanotic skin	e,f. The compensatory response to decreased circulating oxygen is to increase heart and respiratory rates and to decrease circulation to the kidneys (resulting in decreased urine output) and to the extremities (resulting in diminished pulses and skin changes).
7. Administer low-flow (2 L/min) oxygen as needed through a cannula.	7. Supplemental oxygen therapy increases circulating oxygen. Higher flow rates increase CO_2 retention. Use of a nasal cannula rather than a mask minimizes feelings of suffocation (Nelson, Zejdlik & Love, 2002).
8. Assess ability to cough and use of accessory muscles. Suction as needed. Perform assisted coughing techniques to aid in moving secretions to the upper airways.	8. Lost innervation of intercostal muscles (T1–T7) and abdominal muscles (T6–T12) destroys the ability to cough and deep breathe effectively (Nelson, Zejdlik, & Love, 2002).

(continues on page 398)

Interventions continued	**Rationales** continued
9. Auscultate lung fields regularly.	9. Auscultation can detect accumulation of retained secretions and asymmetric breath sounds that may indicate pneumonia, pneumothorax.
10. Monitor serial vital capacities.	10. Ascending edema of spinal cord can cause respiratory difficulty requiring immediate intervention (Hickey, 2001).
11. Monitor for signs of paralytic ileus: a. Decreased or absent bowel sounds b. Abdominal distention	11. Gastric dilatation and ileus can result from depressed reflexes, and hypoxia is a late sign of spinal shock (Nelson, Zejdlik, & Love, 2002).
12. Monitor for signs of urinary retention: a. Bladder distention b. Decreased urine output	12. Urinary retention is caused by bladder atony and contraction of the urinary sphincter during spinal shock. Bladder distention can lead to urinary reflux, pyelonephritis, stone formation, renal insufficiency, and dysreflexia (Nelson, Zejdlik, & Love, 2002).
13. Monitor for signs and symptoms of pyelonephritis: a. Fever, chills b. Costovertebral angle pain if sensation is intact at this level; otherwise vague, referred pain c. Leukocytosis d. Bacteria, pus, and nitrites in urine e. Dysuria, frequency	13. Urinary tract infections can be caused by urinary stasis (Nelson, Zejdlik, & Love, 2002). a. Bacteria can act as a pyrogen by raising the hypothalamic thermostat through the production of endogenous pyrogen that may mediate through prostaglandins. Chills can occur when the temperature set-point of the hypothalamus rapidly changes. b. CVA pain results from distention of the renal capsule. c. Leukocytosis reflects an increase in WBCs to fight infection through phagocytosis. d. Bacteria changes urine's odor and pH because of increased nitrites, a by-product of bacteria. e. Bacteria irritate bladder tissue, causing spasms and frequency.
14. Monitor for early signs and symptoms of renal insufficiency:	14. Repeated infections can alter renal function (Nelson, Zejdlik, & Love, 2002).

(continues on page 399)

Interventions continued	Rationales continued
a. Sustained elevated urine specific gravity b. Elevated urine sodium level c. Sustained insufficient urine output (<30 mL/hr) d. Elevated blood pressure e. Elevated blood urea nitrogen (BUN); serum creatinine, potassium, phosphorus, and prealbumin; and creatinine clearance	a,b. Decreased ability of the renal tubules to reabsorb electrolytes causes increased urine sodium levels and increased specific gravity. c,d. Decreased glomerular filtration rate eventually causes insufficient urine output and stimulates renin production, which raises blood pressure in an attempt to increase blood flow to the kidneys. e. Decreased excretion of urea and creatinine in the urine results in elevated BUN and creatinine levels.
15. Monitor intake and output.	15. Intake and output measurements help to evaluate hydration status.
16. Monitor for signs and symptoms of GI bleeding: a. Shoulder pain (referred pain) b. Frank or occult blood in stool c. Hemoptysis d. Nausea and vomiting e. Drop in hemoglobin f. Increased gastric pH	16. GI bleeding can result from irritation of gastric mucosa as a side effect of corticosteroids or from a stress ulcer caused by vagal stimulation which produces gastric hyperacidity (Hickey, 2001). Also monitor laboratory test results for signs and symptoms of pancreatitis.
17. Provide range of motion to all extremities. 18. Consult physical therapy and occupational therapy.	17,18. Range of motion of all extremities can reduce new bone formation around joints of paralyzed limbs (Hickey, 2001).

▼ Related Physician-Prescribed Interventions

Medications. Muscle relaxants; stool softeners, laxatives, suppositories; anticholinergic drugs; etidronate disodium (Didronel); alpha-adrenergic antagonists; methylprednisolone; heparin (subcutaneous); antibiotics; low-molecular weight heparins (LMSH)

Intravenous Therapy. IV steroid therapy initially post injury, IV fluids during spinal shock phase, IV water antagonists during spinal shock phase (to prevent GI bleeding)

Laboratory Studies. Renal function studies, urodynamic studies, arterial blood gases, joint x-ray films, serum alkaline phosphatase, bone scans, erythrocyte sedimentation rate, antibiotic-resistant organisms (ARO) cultures

Diagnostic Studies. Spinal x-ray films, magnetic resonance imaging (MRI), computed tomography (CT) scan, pulmonary function studies

Therapies. Immobilization devices, myelograms, alternating pressure beds, ultrasound (lower extremities), antiembolic stockings, physical therapy, speech therapy, indwelling catheterization, laminectomy, occupational therapy, spinal fusion, psychological services

🔖 Documentation

Flow records
    Vital signs
    Intake and output
    Respiratory assessment
    Abdominal assessment (bowel sounds, distention)
    Stool and emesis assessment (blood)
    Traction (type, weights)
    Vital capacity
    Muscle testing
Progress notes
    Change in status
    Interventions
    Response to interventions

Nursing Diagnoses

Anxiety Related to Perceived Effects of Injury on Life Style and Unknown Future

Focus Assessment Criteria	Clinical Significance
1. Understanding of injury 2. Knowledge of structure and function of affected organs	1,2. The client's understanding of the disorder can affect his or her anxiety level. The client may be influenced positively or negatively by information from others. Assessing client's knowledge level also helps the nurse plan teaching strategies.
3. Life style, strengths, coping mechanism, and available support systems	3. This helps to identify client's resources for managing stress and anxiety.

Goal

The client will relate increased psychological and physiologic comfort.

Indicators
- Share feelings and fears.
- Discuss feelings with significant others.

Interventions	Rationales
1. Provide opportunities for the client to share feelings and concerns. Maintain a calm, relaxed atmosphere; convey a nonjudgmental attitude; and listen attentively. Identify the client's support systems and coping mechanisms and suggest alternatives as necessary.	1. Sharing feelings openly facilitates trust and helps reduce anxiety (Christman & Kirchhoff, 1992).

2. Explain the following:
  a. The need for frequent assessments
  b. Diagnostic tests
	2. Accurate descriptions of expected sensations and procedures help to ease anxiety and fear (Christman & Kirchhoff, 1992).

(continues on page 401)

Interventions continued	Rationales continued
c. The consequences of spinal shock (flaccid paralysis and absent reflexes) d. Treatment	
3. Attempt to provide consistency with staff assignments.	3. Familiarity may increase opportunities for sharing and provide stability and security.
4. Provide opportunities for family members or significant others to share their concerns.	4. Exploration gives nurse the opportunity to correct misinformation and validate the situation as difficult and frightening.
5. Identify a client at risk for unsuccessful adjustment; look for the following characteristics: a. Poor ego strength b. Ineffective problem-solving strategies c. Lack of motivation d. External focus of control e. Poor health f. Unsatisfactory preinjury sex life g. Lack of positive support systems h. Unstable economic status i. Rejection of counseling j. Poor goal directions	5. A client's successful adjustment is influenced by such factors as previous coping success, achievement of developmental tasks before the injury, the extent to which the disability interferes with goal-directed activity, sense of control, and realistic perception of the situation by self and support persons (Elliott & Frank, 1996; Friedman-Campbell & Hart, 1984).
6. Refer high-risk clients to appropriate agencies.	6. Cognitive aspects of depression are less amenable to pharmacological strategies and warrant psychological interventions (Elliott & Frank, 1996).

 Documentation

Progress notes
   Present emotional status
   Interventions
   Client's and/or family's response to interventions

Grieving Related to Loss of Body Function and Its Effects on Life Style

This diagnosis is not currently on the NANDA list but has been added for clarity and usefulness.

Focus Assessment Criteria	Clinical Significance
1. Signs and symptoms of grief reaction (e.g., crying, withdrawal, anxiety, fear, restlessness, decreased appetite, decreased interest, and participation in activities)	1. The client is experiencing losses related to sexual identity, function, and independence. The grief response may be profound or subtle.

Goal

The client will express grief.

Indicators

• Describe the meaning of loss.
• Report an intent to discuss feelings with significant others.

Interventions	Rationales
1. Provide opportunities for the client and family members to ventilate feelings, discuss the loss openly, and explore the personal meaning of the loss. Explain that grief is a common and healthy reaction.	1. Loss may give rise to feelings of powerlessness, anger, profound sadness, and other grief responses. Open, honest discussions can help the client and family members to accept and cope with the situation and their responses to it.
2. Encourage use of positive coping strategies that have proved successful in the past.	2. Positive coping strategies aid acceptance and problem solving.
3. Encourage the client to express positive self-attributes.	3. Focusing on positive attributes increases self-acceptance and acceptance of the loss.
4. Implement measures to support the family and promote cohesiveness: a. Help them acknowledge and accept losses. b. Explain the grieving process. c. Encourage verbalization of feelings. d. Allow family members to participate in client care.	4. Family cohesiveness is important to client support.
5. Promote grief work with each response: a. Denial: • Encourage acceptance of the situation; do not reinforce denial by giving false reassurance. • Promote hope through assurances of care, comfort, and support. • Explain the use of denial by one family member to other members. • Do not push a person to move past denial until he or she is emotionally ready. b. Isolation: • Convey acceptance by encouraging expressions of grief. • Promote open, honest communication to encourage sharing. • Reinforce the client's self-worth by providing for privacy when desired. • Encourage socialization as feasible (e.g., support groups, church activities).	5. Grieving involves profound emotional responses; interventions depend on the particular response.

(continues on page 403)

Interventions continued	**Rationales** continued
c. Depression: • Reinforce the client's self-esteem. • Employ empathetic sharing and acknowledge grief. • Identify the degree of depression and develop appropriate strategies. d. Anger: • Explain to other family members that anger represents an attempt to control the environment and stems from frustration at the inability to control the disease. • Encourage verbalization of anger. e. Guilt: • Acknowledge the person's expressed self-image. • Encourage identification of the relationship's positive aspects. • Avoid arguing and participating in the person's system of thinking, "I should have . . ." and, "I shouldn't have. . . ." f. Fear: • Focus on the present and maintain a safe and secure environment. • Help the person to explore reasons for and meanings of the fears. g. Rejection: • Provide reassurance by explaining what is happening. • Explain this response to other family members. h. Hysteria: • Reduce environmental stressors. (e.g., limit personnel). • Provide a safe, private area in which to express grief.	

 Documentation

Progress notes
    Present emotional status
    Interventions
Response to nursing interventions

High Risk for Disturbed Self-Concept Related to Effects of Disability on Achieving Developmental Tasks and Life Style

Focus Assessment Criteria	**Clinical Significance**
1. Previous exposure to persons with spinal cord injury	1–4. This information helps the nurse to detect patterns of response due to adaptation.

(continues on page 404)

Focus Assessment Criteria continued	Clinical Significance continued
2. Ability to express feelings about condition 3. Ability to share feelings with family members or significant others 4. Evidence of or others' reports of negative self-concept	It may be helpful to note how the client's support persons view the client's self-concept; they can provide insight into factors that may have had a negative impact on self-concept, and they tend to be sensitive to subtle changes.
5. Participation in self-care 6. Evidence of adapting life style to disabilities	5,6. Participation in self-care and adaptation of goals to disability indicate attempts to cope with the changes (Hamburg & Adams, 1983).

Goal

The client will demonstrate positive coping skills.

Indicators

- Acknowledge changes in body structure and function.
- Communicate feelings about disability
- Participate in self-care.

Interventions	Rationales
1. Contact client frequently and treat him or her with warm, positive regard.	1. Frequent contact by the caregiver indicates acceptance and may facilitate trust. The client may be hesitant to approach the staff because of negative self-concept (Dudas, 1993).
2. Encourage client to express feelings and thoughts about the following: a. Condition b. Progress c. Prognosis d. Effects on life style e. Support system f. Treatments	2. Encouraging client to share feelings can provide a safe outlet for fears and frustrations and can increase self-awareness (Dudas, 1993).
3. Provide reliable information and clarify any misconceptions.	3. Misconceptions can needlessly increase anxiety and damage self-concept. Answer all questions honestly.
4. Help client to identify positive attributes and possible new opportunities.	4. Client may tend to focus only on the change in self-image and not on the positive characteristics that contribute to the whole concept of self. The nurse must re-

(continues on page 405)

Interventions continued	Rationales continued
	inforce these positive aspects and encourage the client to reincorporate them into a new self-concept (Dudas, 1993).
5. Assist with hygiene and grooming as needed.	5. Participation in self-care and planning can aid positive coping.
6. Encourage visitors.	6. Frequent visits by support persons can help the client feel that he or she is still a worthwhile, acceptable person; this should promote a positive self-concept.
7. Help client to identify strategies to increase independence and maintain role responsibilities: a. Prioritizing activities b. Using mobility aids and assistive devices as needed.	7. A strong component of self-concept is the ability to perform functions expected of one's role, thus decreasing dependency and reducing the need for others' involvement.
8. Prepare significant others for physical and emotional changes.	8. Others can give support more freely and more realistically if they are prepared (Dudas, 1993).
9. Discuss with members of client's support system the importance of communicating the client's value and importance to them.	9. This will enhance self-esteem and promote adjustment (Dudas, 1993).
10. Allow the client's support persons to share their feelings regarding the diagnoses and actual or anticipated effects.	10. Spinal cord injury can negatively affect support persons financially, socially, and emotionally.
11. Assess for signs of negative response to changes in appearance: a. Refusal to discuss loss b. Denial of changes c. Decreased self-care ability d. Social isolation e. Refusal to discuss future	11. These signs may indicate that the client is at high risk for unsuccessful adjustment.
12. Refer an at-risk client for professional counseling.	12. Follow-up therapy may be indicated to assist with adjustment.

 Documentation

Progress notes
Present emotional status
Interventions
  Response to interventions

High Risk for Dysreflexia Related to Reflex Stimulation of Sympathetic Nervous System Below the Level of Cord Injury Secondary to Loss of Autonomic Control

Focus Assessment Criteria	Clinical Significance

1. History of dysreflexia:
  a. Triggered by:
    • Bladder distention
    • Bowel distention/impaction
    • Tactile stimulation
    • Skin lesion(s)
    • Sexual activity
    • Menstruation
    • Urinary tract infection
    • Labor and delivery
    • Muscle spasms
    • Urethral stone
    • Constricting clothing
  b. Initial symptoms:
    • Increased systolic and diastolic BP
    • Headache
    • Sweating above the level of injury
    • Chills
    • Metallic taste
    • Nasal congestion
    • Blurred vision
    • Numbness
    • Piloerection or "goose bumps" above the level of injury
    • Apprehension
    • Bradycardia or tachycardia (occasionally)
    • Penile erections
    • Facial flushing
    • Blanching
    • Rash on neck and chest
  c. Current medications: any recent changes in use
	1. With spinal cord injury (T6 or above), the cord activity below the injury is deprived of the controlling effects from the higher centers; this results in poorly controlled responses (Hickey, 2001; Teasell, Malcolm & Delaney, 1996). The uninhibited responses are life-threatening if not reversed. A baseline of history, triggering activities, initial symptoms, and medication use enables the nurse to make subsequent assessments of dysreflexic activity (Lee, Yarmakar, Herz & Sturgill, 1995; Nelson, Zejdlik & Love, 2002).

2. Bladder program: type, problems, any recent changes 3. Bowel program: type, problems, any recent changes	2,3. A distended bowel or bladder can trigger dysreflexia.
4. Knowledge of dysreflexia (if source is not found quickly, call 911)	4. The client and family can be taught how to prevent and treat dysreflexia.

Goal

The client and family will prevent or respond to early signs/symptoms of dysreflexia.

Indicators
• State factors that cause dysreflexia.
• Describe the treatment for dysreflexia.
• Relate when emergency treatment is indicated.

Interventions	Rationales

1. Monitor for signs and symptoms of dysreflexia:
  a. Paroxysmal hypertension (sudden periodic elevated blood pressure: systolic pressure >140 mm Hg, diastolic >90 mm Hg)
  b. Bradycardia or tachycardia
  c. Diaphoresis
  d. Red splotches on skin above the level of injury
  e. Pallor below the level of injury
  f. Headache
	1. Spasms of pelvic viscera and arterioles cause vasoconstriction below the level of injury, producing hypertension and pallor. Afferent impulses triggered by high blood pressure cause vagal stimulation, resulting in bradycardia. Baroreceptors in the aortic arch and carotid sinus respond to the hypertension, triggering superficial vasodilatation, flushing, diaphoresis, and headache (above the level of cord injury) (Nelson, Zejdlik, & Love, 2002; Lee, 1995).

2. If signs of dysreflexia occur, raise the head of the bed, loosen constrictive clothing or restraints, and remove the noxious stimuli as follows:
  a. Bladder distention:
   • Check for distended bladder
   • If catheterized, check the catheter for kinks or compression; empty collection bag; irrigate with only 30 mL of saline solution instilled very slowly; replace the catheter if it will not drain.
   • If not catheterized, insert a catheter using dibucaine hydrochloride ointment (Nupercaine). Then remove the 500 mL clamp for 15 minutes; repeat until the bladder is drained. May have bladder spasm secondary to urinary tract infection. Send urine culture before giving Nupercaine.
  b. Fecal impaction:
   • First, apply Nupercaine to the anus and about 1 inch into the rectum. Wait 5 to 10 minutes before removing stool.
   • Gently check the rectum with a well-lubricated gloved finger.
   • Insert a rectal suppository or gently remove the impaction.
  c. Skin stimulation: Spray the skin lesion triggering dysreflexia with a topical anesthetic agent.
	2. These interventions aim to reduce cerebral hypertension and induce orthostatic hypotension (Nelson, Zejdlik, & Love, 2002).
	
	  a. Bladder distention is the most common cause of dysreflexia. Bladder distention can trigger dysreflexia by stimulating sensory receptors. Nupercaine ointment reduces tissue stimulation. Too rapid removal of urine can result in compensatory hypotension.
	
	  b. Fecal impaction prevents stimulation of sensory receptors. It is the second most common cause.
	
	  c. Dysreflexia can be triggered by stimulation (e.g., of the glans penis or skin lesions).

3. Continue to monitor blood pressure every 3 to 5 minutes.	3. Failure to reverse severe hypertension can result in status epilepticus, cerebrovascular accident, and death (Nelson, Zejdlik, & Love, 2002).
4. Immediately consult the physician for pharmacological treatment if symptoms	4. Use an antihypertensive agent with rapid onset and short duration while the causes

(continues on page 408)

Interventions continued	Rationales continued
or noxious stimuli are not eliminated. Continue to search for cause (e.g., pulmonary embolus).	of autonomic dysreflexia are investigated. Nifedipine and nitrates are the most commonly used agents. Nifedipine used should be in the immediate-release form; sublingual nifedipine may lead to erratic absorption. Other drugs used to treat AD with severe symptoms include hydralazine mecamylamine, diazoxide, and phenoxybenzamine. If 2% nitroglycerin ointment is used, 1″ may be applied to the skin above the level of the SCI. For monitored settings, the use of IV drip of sodium nitroprusside can be used. Nitropaste is used. Blood pressure is monitored.

5. Initiate health teaching and referrals as indicated:
  a. Teach signs and symptoms and treatment of dysreflexia.
  b. Teach when immediate medical intervention is warranted.
  c. Explain what situations can trigger dysreflexia (e.g., menstrual cycle, sexual activity, bladder or bowel routines).
  d. Teach client to watch for early signs and to intervene immediately.
  e. Teach client to observe for early signs of bladder infections and skin lesions (e.g., pressure ulcers or ingrown toenails).
  f. Advise client to consult with the physician for long-term pharmacological management if the client is very vulnerable to dysreflexia.
  g. The unit should have a protocol and an emergency medication tray for autonomic dysreflexia.
	5. Good teaching can help the client and family to successfully prevent or treat dysreflexia at home.

 Documentation

Progress notes
  Episodes of dysreflexia (cause, treatment, response)
Discharge summary record
Client teaching

Interrupted Family Processes Related to Adjustment Requirements, Role Disturbance, and Uncertain Future

Focus Assessment Criteria	Clinical Significance
1. Understanding condition	1–4. The family unit is a system based on interdependence among members and patterns that provide structure and support.
2. Family coping patterns	

(continues on page 409)

Focus Assessment Criteria continued	Clinical Significance continued
3. Current response	Chronic disability disrupts these relationships and patterns.
4. Available resources	

Goal

The client and family members will demonstrate or report a functional system of mutual support.

Indicators
- Verbalize feelings regarding the situation.
- Identify signs of family dysfunction.
- Identify appropriate resources to seek when needed.

Interventions	Rationales
1. Convey an understanding of the situation and its impact on the family.	1. Communicating understanding and a sense of caring and concern facilitates trust and strengthens the nurse's relationship with the client and family.
2. Explore family members' perceptions of the situation. Encourage verbalization of feelings such as guilt, anger, helplessness and blame.	2. Verbalization can provide opportunities for clarification and validation of feelings and concerns this contributes to family unity.
3. Determine if present coping mechanisms are effective.	3. Illness of a family member may cause great changes, which puts the family at high risk for maladaptation.

4. Take steps to promote family strengths:
  a. Acknowledge the assistance of family members.
  b. Involve them in the client's care.
  c. To prevent burnout, encourage time away from caregiving.
  d. Encourage humor. (Refer to Chapter 3, The Ill Adult: Issues and Responses, for more information.)
	4. This can help to maintain the existing family structure and its function as a supportive unit (Clemen-Stone, Eigigasti & McGuire, 2001; Decker, Schultz & Wood, 1989).

5. Assist family to reorganize roles at home, set new priorities, and redistribute responsibilities.	5. Planning and prioritizing can help to maintain family integrity and reduce stress.
6. Prepare family for signs of depression, anxiety, anger, and dependency in the client and other family members.	6. Anticipatory guidance can alert members to potential problems before they occur; this enables prompt intervention at early signs.

(continues on page 410)

Interventions continued	**Rationales** continued
7. Encourage family to call on its social network (e.g., friends, relatives, church members) for emotional and other support.	7. Outside assistance may help to reduce the perception that the family must "go it alone."
8. Identify dysfunctional coping mechanisms such as the following: a. Substance abuse b. Continued denial c. Exploitation of one or more family members d. Separation or avoidance Refer for counseling as necessary.	8. A family with a history of unsuccessful coping may need additional resources. A family with unresolved conflicts prior to diagnosis is at high risk (Clemen-Stone, Eigigasti, & McGuire, 2001; Decker, Schultz, & Wood, 1989).
9. Provide health education and specific information regarding injury, treatments, procedures, and illness symptoms.	9. Thorough education for the family is necessary to assist in maintaining the patient's health and to manage the effects of the disability (Nelson, Zejdlik, & Love, 2002).
10. Direct to community agencies and other sources of assistance (e.g., financial, housekeeping, or direct care) as needed.	10. The family may need assistance to help with management at home.

 Documentation

Progress notes
   Present family functioning
   Interventions
   Family's response to interventions
Discharge summary record
   Referrals if indicated

High Risk for Ineffective Sexuality Pattern Related to Physiologic, Sensory, and Psychological Effects of Disability on Sexuality or Function

Focus Assessment Criteria	**Clinical Significance**
1. Previous sexual patterns 2. Partner availability 3. Upper extremity muscle strength 4. Presence of catheters	1–4. Loss of sensory and motor function can cause erectile problems in men and libido problems in both genders. Sexual options available to the spinal cord-injured client are influenced by sexual value system, previous sexual function, upper-extremity muscle strength, presence of hip flexors and extensors, presence of appliances (e.g., casts and catheters), and availability of a caring partner (Nelson, Zejdlik & Love, 2002).

(continues on page 411)

Focus Assessment Criteria continued	Clinical Significance continued
5. Family planning decisions	5. Cord injuries usually do not affect female fertility. Paraplegic females can become pregnant and deliver vaginally.

Goal

The client will report satisfying sexual activity.

Indicators

• Discuss own feelings and partner's concerns regarding sexual functioning.
• Verbalize intention to discuss concerns with partner before discharge.
• Be knowledgeable of alternative means of sexual satisfaction.

Interventions	Rationales
1. Initiate a discussion regarding concerns associated with sexuality and sexual function. Use the "PLISSIT" model: P-permission, L-limited, I-information, S-sensitivity, S, I-intervention, T-therapy/ treatment.	1. Many clients are reluctant to discuss sexual matters; initiating discussions demonstrates your empathy and concern (Nelson, Zejdlik, & Love, 2002).
2. Provide accurate information on the effect of the cord injury on sexual functioning.	2. Accurate information can prevent false hope or give real hope as appropriate.
3. Reaffirm the need for frank discussion between sexual partners.	3. Both partners have fears and concerns about sexual activity. Repressing these feelings negatively influences the relationship.
4. Explain how the client and partner can use role-playing to bring concerns about sex out in the open.	4. Role-playing helps a person to gain insight by placing self in the position of another and allows more spontaneous sharing of fears and concerns.
5. Discuss alternate means of sexual satisfaction for self and partner (e.g., vibrators, touching, oral-genital techniques, and body massage); consider past sexual experiences before suggesting specific techniques.	5. Client and partner can experience sexual satisfaction and gratification through various alternatives to intercourse (Nelson, Zejdlik, & Love, 2002).
6. Encourage the client to consult with others with spinal cord injuries for an exchange of information; refer client to pertinent literature and organizations.	6. Interacting with others in a similar situation can help to reduce feelings of isolation, provide information on alternative sexual practices, and allow frank sharing of problems and concerns.

(continues on page 412)

Interventions continued	Rationales continued
7. Provide information on managing bowel and bladder programs prior to sexual intercourse.	7. Performing bowel and bladder routines before sex activities decreases incontinence episodes (Nelson, Zejdlik, & Love, 2002).
8. Refer the client and partner to a certified sex or mental health professional if desired.	8. Certain sexual problems require continuing therapy and the advanced knowledge of therapists.
9. Explore birth control options.	9. Because of the risk of thrombophlebitis with the "pill," oral contraceptives are not a good option for an SCI woman.

 Documentation

Progress notes
    Dialogues
Discharge summary record
    Referrals if indicated

Bowel Incontinence: Reflexic Related to Lack of Voluntary Sphincter Control Secondary to Spinal Cord Injury Above the Eleventh Thoracic Vertebra (T11)

Focus Assessment Criteria	Clinical Significance
1. Understanding injury 2. Previous and current bowel patterns 3. Control of rectal sphincter, presence of anal wink and bulbocavernosus reflex 4. Awareness of bowel cues	1–4. Complete central nervous system lesions or trauma occurring above sacral cord segments (S2, S3, S4) (T12-L1-L2 vertebral level) result in a reflexic neurogenic bowel. The ascending sensory signals between the sacral reflex center and the brain are interrupted, resulting in the inability to feel the urge to defecate. Descending motor signals from the brain are also interrupted, causing loss of voluntary control over the anal sphincter. Once spinal shock has abated, the bulbocavernosus reflex usually returns. Because the sacral reflex center is preserved, it is possible to develop a stimulation-response bowel evacuation program using digital stimulation or digital stimulation devices. Fecal incontinence may occur through sacral arc reflex action, although this occurs less frequently than in a reflexic bowel owing to the fact that in a reflexic bowel, the external anal sphincter usually remains in the contracted state until stimulated to relax (Teasell, Malcolm & Delaney, 1996).

Goal
The client will evacuate a soft formed stool every other day or every third day.

Interventions	Rationales
1. Assess previous bowel elimination patterns, diet, and life style.	1. This assessment enables the nurse to plan a bowel program to meet the client's habits and needs.
2. Determine present neurological and physiological statuses and functional levels.	2. Establishing an appropriate bowel program in accordance with the client's functional level and ability helps to reduce frustration.
3. Plan a consistent, appropriate time for elimination. Institute a daily bowel program for 5 days or until a pattern develops, then an alternate-day program (morning or evening).	3. A routine evacuation schedule decreases or eliminates the chance of involuntary stool passage.
4. Provide privacy and a nonstressful environment.	4. Privacy decreases anxiety and promotes self-image and esteem.
5. Position in an upright or sitting position if functionally able. If not functionally able (quadriplegic), position in left side-lying position; use digital stimulation—gloves, lubricant, or index finger (adults).	5. Upright positioning facilitates movement of stool by enlisting the aid of gravity and by aiding emptying of the descending colon into the sigmoid colon.
6. For a functionally able client, use assistive devices (e.g., dil stick, digital stimulator, raised commode seat, and lubricant and gloves as appropriate).	6. A dil stick and digital stimulator stimulate the rectal sphincter and lower colon, initiating peristalsis for movement of fecal material.
7. For a client with upper extremity mobility and abdominal musculature innervation, teach bowel elimination facilitation techniques as appropriate: a. Valsalva's maneuver b. Forward bends c. Sitting push-ups d. Abdominal massage in clockwise manner.	7. These techniques increase intra-abdominal pressure to facilitate passage of stool at evacuation time. a. Do not teach Valsalva's maneuver if person has a cardiac problem (Nelson, Zejdlik, & Love, 2002).
8. Assist with or provide equipment needed for hygiene measures as necessary.	8. Good hygiene helps to prevent skin breakdown.
9. Maintain an elimination record or a flow sheet of the bowel schedule that includes time, stool characteristics, assistive method(s) used, and number of involuntary stools (if any).	9. Ongoing documentation of elimination schedule and results provides data helpful to bowel program management.

(continues on page 414)

Interventions continued	**Rationales** continued
10. Provide reassurance and protection from embarrassment while establishing the bowel program.	10. Reassurance decreases anxiety and promotes self-esteem.
11. Initiate a nutritional consultation; provide a diet high in fluid and fiber content. Monitor fluid intake and output.	11. Frequency and consistency of stool are related to fluid and food intake. Fiber increases fecal bulk and enhances water absorption into stool. Adequate dietary fiber and fluid intake promote firm but soft, well-formed stools and decrease the risk of hard, dry, constipated stools.
12. Provide physical activity and exercise appropriate to the client's functional ability and endurance.	12. Physical activity promotes peristalsis, aids digestion, and facilitates elimination.
13. Teach appropriate use of stool softeners, laxatives, and suppositories; and explain the hazards of enemas.	13. Laxatives upset a bowel program because they cause much of the bowel to empty and can cause unscheduled bowel movements. With constant laxative use, the colon loses tone and bowel retraining becomes difficult. Chronic use of bowel aids can lead to inconsistent stool consistency, which interferes with the scheduled bowel program and bowel management. Stool softeners may not be necessary if diet and fluid intake are adequate. Enemas lead to overstretching of the bowel and loss of bowel tone, contributing to further constipation.
14. Explain the signs and symptoms of fecal impaction and constipation.	14. Fecal impaction and constipation may lead to autonomic dysreflexia in a client with injury at T7 or higher, owing to bowel overdistention. Chronic constipation can lead to overdistention of the bowel with further loss of bowel tone. Unrelieved constipation may result in fecal impaction. Early intervention in diet and fluid intake, bowel evacuation methods, and schedules helps to prevent constipation, further loss of bowel tone, and fecal impaction.
15. Initiate teaching of a bowel program as soon as the client is able to sit up in a wheelchair for 2 to 4 hours. If the client is functionally able, encourage independence with the bowel program; if client is quadriplegic with limited hand function, incorporate assistive devices or attendant care as needed.	15. Teaching bowel management techniques, bowel complications, and the impact of diet, fluids, and exercise on elimination can help to promote independent functioning or help the client to instruct others in specific care measures that promote adequate elimination and prevent complications.

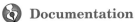 **Documentation**

Flow records
  Stool results (time, method used, involuntary stools)
Discharge summary record
  Client teaching
    Outcome achievement or status

Bowel Incontinence: Areflexic Related to Lack of Voluntary Sphincter Secondary to Spinal Cord Injury Involving Sacral Reflex Arc (S2–S4)

Focus Assessment Criteria	Clinical Significance
1. Understanding injury	1. Complete spinal cord injury, spinal cord lesions, neurologic disease, or congenital defects causing an interruption of the sacral reflex arc (at the sacral segments S2, S3, S4) result in an areflexic (autonomous) or flaccid bowel. Flaccid paralysis at this level, known as an LMN lesion, results in loss of the defecation reflex, loss of sphincter control (flaccid anal sphincter), and absence of the bulbocavernosus reflex. Lower motor neuron dysfunction may be temporary as in spinal shock or permanent when there is an injury (generally associated with fractures at or below the T12-L1 vertebrae) (Nelson, Zejdlik, & Love, 2002).
2. Previous and present bowel patterns 3. Dietary patterns: food and fluid intake	2,3. Because of an interrupted sacral reflex arc and a flaccid anal sphincter, bowel incontinence can occur without rectal stimulation whenever stool is present in the rectal vault. The stool may leak out if too soft or remain (if not extracted), predisposing the client to fecal impaction or constipation. Some intrinsic contractile abilities of the colon remain, but peristalsis is sluggish, leading to stool retention with contents present in the rectal vault.
4. Awareness of bowel cues	4. Interruption of the sensory and motor pathways to the brain usually results in loss of cerebral awareness and control of elimination.

Goal

The client will evacuate a firm, formed stool every day.

Indicator

• Relate bowel elimination techniques.

Interventions	Rationales
1. Assess previous bowel elimination patterns, diet, and life style.	1. This assessment enables the nurse to plan a bowel program to meet the client's habits and needs.
2. Determine present neurologic and physiologic statuses and functional levels.	2. Establishing an appropriate bowel program in accordance with the client's functional level and ability helps to reduce frustration.
3. Plan a consistent, appropriate time for elimination. Institute a *daily* bowel program.	3. A routine evacuation schedule decreases or eliminates the chance of involuntary stool passage. Evacuating any stool in rectum before periods of activity can prevent accidents. A major evacuation should be performed daily (Nelson, Zejdlik, & Love, 2002).
4. Provide privacy and a nonstressful environment.	4. Privacy decreases anxiety and promotes self-image and esteem.
5. Position in an upright or sitting position as soon as his or her condition warrants.	5. Upright positioning facilitates movement of stool by enlisting the aid of gravity and by aiding emptying of the descending colon into the sigmoid colon.
6. Digitally (manually) empty the rectum with a gloved and well-lubricated finger.	6. Techniques used to trigger a stimulus–response reflex, such as digital stimulation or suppository administration, are not effective with an areflexic bowel because of the absence of the sacral reflex arc (Mitchell, 1988).
7. Teach bowel elimination facilitation techniques: a. Valsalva's maneuver b. Forward bends c. Sitting push-ups d. Abdominal massage in clockwise manner	7. These techniques increase intra-abdominal pressure to facilitate stool passage at evacuation time. Upper-extremity function should be intact with this level of lesion, and thus the client can assume responsibility for the procedure. a. Do not teach Valsalva's maneuver if patient has a cardiac problem (Nelson, Zejdlik, & Love, 2002).
8. Assist with or provide equipment needed for hygiene measures as necessary.	8. Good hygiene helps to prevent skin breakdown.

(continues on page 417)

Interventions continued	**Rationales** continued
9. Maintain an elimination record or a flow sheet of the bowel schedule that includes time, stool characteristics, assistive method(s) used, and number of involuntary stools, if any.	9. Ongoing documentation of elimination schedule and results provides data helpful to bowel program management.
10. Provide reassurance and protection from embarrassment while establishing the bowel program.	10. Reassurance decreases anxiety and promotes self-esteem.
11. Initiate a nutritional consultation; provide a diet high in fluid and fiber content. Monitor fluid intake and output.	11. Frequency and consistency of stool are related to fluid and food intake. Fiber increases fecal bulk and enhances water absorption into the stool. Adequate dietary fiber and fluid intake promote firm but soft, well-formed stools and decrease the risk of hard, dry, constipated stools.
12. Provide physical activity and exercise appropriate to the client's functional ability and endurance.	12. Physical activity promotes peristalsis, aids digestion, and facilitates elimination.
13. Teach appropriate use of stool softeners and laxatives; explain the hazards of enemas.	13. Laxatives upset a bowel program because they cause much of the bowel to empty and can cause unscheduled bowel movements. With constant laxative use, the colon loses tone and bowel retraining becomes difficult. Chronic use of bowel aids can lead to inconsistent stool consistency, which interferes with the scheduled bowel program and bowel management. Stool softeners may not be necessary if diet and fluid intake are adequate. Enemas lead to overstretching of the bowel and loss of bowel tone, contributing to further constipation.
14. Explain the signs and symptoms of fecal impaction and constipation.	14. Bowel motility is decreased in LMN cord damage; decreased stool movement through the colon can result in increased fluid absorption from stool, resulting in hard, dry stools and constipation. Unrelieved constipation may result in fecal impaction. Early intervention in diet and fluid intake, bowel evacuation methods, and schedules help to prevent constipation, further loss of bowel tone, and fecal impaction.

(continues on page 418)

Interventions continued	Rationales continued
15. Initiate teaching of a bowel program when the client is mobile (wheelchair or ambulation). Encourage independence with the bowel program.	15. Teaching bowel management techniques, bowel complications, and the impact of diet, fluids, and exercise on elimination can help to promote independent functioning or help the client to instruct others in specific care measures that promote adequate elimination and prevent complications.

Documentation

Flow records
  Consistency of stool
  Amount of stool
  Time of evacuation
  Time and number of involuntary stools if any
  Any leakage of stool from rectum
  Bowel sounds
  Intake and output
  Assistive devices if any
Progress notes
  Unsatisfactory results/toleration of procedure
  Evidence of hemorrhoids, bleeding, abnormal sacral skin appearance
Discharge summary record
Client teaching

High Risk for Ineffective Therapeutic Regimen Management Related to Insufficient Knowledge of the Effects of Altered Skin, Bowel, Bladder, Respiratory, Thermoregulatory, and Sexual Function and Their Management; Signs and Symptoms of Complications; Follow-up Care; and Community Resources

Focus Assessment Criteria	Clinical Significance
1. Readiness and ability to learn and retain information	1. A client or family who fails to achieve learning goals requires a referral for assistance postdischarge.

Goals

The goals for this diagnosis represent those associated with discharge planning. Refer to the discharge criteria.

Interventions	Rationales
1. Reinforce the effects of injury on bowel, bladder, thermoregulation, respiratory system, and integumentary function.	1. This information may encourage the client and family to comply with the therapeutic regimen.
2. Assist in formulating and accepting realistic short- and long-term goals.	2. Mutual goal setting reinforces the client's sense of control over life.

(continues on page 419)

Interventions continued	**Rationales** continued
3. Evaluate the client's and family member's or significant other's ability to perform the following: a. Skin care and assessment b. Bowel program c. Bladder program d. Proper positioning e. Transfer techniques f. Application of abdominal binder, anti-embolic hose, splints, and protectors g. Range-of-motion exercises (active and passive) h. Assisted coughing techniques	3. These skills are essential to an effective home management program.
4. Reinforce the teaching about dysreflexia and its treatment.	4. Reinforcement promotes feelings of competency and confidence.
5. Explain the reasons for temperature fluctuation and risks of hypothermia and hyperthermia.	5. Interruption in the sympathetic system disrupts the vasoconstriction or vasodilatation response to temperature changes. Also diaphoresis is absent below the level of cord injury. As a result, the client's body assumes the temperature of the environment (poikilothermia).
6. Explain the importance of a well-balanced diet with caloric intake appropriate for activity level.	6. A well-balanced diet is needed to maintain tissue integrity, prevent complications (e.g., skin problems, infection, osteoporosis), and prevent weight gain.
7. Instruct to report the following: a. Cloudy, foul-smelling urine b. Unresolved signs of dysreflexia c. Fever, chills d. Green, purulent, or rust-colored sputum e. Nausea and vomiting f. Persistent skin lesion or irritation g. Swelling and redness of lower extremities h. Increased restriction of movement i. Unsatisfactory bowel or bladder results	7. Early detection of complications enables prompt interventions to prevent debilitating results. Complications can include infections (urinary tract, respiratory, or GI), thrombophlebitis, pressure ulcers, contractures, and dysreflexia.
8. Emphasize the need to participate in the scheduled rehabilitation plan.	8. With training and assistance, most spinal cord-injured clients can attain some degree of independence in activities of daily living.
9. Initiate a referral for assistance with home care (e.g., community nurses, social service).	9. Regardless of the success experienced in the hospital, the client and family need assistance with adjustment postdischarge.

(continues on page 420)

Interventions continued	**Rationales** continued
10. Provide information on self-help sessions and hand out printed material such as the following: a. National Spinal Cord Injury Association, 600 West Cummings Park, Suite 2000, Woburn, MA 01801, 1-800-962-9629 b. *Yes, You Can! A Guide To Self-Care for Persons with Spinal Cord Injury* Paralyzed Veterans of America, 801 Eighteenth Street, N.W., Washington, DC 20006, 1-800-424-8200 c. Spinal Network, P.O. Box 4162, Boulder, CO 80306, 1-800-338-5412	10. Specialized organizations and resources can provide timely information on a variety of related issues or problems.

 Documentation

Discharge summary record
  Client teaching
  Outcome achievement or status
  Referrals if indicated

Sensory Disorders

GLAUCOMA

Glaucoma involves an intraocular pressure increase resulting from pathologic changes at the irido-corneal angle that prevent the normal outflow of aqueous humor. This increased pressure causes progressive structural or functional damage to the optic nerve and may eventually lead to blindness. This process is asymptomatic and preventable in most individuals.

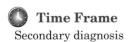 **Time Frame**

Secondary diagnosis

DIAGNOSTIC CLUSTER*	
Collaborative Problems	
PC: Increased Intraocular Pressure	
Nursing Diagnoses	**Refer to**
• Anxiety related to actual or potential vision loss and perceived impact of chronic illness on life style	
• High Risk for Noncompliance related to negative side effects of prescribed therapy versus the belief that no treatment is needed without the presence of symptoms	
• High Risk for Ineffective Therapeutic Regimen Management related to insufficient knowledge of disease process, current clinical status, and treatment plan	
• High Risk for Injury related to visual limitations	• Enucleation
• High Risk for Loneliness related to reduced peripheral vision and altered visual acuity	• Enucleation
• High Risk for Disturbed Self-Concept related to effects of visual limitations	• Enucleation

*This medical condition was not included in the validation study.

Discharge Criteria

Before discharge, the client or family will

1. Describe the causes and effects of glaucoma.
2. Identify present visual impairments if any.
3. Describe the need for daily medications and regular follow-up.
4. State the signs and symptoms that must be reported to a health care professional.

Collaborative Problems

Potential Complication: Increased Intraocular Pressure

Nursing Goal

The nurse will detect early signs and symptoms of increased intraocular pressure and collaboratively intervene to stabilize client.

Indicators
- Intact color vision
- Clear vision
- Reports of no halos around lights

Interventions	Rationale

1. Teach client to report the following:
  a. Difficulty perceiving changes in colors
  b. Blurred vision
  c. Persistent aching in eyes
  d. Intense eye pain
  e. Sudden decrease in or loss of vision
  f. Halos around lights (blue, violet, yellow, red)
	1. If aqueous humor production exceeds its outflow into the Schlemm's canal to the venous system, increased intraocular pressure will result. If untreated, this can lead to compression of nerve fibers and blood vessels in the optic disc and possible permanent damage. (Porth, 2002)

 Related Physician-Prescribed Interventions

Medications. Alpha-adrenergic agonists, cholinergic (miotics), adrenergic agonists, beta blockers, prostaglandin analogs

Diagnostic Studies. Tonometry, perimetry slit-lamp examination, argon laser trabeculoplasty

Therapies. Laser peripheral iridectomy, filtering surgery, drainage implant surgery, carbonic anhydrase inhibitors, visual field test, gonioscopy, ophthalmoscopy

 Documentation

Progress notes
  Complaints of visual or eye problems

Nursing Diagnoses

Anxiety Related to Actual or Potential Vision Loss and Perceived Impact of Chronic Illness on Life Style

Focus Assessment Criteria	Clinical Significance
1. Verbal and nonverbal indicators of anxiety 2. Perception of illness	1–5. The client diagnosed with glaucoma frequently experiences anxiety and fear. Many people associate glaucoma with

(continues on page 425)

Focus Assessment Criteria continued	Clinical Significance continued
3. Understanding of information presented 4. Available support systems 5. Coping mechanisms	blindness, fear of dependence on others, and life style changes. Because few symptoms are associated with the more common forms of the disease, some vision loss may already have occurred by the time of diagnosis. Client may express concerns regarding vision loss and how well the treatment regimen is maintaining intraocular pressure within an acceptable range.

Goal

The client will report increased psychological comfort.

Indicators

• Verbalize his or her concerns and fears.
• Identify one method to reduce anxiety.

Interventions	Rationales
1. Explore client's perception of the condition and its effects on his or her life style and self-concept.	1. Because each person manifests anxiety or fear in a unique manner, the nurse must be alert to subtle changes in the client's behavior. In addition, each client views the disease differently. A client with declining vision may focus only on negative aspects, especially if glaucoma threatens his or her self-concept. For example, to a pilot the diagnosis may mean loss of the work role, but a retired gardener may perceive the diagnosis as less threatening to her or his role. The nurse should attempt to move the client from this phase toward a broadening view of self that incorporates positive role aspects.
2. Provide accurate information and correct any misconceptions.	2. Common misconceptions, such as "all people with glaucoma go blind," "increased intraocular pressure is like high blood pressure," and "the side effects of the medications are worse than the disease," can create or intensify anxiety. Accurate information on disease progression, treatments, and necessary life style changes usually reduces client anxiety.
3. Assist client to identify and use past successful coping mechanisms and support systems.	3. Examining past coping mechanisms and support systems provides the nurse with insight into previous behaviors and a source of data from which to guide future development of coping skills.

(continues on page 426)

Interventions continued	Rationales continued

4. Discuss strategies for socialization and role development:
  a. Continued involvement in previously enjoyed activities
  b. Investigation of possible new roles and activities
	4. Increased socialization can promote self-esteem and reduce anxiety.

5. Refer to outside agencies as appropriate:
  a. Glaucoma Research Foundation
  b. Sight Center/Services for Visually Impaired
  c. Support groups
	5. Referrals to outside agencies may decrease client anxiety by providing other sources of information and support and by enabling the client to interact with others experiencing similar problems.

 Documentation

Progress notes
  Verbal and nonverbal indicators of anxiety
  Interventions
  Client response to interventions
Discharge summary record
  Referrals if indicated

High Risk for Noncompliance Related to Negative Side Effects of Prescribed Therapy Versus the Belief that No Treatment is Needed Without the Presence of Symptoms

Focus Assessment Criteria	Clinical Significance
1. Perception and understanding of glaucoma	1. Assessing client's perception of glaucoma and its seriousness can help to predict compliance or noncompliance.

Goal

The client will verbalize the intent to comply with the prescribed treatment after discharge.

Indicators

• Identify source(s) of support for assisting with compliance.
• Verbalize potential complications of noncompliance

Interventions	Rationales

1. Identify factors that may predict non-compliance:
  a. Lack of knowledge
  b. Noncompliance (previous history of)
  c. Failure to perceive the seriousness or chronicity of glaucoma
  d. Belief that the condition resolves itself
	1. Openly addressing the barriers to compliance may reduce noncompliance.

(continues on page 427)

Interventions continued	Rationales continued
2. Stress the importance of adhering to the treatment regimen and of notifying a health care professional if unable to do so.	2. Client may require frequent motivation to adhere to a sometimes complex routine. If some vision loss has occurred, he or she may question the need for continued treatment that does not seem effective. The nurse should reinforce the medication as a mechanism for saving sight, even though it cannot restore sight that has already been lost. Conversely a client with no symptoms also may not perceive the point of medication therapy. The nurse must explain that medication still is important to prevent vision loss.
3. Explain out that elevated intraocular pressure may produce no symptoms.	3. Lack of symptoms often encourages noncompliance.
4. Discuss the effects of the client's vision loss or blindness on family members and significant others.	4. Emphasizing the potential impact of vision loss on the client's support persons (e.g., loss of family income, role changes, possible family dysfunction) may encourage compliance.
5. Include family members and significant others in teaching sessions as appropriate.	5. Family members and significant others who understand the disorder and the treatment regimen may help the client to achieve compliance. (They should not be charged with "policing" the client, however.)
6. Discuss strategies to improve compliance with the treatment regimen. If noncompliance is related to financial concerns, do the following: a. Explore available funding sources (e.g., Lions Club, other civic organizations, social service agencies). b. Refer for governmental assistance as appropriate. c. Compare costs of medications at various pharmacies and encourage patronizing the one with the lowest prices. d. If noncompliance is related to memory impairment, do the following: • Explore mechanisms for cueing (e.g., calendar, notes, reminder calls from family, association of administration with other events). • Develop a set time schedule for administration.	6. To be effective, the regimen must meet the client's individual needs. Involving the client in planning the regimen can help to ensure compliance.

(continues on page 428)

Interventions continued	**Rationales** continued
• Simplify the regimen as much as possible. • Provide written instructions. e. If noncompliance is related to medication's side effects, do the following: • Discuss side effects with the physician, who may change the prescription. • Help client to minimize side effects if prescription cannot be changed; for example, drops may be administered at times when their adverse effect on vision is minimized, such as before bedtime.	
7. Emphasize that ultimately it is the client's choice and responsibility to adhere to the treatment plan.	7. Stressing the client's decision-making ability and responsibility can strengthen feelings of control and self-determination that can promote compliance.

 Documentation

Progress notes
  Noncompliant behavior
Discharge summary record
  Client teaching
  Response to teaching

High Risk for Ineffective Therapeutic Regimen Management Related to Insufficient Knowledge of Disease Process, Current Clinical Status, and Treatment Plan

Focus Assessment Criteria	**Clinical Significance**
1. Knowledge of disease at time of diagnosis and at periodic intervals thereafter	1. Validating the client's knowledge of the disease process enables the nurse to determine the appropriate information to present. A newly diagnosed client may have little information about the disease; a client with long-standing glaucoma should be evaluated and updated periodically about new information generated by ongoing research.
2. Readiness and ability to learn and retain information	2. In a recently diagnosed client, anxiety and denial may impair his or her ability to process information. If such symptoms are noted, reschedule another time to discuss this information.
3. Details and amount of information desired	3. Clients differ in the amount of information they find helpful. Detailed instruction may be overwhelming to one, yet allay the anxieties of another.

Goals

The goals for this diagnosis represent those associated with discharge planning. Refer to the discharge criteria.

Interventions	Rationales
1. Present information necessary for self-care by using a variety of instructional aids and teaching methods: a. Pamphlets b. Audiovisual programs c. Demonstrations	1. a. Pamphlets provide material to review later and are of great benefit if the client is experiencing anxiety and a resulting decreased learning retention. b. Audiovisual programs enable client to stop the presentation at any time and to review the material later or with family. c. Demonstration provides both visual and verbal reinforcement.
2. Discuss the client's current clinical status.	2. Advising client of the latest assessment data provides him or her with information on which to base decisions. It also indicates how well self-care activities are reducing or maintaining intraocular pressure.
3. Describe the dosage schedule, route of administration, and possible side effects of all prescribed medications.	3. Client is more likely to comply with a medication regimen when he or she understands it and its importance. If not advised otherwise, the client may view side effects of glaucoma medications as normal and may not report them.
4. Reiterate plans for follow-up care and testing.	4. Follow-up care enables evaluation of treatment efficacy. Side effects of medications may create a potential for injury. For example, miotics slow pupillary response, predisposing the patient to injury when moving from bright sunlight to a darkened room.
5. Reinforce the need to carry an identification card that specifies the client's diagnosis of glaucoma (crucial in cases of angle closure glaucoma).	5. In a medical emergency such as cardiac arrest, health care providers need to recognize a client with glaucoma to avoid administering atropine or similar-acting agents that can cause a dangerous elevation in intraocular pressure.
6. If peripheral visual losses have occurred, teach the client to scan the environment.	6. Accommodating for peripheral vision losses can prevent injury.

(continues on page 430)

Interventions continued	Rationales continued
7. Explore with client and family members or significant others whether or not vision losses are interfering with activities (e.g., driving, socializing, self-care).	7. Owing to the nature of the disease, the glaucoma client may lose peripheral vision over time. Side effects of glaucoma medications may further reduce visual ability especially in poorly illuminated environments. As vision declines, the client may become uneasy in social situations. Rather than risk detection of reduced acuity, he or she may choose to withdraw from social situations.
8. Provide information on community resources for visually impaired persons, if indicated (e.g., Visually Impaired Society, Bureau of Visually Impaired).	8. Such resources can provide needed assistance with home management and self-care.

 Documentation

Discharge summary record
   Material presented
   Teaching methods used
   Response to teaching

Hematologic Disorders

SICKLE CELL DISEASE

Sickle cell disease (SCD) is an incurable genetic disorder affecting approximately 1 of every 375 African Americans (U.S. Department of Health, 1992). The term *sickle cell disease* actually represents a group of disorders characterized by the production of hemoglobin S. Under certain conditions, this hemoglobin leads to anemia and acute and chronic tissue damage secondary to the sickling of the abnormal red cells. Hemoglobin S (Hb S) molecules tend to bond to one another and to hemoglobin A, forming long aggregates or tactoids. These aggregates increase the viscosity of blood, causing stasis in blood flow. The low oxygen tension concentration of Hb S causes the cells to assume a sickle rather than biconcave shape. This hemoglobin damages erythrocyte membranes, leading to erythrocyte rupture and chronic hemolytic anemia (Porth, 2002).

Symptoms of sickle cell anemia result from thrombosis and infarction, leading to vascular occlusion by the sickled cells and the hemolytic anemia. These episodes are called *sickle cell crisis*. The incidence of sickle cell crisis varies among clients. Some report an incident once a year, whereas others report more than one each month.

The disease in the United States is primarily seen in African Americans but also may be found in people of Mediterranean, Caribbean, South and Central American, and East Indian descent (U.S. Department of Health, 1992). This chronic disease leaves its victims not only debilitated but also with a shortened life span. Presently the disease has no cure but some options are available for altering its course.

Clients can carry the sickle cell trait but not have the disease. These asymptomatic people have reported some sickling symptoms in low oxygen (e.g., unpressurized airplanes, high altitudes, scuba diving).

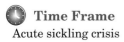 **Time Frame**
Acute sickling crisis

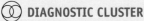 **DIAGNOSTIC CLUSTER**

Collaborative Problems

△ PC: Acute Chest Syndrome
△ PC: Infection
* Anemia
* Vaso-occlusive Crisis
* Aplastic Crisis
* Leg Ulcers
* Neurologic Dysfunction
* Splenic Dysfunction
* Avascular Necrosis of Femoral/Humeral Heads
* Priapism

Nursing Diagnoses

▲ Acute Pain related to viscous blood and tissue hypoxia
△ High Risk for Ineffective Therapeutic Regimen Management related to insufficient knowledge of disease process, risk factors for sickling crisis, pain management, signs and symptoms of complications, genetic counseling, and family planning services
* Powerlessness related to future development of complications of SCD (refer to Diabetes Mellitus)

▲ This diagnosis was reported to be monitored for or managed frequently (75%–100%).
△ This diagnosis was reported to be monitored for or managed often (50%–74%).
* This diagnosis was not included in the validation study.

Discharge Criteria

Before discharge, the client or family will

1. Identify precipitating factors of present crisis if possible.
2. Plan one change in life style to reduce crisis or to improve health.
3. Describe signs and symptoms that must be reported to a health care professional.
4. Describe necessary health maintenance and follow-up care.

Collaborative Problems

Potential Complication: Anemia

Potential Complication: Sickle Cell Crisis

Potential Complication: Acute Chest Syndrome

Potential Complication: Infection

Potential Complication: Leg Ulcers

Potential Complication: Neurologic Dysfunction

Potential Complication: Splenic Dysfunction

Nursing Goal

The nurse will detect early signs and symptoms of (a) anemia, (b) vaso-occlusive crisis, (c) acute chest syndrome, (d) aplastic anemia, (e) infection, (f) leg ulcers, (g) neurologic dysfunction, (h) splenic dysfunction, (i) priapism, and (j) avascular necrosis (femoral/humeral heads) and collaboratively intervene to stabilize client.

Indicators
- Hemoglobin (a, b, d)
  - Males: 13–18 gm/dL
  - Females: 12–16 gm/dL
- Hematocrit (a, b, d)
  - Males: 42–50%
  - Females: 40–48%
- Red blood cells (a, b, d)
  - Males: 4.6–5.9 million/mm^3
  - Females: 4.2–5.4 million/mm^3
- Platelets 150,000–400,000/mm^3 (e)
- White blood cells 4,300–10,800/mm^3 (e)
- Oxygen saturation >95% (a, b, c, d)
- No or minimal bone pain (b, e, j)
- No or minimal abdominal pain (b, e, h)
- No or minimal chest pain (c)
- No or minimal fatigue (a, b, e)
- Pinkish, ruddy, brownish, or olive skin tones (a, b)
- No or minimal headache (b, g)
- Clear, oriented (b, g)
- Clear speech (b, g)
- Pulse rate 60–100 beats/min (a, b, c, g, h)
- Respirations 16–20 breaths/min (b, c, e, g)
- B/P >90/60, <140/90 mm Hg (a, b, c, g, h)
- Temperature 98–99.5°F (b, a, e, f, j)
- Urine output >30 ml/m (b, c, h)
- Urine specific gravity 1.005–1.030 (b, c, h)
- Flaccid penis (i)

Interventions	Rationales

1. Monitor for signs and symptoms of anemia.
  a. Lethargy
  b. Weakness
  c. Fatigue
  d. Increased pallor
  e. Dyspnea on exertion
	1. Because anemia is common with most of these clients, low hemoglobins are relatively tolerated; therefore, changes should be described in reference to person's baseline or acute symptoms (Porth, 2002).

2. Monitor laboratory values including complete blood cell count (CBC) with reticulocyte count.	2. Elevated reticulocytes (normal level about 1%) represent active erythropoiesis. Lack of elevation with anemia may represent a problem (Porth, 2002).

3. Monitor for vaso-occlusive crisis:
  a. Abdominal pain
  b. Chest pain
  c. Bones, joints
	3. Sickled cells block capillaries and cause pain by infarction.

4. Obtain:
  a. Chest x-ray
  b. Abdominal x-ray
  c. CBC with differentiation
  d. Electrolytes
  e. BUN
  f. Liver function test
	4. Other causes of pain (e.g., appendicitis) must be ruled out.

5. Monitor:
  a. Oxygen saturation with pulse oximetry
 	
  b. Hydration status (urine output, specific gravity)
 	
  c. Level of consciousness
	5.
	  a. O_2 should be administered only if oxygen saturation is less than 95%.
	  b. Increased hydration is needed to mobilize clustered cells and to improve tissue perfusion.
	  c. Glasgow coma scale can be used to detect cerebral infarction.

6. Aggressively hydrate client (1.5 × maintenance volume). Avoid IV therapy if possible.	6. Hydration can disrupt the clustered cells and improve hypoxemia.

7. Monitor for signs and symptoms of acute chest syndrome:
  a. Fever
  b. Acute chest pain
  c. Cough
	7. Acute chest syndrome is the term used to represent the group of symptoms, namely, acute pleuritic chest pain, fever, leukocytosis, and infiltrates on chest X-ray seen in SCD. This represents a medical emergency and may be caused by "sickling" leading to pulmonary infarction (Porth, 2002).

8. Teach client how to use incentive spirometer and its importance.	8. Incentive spirometry has been shown to help prevent acute chest syndrome (Rucknagel, 1996).

(continues on page 436)

Interventions continued	**Rationales** continued

9. Monitor for signs and symptoms of infection:
   a. Fever
   b. Pain
   c. Chills
   d. Increased white blood cells
	9. Bacterial infection is one major cause of morbidity and mortality. Decreased functioning of the spleen (asplenia) results from sickle cell anemia. The loss of the spleen's ability to filter and to destroy various infectious organisms increases the risk of infection (Newcombe, 2002).

10. Monitor for aplastic crisis:
   a. CBC with differential
   b. Pallor
   c. Tachycardia
	10. With infection (e.g., B19 parvovirus), production of RBCs pauses temporarily, causing even more severe acute anemia (Newcombe, 2002).

11. Monitor for signs and symptoms of leg ulcers:
   a. Hyperpigmentation
   b. Skin wrinkling
   c. Pruritus, tenderness
	11. Leg ulcers can occur in 50% to 75% of older children and adults with sickle cell anemia. Minor leg trauma can result in localized edema and compression of the tissue around the injury. Capillary blood flow is decreased, causing increased arterial pressure. This increased pressure causes some arterial blood carrying oxygen to the tissue to be directed to the veins without reaching the injured area. Skin grafting may be needed (Chung, Cackovic, & Kerstein, 1996).

12. Monitor for changes in neurologic function:
   a. Speech disturbances
   b. Sudden headache
   c. Numbness, tingling
	12. Cerebral infarction and intracranial hemorrhage are complications of SCD. Occlusion of nutrient arteries to major cerebral arteries causes progressive wall damage and eventual occlusion of the major vessel. Intracerebral hemorrhage may be secondary to hypoxic necrosis of vessel walls (Porth, 2002).

13. Monitor for splenic dysfunction.	13. The spleen is responsible for filtering blood to remove old bacteria. Sluggish circulation and increased viscosity of sickle cells causes splenic blockage. The spleen's normal acidic and anoxic environment stimulates sickling, which increases blood flow obstruction.

14. Monitor for splenic sequestration crisis:
   a. Sudden onset of lassitude
   b. Very pale, listless
	14. Increased blood obstruction from the spleen together with rapid sickling can cause sudden pooling of blood into

(continues on page 437)

Interventions continued	Rationales continued
c. Rapid pulse d. Shallow respirations e. Low blood pressure	the spleen. This causes intravascular hypovolemia and hypoxia progressing to shock.
15. Intervene for priapism. a. Provide analgesics, sedation. b. Maintain hydration. c. Apply ice packs to penis. d. Prepare for needle aspiration of blood from corpora cavernosa. e. Prepare for surgical intervention if previous interventions are unsuccessful.	15. Sickled cells impairing blood flow cause priapism (involuntary, prolonged, abnormal, and painful erection). Persistent stasis priapism not resolved in 24 to 48 hours can cause permanent erectile dysfunction (Waterbury, 2003). a. Sedation may cause tissue relaxation and improve perfusion. b. Hydration can mobilize cluster cells. c. Icing can reduce edema and improve perfusion. d. Removal of clustered sickle cells can improve circulation. e. Shunting by incision of dorsal arteries of penis may be needed to prevent tissue necrosis.
16. Monitor for avascular necrosis: a. Bone pain (hip, leg) b. Fever c. Limited movement	16. Avascular necrosis is death of tissue from decreased circulation secondary to clustered sickled cells.
17. If avascular necrosis is suspected, prepare for: a. X-rays b. Surgical intervention	17. X-rays will show calcium loss and structural collapse. Surgical interventions will attempt to revitalize the bone (Maher, 1998).

◤ Related Physician-Prescribed Interventions

Medications. Anti-sickling agents, analgesics, folic acid, hydroxyurea

Intravenous Therapy. Exchange transfusions

Laboratory Studies. CBC, liver function tests, hemoglobin electrophoresis, serum iron, erythrocyte sedimentation rate, arterial blood gases

Diagnostic Studies. Depend on complications

Therapies. Depend on complications, bone marrow/stem cell transplantation, recombinant human erythropoietin (r-HuEPO), L-arginine therapy, steroid therapy

Documentation
Flow records
  Skin assessment
  Neurologic
  Vital signs

Progress notes
  Abnormal findings
  Interventions
  Evaluation

Nursing Diagnoses

Acute Pain Related to Viscous Blood and Tissue Hypoxia

Focus Assessment Criteria	Clinical Significance

1. Pain
  a. Description
  b. Location
  c. Duration
  d. Intensity (1–10)
	1. Painful episodes related to SCD vary in duration, frequency, and character.

Goal

The client will report decreased pain after pain-relief measures.

Indicators

• Relate factors that increase pain.
• Relate factors that can precipitate pain.

Interventions	Rationales
1. Explore with client if the painful episode is "typical" or "unusual."	1. Most clients have a distinctive, unique pattern of pain. Changes may indicate another complication (e.g., infection, abdominal surgical emergency).
2. Assess for any signs of infection (e.g., respiratory, urinary, vaginal).	2. Painful events often occur with infection.
3. Aggressively manage acute pain episodes. Consult with physician or advanced practice nurse.	3. The pain of SCD, like the pain of cancer, should be treated based on client's tolerance and discretion (Waterbury, 2003).
4. Provide narcotic analgesic every 2 hours (not PRN). Consider patient-controlled analgesic.	4. People with sickle cells metabolize narcotics rapidly (Waterbury, 2003).
5. Provide an initial bolus dose of a narcotic analgesic (e.g., morphine) followed by continuous low-dose narcotic or dosing at fixed intervals.	5. A continuous serum level of narcotic is needed to control pain (Jenkins, 2002).

(continues on page 439)

Interventions continued	Rationales continued
6. Avoid meperidine (Demerol).	6. Meperidine contains the metabolite normeperide that the kidney must excrete and increased levels are associated with increased seizures (Jenkins, 2002).
7. After the acute pain crisis, taper narcotics.	7. This will help to minimize physical dependence (Jenkins, 2002).
8. In addition to analgesics, provide relaxation therapy, self-hypnosis, and massage therapy.	8. These can be useful adjuncts to a pain management program.
9. Refer to High Risk for Ineffective Therapeutic Regimen Management of Chronic Pain postdischarge.	9. Using an objective scoring system helps to evaluate a subjective experience.
10. Assess level of pain using 0 to 10 scale before and after analgesics.	10. The pain of sickling should decrease. A decrease in the pain score of 2 or more points is an indication to reduce the narcotic analgesic (Ballas & Delengowski, 1993).
11. Evaluate whether or not pain is decreasing.	

 Documentation

Medication administration record
 Type, route, and dosage of all medications
Progress notes
 Status of pain
 Degree of relief from pain-relief measures

High Risk for Ineffective Therapeutic Regimen Management Related to Insufficient Knowledge of Disease Process, Risk Factors for Sickling Crisis, Pain Management, Signs and Symptoms of Complications, Genetic Counseling, and Family Planning Services

Focus Assessment Criteria	Clinical Significance
1. Readiness and ability to learn and to retain information	1. A client or family who fails to achieve learning goals requires a referral for assistance postdischarge.

Goals

The goals for this diagnosis represent those associated with discharge planning. Refer to the discharge criteria.

Interventions	Rationales
1. Review present situation, disease process, and treatment (Marchiondo & Thompson, 1996).	1. Even though the client has had the disease since childhood, the nurse should evaluate present knowledge.

2. Discuss precipitating factors.
  a. High altitude (more than 7,000 feet above sea level)
  b. Unpressurized aircraft
  c. Dehydration (e.g. diaphoresis, diarrhea, vomiting)
  d. Strenuous physical activity
  e. Cold temperatures (e.g., iced liquids)
 	
  f. Infection (e.g., respiratory, urinary, vaginal)
  g. Ingestion of alcohol
  h. Cigarette smoking
	2.
	  a,b. Decreased oxygen tension can cause red blood cells to sickle.
	
	  c,d. Any situation that causes dehydration or increases blood viscosity can precipitate sickling.
	  e. Cold causes peripheral vasoconstriction, which slows circulation.
	  f. The exact mechanism is unknown.
	
	  g. Alcohol use promotes dehydration.
	  h. Nicotine interferes with oxygen exchange.

3. Emphasize the need to drink at least 16 cups (8 oz) of fluid daily and to increase to 24 to 32 cups during a painful crisis or when at risk for dehydration.	3. Dehydration must be prevented to prevent a sickling crisis (Marchiondo & Thompson, 1996).

4. Discuss the importance of maintaining optimal health.
  a. Regular health care professional examinations (e.g. ophthalmic, general)
  b. Good nutrition
  c. Stress reduction methods
  d. Dental hygiene
  e. Immunization
	4. Adhering to a health maintenance plan can reduce risk factors that contribute to crisis.

5. Explain the importance of an eye examination every 6 to 12 months.	5. SCD can cause retinopathy by plugging small retinal vessels and causing neovascularization (Lawton, 1996).
6. Explain the susceptibility to infection.	6. Certain organisms (e.g., salmonella) thrive in diminished oxygen status. Phagocytosis, which is dependent on oxygen, is inhibited with SCD (Porth, 2002).

7. Stress the importance of reporting signs and symptoms of infection early.
  a. Persistent cough
  b. Fever
  c. Foul-smelling vaginal drainage
  d. Cloudy, reddish, or foul-smelling urine
  e. Increased redness of wound
  g. Purulent drainage
	7. Early recognition and treatment may prevent a crisis.

(continues on page 441)

Interventions continued	**Rationales** continued
8. After crisis, attempt to help person identify some warning signs that occur day or hours before crisis.	8. Most clients with SCD experience a prodromal stage (a gradual build up of symptoms for days before a crisis). More commonly, however, symptoms begin less then 1 hour before crisis (Newcombe, 2002).
9. Instruct client to provide prompt treatment of cuts, insect bites, and so on.	9. Decreased peripheral circulation increases the risk for infection.

10. Instruct to report:
   a. Any acute illness
   b. Severe joint or bone pain
   c. Chest pain
   d. Abdominal pain
   e. Headaches, dizziness
   f. Gastric distress
	10. These symptoms may indicate vaso-occlusion in varied sites from sickling. Some illnesses may predispose client to dehydration.

11. Provide access to training for new coping strategies:
   a. Relaxation breathing
   b. Imagery
   c. Calming self statements
   d. Mental counting technique
   e. Focus on physical surroundings
   f. Reinterpretation of pain sensations
	11. Individuals who practiced selected coping strategies during pain episodes had less need for ER management (Gil et al., 2000).

12. Advise client to practice coping strategies daily regardless of pain level.	12. Practice is needed to improve efficiency of the strategy when it is needed (Gil et al., 2000).
13. Explore client's knowledge regarding the genetic aspects of the disease. Refer to appropriate resource (e.g., genetic counseling).	13. This disease is hereditary. The incidence of offspring inheriting SCD is related to parents as carriers or noncarriers of the hemoglobin genotype AS.
14. Explore with client the effects of SCD on family, roles, occupation, and personal goals.	14. Clients with SCD experience it personally and have witnessed its effects on others. This chronic disease regularly challenges client and family functioning. Adults are at risk for poor psychological adjustment.
15. Refer to community support groups and appropriate agencies (e.g., National Association for Sickle Cell Disease).	15. Successful coping is promoted by witnessing others successfully coping and others believing that they will be successful (Bandura, 1982).

 Documentation

Discharge summary record
   Client teaching
   Outcome achievement
   Referrals if indicated

Integumentary Disorders

PRESSURE ULCERS

Pressure ulcers are localized areas of cellular necrosis that tend to occur from prolonged compression of soft tissue between a bony prominence and a firm surface—most commonly as a result of immobility. Extrinsic factors that exert mechanical force on soft tissue include pressure, shear, friction, and maceration. Intrinsic factors that determine susceptibility to tissue breakdown include malnutrition, anemia, loss of sensation, impaired mobility, advanced age, decreased mental status, incontinence, and infection. Extrinsic and intrinsic factors interact to produce ischemia and necrosis of soft tissue in susceptible persons (Agency for Health Care Policy Research [AHCPR], 1994; Maklebust & Sieggreen, 2001).

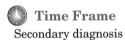 **Time Frame**
Secondary diagnosis

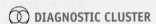 **DIAGNOSTIC CLUSTER**

Collaborative Problems

▲ PC: Sepsis

Nursing Diagnoses

▲ Impaired Tissue Integrity related to mechanical destruction of tissue secondary to pressure, shear, or friction
▲ Impaired Physical Mobility related to imposed restrictions, deconditioned status, loss of motor control, or altered mental status
▲ Imbalanced Nutrition: Less Than Body Requirements related to insufficient oral intake
▲ High Risk for Infection related to exposure of ulcer base to fecal/urinary drainage
△ High Risk for Ineffective Therapeutic Regimen Management related to insufficient knowledge of etiology, prevention, treatment, and home care

Related Nursing Care Plan

Immobility or Unconsciousness

▲ This diagnosis was reported to be monitored for or managed frequently (75%–100%).
△ This diagnosis was reported to be monitored for or managed often (50%–74%).

Discharge Criteria

Before discharge, the client or family will

1. Identify factors that contribute to ulcer development.
2. Demonstrate the ability to perform skills necessary to prevent and treat pressure ulcers.
3. State the intent to continue prevention and treatment strategies at home (e.g., activity, nutrition).

Collaborative Problems

Potential Complication: Sepsis

Nursing Goal
The nurse will monitor for signs/symptoms of sepsis and collaboratively intervene to stabilize the client.

445

Indicators

- Temperature 98–99.5°F
- Heart rate 60–100 beats/min
- Blood pressure >90/60, <140/90 mm Hg
- Respirations 16–20 breaths/min
- Urine output >30 ml/hr
- Clear urine
- Negative blood culture
- White blood count 4300–10,800 mm
- Oriented, alert

Interventions	Rationales

1. Monitor for signs and symptoms of sepsis:
  a. Temperature >101°F or <98.6°F
  b. Tachycardia (>90 beats/min) and tachypnea (>20 breaths/min)
  c. Pale, cool skin
  d. Decreased urine output
  e. WBCs and bacteria in urine
  f. Positive blood culture
  g. Elevated white blood count >12,000 cells/mm³ or decreased WBC <4,000 cells/mm³
 	
  h. Confusion, changes in mentation
	1. Gram-positive and gram-negative organisms can invade open wounds; debilitated clients are more vulnerable. Response to sepsis results in massive vasodilatation with hypovolemia, resulting in tissue hypoxia and decreased renal function and cardiac output. This in turn triggers a compensatory response of increased heart rate and respirations to correct hypoxia and acidosis. Bacteria in urine or blood indicate infection.
	  h. These may be the only signs in older adults.

 Related Physician-Prescribed Interventions

Medications. Topical antibiotics, proteolytic enzymes, pharmacologic therapy depending on laboratory results

Intravenous Therapy. Intravenous antibiotics

Laboratory Studies. Tissue cultures, blood cultures

Therapies. Topical skin barriers; wound care; pressure-relief systems (air-fluidized bed, low-air-loss bed, kinetic bed); ulcer care; folic acid; thiamine

 Documentation

Flow records
  Vital signs

Nursing Diagnoses

Impaired Tissue Integrity Related to Mechanical Destruction of Tissue Secondary to Pressure, Shear, or Friction

Focus Assessment Criteria	Clinical Significance
1. Skin condition (lesions, circulation) 2. Systemic disorders (e.g., diabetes mellitus) 3. Chemical irritants (e.g., incontinence) 4. Mechanical irritants (e.g., casts) 5. Nutritional or fluid deficits 6. Level of consciousness 7. Ability to move in bed and out of bed	1–7. Contributing factors to tissue destruction can be intrinsic (e.g., vulnerable skin, systemic disorders) or extrinsic (e.g., mechanical, chemical). The more factors present, the more vulnerable the client.

Goal
The client will demonstrate progressive healing of tissue.

Indicators
- Participate in risk assessment.
- Express willingness to participate in prevention of pressure ulcers.
- Describe etiology and prevention measures.
- Explain rationale for interventions.

Interventions	Rationales
1. Apply pressure ulcer prevention principles:	1. Principles of pressure ulcer prevention include reducing or rotating pressure on soft tissue. If pressure on soft tissue exceeds intracapillary pressure (approximately 32 mm Hg), capillary occlusion and resulting hypoxia can cause tissue damage.
a. Encourage range-of-motion (ROM) exercise and weight-bearing mobility when possible.	a,b. Exercise and mobility increase blood flow to all areas.
b. Promote optimal mobility (AHCPR, 1994). (Refer to the Impaired Mobility care plan for more information.)	
c. Keep the bed as flat as possible (lower than 30 degrees) and support feet with a foot board (AHCPR, 1994).	c. These measures help to prevent shear, the pressure created when two adjacent tissue layers move in opposition. If a bony prominence slides across the subcutaneous tissue, the subepidermal capillaries may become bent and pinched, resulting in decreased tissue perfusion.
d. Avoid using a knee gatch.	d. A knee gatch may promote blood pooling and decrease circulation in the lower extremities.
e. Use foam blocks or pillows to provide a bridging effect to support the body above and below the high-risk or ulcerated area; this prevents the affected area from touching the bed surface. Do not use foam donuts or inflatable rings (AHCPR, 1994: Crewe, 1987).	e. This measure helps to distribute pressure to a larger area.
f. Alternate or reduce pressure on the skin surface with devices such as these: • Air mattresses • Low-air-loss beds • Air-fluidized beds • Vascular boots or pillow under calf to suspend heels off of bed surface	f. Foam mattresses (e.g., egg-crate type) are for comfort; generally they do not provide adequate pressure relief. Special air mattresses and air beds redistribute the body weight evenly across the body surface (Maklebust, 1996).
g. Use sufficient personnel to lift the client up in bed or a chair without sliding or pulling the skin surface. Use long sleeves or stockings to reduce friction on elbows and heels.	g. Proper transfer technique reduces friction forces that can rub away or abrade skin.
h. Instruct a sitting client to lift himself or herself using the chair arms every 10 minutes, if possible, or assist client in rising up off the chair every 10 to 20 minutes depending on risk factors present.	h. This measure allows periodic reperfusion of ischemic areas.

(continues on page 448)

Interventions continued	Rationales continued
i. Do not elevate legs unless calves are supported. Support calves and align hip and knee bone to avoid shifting weight to ischial tuberosities while chair sitting. j. Pad the chair with a pressure-relieving device. k. Inspect other areas at risk for developing ulcers with each position change: • Ears • Elbows • Occiput • Trochanter • Heels • Ischia • Sacrum • Scapula • Scrotum	i. Supporting the calves reduces pressure over the ischial tuberosities (AHCPR, 1994). j. Ischial tuberosities are prime areas for pressure ulcer development. Air cushions provide better pressure relief than foam cushions. k. A client with one pressure ulcer is at increased risk for developing others.
2. Observe for erythema and blanching, and palpate surrounding area for warmth and tissue sponginess with each position change.	2. Warmth and sponginess are signs of tissue damage.
3. Compensate for sensory deficits: a. Inspect skin every 2 hours for signs of injury. b. Teach client and family members to inspect the skin frequently. Show client how to use a mirror to inspect hard-to-see areas.	3. a. An immobilized client may have impaired sensation; this interferes with the ability to perceive pain from skin damage. b. Regular skin inspection enables early detection of damage. Client's involvement promotes responsibility for self-care.
4. Identify the stage of pressure ulcer development: a. Stage I: nonblanchable erythema of intact skin b. Stage II: ulceration of epidermis or dermis not involving underlying subcutaneous fat c. Stage III: ulceration involving subcutaneous fat or fascia d. Unstageable Stage IV: extensive ulceration penetrating muscle and bone	4. Staging is a communication tool that denotes the anatomic depth of tissue involvement.
5. Reduce or eliminate factors that contribute to extension of existing pressure ulcers: a. Wash area surrounding ulcer gently with a mild soap, rinse area thoroughly to remove soap, and pat dry.	5. Mechanical or chemical forces contribute to pressure ulcer deterioration. a. Soap is an irritant and dries skin.

(continues on page 449)

Interventions continued	**Rationales** continued
b. Do not massage any reddened areas (AHCPR, 1994; Ek, 1982).	b. Vigorous massage angulates and tears the vessels. Massaging over reddened areas may cause breaking of capillaries and traumatize skin (Maklebust & Sieggreen, 2001).
c. Institute one or a combination of the following: • Apply a thin coat of liquid copolymer skin sealant. • Cover area with a moisture-permeable film dressing. • Cover area with a hydroactive wafer barrier and secure with strips of 1-inch microscope tape; leave in place for 4 to 5 days.	c. Healthy skin should be protected.
6. Devise a plan for pressure ulcers using moist wound healing principles as follows:	6. When wounds are semi-occluded and the wound's surface remains moist, epidermal cells migrate more rapidly over the surface (Maklebust & Sieggreen, 2001).
a. Avoid breaking blisters.	a. Blisters indicate stage II pressure ulcers; the fluid contained in the blister provides an environment for formation of granulation tissue.
b. Flush ulcer base with sterile saline solution. If it is infected, use forceful irrigation.	b. Irrigation with normal saline solution may aid in removing dead cells and reducing bacterial count. Forceful irrigation should not be used in the presence of granulation tissue and new epithelium.
c. Avoid using wound cleaners and topical antiseptics (Agency for Health Care Policy and Research [AHCPR], 1992).	c. These products may be cytotoxic to tissue.
d. Consult with a surgeon or wound specialist to debride necrotic tissue mechanically or surgically.	d. A necrotic ulcer does not heal until the necrotic tissue is removed.
e. Cover pressure ulcers with broken skin with a dressing that maintains a moist environment over the ulcer base (e.g., film dressing, hydrocolloid wafer dressing, absorption dressing, moist gauze dressing).	e. Moist wounds heal faster (AHCPR, 1994).
f. Avoid drying agents (e.g., heat lamps, Maalox, Milk of Magnesia) (Maklebust, 1987).	f. Heat creates an increased oxygen demand. Heat lamps are contraindicated in pressure ulcers as the lamps increase the oxygen demand to tissue that is already stressed (Maklebust & Sieggreen, 2001).
7. Consult with a nurse specialist or physician for treatment of deep or infected pressure ulcers.	7. Expert consultation may be needed for more specific interventions. a. Notify interdisciplinary team of wound.

Documentation

Flow records
  Size of ulcer base (length, width, depth)
  Ulcer characteristics: granulation, epithelialization, necrotic tissue, undermined areas, sinus tracts, drainage, surrounding erythema, induration
  Treatment
  Unsatisfactory response

Impaired Physical Mobility Related to Imposed Restrictions, Deconditioned Status, Loss of Motor Control, or Altered Mental Status

Focus Assessment Criteria	Clinical Significance
1. Ability to move within the environment, e.g., in bed, transfer from bed to chair 2. Ability of the primary caregiver to move and turn the client in bed, transfer client from bed to chair, etc.	1,2. Impaired physical mobility forces the client to maintain the same body posture for long periods. Constant unrelieved pressure causes ischemia in compressed tissue, the primary cause of soft tissue ulceration.

Goal

The client will demonstrate increased mobility as (specify).

Indicators

- Shift body weight at least every 2 hours.
- Demonstrate reduced interface pressure over the ulcer to less than 32 mm Hg.
- Show intact skin without nonblanchable erythema.

Interventions	Rationales
1. Encourage the highest level of mobility. Provide devices such as an overhead or partial side rails, if possible, to facilitate independent movement (AHCPR, 1994).	1. Regular movement relieves constant pressure over a bony prominence.

2. Promote optimal circulation while in bed.
  a. If client cannot turn self, reposition every 2 hours. Use a "turn clock" to indicate the appropriate position for each full-body turn (Maklebust & Sieggreen, 2001).
  b. Make minor shifts in body position between full turns.
  c. Examine bony prominences with each repositioning. If reddened areas do not fade within 30 minutes after repositioning, turn the client more frequently.
  d. Position the client in a 30-degree, laterally inclined position. Do *not* use high Fowler's position (AHCPR, 1994).
  e. Use a pressure-relief device to augment the turning schedule.
	2.
	  a. Intermittent pressure relief lets blood reenter capillaries that compression had deprived of blood and oxygen.
	
	  b. Minor shifts in body weight aid reperfusion of compressed areas.
	  c. Reactive hyperemia may be insufficient to compensate for local ischemia.
	
	  d. This position relieves pressure over the trochanter and sacrum simultaneously. High Fowler's position increases sacral shear.
	  e. Pressure-reducing devices may increase the time intervals between necessary repositioning.

(continues on page 451)

Interventions continued	Rationales continued
f. Do not use foam donuts or rubber rings (AHCPR, 1994).	f. These devices compress the surrounding vasculature, increasing the area of ischemia.
g. Pay particular attention to the heels.	g. Studies demonstrate that the heels are extremely vulnerable to breakdown because of the high concentration of body weight over their relatively small surface.
h. *Do not* massage reddened areas.	h. Vigorous massage can angulate and break capillaries (AHCPR, 1994).

 Documentation

Flow record
   Degree of mobility
   Frequency of repositioning
   Actual body position (e.g., left side, supine, right side, prone, 30-degree laterally inclined on left or right)
   Pressure relief devices used
Progress notes
   Abnormal local tissue response to repositioning

Imbalanced Nutrition: Less Than Body Requirements Related to Insufficient Oral Intake

Focus Assessment Criteria	Clinical Significance

1. Dietary history
 	
2. Present nutritional status
  a. Weight
  b. Nutritional intake (e.g., ability to eat, dentition, nausea/vomiting)
  c. Laboratory values: hemoglobin, serum prealbumin, C-reactive protein, nitrogen balance, serum transferrin (Bagley, 1996)
	1,2. Poor general nutrition commonly leads to weight loss and muscle atrophy. Reduction of subcutaneous fat and muscle tissue eliminates some of the padding between the skin and underlying bony prominences, increasing the susceptibility to pressure ulcers. Poor nutrition also decreases resistance to infection and interferes with wound healing.
	
	   Adequate hemoglobin is required to transport oxygen to cells. Hemoglobin and serum pre-albumin levels often provide good clues to overall nutritional status. Decreased albumin levels may result from inadequate protein intake or protein loss from a draining ulcer. (Protein is essential to new tissue synthesis.) Studies show a threefold increase in pressure ulcer incidence with every 1-g decrease in serum albumin level. Serum transferrin also evaluates protein levels but is a more costly procedure (Bagley, 1996; Bergstrom, 1992).

3. Loss of nitrogen from wound drainage	3. Daily drainage from wounds may contain up to 100 g of protein. Replacement therapy may be necessary (Bagley, 1996).

Goal

The client will ingest daily nutritional requirements in accordance with activity level and metabolic needs.

Indicators

- Relate importance of good nutrition.
- Identify deficiencies in daily intake.
- Relate methods to increase appetite.

Interventions	Rationale
1. Refer to the nursing diagnosis Imbalanced Nutrition: Less than Body Requirements in the Thermal Injury care plan for specific interventions and rationales.	

🔊 Documentation

Flow records
  Actual nutritional intake
  Twice-weekly weights
  Status of wounds
  Amount of wound drainage
  Serum albumin levels

High Risk for Infection Related to Exposure of Ulcer Base to Fecal/Urinary Drainage

Focus Assessment Criteria	Clinical Significance
1. Skin and ulcer base for exposure to urine or feces	1. Irritation, denuded skin, and infection exacerbate ulcers. The proximity of pelvic pressure ulcers to fecal and urinary drainage increases the risk of infection in these areas.

Goal

The client will report risk factors associated with infection and precautions needed.

Indicators

- Demonstrate meticulous handwashing and skin hygiene technique by the time of discharge.
- Describe methods of transmission of infection.
- Describe the influence of nutrition on prevention of infection.

Interventions	Rationales
1. Teach the importance of good skin hygiene. Use emollients if skin is dry, but do not leave skin "wet" from too much lotion or cream.	1. Dry skin is susceptible to cracking and infection. Excessive emollient use can lead to maceration.
2. Protect skin from exposure to urine/feces	2. Contact with urine and stool can cause skin maceration. Feces may be more ulcerogenic

(continues on page 453)

Interventions continued	**Rationales** continued
a. Cleanse skin thoroughly after each incontinent episode using a liquid soap that does not alter skin pH. b. Collect feces and urine in an appropriate containment device (e.g., condom catheter, fecal incontinence pouch, polymer-filled incontinent pads), or apply a skin sealant, cream, or emollient to act as a barrier to urine and feces.	than urine owing to bacteria and toxins in stool.
3. Consider using occlusive dressings on clean superficial ulcers but never on deep ulcers.	3. Occlusive dressings protect superficial wounds from urine and feces but can trap bacteria in deep wounds.
4. Ensure meticulous handwashing to prevent infection transmission.	4. Improper handwashing by caregivers is the primary source of infection transmission in hospitalized clients.
5. Use good technique during all dressing changes.	5. Good technique reduces the entry of pathogenic organisms into the wound.
6. Flush the ulcer base with sterile saline solution.	6. Infection produces necrotic debris with secretions that provide an excellent medium for microorganism growth. Flushing helps to remove necrotic debris and dilutes the bacterial count. An infected partial-thickness wound may progress to wound sepsis with increasing necrosis then eventually to a full-thickness lesion.
7. Use new gloves for each dressing change on a client with multiple pressure ulcers (AHCPR, 1994).	7. Each ulcer may be contaminated with different organisms; this measure helps to prevent cross-infection.
8. Monitor for signs of local wound infection (e.g., purulent drainage, cellulitis).	8. Infected ulcers require additional interventions.

 Documentation

Flow records
    Skin condition (e.g., redness, maceration, denuded areas)
    Amount and frequency of incontinence
    Skin care and hygiene measures
    Containment devices used
Progress notes
    Change in skin condition

High Risk for Ineffective Therapeutic Regimen Management Related to Insufficient Knowledge of Etiology, Prevention, Treatment, and Home Care

Focus Assessment Criteria	Clinical Significance
1. Ability of the client or family members to perform necessary turning, lifting, bathing, food purchase and preparation, and other necessary care activities 2. Available support systems for sharing caretaking responsibilities 3. Readiness and ability to learn pressure ulcer prevention and care techniques (Maklebust, 1996).	1–3. An assessment of client and family learning needs allows the nurse to plan appropriate teaching strategies. About 80% of healed pressure ulcers recur, many because of failure to maintain a regimen for ulcer prevention.

Goals

The goals for this diagnosis represent those associated with discharge planning. Refer to the discharge criteria.

Interventions	Rationales

1. Teach measures to prevent pressure ulcers (AHCPR, 1992)
  a. Adequate nutrition
  b. Mobility
  c. Turning and pressure relief
  d. Small shifts in body weight
  e. Active and passive range of motion
  f. Skin care
  g. Skin protection from urine and feces
  h. Recognition of tissue damage
	1. Preventing pressure ulcers is much easier than treating them.

2. Teach methods of treating pressure ulcers:
  a. Use of pressure ulcer prevention principles
  b. Wound care specific to each ulcer
  c. How to evaluate effectiveness of current treatment
	2. These specific instructions help the client and family learn to promote healing and prevent infection.

3. Ask family members to determine the amount of assistance they need in caring for the client.	3. This assessment is required to determine if the family can provide necessary care and assistance.
4. Determine equipment and supply needs (e.g., pressure relief devices, wheelchair cushion, dressings). Consult with social services, if necessary, for assistance in obtaining needed equipment and supplies.	4. Equipment and supplies should be arranged for before discharge.

(continues on page 455)

Interventions continued	Rationales continued
5. If appropriate, refer the client and family to a home health agency for ongoing assessment and evaluation of complex care.	5. Ongoing assessment and teaching may be necessary to sustain the complex level of care.
6. Encourage available caregivers to share the chores of client care.	6. Role fatigue and burnout may occur when one person devotes an inordinate amount of time to caregiving. Periodic relief or assistance can help to prevent this situation.
7. Stress the need to continue wound care and maintain adequate nutrition at home. (Refer to the nursing diagnoses Impaired Tissue Integrity in this care plan and Imbalanced Nutrition in the Thermal Injury care plan for specific information.)	7. Strategies must be continued at home for complete healing to occur.

 Documentation

Discharge summary record
   Client teaching
   Outcome achievement or status
   Referrals if indicated

THERMAL INJURIES

Thermal injuries, or burns, are classified according to cause as thermal (e.g., fire, steam, hot liquids), chemical (e.g., acid and oven cleaners), electrical, or radiation (e.g., sun and x-rays). Severity of a burn is determined by the percentage of burn wound and its size and depth. Burns are classified as partial thickness or full thickness. Partial-thickness burns are subcategorized as superficial (involving the first two to three layers of the five layers of epidermis), moderate partial-thickness (involving the upper third of dermis), and deep dermal partial-thickness (involving the entire epidermal layer and part of the dermis). A full-thickness burn involves destruction of all layers of the skin including subcutaneous tissue (Porth, 2002). This care plan focuses on the period of hospitalization after emergency treatment on admission and before admission to a rehabilitation unit.

 Time Frame

Acute episode (post emergency room)

⊗ DIAGNOSTIC CLUSTER

Collaborative Problems

* PC: Hypoxia
▲ PC: Hypovolemia/Shock
▲ PC: Electrolyte Imbalance
△ PC: Metabolic Acidosis
* PC: Compartmental Syndrome
△ PC: Paralytic Ileus
△ PC: Curling's Ulcer
△ PC: Renal Insufficiency
△ PC: Negative Nitrogen Balance
* PC: Cellulitis/Infection
▲ PC: Graft Rejection
▲ PC: Sepsis

Nursing Diagnoses

▲ Anxiety related to sudden injury, treatments, uncertainty of outcome, and pain

---

▲ Pain related to thermal injury treatments and immobility

▲ High Risk for Imbalanced Nutrition: Less than Body Requirements related to increased protein, calorie, and vitamin requirements for wound healing and

---

(continues on page 457)

Nursing Diagnoses continued

decreased intake secondary to pain, decreased mobility and activity, and possibly nausea and vomiting

△ High Risk for Disturbed Self-Concept related to effects of burn on appearance, increased dependence on others, and disruption of life style and role responsibilities

△ Deficient Diversional Activity related to prolonged hospitalization, physical limitations, and monotony of confinement

* Impaired Physical Mobility related to painful burn wounds

△ High Risk for Ineffective Therapeutic Regimen Management related to insufficient knowledge of wound care, healed skin care, nutritional requirements, management of pain and itching, burn prevention, and follow-up care

△ Disuse Syndrome related to effects of immobility and pain on muscle and joint function	Immobility or Unconsciousness
△ Self-Care Deficit (specify) related to impaired range-of-motion ability secondary to pain	Immobility or Unconsciousness
▲ High Risk for Infection related to loss of protective layer secondary to thermal injury	Pressure Ulcers

Related Care Plan

Immobility or Unconsciousness

▲ This diagnosis was reported to be monitored for or managed frequently (75%–100%).
△ This diagnosis was reported to be monitored for or managed often (50%–74%).
* This diagnosis was not included in the validation study.

Discharge Criteria

Before discharge, the client or family will

1. Relate an intent to discuss feelings and concerns with significant others after discharge.
2. Relate the need to comply with the prescribed dietary and daily exercise program and the consequences of noncompliance

3. Demonstrate correct wound care.
4. Describe methods to decrease the risk of infection.
5. State the signs and symptoms that must be reported to a health care professional.
6. Relate an intent to adhere to the follow-up schedule.
7. Describe community resources available for assistance at home.

Collaborative Problems

Potential Complication: Hypoxia

Potential Complication: Hypovolemia/Shock

Potential Complication: Electrolyte Imbalance

Potential Complication: Metabolic Acidosis

Potential Complication: Compartmental Syndrome

Potential Complication: Paralytic Ileus

Potential Complication: Curling's Ulcer

Potential Complication: Renal Insufficiency

Potential Complication: Negative Nitrogen Balance

Potential Complication: Cellulitis/Infection

Potential Complication: Graft Rejection

Potential Complication: Sepsis

Nursing Goal

The nurse will detect early signs and symptoms of (a) hypoxia, (b) inhalation injury, (c) hypovolemia/shock, (d) electrolyte imbalances, (f) metabolic acidosis, (g) compartmental syndrome, (h) paralytic ileus, (i) Curling's ulcer, (j) renal insufficiency, (k) negative nitrogen balance, (l) infection/cellulites, (m) graft rejection, (n) sepsis, and (o) thromboembolism and collaboratively intervene to stabilize client.

Indicators
- Temperature 98–99.5°F (k, m, n)
- Respiratory rate 16–20 breaths/min (a, b, c, e, m)
- Normal breath sounds, no adventitious sounds (a, b, c)
- Normal relaxed, quiet, even breathing (a, b, c)
- Peripheral pulses full, bounding (c, f)
- Pulse 60–100 beats/min (a, b, c, n)
- Blood pressure >90/60, <140/90 mm Hg (a, b, c)
- SAO_2 arterial oxygen saturation (pulse oximeter) >95% (a, b, c, d, e, n)
- $PaCO_2$ arterial carbon dioxide 35–45 mm Hg (a, b, c, d, e, n)
- Serum pH 7.35–7.45 (a, b, c, d, e, m)
- Serum carboxyhemoglobin, low or none (a, b)
- EKG—normal sinus rhythm (d)
- Warm, dry skin (a, c)
- Pinkish, ruddy-brownish, or olive skin tones (c, f)
- Calm, oriented (a, b, c)
- No nausea or vomiting (c, d, e, h)
- No headache or dizziness (d, e)
- No hoarseness or voice changes (b)
- No bloody, purulent, or sooty sputum (b, k)
- Urine output >30 ml/hour (a, c, e, i, j, n)
- Urine specific gravity 1.005–1.030 (a, c, e, i, j, n)
- Pale yellow urine (i)

- Blood urea nitrogen 5–25 mg/dL (i)
- Serum pre-albumin 20–50 mg/dL (i)
- Red blood cells (a)
  ○ Male 4.6–5.9 million/mm³
  ○ Female 4.2–5.4 million/mm³
- White blood count 4,300–10,800 mm³ (k, m)
- Serum potassium 3.5–5.0 mEq/L (d, i)
- Creatinine clearance (i)
  ○ Male 95–135 ml/mm
  ○ Female 85–125 ml/mm
- Serum sodium 135–145 mEq/L (d, i)
- No extremity edema (k, n, f, m, o)
- Capillary refill <3 seconds (c, f, m, o)
- Bowel sounds present in all quadrants
- Stool occult blood-negative (h)
- Wounds without increased redness or purulent drainage (k, n)
- Negative Homans' sign (o)
- No calf tenderness, unusual warmth or redness (o)
- Usual weight (j)
- No c/o of membranes (f)
- No pain with stretching of toes/fingers (f)

Interventions	Rationales
1. Assess and monitor respiratory function: breath sounds, rate and rhythm of respiration, pulse oximeter, and hemoglobin. Initiate pulse oximetry.	1. Three separate oxygenation complications are associated with smoke inhalation: carbon monoxide poisoning, laryngeal swelling and upper airway obstruction, and chemical pneumonia (Carrougher, 1998).
2. Assess for risk factors of inhalation injury: a. Facial burns b. Singed eyebrows/nasal hair c. History of confinement in burning environment d. Bloody or sooty sputum e. Hoarseness, voice change, dry cough, stridor f. Labored breathing or rapid breathing	2. Inhalation injury produces the inflammatory response, which leads to erythema, edema, possible de-epithelialization of the respiratory mucosa, and increased secretions, possibly resulting in respiratory compromise. This can cause pulmonary edema, atelectasis, pneumonia, and adult respiratory distress syndrome.
3. Monitor arterial blood gases and carboxyhemoglobin. 4. Monitor for signs and symptoms of the following: a. Carbon monoxide poisoning • headache, dizziness • Nausea, vomiting • Dyspnea • Cherry-red skin	3,4. High levels of carbon monoxide cause a decreased oxygen-carrying capacity of hemoglobin molecules (Carrougher, 1998).

(continues on page 460)

Interventions continued	**Rationales** continued
b. Upper airway obstruction • Increased respiratory rate • Decreased depth of breathing • Hoarseness c. Chemical pneumonitis • Increased pH • Decreased partial pressure of carbon dioxide • Increased respiratory rate	
5. Encourage turning, deep breathing, and coughing every 2 hours. Percuss and suction client as needed.	5. Inhalation injury causes increased mucus production because of irritation of airway mucosa. In lower airway injury, the inactivation of cilia causes a decreased ability to clear secretions. Also, inactivation of surfactant can lead to alveolar collapse and atelectasis (Stillwell, 1996).
6. Consider positioning client (based on chest X-ray results) to maximize oxygenation.	6. Position of person should be dependent on need to perfuse alveoli or enhance bronchial drainage.
7. Monitor for signs of pulmonary infection. a. Chest x-ray results b. Sputum production: color and amount c. Temperature, white blood cell count, and sputum culture reports	7. Inhalation injury alters the client's defense mechanism, placing him or her at risk for infection. Elevated bands are an early indication of infection. Chest x-ray results and sputum are monitored for changes indicating infection (Thelan, Lough, Urden, & Stacy, 1998).
8. Monitor trends in peak airway pressure when client is intubated and mechanically ventilated.	8. Elevated peak airway pressures that do not decrease after suctioning may be an early indication of pulmonary edema or adult respiratory distress syndrome.
9. Calculate fluid resuscitation for the first 24 hours using the Consensus Formula, and use as a guide in evaluating client fluid status: 3–4 mL LR × kg wt × % burn	9. Because fluid requirements vary for each client, it is necessary to calculate an estimated volume to assist in administration of fluids and evaluation of fluid status and burn injury (Greenfield, 1998).
10. Monitor intake and output: a. Maintain urine output at 0.5 to 1 mL/kg/hr.	10. Urine output is the best indicator of adequate fluid resuscitation. Intravenous fluid rates may need to be adjusted frequently throughout the first 24 hours to achieve a urine output at 0.5 to

(continues on page 461)

Interventions continued	**Rationales** continued
b. Maintain and adjust intravenous fluid rates according to orders and urine output. c. Monitor urine color.	1 mL/kg/ hr and perfuse the kidneys. Burn injury causes vasoconstriction of the renal artery. Port wine-colored urine is an indication of cell degradation products and myoglobin in the urine. Intravenous fluids need to be increased to prevent precipitation in the renal tubules and acute tubular necrosis (Thelan et al., 1998).

11. Monitor for signs and symptoms of hypovolemia/shock:
  a. Urine output <30 mL/hr
  b. Increasing pulse rate with a low, normal, or slightly decreased blood pressure
  c. Restlessness, agitation, and change in mentation
  d. Increasing respiratory rate
  e. Diminished peripheral pulses
  f. Cool, pale, or mottled skin
  g. Decreased serum pH
  h. Elevated hematocrit
	11. In the immediate period after the burn, the body releases large amounts of vaso-active substances, which increases capillary permeability. Serum, proteins, and electrolytes leak into damaged and normal tissue, resulting in severe hypovolemia and edema (a phenomenon known as third spacing). Circulating blood volume can be reduced by 50%. Capillary integrity is generally re-established at any time from 12 to 48 hours postburn. The compensatory response to decreased circulatory volume is to increase blood oxygen by increasing heart and respiratory rates and decreasing circulation to extremities (manifested by decreased pulses and cool skin). Diminished cerebral oxygenation can cause changes in mentation (Greenfield, 1998).

12. Encourage oral fluids (e.g., juices or Gatorade) if the client is able to tolerate.	12. Clients with smaller percentage burns (generally <25% PT and FT) can often be resuscitated orally (Greenfield, 1998).
13. Avoid free water orally during the first 48 to 72 hours.	13. Free water is hypotonic. As a result of the fluid shifts, excess free water tends to move into the cell, causing cellular swelling and death (Thelan, 1998).
14. Obtain daily weights. Ensure accuracy by weighing client after dressing change or hydrotherapy (when dressings are dry). (If a litter scale or specialty bed weight is obtained, use the same number of linens each time. Remove all extremity splints for weight.)	14. Accurate daily weights provide data to aid in determining fluid status (Greenfield, 1998).

(continues on page 462)

Interventions continued	**Rationales** continued
15. Monitor fluid status continuously. Assess mucous membranes, peripheral pulses, color, and temperature of unburned areas, wound drainage, and nasogastric drainage.	15. The burn patient is at risk for fluid imbalance throughout hospitalization because of large open wounds and numerous surgical procedures to achieve wound coverage (Thelan et al., 1998).
16. Monitor laboratory study results: electrolytes, glucose, arterial blood gases, blood urea nitrogen (BUN), serum prealbumin, hematocrit, hemoglobin, carboxyhemoglobin, red blood cell count, and white blood count.	16. A major burn affects all body systems either through direct burn damage or through compensatory mechanisms that attempt to maintain homeostasis. All body-system functioning must be assessed frequently for status and response to treatment.
17. Monitor for signs and symptoms of electrolyte imbalances: a. Hyperkalemia (serum potassium >5.5 mEq/L): • Irregular pulse or dysrhythmias such as premature ventricular contractions • Weakness or paralysis • Muscle irritability • Paresthesias • Nausea, abdominal cramps, or diarrhea b. Hypokalemia: • Dysrhythmias such as premature contractions or tachyarrhythmias • Muscle weakness progressing to muscle paralysis • Electrocardiogram changes such as T-wave inversion, ST depression c. Hyponatremia (serum sodium <135 mEq/L): • Lethargy, coma • Weakness • Abdominal pain • Muscle twitching and convulsions	17. a,b. During the emergent period, damaged cells release potassium into the circulation. In addition, sodium potassium pump activity is altered due to hypoxia. If fluid resuscitation is inadequate or renal blood flow is compromised, serum potassium levels rise. However, once fluid resuscitation is adequate, potassium will be excreted in the urine with a subsequent decrease in serum potassium. Generally a hypokalemia is seen more often because of increased awareness of adequate fluid resuscitation. Fluctuations in potassium affect neuromuscular transmission and can cause such complications as cardiac dysrhythmias and reduced action of gastrointestinal (GI) smooth muscles (Thelan et al., 1998). c. Sodium losses result from denuded skin areas and the shift into interstitial spaces during periods of increased capillary permeability. Cellular edema, caused by osmosis, produces changes in sensorium, weakness, and muscle cramps (Greenfield, 1998).
18. Monitor for signs and symptoms of metabolic acidosis: a. Decreased serum pH and negative base excess b. Rapid, shallow respirations c. Behavioral changes and drowsiness d. Headache e. Nausea and vomiting	18. Metabolic acidosis can result from fixed acids released from damaged cells, hyperkalemia, or reduced renal tubular function. Excessive ketone bodies cause headaches, nausea, abdominal pain, and vomiting. Respiratory rate and depth increase in an attempt to increase excretion of carbon dioxide and reduce acidosis. Acidosis affects the central nervous system and can increase neuromuscular irritability (Thelan et al., 1998).

(continues on page 463)

Interventions continued	**Rationales** continued
19. Monitor for signs and symptoms of compartmental syndrome in extremities with circumferential burns: (Tumbarello, 2000) a. Diminishing pulses—if hands and fingers are burned, assess palmar arch pulse and pulses along medial or lateral aspect of fingers b. Coolness, pallor c. Mottled or cyanotic skin d. Pressure resulting from significant edema e. Pain with passive stretch movement of toes or fingers f. Delayed capillary refill >3 seconds g. Numbness of peripheral pulses	19. The tight, leathery eschar of a full-thickness burn, together with the increasing interstitial edema resulting from third spacing and fluid resuscitation, place an extremity with a circumferential injury at risk for neurovascular compromise. An escharotomy (a linear incision down through the eschar of a full-thickness burn until punctate bleeding is reached) or fasciotomy is the surgical procedure necessary to restore circulation.
20. Elevate affected extremities at heart level or leave in a neutral position.	20. Edema impairs circulation: however, if the extremity is elevated above heart level, this may decrease arterial blood flow. In a partial-thickness burn, edema may diminish blood flow and thus increase the depth of the burn wound (Thelan et al., 1998).
21. Monitor with Doppler ultrasound dense hourly.	21. Doppler assessments will detect early changes in circulation.
22. Assess and monitor escharotomy sites: a. Return of adequate pulse b. Normal capillary refill, color, and skin temperature c. Bleeding	22. A successful escharotomy will produce immediate return of pulses. Escharotomies are most often performed during the emergent period when circulating volume is diminished and there is minimal bleeding from the site. However, when volume is restored, bleeding may increase (Thelan et al., 1998).
23. Encourage active range-of-motion exercises and self-care activities if appropriate for client.	23. Activity enhances mobilization of fluid and minimizes edema.
24. Monitor for nausea and vomiting.	24. During the emergent period, nausea and vomiting may develop because of gastric dilatation as a result of hypoperfusion to the GI tract. Treatment involves not giving the client anything by mouth and inserting a nasogastric tube (Greenfield, 1998).

(continues on page 464)

Interventions continued	Rationales continued

25. Monitor for signs and symptoms of paralytic ileus:
  a. Nausea and vomiting
  b. Absent bowel sounds
  c. Abdominal distention
	25. Hypoperfusion of the GI tract can also lead to paralytic ileus and is especially associated with a major burn. Treatment involves inserting a nasogastric tube and ensuring adequate fluid resuscitation (Greenfield, 1998).

26. If bowel sounds absent, initiate insertion of NG tube.	26. This reduces gastric distention and prevents vomiting.

27. Monitor for signs and symptoms of Curling's ulcer:
  a. Blood in vomitus or nasogastric drainage
  b. Tarry stools
  c. Pain
	27. Curling's ulcer is a gastroduodenal ulcer known to develop early in a large percentage of burn injuries. Its etiology is associated with the stress response and hypoperfusion of the GI tract. Treatment involves administration of histamine blockers and antacid early post burn (Greenfield, 1998).

28. Monitor for early signs and symptoms of renal insufficiency:
 	
  a. Sustained elevated urine specific gravity
  b. Elevated urine sodium
 	
  c. Sustained insufficient urine output (<30 mL/hr)
 	
  d. Elevated BUN, serum creatinine, potassium, phosphorus, and ammonia, and decreased creatinine clearance
	28. Decreased renal blood flow results from hypotension and secretion of antidiuretic hormone and aldosterone. In addition, nephrons can be blocked by free hemoglobin increased by red blood cell destruction (Carrougher, 1998).
	a,b. Decreased ability of the renal tubules to reabsorb electrolytes results in increased urine sodium levels and urine specific gravity.
	c. Decreased glomerular filtration rate eventually leads to insufficient urine output.
	d. These changes result from decreased excretion of urea and creatinine in urine.

29. Monitor for signs of negative nitrogen balance:
  a. Weight loss
  b. 24-hour urine nitrogen balance below zero
	29. Burns produce a hypermetabolic response due to increased heat loss from wounds and an increase in beta-adrenergic activity, causing the need for additional nutrients to prevent negative nitrogen balance (Thelan et al., 1998).

30. Institute daily calorie counts when the client is able to tolerate a diet.	30. An accurate calorie and protein intake can be calculated to assure that the client's intake is meeting his nutritional requirements (Thelan et al., 1998).

(continues on page 465)

Interventions continued	**Rationales** continued
31. Offer high-protein, high-calorie snacks at regular intervals. Determine the client's food preferences and eating patterns before injury.	31. Because the burn patient's appetite is often decreased because of inactivity, it is often difficult to meet nutritional requirements at mealtime alone (Schuman, 1991).
32. Consult with the physician on the need for total parenteral nutrition on tube feedings.	32. When a client sustains a major burn injury, total parenteral nutrition is instituted within 2 to 4 days when the patient's fluid and electrolytes are stabilized. Often, duodenal feeding tubes are used until the client is able to take in adequate protein and calories orally.
33. Monitor for signs and symptoms of wound infection and cellulitis: a. Increased thick yellow or green drainage b. Foul-smelling drainage c. Spotty, black areas underneath eschar d. Soft, sloughing eschar e. Increased swelling f. Increased redness around periphery of wound	33. Initially large amounts of serum drainage are expected from a burn wound. About 4 to 5 days postburn, normal drainage consists of moderate amounts of yellow drainage. It is also normal to observe a small amount of erythema at the edge of the wound; however, when this increases in intensity and width, cellulitis may have developed. Cellulitis is caused by streptococcus, and streptococcus will dissolve an autograft.
34. Provide hydrotherapy, dressing changes daily or b.i.d., depending on status of wounds: a. Premedicate client. b. Assess wounds. c. Cleanse with antiseptic soap (e.g., Hibiclens). d. Debride loose eschar or debris. e. Apply antimicrobial cream, synthetic dressing, and so forth as ordered by physician.	34. Initially, burn wounds are cleansed twice daily until drainage decreases and the wound begins to heal. Generally, antimicrobial cream is applied to all burn wounds initially. When drainage decreases and wound begins to heal, a synthetic dressing may be applied. Various synthetic and biosynthetic dressings are used as autograft dressing; the selection often depends on physician preference.
35. Monitor for signs of graft loss or infection: a. Sloughing b. Continued pale white-yellow or gray appearance c. No blanching or capillary refill d. Increased drainage	35. Autografts (skin taken from the client's own body) are used to provide permanent wound coverage. Skin substitutes (biologic or synthetic) are used until autograft is possible (Thelan et al., 1998).
36. Teach the client to do the following: a. Avoid movement of grafted area, especially if graft is over a joint. b. Avoid pressure on the graft. c. Elevate the involved body part. d. Turn in bed carefully to avoid shearing of graft.	36. Excessive movement and pressure may interfere with revascularization. Elevation facilitates venous return and minimizes edema.

(continues on page 466)

Interventions continued	Rationales continued
37. Provide donor site care according to type of dressing.	37. Donor site care may vary depending on dressing. The donor site is a partial-thickness wound and generally takes about 10 to 14 days to heal.

38. Monitor for signs and symptoms of sepsis (American College of Chest Physicians/Society of Critical Care Medicine [ACCP/SCCM] Consensus Conference Committee, 1992):
  a. Temperature <38°C or <36°C
  b. Heart rate <90 beats/min
  c. Respiratory rate >20 breaths+/min or $PaCO_2$ <32 torr (<4.3 kPa)
  d. White blood cell (WBC) count > 12,000 cells/mm³, <4000 cells/mm³, or >10% immature (band) forms
	38. The skin provides a physical barrier that protects the body from infection. When a burn injury occurs, organisms invade open wounds. Also, the burn injury alters the immune response. Bacteria in urine, sputum, or blood indicates infection. Sepsis results in massive vasodilatation with hypovolemia; this leads to tissue hypoxia and results in decreased renal function and decreased cardiac output. The compensatory response of increased heart rate and respiration attempts to correct hypoxia and acidosis.

39. Monitor for signs and symptoms of thromboembolism:
  a. Positive Homans' sign (dorsiflexion of the foot causes pain)
  b. Calf tenderness, unusual warmth, or redness
  c. Low-grade fever
  d. Extremity edema
	39. Hypovolemia increases blood viscosity because of hemoconcentration. Immobility reduces vasomotor tone resulting in decreased venous return with peripheral blood pooling (Caswell, 1993).
	  a. Positive Homans' sign indicates insufficient circulation.
	  b,c. These signs and symptoms point to inflammation.

40. Encourage client to perform leg exercises. Discourage placing pillows under the knees, use of a knee gatch, crossing the legs, and prolonged sitting.	40. These measures help to increase venous return and prevent venous stasis (Caswell, 1993).
41. Ambulate as soon as possible with at least 5 minutes of walking each waking hour. Avoid prolonged chair sitting with legs dependent.	41. Walking contracts leg muscles, stimulates the venous pump, and reduces stasis (Caswell, 1993).

 Related Physician-Prescribed Interventions

Medications. Antacids, antibiotics, histamine inhibitors

Intravenous Therapy. Hyperalimentation; replacement therapy (fluids, electrolytes, plasma, and albumin); blood products

Laboratory Studies. Complete blood count, serum glucose, WBC count, serum prealbumin, serum electrolytes, alkaline phosphatase, wound cultures

Diagnostic Studies. Serial chest x-ray films

Therapies. Pressure-relief beds; grafts (autograft, biologic, synthetic); whirlpool; analgesics; topical agents (silver sulfadiazine, mafenide acetate, silver nitrate); blood cultures; sputum cultures; urine culture; serum osmolarity; urine osmolarity; BUN; stools for occult blood; wound care/dressings; debridement; autografts

🕊 Documentation

Flow records
    Vital signs
    Respiratory assessment
    Weight
    Edema (sites, amount)
    Urine specific gravity
    Intake and output (calories, amounts)
    Occult blood tests
    Bowel sounds
Progress notes
    Complaints of nausea, vomiting, muscle cramps
    Changes in behavior or sensorium
    Treatments
    Condition of graft and donor sites (appearance, evidence of epithelialization, exudates, odor)

Nursing Diagnoses

Anxiety Related to Sudden Injury, Treatment, Uncertainty of Outcome, and Pain

Focus Assessment Criteria	Clinical Significance

1. Anxiety level
  a. Mild: broad perceptual field, relaxed facial expression, lack of muscle tension, learning ability intact
  b. Moderate: narrowed perceptual field, increased respiratory and pulse rate, visible nervousness, problem-solving ability intact
  c. Severe: distorted sense of time, inattentiveness, greatly reduced perception, hyperventilation, complaints of headache and dizziness.
  d. Panic: distorted perception: profound confusion; possible incoherence, vomiting, and violence; learning impossible
	1. Anxiety level varies depending on the client's perception of burn severity and on successful or unsuccessful coping.

2. Personal stressors 3. Specific concerns and fears	2,3. A seriously burned client may have many legitimate fears such as pain, death, abandonment, dependency, and disfigurement. Recognizing and expressing fears may help to reduce anxiety.
4. Available support systems	4. Client needs much support during the acute and rehabilitative periods.

Goal

The client will report reduced anxiety to a mild-moderate level.

Indicators

- Effectively communicate feelings regarding injuries.
- Describes usual patterns with coping with stress.

Interventions	Rationales

1. Help client to reduce anxiety:
  a. Provide constant comfort and reassurance.
  b. Stay with client as much as possible.
  c. Speak in a calm, soothing voice.
  d. Identify and support effective coping mechanisms.
  e. Convey your understanding and empathy.
  f. Encourage client to verbalize fears and concerns.
	1. An anxious client has a narrowed perceptual field and a diminished ability to learn. He or she may experience muscle tension, pain, and sleep disturbances, and tend to overreact to situations. Anxiety tends to feed on itself and can catch the client in a widening spiral of tension and physical and emotional pain; thus, anxiety reduction is essential to effective client care (Redman & Thomas, 1992).

2. If anxiety is mild to moderate, take the opportunity to provide client teaching about procedures.	2. Accurate information about what to expect may help to reduce anxiety associated with the unknown.
3. Encourage family and friends to verbalize their fears and concerns to staff. Prepare them for initial visit by discussing the client's appearance and any invasive lines or other care measures they may see.	3. Discussions to help clarify misconceptions and allow sharing. Descriptions of what to expect help to prevent a shocked response that may trigger anxiety in the patient.
4. Encourage use of relaxation techniques.	4. Relaxation exercises provide control over the body's response to stress and can help to reduce anxiety.
5. Notify physician immediately if anxiety reaches the severe or panic level.	5. Severe to panic anxiety can lead to injury or other problems and makes learning and compliance with treatment impossible.

 Documentation

Progress notes
Present emotional status
Response to nursing interventions

Pain Related to Thermal Injury Treatments and Immobility

Focus Assessment Criteria	Clinical Significance

1. Source of pain:
  a. Burn area
  b. Donor site
  c. Invasive lines
	1. Burn pain stems from nerve and tissue destruction; other pain may develop from complications (e.g., ileus, electrolyte imbalance, thrombus) or from treatment.

(continues on page 469)

Focus Assessment Criteria continued	Clinical Significance continued

d. Pressure ulcer
   e. Abdomen
   f. Muscle
	Distinguishing the source of pain guides pain relief interventions.

2. Client's perception of pain severity, based on a scale of 0 to 10 (0 = no pain; 10 = most severe pain), rated as follows:
   a. At its best
   b. At its worst
   c. After each pain relief intervention
	2. This scale provides a good method of evaluating the subjective experience of pain.

3. Physical signs of pain (e.g., increased pulse rate and respirations, elevated blood pressure, restlessness, facial grimacing, guarding)	3. In some clients, objective signs may be more reliable indicators of pain; for whatever reason, some clients are reluctant to express pain or request pain relief medications.

Goal

The client will report progressive reduction of pain and relief after pain relief measures.

Indicators
* Relate factors that increase pain.
* Relate effective interventions.

Interventions	Rationales
1. Convey that you acknowledge and accept client's pain.	1. A client who feels that he or she must convince skeptical caregivers of the seriousness of his or her pain experiences increased anxiety that can increase pain.

2. Provide accurate information:
   a. Explain the cause of pain if known.
   b. Explain how long the pain should last if known.
   c. If indicated, reassure client that narcotic addiction is not likely to develop from the pain relief regimen.
	2. A client who understands and is prepared for pain by detailed explanations tends to experience less stress—and consequently less pain—than a client who receives vague or no explanations.

3. Provide privacy for client during acute pain episodes.	3. Privacy reduces embarrassment and anxiety and enables more effective coping.
4. Collaborate with client to identify effective pain relief measures. This should include a measure to be used during dressing changes.	4. Client can provide valuable insight to the pain and its relief. Burn pain cannot be resolved entirely until the wound is completely healed. Distraction stimulates

(continues on page 470)

Interventions continued	**Rationales** continued
a. Distraction b. Breathing exercises c. Relaxation techniques	the thalamus, midbrain, and brain stem; this increases production of endorphins and alters pain transmission. Distraction techniques have been demonstrated to reduce pain and anxiety during dressing change (Miller, 1992). Breathing exercises and relaxation techniques decrease oxygen consumption, respiratory rate, heart rate, and muscle tension that interrupt the cycle of pain—anxiety—muscle tension.
5. Provide optimal pain relief with prescribed analgesics (Agency for Health Care Policy and Research [AHCPR], 1992): a. Consult with a pharmacist for possible adverse interactions with other medications the client is taking, such as muscle relaxants and tranquilizers. b. Use a preventive approach to pain medication; administer before treatment procedures or activity and instruct the client to request PRN pain medications before pain becomes severe. c. Assess vital signs, especially respiratory rate, before and after administration. d. About ½ hour after administration, assess pain relief.	5. a. Some medications potentiate the effects of narcotics. b. The preventive approach (e.g., every 4 hours) may reduce the total 24-hour drug dose as compared with the PRN approach and may reduce the client's anxiety associated with having to ask for and wait for PRN medications (AHCPR, 1992). c. Narcotics depress the brain's respiratory center. d. Response to analgesics can vary with stress levels, fatigue, and pain intensity.
6. Explain the prescribed burn wound care and its advantages and disadvantages. a. Open method: no dressings with frequent reapplication of ointment. Advantages: no dressings, hastened eschar separation reduces infection. Disadvantages: requires frequent reapplication; increased heat loss. b. Semiclosed method: dressings with antimicrobials changed once or twice a day. Advantages: dressing removal debrides wounds; heat loss is reduced; wounds are not always visible. Disadvantages: dressing changes are required; debridement is painful. c. Closed method: occlusive dressings not changed for up to 72 hours. Advantages: fewer dressing changes; others the same as semiclosed. Disadvantages: wounds cannot be inspected daily; dressings can be too tight or too loose.	6. Explaining the method and its advantages and disadvantages can help the client to recognize and report any problems or complications.

(continues on page 471)

Interventions continued	Rationales continued

7. Take steps to reduce pain during dressing changes:
 	
  a. Administer analgesics 30 minutes before treatment. Consider additional intravenous boluses during treatment if needed.
  b. Encourage client to use relaxation techniques or distraction (effective pain relief measure identified in intervention 4).
  c. Regulate the amount of debridement or staple removal to be done with each dressing change.
  d. Inform client when process will be painful.
  e. Handle carefully wounds that are healing and, therefore, are more sensitive to pain.
  f. Moisten adherent dressings on skin graft or healing wounds with decreased drainage.
  g. Use heat lights if client's body temperature allows.
  h. Encourage client to become involved in wound care when appropriate.
	7. Dressing changes are painful because of manipulation of wounds, exposure to air, and associated debridement.
	  a. Early administration allows full drug effects during the dressing change.
	
	  f. These wounds do not require debridement with dressing removal. Wet dressings facilitate removal and reduce discomfort and bleeding.
	
	  h. Client involvement allows client a sense of control.

8. Reduce exposure time during treatments.	8. Loss of insulating skin surface increases heat loss. Exposure of wound surface to air often causes burning sensation.
9. Collaborate with client to evaluate effectiveness of medication and nonpharmacologic measures to minimize pain during hydrotherapy.	9. Client's participation enhances cooperation and success.

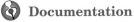 Documentation

Medication administration record
  Type, dosage, schedule, and route of all medications administered
Progress notes
  Pain relief measures
  Unsatisfactory pain relief from these measures

High Risk for Imbalanced Nutrition: Less Than Body Requirements Related to Increased Protein, Calorie, and Vitamin Requirements for Wound Healing and Decreased Intake Secondary to Pain, Decreased Mobility and Activity, and Possibly Nausea and Vomiting

Focus Assessment Criteria	Clinical Significance
1. Intake (caloric count, types of foods)	1. The hypermetabolic response to tissue injury results in vitamin, mineral, and trace element reductions and changes in carbohydrate, fat, and protein metabolism (Porth, 2002).

(continues on page 472)

Focus Assessment Criteria continued	**Clinical Significance** continued
2. Daily weight, laboratory values: serum albumin, protein, urine nitrogen (24 hours)	2. Daily weights and laboratory studies enable early detection of negative nitrogen balance.

3. Presence of the following:
  a. Bowel sounds
  b. Nausea
  c. Vomiting
  d. Flatus
	3. Medications and immobility can disrupt GI function.

Goal

The client will resume ingesting the daily nutritional requirements.

Indicators

- Select from the basic four food groups.
- Consume 2000 to 3000 mL of fluids/day.
- Consume adequate vitamins, fiber, and minerals.
- Maintain or gain weight.

Interventions	**Rationales**
1. Discuss the nutritional requirements and dietary sources.	1. Major complications of trauma and sepsis increase the metabolic rate from 10% to 50%. In the presence of insufficient protein, the body breaks down its own endogenous protein stores (Porth, 2002).
a. Calories a day: 2500–3000 b. Protein: 100–125 g; sources: dairy, meat, poultry, fish, and legumes	a,b. Increased caloric and protein intake is needed to enhance the body's protein-sparing capacity.
c. B-complex vitamins; sources: meat, nuts, and fortified cereals	c. B-complex vitamins are required for metabolism of CHO, fat, and protein.
d. Vitamin C: 75–300 mg; sources: green vegetables and citrus fruits	d. Vitamin C is essential for collagen formation and wound healing.
e. Phosphorus, magnesium, and vitamin D; sources: multivitamins	e. These nutrients are required for healing.
2. Consult with a nutritionist to establish daily caloric and food type requirements.	2. Meeting a burn client's special nutritional needs requires expert consultation.
3. Determine client's food preferences and eating patterns before injury. Collaborate with client to establish a mutually acceptable nutrition plan if appropriate.	3. Knowledge of client's eating habits prior to injury and her or his input and acceptance of meal plan will increase success in meeting nutritional requirements.
4. Explain the causes of anorexia and nausea.	4. Pain, fatigue, analgesics, and immobility can contribute to anorexia and nausea. Explanations can reduce the anxiety associated with the unknown.

(continues on page 473)

Interventions continued	**Rationales** continued
5. Provide rest period for client before meals and after therapies such as rehabilitation.	5. Fatigue further diminishes a decreased desire to eat.
6. Offer frequent small feedings (six per day plus snacks) rather than infrequent large meals.	6. Distributing the caloric intake over the day helps increase total intake.
7. Restrict liquids with meals and 1 hour before and after meals.	7. Overdistending the stomach decreases appetite and intake.
8. Maintain good oral hygiene before and after meals.	8. Accumulation of food particles can contribute to foul odors and taste that diminish appetite.
9. Arrange to have foods with the highest protein and calorie content served at the times when the client usually feels most like eating.	9. This measure may improve protein and calorie intake.
10. Prevent pain from interfering with eating: a. Plan care so that painful procedures are not done immediately before meals. b. Provide pain medication ½ hour before meals, as ordered.	10. Pain causes fatigue, which can reduce appetite.
11. Take steps to prevent nausea and vomiting: a. Frequently provide small amounts of ice chips or cool clear liquid (e.g., dilute tea, Jello water, flat ginger ale, or cola), unless vomiting persists. b. Eliminate unpleasant sights and odors. c. Provide good oral care after vomiting. d. Encourage deep breathing. e. Restrict liquids before meals. f. Avoid having the client lie down for at least 2 hours after meals. (A client who must rest should sit or recline so the head is at least 4 inches higher than the feet.) g. Administer antiemetics before meals if indicated.	11. Control of nausea and vomiting improves nutritional status. a. Frequent intake of small amounts of fluid helps to prevent overdistention. b. This diminishes visual and olfactory stimulation of the vomiting center. c. Good oral hygiene can reduce nausea. d. Deep breathing can suppress the vomiting reflex. e. Restricting liquids can prevent overdistention. f. Sitting reduces gastric pressure. g. Antiemetics prior to meals can prevent nausea and vomiting.
12. Encourage client to try commercial supplements available in many forms (liquids, powder, pudding); keep switching brands until some are acceptable to the individual in taste and consistency.	12. These supplements can substantially increase caloric intake without the need to consume large quantities of food.

(continues on page 474)

Interventions continued	Rationales continued

13. Teach client techniques to enhance nutritional content of food:
  a. Add powdered milk or egg to milk-shakes, gravies, sauces, puddings, cereals, etc. to increase protein and calorie content.
  b. Add blenderized or baby foods to meat juices or soups.
  c. Use fortified milk: 1 cup nonfat dry milk added to 1 quart fresh milk.
  d. Use milk, half-and-half, or soy milk instead of water when making soups and sauces.
  e. Add cheese or diced meat to foods whenever able.
  f. Spread cream cheese or peanut butter on toast, crackers, celery sticks.
  g. Add extra butter or margarine to foods.
  h. Use mayonnaise instead of salad dressing.
  i. Add raisins, dates, nuts, and brown sugar to hot and cold cereals.
  j. Keep snacks readily available.
	13. Simple food additives can increase calorie, protein, carbohydrate, and fat intake.

14. If client still has insufficient nutritional intake, consult with physician for alternative strategies.	14. Client may require high-protein supplements, tube feedings, or total parenteral nutrition.

 Documentation

Flow records
  Weight
  Intake (type, amount)

High Risk for Disturbed Self-Concept Related to Effects of Burn on Appearance, Increased Dependence on Others, and Disruption of Life Style and Role Responsibilities

Focus Assessment Criteria	Clinical Significance
1. Experience with or previous exposure to persons with burns	1–5. The psychosocial recovery after burn injury may require learning new skills and coping with feelings of fear, guilt, anger, and depression (Greenfield, 1998).
2. Ability to visualize burned area	
3. Ability to express feelings about appearance	
4. Ability to share feelings about appearance with family members and significant others	
5. Participation in self-care activities	

Goal
The client will demonstrate healthy adaptation and coping skills.

Indicators
- Communicate his or her feelings about the burns.
- Participate in self-care.

Interventions	Rationales
1. Contact the client often and treat him or her with warm, positive regard.	1. Frequent client contact indicates acceptance and may facilitate trust. Client may be hesitant to approach staff because of a poor self-concept.
2. Incorporate emotional support into technical self-care sessions. Encourage narration, visualization, participation, and exploration.	2. These activities promote exploration of feelings and resolution of emotional conflicts during acquisition of technical skills. Four stages of psychological adjustment have been identified. a. Narration: The person recounts the injury experience and reveals an understanding of how and why he or she is in this situation. b. Visualization and verbalization: The person looks at and expresses feelings about the injury. c. Participation: The person progresses from observer to assistant then to independent practitioner of the medical aspects of wound care. d. Exploration: The person begins to explore methods of incorporating appearance changes into his or her life style.
3. Encourage client to look at burned areas.	3. Client begins the adaptation process by acknowledging the injury and loss.
4. Encourage client to verbalize feelings and perceptions of life style effects. Validate client's perceptions and assure him or her that his or her responses are normal and appropriate.	4. Validating the client's feelings and perceptions increases self-awareness and boosts self-concept.
5. Have client participate in care as much as possible. Provide feedback on progress and reinforce positive behavior and proper techniques.	5. Participation in care can improve the client's self-esteem and sense of control; feedback and reinforcement encourage continued participation.
6. Have client demonstrate wound care and teach procedure independently to a support person.	6. Evaluation of a return demonstration helps the nurse to identify need for further teaching and supervision.

(continues on page 476)

Interventions continued	Rationales continued
7. Involve family members or significant other(s) in learning wound care.	7. Acceptance of support persons is one of the most important factors in the client's acceptance of body image changes.
8. Encourage client to verbalize positive self-attributes.	8. Evidence that the client will pursue personal goals and maintain his or her life style reflects positive adjustment.
9. Encourage contact with others on the unit.	9. Such contacts give client the opportunity to test the response of others to his or her injuries and possible altered appearance.
10. Offer constant verbal encouragement to achieve short-term goals.	10. This enhances the client's level of hope.

11. Identify a client at risk for unsuccessful adjustment; look for these characteristics:
 	
  a. Poor ego strength
  b. Ineffective problem-solving ability
 	
  c. Learning difficulty
 	
  d. Lack of motivation
  e. External focus of control
  f. Poor health
  g. Unsatisfactory preinjury sex life
  h. Lack of positive support systems
  i. Rejection of counseling
	11. Successful adjustment to changes in appearance are influenced by factors such as the following:
	  a. Previous successful coping
	  b. Achievement of developmental tasks preinjury
	  c. Extent to which injury interferes with goal-directed activity
	  d. Sense of control
	  e. Realistic self-perception and realistic perception from support persons

12. Refer an at-risk client for professional counseling.	12. The client may need follow-up therapy to aid in successful adjustment.

 Documentation

Progress notes
Present emotional status
Interventions
Client's or family's response to nursing interventions

Deficient Diversional Activity Related to Prolonged Hospitalization, Physical Limitations, and Monotony of Confinement

Focus Assessment Criteria	Clinical Significance
1. Current activity level 2. Past activity pattern 3. Motivation	1–3. Previous activity levels and motivation influence the client's response to reduced activity levels.

Goal

The client will engage in a diversional activity.

Indicators

- Relate feelings of boredom and discuss methods of finding diversional activities.
- Relate methods of coping with feelings of anger or depression caused by boredom.

Interventions	Rationales
1. Validate the client's boredom.	1. Acknowledgment may increase motivation to increase stimulation.
2. Explore the client's likes and dislikes.	2. Exploration may help to identify possible recreational activities.
3. Vary the client's routine when possible.	3. Monotony contributes to boredom.
4. Encourage visitors, telephone calls, and letter writing if appropriate.	4. Visitors provide social interaction and mental stimulation.
5. To reduce boredom, use various strategies to vary the physical environment and the daily routine: a. Update bulletin boards, change pictures on the walls, rearrange furniture. b. Maintain a pleasant, cheerful environment. Position client near a window if possible. If appropriate, provide a goldfish bowl for visual variety. c. Provide a variety of reading materials (or "books on tape" if impairment hinders reading ability) and a television and radio. d. Discourage excessive television watching. e. Plan some "special" activity daily to give client something to look forward to each day. f. Consider enlisting a volunteer to read to the client or play board games or card games. g. Encourage client to devise his or her own strategies to combat boredom.	5. Creative strategies to vary the environment and daily routine can reduce boredom.
6. If feasible	6. Such work provides opportunities to assist others and reduces feelings of dependency and isolation.
7. Encourage staff and visitors to discuss experiences	7. Initiating such discussions validates that client has interests and opinions and also involves client in subjects beyond personal concerns.

Documentation
Progress notes
Activities
Participation in self-care activities

Impaired Physical Mobility Related to Painful Burn Wounds

Focus Assessment Criteria	Clinical Significance
1. Ability to perform active range-of-motion exercises	1–4. This information helps the nurse to evaluate the client's degree of immobility and tolerance for activities to increase mobility.
2. Extent of range and strength of affected extremities	
3. Ability to perform self-care activities	
4. Level of tolerance: blood pressure, heart rate, respiratory rate, and fatigue	

Goal

The client will participate in self-care activities.

Indicators

- Experience minimal immobility as a result of the burn injury.
- Adapt physically to undesirable outcome of the burn injury.

Interventions	Rationales
1. Determine client's preburn level of activity, tolerance, and use of assistive devices.	1. Knowledge of preburn activity allows for reasonable expectations related to outcome of program.
2. Collaborate with physical therapist and occupational therapist to plan an exercise and activity program conducive to increasing range of affected extremities.	2. Consultation allows for expert evaluation and interventions to be reinforced by all team members.
3. Plan for a team meeting with client to discuss the exercise and activity program, its purpose, and expectations of therapists, nursing, and client.	3. Knowledge and understanding of program enhances client cooperation and program effectiveness.
4. Perform passive range-of-motion exercises as recommended by therapists.	4–6. Burn patients require frequent exercising to remain mobile. Although therapists are primarily responsible for rehabilitation, it is also necessary for nurses to assist with follow-up.
5. Continue splinting of affected extremities as recommended by therapist.	5. Splinting is required to maintain position of function rather than position of comfort for affected extremity.

(continues on page 479)

Interventions continued	Rationales continued
6. Encourage client to perform active range-of-motion exercises independently at regular intervals throughout the day.	
7. Apply pressure dressings (ace wraps or Tubigrip) or pressure garments as recommended by therapists.	7. Pressure garments are worn when wounds are healed and edema has subsided. These dressings and garments promote collagen breakdown and thus minimize hypertrophic scarring by exerting a controlled amount of pressure over the affected areas. Ace wraps can be used before the wound is healed. Pressure garments must be worn at all times.
8. Encourage self-care activities. Collaborate with therapist and client to determine methods or devices that would facilitate self-care.	8. Performance of self-care activities builds client's self-esteem and helps him or her to realize improvement and recovery.

High Risk for Ineffective Therapeutic Regimen Management Related to Insufficient Knowledge of Wound Care, Healed Skin Care, Nutritional Requirements, Management of Pain and Itching, Burn Prevention, and Follow-up Care

Focus Assessment Criteria	Clinical Significance
1. Readiness and ability to learn and retain information	1. A client or family failing to meet learning goals requires a referral for assistance postdischarge.
2. Ability to perform self-care activities independently	

Goals

The goals for this diagnosis represent those associated with discharge planning. Refer to the discharge criteria.

Interventions	Rationales
1. Explain the appearance of the burn wound at various stages of healing.	1. Knowledge of healing process provides the client with reasonable expectations.
2. Instruct and demonstrate wound care to the client and a significant other. Be clear and simple. Also provide written information.	2. Knowledge and understanding of process enhances cooperation.

(continues on page 480)

Interventions continued	Rationales continued
3. Allow for return demonstration of wound care by client and significant other.	3. Evaluation of a return demonstration helps the nurse identify the need for further teaching and supervision.

4. Discuss skin care measures:
  a. Apply lubricant (e.g., cocoa butter) frequently to healed and unaffected skin.
 	
  b. Use sunscreen.
 	
  c. Wear loose-fitting cotton garments next to skin.
  d. Avoid harsh soaps and hot water.
	4. Healing skin is more vulnerable to injury.
	  a. Lubricants relieve pruritus of dry skin. (Grafted skin areas do not contain sweat or oil glands.)
	  b. Burned and grafted skin tans unevenly, and burned skin is more vulnerable to skin cancer.
	  c. Cotton garments reduce itching and abrasion.
	  d. Healed burned skin may be hypersensitive.

5. Instruct client and family to watch for and report the following:
  a. Change in healed areas
  b. Change in wound drainage or color
  c. Fever or chills
  d. Weight loss
	5. Healing burns are prone to infection and require optimal nutrition.
	  a. Changes may point to infection or graft rejection.
	  b,c. These signs may indicate infection.
	  d. Weight loss indicates that intake is insufficient to meet metabolic needs.

6. Describe the action of pressure garments (e.g., Jobst) and the need to wear them 23 hours a day (1 hour to launder).	6. Constant pressure on the wound throughout scar maturation (usually 1 year) can retard scar growth.
7. Explain the importance of continuing range-of-motion exercises at home.	7. As the burn heals, hypertrophic scar tissue formation causes some shortening or contraction. Daily exercise can help reduce severity.
8. Explain the need to maintain adequate nutrition after discharge. (Refer to the nursing diagnosis Imbalanced Nutrition in this care plan for specific instructions.)	8. Burn healing requires increased protein and carbohydrate intake.
9. Describe available community resources (e.g., home care, vocational rehabilitation, financial assistance).	9. Such resources may assist in recovery.

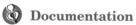 **Documentation**
Discharge summary record
Client teaching
Outcome achievement or status
Referrals if indicated

Musculoskeletal and Connective-Tissue Disorders

FRACTURES

Fractures are breaks in the continuity of bone. They result from external pressure greater than the bone can absorb. When the fracture displaces the bone, it also damages surrounding structures (muscles, tendons, nerves, and blood vessels). Traumatic injuries cause most fractures. Pathologic fractures occur without trauma in bones weakened from excessive demineralization.

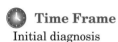 **Time Frame**
Initial diagnosis

 DIAGNOSTIC CLUSTER

Collaborative Problems

▲ PC: Neurovascular Compromise
* PC: Compartmental Syndrome
▲ PC: Fat Embolism
▲ PC: Hemorrhage/Hematoma Formation
▲ PC: Thromboembolism

Nursing Diagnoses	Refer to
▲ Pain related to tissue trauma secondary to fracture	
△ High Risk for Ineffective Therapeutic Regimen Management related to insufficient knowledge of condition, signs and symptoms of complications, activity restrictions	
▲ Self-Care Deficit (specify) related to limitation of movement secondary to fracture	Casts
△ High Risk for Ineffective Respiratory Function related to immobility secondary to traction or fixation devices	Immobility or Unconsciousness

Related Care Plan

Casts

▲ This diagnosis was reported to be monitored for or managed frequently (75%–100%).
△ This diagnosis was reported to be monitored for or managed often (50%–74%).
* This diagnosis was not included in the validation study.

Discharge Criteria

Before discharge, the client or family will

1. Describe necessary precautions during activity.
2. State signs and symptoms that must be reported to a health care professional.
3. Demonstrate the ability to provide self-care or report available assistance at home.

Collaborative Problems

Potential Complication: Neurovascular Compromise

Potential Complication: Compartmental Syndrome

Potential Complication: Fat Embolism

Potential Complication: Hemorrhage/Hematoma Formation

Potential Complication: Thromboembolism

Nursing Goal

The nurse will detect early signs and symptoms of (a) neurovascular compromise, (b) compartmental syndrome, (c) fat embolism, and (d) cardiovascular alterations and collaboratively intervene to stabilize the client.

Indicators
- Pedal pulses 2+, equal (a, b, d)
- Capillary refill <3 seconds (a, b, d)
- Warm extremities (a, b, d)
- No c/o paresthesia, tingling (a, b, d)
- Pain relieved by medications (b)
- Minimal swelling (a, b, d)
- Ability to move toes or fingers (b)
- BP >90/60, <140/90 mm Hg (d)
- Pulse 60–100 beats/min (d)
- Respirations 16–20 breaths/min (d)
- Temperature 98–99.5°F (c)
- Oriented, calm, alert (c, d)
- Urine output >30ml/hr (c, d)
- Negative Homan's sign (a, b)

Interventions	Rationales
1. Monitor for signs and symptoms of neurovascular compromise, comparing findings on affected limb to other limb: a. Diminished or absent pedal pulses b. Numbness or tingling c. Capillary refill time > 3 seconds d. Pallor, blanching, cyanosis, coolness e. Inability to flex or extend extremity	1. Trauma causes tissue edema and blood loss that reduce tissue perfusion. Inadequate circulation and edema damage peripheral nerves resulting in decreased sensation, movement, and circulation (Porth, 2002).
2. Monitor for signs of compartmental syndrome (Slye, 1991; Pellino, 1998).	2. Compartmental syndrome is when increased pressure in a limited space

(continues on page 485)

Interventions continued	**Rationales** continued
	compromises circulation and function. Some causes of increased pressure are bleeding, edema, traction, and casts (Snyder, 1998; Tumbarello, 2000).
a. Early signs: • Unrelieved or increasing pain • Pain with passive stretch of toes or fingers • Mottled or cyanotic skin • Excessive swelling • Poor capillary refill • Paresthesia • Inability to move toes or fingers	a. Pain and paresthesia indicate compression of nerves and increasing pressure within muscle compartment. Passive stretching of muscles decreases muscle compartment, thus increasing pain. Poor capillary refill, or mottled or cyanotic skin, indicates obstructed capillary blood flow.
b. Late signs: • Pallor • Diminished or absent pulse • Cold skin	b. Arterial occlusion will produce these late signs.
3. Assess peripheral nerve function at least every hour for first 24 hours.	3. Peripheral neurovascular compromise may be the first sign (Tumbarello, 2000).
4. For injured arms (Ross, 1991; Pellino, 1998): a. Assess for movement ability: • Hyperextension of thumbs, wrist, and four fingers • Abduction (fanning out of) all fingers • Ability to touch thumb to small finger b. Assess sensation with pressure from a sharp point: • Web space between thumb and index finger • Distal fat pad of small finger • Distal surface of the index finger	4. These specific assessment techniques will detect changes in sensation and movement (Snyder, 1998; Tumbarello, 2000).
5. For injured legs (Ross, 1991; Pellino, 1998): a. Assess for movement ability: • Dorsiflex (upward movement) ankle and extend toes at metatarsophalangeal joints • Plantarflex (downward movement) ankle and toes b. Assess sensations with pressure from a sharp point: • Web space between great toe and second toe • Medial and lateral surfaces of the sole (upper third)	5. Crush syndrome a. Inspection and palpation, tense swollen extremity may be present. • Swelling may be absent in the presence of dehydration and peripheral vasoconstriction from shock. • Cool, clammy skin with hypovolemia • Accompanying skin changes; erythema, bullae, vesicles b. Alteration in urinary output (Core Curriculum, 2001)

(continues on page 486)

Interventions continued	**Rationales** continued
6. Instruct to report unusual, new, or different sensations (e.g., tingling, numbness, or decreased ability to move toes or fingers, "pins/needles," "feels asleep").	6. Early detection of compromise can prevent serious impairment (Snyder, 1998).

7. Reduce edema or its effects on function:
   a. Remove jewelry from affected limb.
   b. Elevate limbs unless contraindicated.
   c. Move fingers or toes of affected limb two to four times/hour.
   d. Apply ice bags around injured site. Place a cloth between ice bag and skin.
   e. Monitor drainage (characteristics and amount) from wounds or incisional site.
   f. Maintain patency of the wound drainage system.
	7. Edema reduction can deter compartmental syndrome.

8. Notify the physician if the following occur:
   a. Change in sensation
   b. Change in movement ability
   c. Pale, mottled, or cyanotic skin
   d. Slowed capillary refill (more than 3 seconds).
   e. Diminished or absent pulse
   f. Increasing pain or pain not controlled by medication
   g. Pain with passive stretching of muscle
   h. Pain increased with elevation
	8. A decompressive fasciotomy may be needed (Core Curriculum, 2001; Slye, 1991).

9. If preceding signs or symptoms occur, discontinue elevation and ice application.	9. These measures will decrease tissue pressure and restore local blood flow (Slye, 1991).

10. Monitor for signs and symptoms of fat embolism (Hager & Brnich, 1998).
 	
   a. Tachypnea >30 breaths/min
 	
   b. Sudden onset of chest pain or dyspnea
 	
   c. Restlessness, apprehension
 	
   d. Confusion
 	
   e. Elevated temperature >103°F
 	
   f. Increased pulse rate >140 beats/min
   g. Petechial rash (12–96 hours postoperatively)
	10. A fracture can release bone marrow into the bloodstream where it forms an embolism that can obstruct circulation (distal, cerebral, or pulmonary). Symptoms depend on the site of obstruction.
	   a–d. These changes are the result of hypoxemia. Fatty acids attract red blood cells and platelets to form microaggregates that impair circulation to vital organs (e.g., brain). Fatty globules passing through the pulmonary vasculature cause a chemical reaction that decreases lung compliance and ventilation/perfusion ratio.
	   e. Temperature increases are a response to circulating fatty acids.
	   f. Refer to a to d rationale.
	   g. This rash is the result of capillary fragility. Common sites are conjunctiva, axilla, chest, and neck.

(continues on page 487)

Interventions continued	**Rationales** continued
11. Minimize movement of a fractured extremity for the first 3 days after the injury.	11. Immobilization minimizes further tissue trauma and reduces the risk of embolism dislodgment (Core Curriculum, 2001; Slye, 1991).
12. Ensure adequate hydration.	12. Optimal hydration will dilute the irritating fatty acids through the system (Core Curriculum, 2001; Slye, 1991).
13. Monitor intake/output, urine color, and specific gravity.	13. These data will reflect hydration status.

14. Monitor for signs and symptoms of hemorrhage/shock:
  a. Increasing pulse rate with normal or slightly decreased blood pressure
  b. Urine output <30 mL/hr
  c. Restlessness, agitation, change in mentation
  d. Increasing respiratory rate
  e. Diminished peripheral pulses
  f. Cool, pale, or cyanotic skin
  g. Thirst
	14. Bone is very vascular; blood loss can be substantial, especially with multiple fractures and fractures of the pelvis and femur. The compensatory response to decreased circulatory volume involves increasing blood oxygen by raising heart and respiratory rates and decreasing circulation to the extremities (marked by decreased pulses, cool skin). Diminished cerebral oxygenation can cause altered mentation.

15. Monitor for signs and symptoms of thrombophlebitis:
  a. Positive Homans' sign (Dorsiflexion of the foot causes pain from insufficient circulation.)
  b. Calf tenderness, unusual warmth, redness
  c. Low-grade fever
  d. Extremity edema
	15. Three factors increase the incidence of clot formation: stasis, coagulation abnormalities and vessel damage. Clients with fractures are immobile and sustain vessel damage from trauma. A decrease in fibrinolytic activity occurs after surgery, beginning 24 hours post-operative with the lowest point on day 3 (Carroll, 1993).

16. In leg fracture, encourage exercises of the unaffected leg. Discourage placing pillows under the knees, using a knee gatch, crossing the legs, and prolonged sitting.	16. Leg exercises help to increase venous return; avoiding external pressure helps to prevent venous stasis (Carroll, 1993).
17. Ambulate as soon as possible with at least 5 minutes of walking each waking hour. Avoid prolonged chair sitting with legs dependent.	17. Walking contracts leg muscles, stimulates the venous pump, and reduces stasis (Core Curriculum, 2001).
18. For high-risk clients, consult with physician for use of (Snyder, 1998):	18. High-risk persons are those over 40 years old, obese with multiple trauma, or history of circulation deficits and on estrogen

(continues on page 488)

Interventions continued	Rationales continued
	therapy as well as those who have systemic infection or are cigarette smokers (Carroll, 1993; Snyder, 1998).
a. Sequential compression stockings	a. These stockings reduce venous stasis by applying a graded degree of compression to the ankle and the calf.
b. Low-dose heparin	b. Low-dose heparin reduces the coagulability of the blood by acting as antagonist to thrombin and prevents the conversion of fibrinogen to fibrin.
c. Low-dose dextran	c. Dextran decreases blood viscosity and reduces platelet aggregation. In addition, clots formed in the presence of dextran are more susceptible to fibrinolysis.
19. Monitor for heparin-induced thrombocytopenia (Core Curriculum, 2001, p. 176).	19. Heparin causes platelet sequestration.

 Related Physician-Prescribed Interventions

Medications. Analgesics, anticoagulants, muscle relaxants

Laboratory Studies. Complete blood count, blood chemistry studies

Diagnostic Studies. X-ray examinations, tomograms, bone scans

Therapies. Casts; wound care; traction (skin, skeletal); compression stockings; oxygen; surgery (internal fixation)

 Documentation

Flow records
  Vital signs
  Pulses, color, warmth, sensation, movement of distal areas
  Intake and output
Progress notes
  Unusual complaints

Nursing Diagnoses

Pain Related to Tissue Trauma Secondary to Fracture

Focus Assessment Criteria	Clinical Significance

1. Source of pain:
  a. Fracture
  b. Edema
  c. Poor alignment
  d. Splint or traction
  e. Cast
	1. Pain following fracture can result from destruction of nerves and tissue by trauma, tissue edema during healing, poor alignment, and poorly fitted splints, traction devices, or casts. Assess client carefully to differentiate fracture pain from other possible causes.

(continues on page 489)

Focus Assessment Criteria continued	Clinical Significance continued

2. Client's perception of pain severity based on a scale of 0 to 10 (0 = no pain; 10 = worst pain), rated as follows:
  a. At its best
  b. At its worst
  c. After each pain relief measure
	2. Such a rating scale enables nurse to assess the subjective experience of pain.

3. Physical signs of pain: increased heart rate, respirations, and blood pressure; restlessness; facial grimacing; guarding	3. Objective data may be more reliable indicators of pain in certain clients. Some clients are reluctant to admit the extent of pain or to request pain medication.

Goal

The client will report progressive reduction of pain and relief after pain-relief measures.

Indicators
- Relate factors that increase pain.
- Relate interventions that are effective.

Interventions	Rationales
1. Refer to the General Surgery care plan, Appendix II, for general pain relief interventions.	1. Rationale is self-evident.
2. Immobilize the injured part as much as possible, using splints when indicated.	2. Immobilization reduces pain and displacement.
3. Teach client to change position slowly.	3. Slow movements decrease muscle spasms.
4. Elevate an injured extremity unless contraindicated.	4. Elevation reduces edema and the resulting pain from compression.
5. Investigate pain not relieved by pain medications or other relief measures.	5. Unrelenting pain can indicate neurovascular compression from embolism, edema, or bleeding (Core Curriculum, 2001).

 Documentation

Medication administration record
   Type, dosage, route of all medications administered
Progress notes
   Unrelieved pain and actions taken

High Risk for Ineffective Therapeutic Regimen Management Related to Insufficient Knowledge of Condition, Signs and Symptoms of Complications, and Activity Restrictions

Focus Assessment Criteria	Clinical Significance
1. Readiness and ability to learn and to retain information	1. A client or family who fails to achieve learning goals requires a referral for assistance post-discharge.

Goals

The goals for this diagnosis represent those associated with discharge planning. Refer to the discharge criteria.

Interventions	Rationales
1. Teach client to watch for and to report the following immediately: a. Severe pain b. Tingling, numbness c. Skin discoloration d. Cool extremities	1. These signs may indicate neurovascular compression, a condition requiring immediate medical intervention.
2. Explain the risks of infection and signs of osteomyelitis: a. Chills, high fever b. Rapid pulse c. Malaise d. Painful, tender extremity	2. Bone infections can occur during the first 3 months after fracture.
3. Explain activity restrictions.	3. Resting the affected limb promotes healing.
4. Instruct on proper ambulation techniques as appropriate.	4. Improper use of assistive devices can cause injuries.
5. Refer to Cast care plan	

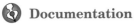 Documentation

Discharge summary record
   Client teaching
   Outcome achievement or status

INFLAMMATORY JOINT DISEASE (RHEUMATOID ARTHRITIS, INFECTIOUS ARTHRITIS)

Rheumatoid arthritis is a systemic disease characterized primarily by chronic inflammation with destructive synovitis in multiple diarthrodial joints. The etiology is unknown. The joints involved are usually symmetrically affected, with the small bones of hands and feet affected first. The disease is characterized by cycles of exacerbations and remission. Extra-articular involvement of rheumatoid arthritis can include muscle atrophy, anemia, osteoporosis, and skin, ocular, vascular, pulmonary, and cardiac symptoms. Because many consequences of arthritis cannot be measured (e.g., functional, social, leisure), the impact of arthritis is often underestimated (Holmes, 1998).

Infectious arthritis is an inflammation of a joint resulting from a viral, bacterial, or fungal organism invading the synovium and synovial fluid. Individuals at risk for this opportunistic disease are those immunocompromised by a chronic disease or by medications.

 Time Frame

Initial diagnosis
Secondary diagnosis

⊗ DIAGNOSTIC CLUSTER*

Collaborative Problems	Refer to
PC: Septic Arthritis	
PC: Sjögren's Syndrome	
PC: Neuropathy	
PC: Anemia, Leukopenia	Inflammatory Bowel Disease

Nursing Diagnoses	Refer to
Fatigue related to decreased mobility, stiffness	
High Risk for Impaired Oral Mucous Membrane related to effects of medications or Sjögren's syndrome	
Disturbed Sleep Pattern related to pain or secondary to fibrositis	
High Risk for Loneliness related to ambulation difficulties and fatigue	
(Specify) Self-Care Deficit related to limitations secondary to disease process	

491

Nursing Diagnoses continued	Refer to continued
Ineffective Sexuality Patterns related to pain, fatigue, difficulty in assuming positions, and lack of adequate lubrication (female) secondary to disease process	
Impaired Physical Mobility related to pain and limited joint motion	
Chronic Pain related to inflammation of joints and juxta-articular structures	
High Risk for Ineffective Therapeutic Regimen Management related to insufficient knowledge of condition, pharmacologic therapy, home care, stress management, and quackery	
Interrupted Family Processes related to difficulty/inability of ill person to assume role responsibilities secondary to fatigue and limited motion	Multiple Sclerosis
Powerlessness related to physical and psychological changes imposed by the disease	Chronic Obstructive Pulmonary Disease
Related Care Plans Corticosteroid Therapy Raynaud's Disease	

* This medical condition was not included in the validation study.

Discharge Criteria

Before discharge, the client or family will

1. Identify components of a standard treatment program for inflammatory arthritis.
2. Relate proper use of medications and other treatment modalities.
3. Identify characteristics common to "quack" cures.
4. Identify factors that restrict self-care and home maintenance.
5. Relate signs and symptoms that must be reported to a health care professional.

Collaborative Problems

Potential Complication: Septic Arthritis

Potential Complication: Sjögren's Syndrome

Potential Complication: Neuropathy

Nursing Goal

The nurse will detect early signs/symptoms of (a) septic arthritis, (b) Sjögren's syndrome, (c) neuropathy, and (d) anemia and collaboratively intervene to stabilize the client.

Indicators

- Temperature 98–99.5°F (a)
- No change in usual level of pain (a)
- No change in usual level of fatigue (a)
- Moist, mucous membranes (b)
- No c/o paresthesias and numbness (c)
- Hemoglobin (d)
    - Male: 14–18 g/dL
    - Female: 12–16 g/dL
- WBC 4300–10,800 mm (a)

Interventions	Rationales
1. Monitor for septic signs and symptoms of arthritis: a. Warm, painful, swollen joints b. Decreased range of motion c. Fever, chills, and fatigue	1. The chronic inflammation of arthritis increases the risk of joints becoming infected from infections in other body parts.
2. Explain the need to splint or support and rest the inflamed joint.	2. Reducing movement can decrease permanent damage to articular cartilage.
3. Monitor for signs and symptoms of Sjögren's syndrome: a. Dry mucous membranes (mouth, vagina) b. Nasal crusting and epistaxis c. Decreased salivary and lacrimal gland secretions d. Nonproductive cough	3. The etiology of this syndrome is unknown. It is characterized by faulty secretion of lacrimal, salivary, gastric, and sweat glands.
4. Monitor for symptoms of neuropathy: a. Paresthesias b. Numbness	4. Swelling and actual joint changes can cause nerve entrapment.
5. Provide and explain the importance of disease-modifying antirheumatic medications. Monitor for adverse effects.	5. Refer to a pharmacological reference for specific information.

◢ Related Physician-Prescribed Interventions

Medications. Acetylsalicylates, immunosuppressives, corticosteroids, etanercept, cyclosporin A, cyclophosphamide, hydroxychloride, hydroxyquine, d-Penicillamine, nonsteroidal anti-inflammatory agents, gold salts, sulfasalazine

Laboratory Studies. WBC count, sedimentation rate, agglutination reactions, rheumatoid factor, immunoglobins

Diagnostic Studies. X-ray films, radionuclide scans, direct arthroscopy, synovial fluid aspirate, bone scan

Therapies. Physical therapy, aqua therapy

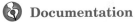 **Documentation**
Progress notes
   Changes in range of motion
   Complaints

Nursing Diagnoses

Fatigue Related to Decreased Mobility, Stiffness

Focus Assessment Criteria	Clinical Significance
1. Fatigue pattern (morning, evening, transient, constant)	1. Inflammation produces joint symptoms such as pain and stiffness that result in fatigue. Identifying periods of decreased fatigue can assist in scheduling activities.
2. Effects of fatigue on activities of daily living (ADLs), role responsibilities, recreation, relationships	2. Fatigue can negatively influence a client's ability for reciprocity—returning support to one's support persons—which is vital for balanced and healthy relationships.

Goal

The client will report less fatigue.

Indicators
- Identify daily patterns of fatigue.
- Identify signs and symptoms of increased disease activity that affect activity tolerance.
- Identify principles of energy conservation.

Interventions	Rationales

1. Discuss the causes of fatigue (Crosby, 1991):
  a. Joint pain
  b. Decreased sleep efficiency
  c. Increased effort required for ADL
	1. Persons with rheumatoid arthritis report that their fatigue was related to joint pain. In addition, findings reported that clients with flare were observed to awaken more often and take longer to walk and perform activities than nonflare clients and the control group (Crosby, 1991).

2. Assist in identifying energy patterns; have the client rate his or her fatigue on a scale of 0 to 10 (0 = not tired; 10 = total exhaustion) every hour for a 24-hour period.	2. Identifying times of peak energy and exhaustion can aid in planning activities to maximize energy conservation and productivity.

(continues on page 495)

Interventions continued	Rationales continued

3. Allow client to express feelings regarding the effects of fatigue on his or her life (Carpenito, 1997):
  a. Identify difficult activities.
  b. Identify activities that interfere with role responsibilities.
  c. Identify frustrations.
	3. In many chronic diseases, fatigue is the most common, disruptive, and distressful symptom experienced because it interferes with self-care activities (Hart, Freel & Milde, 1990). Exploring with client the effects of fatigue on his or her life will help both the nurse and client to plan interventions.

4. Assist individual to identify strengths, abilities, and interests (Carpenito, 1997):
  a. Identify client's values and interests.
  b. Identify client's areas of success and usefulness; emphasize past accomplishments.
  c. Use this information to develop goals with the client.
  d. Assist client to identify sources of hope (e.g., relationships, faith, things to accomplish).
  e. Assist client to develop realistic short-term and long-term goals (progress from simple to more complex; client may use a "goal poster" to indicate type and time for achieving specific goals).
	4. Focusing client on strengths and abilities may provide him or her with insight of positive events and decrease overgeneralizing the severity of disease, which can lead to depression (Holmes, 1998).

5. Help client to schedule and coordinate procedures and activities to accommodate energy patterns.
  a. Promote participation in a fitness/ conditioning program to increase maximize endurance.
 	
6. Explain the purpose of pacing and prioritization (Carpenito, 1997):
  a. Assist individual to identify priorities and to eliminate nonessential activities.
  b. Plan each day to avoid energy- and time-consuming nonessential decision making.
  c. Organize work with items within easy reach.
  d. Distribute difficult tasks throughout the week.
  e. Rest before difficult tasks and stop before fatigue ensues.
	5,6. Client requires rest periods before or after some activities. Planning can provide for adequate rest and reduce unnecessary energy expenditure.

7. Teach energy conservation techniques (Carpenito, 1997):
  a. Modify the environment:
    • Replace steps with ramps.
    • Install grab rails.
	7. Such strategies can enable continuation of activities and contribute to positive self-esteem.

(continues on page 496)

Interventions continued	**Rationales** continued
• Elevate chairs 3 to 4 inches. • Organize kitchen or work areas. • Reduce trips up and down stairs (e.g., put a commode on first floor). b. Plan small, frequent meals to decrease energy required for digestion. c. Use taxi instead of driving self. d. Delegate housework (e.g., employ a high school student for a few hours after school).	
8. Explain the effects of conflict and stress on energy levels and assist client to learn effective coping skills (Carpenito, 1997): a. Teach client the importance of mutuality in sharing concerns. b. Explain the benefits of distraction from negative events. c. Teach client the value of confronting issues. d. Teach and assist client with relaxation techniques before anticipated stressful events. Encourage mental imagery to promote positive thought processes. e. Allow client time to reminisce to gain insight into past experiences. f. Teach client to maximize aesthetic experiences (e.g., smell of coffee, back rub, or feel the warmth of the sun or a breeze). g. Teach client to anticipate experiences he or she takes delight in each day (e.g., walking, reading favorite book, or writing letter).	8. There are many stressors related to chronic illness (e.g., pain, threats to independence, self-concept, future plans, and fulfillment of roles). Clients who learn self-help responses face definable, manageable adversities by maintaining control of everyday problems (Braden, 1990).
9. Teach client to identify signs and symptoms that indicate increased disease activity and to decrease activities accordingly: a. Fever b. Weight loss c. Worsening fatigue d. Increased joint symptoms	9. During periods of increased disease activity, rest requirements increase to 10 to 12 hr/day.

 Documentation

Progress notes
  Fatigue pattern assessment
Discharge summary record
  Client teaching

High Risk for Impaired Oral Mucous Membrane Related to Effects of Medications or Sjögren's Syndrome

Focus Assessment Criteria	Clinical Significance

1. Contributing factors:
  a. Immunosuppressive drugs
  b. Disease-modifying agents
  c. Sjögren's syndrome
	1. Medications used in the treatment of inflammatory joint disease can result in oral ulcers or stomatitis. The presence of either or both of these conditions may require the health care provider to hold or reduce the dose.

2. Knowledge of signs and symptoms of oral ulcers and stomatitis	2. The client's understanding enables monitoring and early detection of complications.

Goal

The client will continue to have intact oral mucus membrane.

Indicators

- Identify factors contributing to altered oral mucosa.
- Relate the need to report oral ulcers or stomatitis to a health care provider.
- Identify strategies for maintaining moist oral mucosa.
- Relate the need for frequent, regular dental care for Sjögren's syndrome sequelae.

Interventions	Rationales
1. Teach client to inspect the mouth during daily oral hygiene activities and to report ulcers or stomatitis to a health care provider.	1. Early detection of these problems enables prompt intervention to prevent serious complications.
2. Teach client to drink adequate amounts of nonsugared liquids.	2. Well-hydrated oral tissue is more resistant to breakdown.
3. Teach the importance of regular dental care.	3. Secondary Sjögren's syndrome can result in excessively dry oral mucosa and predispose client to tooth decay and gum disease.
4. Refer individual to Sjögren's Syndrome Foundation, 29 Gateway Drive, Great Neck, NY 11201.	4. This organization can provide more detailed information on the condition and its management.

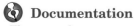 **Documentation**

Flow records
  Oral assessments
Discharge summary record
  Client teaching
  Outcome achievement or status

Disturbed Sleep Pattern Related to Pain or Secondary to Fibrositis

Focus Assessment Criteria	Clinical Significance
1. Usual sleep requirements, pattern, night-time awakenings	1. The amount of sleep a client needs varies with age and life style. Nighttime awakening can disrupt the sleep cycle. Assessment can help to determine individual needs.
2. Presence of pain at night	2. Pain can have a negative impact on sleep.
3. Presence of secondary fibrositis marked by the following: a. Difficulty maintaining sleep or non-restorative sleep b. Characteristic: locally tender body points	3. A syndrome characterized by difficulty maintaining sleep and the presence of locally tender nonarticular body points; fibrositis is often associated with inflammatory joint disease.

Goal

The client will

Indicators

• Describe factors that inhibit sleep.
• Identify techniques to facilitate sleep.
• Demonstrate an optimal balance of activity and rest.

Interventions	Rationales
1. Discuss sleep patterns and requirements: a. Explain that they vary with age, activity level, and other factors. b. Discourage comparing sleep habits with others. c. Discourage focusing on hours slept; instead focus on whether or not client feels rested and restored after sleep. d. Encourage alternate activities if sleep is difficult (e.g., reading or needle-point).	1. Sleep deprivation results in impaired cognitive functioning (e.g., memory, concentration, and judgment) and perception, reduced emotional control, increased suspicion, irritability, and disorientation. It also lowers the pain threshold and decreases production of catecholamines, corticosteroids, and hormones (Cohen & Merritt, 1992).
2. Encourage client to take a warm bath or shower before bedtime; showering first thing in the morning may be beneficial to reduce morning stiffness.	2. Warm water increases circulation to inflamed joints and relaxes muscles.
3. Encourage performance of a bedtime ritual such as hygiene activity, reading, or a having a warm drink.	3. A bedtime ritual helps to promote relaxation and prepare for sleep.

(continues on page 499)

Interventions continued	Rationales continued
4. Initiate pain relief measures before bedtime if appropriate. (Refer to the nursing diagnosis Chronic Pain in this care plan for more details.)	4. A client with inflammatory joint disease often experiences worsening symptoms at night.
5. Encourage proper positioning of joints: a. Pillows for limb position b. Cervical pillow	5. Proper positioning may help to prevent pain during sleep and awakenings.
6. Encourage a balance of activity and rest. a. Encourage afternoon nap as needed to minimize fatigue	6. Regular physical exercise also seems helpful in controlling the symptoms of fibrositis (Holmes, 1998).
7. Provide for uninterrupted sleep to enable completion of a sleep cycle (e.g., use a fan on low setting to drown out sounds).	7. A sleep cycle has an interval of 70 to 100 minutes. Most persons need to complete 4 to 5 cycles each night to feel rested (Cohen & Merritt, 1992).

 Documentation

Progress notes
  Sleep patterns
  Reports of feeling rested in the morning

High Risk for Loneliness Related to Ambulation Difficulties and Fatigue

Focus Assessment Criteria	Clinical Significance
1. Previous and present social patterns 2. Anticipated changes, desire for an increase	1,2. Chronic illness can contribute to social isolation because of lack of energy, decreased mobility, discomforts, fear of exposure to pathogens, and distancing by previous friends who are uncomfortable with the ill person's disabilities (Miller, 1995).

Goal

The client will report continued satisfactory social patterns.

Indicators
- Identify factors that contribute to isolation.
- Identify strategies to increase social interaction.
- Identify appropriate diversional activities.

Interventions	Rationales
1. Encourage client to share feelings and to evaluate socialization patterns.	1. Only client can determine whether socialization patterns are satisfactory or unsatisfactory. Some persons like to spend much of their time alone; others do not.

2. Discuss ways to initiate social contacts:
  a. Inviting a neighbor (adult or child) over for coffee or a snack 1 or 2 days a week
  b. Calling friends and relatives weekly
  c. Participating in social clubs (e.g., book discussion groups)
  d. Volunteering at the library, hospital, or other organizations
	2. Preoccupation with one's own life, problems, and responsibilities often prevents a person from socializing regularly with neighbors or relatives. Initiating contacts may be needed to break established patterns of isolation.

3. Discuss the advantages of using leisure time for personal enrichment (e.g., reading or crafts).	3. Diversional activities can make a person more interesting to others.
4. Discourage excessive TV watching.	4. Other than educational documentaries, TV encourages passive participation and usually does not challenge the intellect.

5. Discuss possible options to increase social activities:
  a. Exercise groups (e.g., YWCA/YMCA)
  b. Senior centers and church groups
  c. Foster grandparent program
  d. Day care centers for the elderly
  e. Retirement communities
  f. House sharing
  g. College classes open to older persons
  h. Pets
  i. Telephone contact
  j. Arthritis support groups
	5. Socialization can promote positive self-esteem and coping.

6. Discuss effects of disease on person's body image and self-esteem.	6. Verbalization of fears can lead to a more positive approach in the management of the disease and may promote a positive self-concept.

7. Identify barriers to social contact:
  a. Lack of transportation
  b. Pain
  c. Decreased mobility
	7. Mobility problems commonly hinder socialization, but many associated difficulties can be overcome with planning.

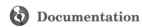 **Documentation**

Progress notes
  Feelings regarding social contacts
Discharge summary record
  Client teaching
  Response to teaching

(Specify) Self-Care Deficit Related to Limitations Secondary to Disease Process

Focus Assessment Criteria	Clinical Significance
1. Extent of disability in self-care activities 2. Need for and ability to use assistive devices	1,2. Inflammatory joint disease can result in temporary or permanent loss of joint function or deformity. This functional loss can impair the client's ability to perform self-care activities.

Goal

The client will demonstrate increased functioning in activities of daily living.

Indicators

• Identify the highest possible level of functioning in the following activities: bathing, dressing, feeding, and toileting.
• Demonstrate the ability to use assistive devices.

Interventions	Rationales
1. Refer to occupational therapy for instruction in energy conservation techniques and use of assistive devices.	1. Occupational therapy can provide specific instruction and further assistance.
2. Provide pain relief before the client undertakes self-care activities. (Refer to the nursing diagnosis Chronic Pain in this care plan for more information.)	2. Unrelieved pain can hinder self-care.
3. Provide privacy and an environment conducive to performance of each activity.	3. A comfortable, secure environment can reduce anxiety and enhance self-care abilities.
4. Schedule activities to provide for adequate rest periods.	4. Exhaustion decreases motivation for self-care activities.

5. Teach about the variety of assistive devices available for use in the home:
a. Bathing:
  • Grip bars in shower and bath
  • Bath seat
  • Washing mitt
  • Long-handled washing appliances
  • Built-up toothbrush
  • Dental floss holder
b. Dressing:
  • Long-handled zipper device
  • Buttoning device
	5. Assistive devices can improve self-care ability and increase the client's sense of control over his or her life.

(continues on page 502)

Interventions continued	Rationales continued

• Stocking/sock device
   • Long-handled shoe horns
   • Reacher
   • Elastic shoe strings
  c. Feeding:
   • Built-up utensils
   • Plate guard
   • Straw holder
  d. Toileting:
   • Raised toilet seat
   • Grip handle around toilet	

6. Explain available self-help reference materials, such as those from the Arthritis Foundation.	6. Promoting self-help promotes self-esteem.
7. Discuss with family members or significant others the changing family processes resulting from client's illness.	7. Disability associated with inflammatory joint disease can interfere with client's ability to care for self, family, and home; this disrupts family functioning.
8. Discuss importance of promoting the client's self-care at an appropriate level.	8. Maximum self-care promotes positive self-esteem and reduces feelings of powerlessness; this can contribute to effective family functioning.

 Documentation

Progress notes
  Type of assistance needed

Ineffective Sexuality Patterns Related to Pain, Fatigue, Difficulty in Assuming Position, Lack of Adequate Lubrication (Female) Secondary to Disease Process

Focus Assessment Criteria	Clinical Significance
1. Usual sexual activity pattern 2. Client's perception of problem	1,2. Sexual expression is essential for complete well-being and should be nurtured in all clients. An assessment to determine patterns and gratification helps to guide interventions (Miller, 1999).

3. Signal symptoms of secondary Sjögren's syndrome:
  a. Dry eyes
  b. Dry nasal mucosa
  c. Dry oral mucosa
  d. Dry vagina
  e. Recurrent parotiditis
	3. Sjögren's syndrome causes a decrease in the body's ability to secrete lubricating fluids; vaginal dryness may inhibit sexual activity.

Goal

The client will relate the intent to practice strategies to improve sexual functioning.

Indicators

• Identify factors that compromise sexual function.
• Identify strategies and techniques to facilitate and enhance sexual pleasure and expression.

Interventions	Rationales
1. Encourage client or couple to identify alternative sexual behaviors that may be used for sexual expression during periods of increased disease activity (e.g., touching, body massage).	1. Sexual expression is not limited to intercourse but encompasses many means of self-pleasure and giving pleasure to others (Miller, 1999).
2. Teach client or couple positions that minimize pain and joint stress during sexual intercourse (e.g., client on bottom, side-lying. Refer them to the Arthritis Foundation pamphlet *Living and Loving* for more information).	2. Inflammatory joint disease can result in loss of joint motion, owing to damage to both articular and juxta-articular structures (muscle, tendon, ligaments). Positions that lessen strain on the client's joints can enhance sexual pleasure (Holmes, 1998).
3. Identify times when sexual activity may be more painful—most commonly in the early morning—and encourage having sex at other times. a. Encourage use of analgesics prior to sexual activity.	3. Inflammatory joint disease is often associated with prolonged morning stiffness.
4. Identify products that can be used to replace or supplement natural vaginal lubrication (e.g., water-soluble lubricants [KY jelly, Surgilube]).	4. Inflammatory joint disease is sometimes associated with Sjögren's syndrome, which is characterized by a decreased ability to secrete lubricating fluids (e.g., tears, saliva, or vaginal secretions). Use of a lubricant can decrease pain on intercourse.
5. Discuss the need to plan for sexual activity (e.g., schedule it for a certain time of day or take a hot shower or bath before activity).	5. Planning sexual activity allows the client to prepare beforehand, which can increase pleasure for both client and partner.

 Documentation

Progress notes
   Client teaching
   Discussions

Impaired Physical Mobility Related to Pain and Limited Joint Motion

Focus Assessment Criteria	Clinical Significance

1. Presence and degree of pain
 	
2. Function and mobility of joints:
   a. Limitations in range of motion
   b. Presence of deformities
 	
3. Muscle strength
	1–3. The chronic inflammation associated with inflammatory joint disease results in damage to articular and juxta-articular structures such as bone demineralization, tendon and ligament laxity, and muscle wasting. This damage can result in impaired mobility.

Goal

The client will maintain and when possible increase strength and endurance in limbs.

Indicators
- Describe the rationale for interventions.
- Minimize joint stress and injury.
- Demonstrate correct performance of exercises.

Interventions	Rationales

1. Provide pain relief as necessary. (Refer to the nursing diagnosis Chronic Pain in this care plan for specific interventions.)
   a. Teach client the use of orthotic devices and ambulatory aids.
   b. Teach client the need to achieve ideal body weight to facilitate mobility.
	1. Pain can contribute to decreased mobility.

2. Encourage compliance with a prescribed exercise program, which may include the following exercises:
   a. Range of motion (ROM)
   b. Muscle strengthening
   c. Endurance
	2. A regular exercise program including ROM, isometrics, and selected aerobic activities can help to maintain integrity of joint function, increase strength, and decrease pain and fatigue (Holmes, 1998).

3. Encourage an amount of exercise consistent with the degree of disease activity.	3. During periods of acute inflammation, the individual may immobilize the joints in the most comfortable position; this is usually partial flexion. Continued immobilization can result in joint stiffness and muscle weakness (extensor groups) that can quickly lead to contractures and more pain (Holmes, 1998).

(continues on page 505)

Interventions continued	**Rationales** continued

4. Teach the client to perform all the following steps: (Holmes, 1998):
   a. Warm-up: Before exercising, take a warm bath or shower or use warm soaks or a heating pad on affected areas. Then perform gentle stretching.
 	
   b. Gentle ROM without passive pressure at least once daily.
   c. Isometric and strengthening exercises: Contract muscle group for a count of eight, then relax for two counts. Perform 10 repetitions, three to four times a day on the quadriceps, abdominal muscles, gluteals, and deltoids.
   d. Endurance/aerobic exercise: Begin with a 5- to 10-minute period and gradually increase time. Appropriate activities include walking, swimming, and light racquet games (badminton, ping-pong). Inappropriate activities include heavy racquet sports (tennis, squash, racquetball), contact sports (football, hockey), and weight-lifting or progressive resistance exercise.
   e. Cool-down period: For 5 to 10 minutes, progressively slow movements of extremities or slow walking pace.
	4.
	
	   a. A warm-up period of local heat or gentle stretching prior to strengthening and endurance exercises allows muscles gradually to become ready for more intense work. (Holmes, 1998).
	   b. Gentle ROM prevents injury to joint tissue (Holmes, 1998).
	   c. Isometric and other strengthening exercises can improve function (Holmes, 1998).
	
	   d. Exercises that jar or bang joints are contraindicated.
	
	   e. A cool-down period after more intense exercise allows muscle waste products to be removed and permits the body to return gradually to its preexercise state.

5. If client complains of postexercise pain persisting longer than $1\frac{1}{2}$ to 2 hours, instruct him or her to do as follows:
   a. Decrease repetitions the next day.
   b. For severe soreness the next day, attempt ROM at least once after local heat application to affected joints.
	5. Exhaustion and pain decrease motivation to continue in an exercise program.

6. Refer to physical therapy as necessary.	6. Assistance may be needed for development of an in-depth instruction in a physical activity program.
7. Refer to community-based exercise groups for people with arthritis (e.g., Arthritis Foundation Aquatic Exercise).	7. Such a program can provide exercise and socialization. Arthritis Foundation Aquatic Exercise provides warm water therapy.

 Documentation

Flow records
   Exercises (type, frequency)

Chronic Pain Related to Inflammation of Joints and Juxta-articular Structures

Focus Assessment Criteria	Clinical Significance
1. Joints affected and the presence of associated warmth, swelling, and erythema 2. Range of motion in affected joints	1,2. Inflammatory joint disease is characterized by an activation of the body's inflammatory response. Stable prostaglandins, thromboxanes, and prostacyclin are mediators of inflammation. Experimental data show that although these mediators are incapable of provoking pain directly, they do produce hyperalgesia and act synergistically with other inflammation mediators to augment pain. These substances also act on small blood vessels, producing vasodilation and changes in vascular permeability that result in erythema, warmth, and swelling (Burrage, 1999).
3. Fatigue, quality of sleep, nutritional intake, and limitations 4. Techniques used: heat, cold, and menthol rubs	3,4. Exploring the effects of pain on client's life and strategies used to manage pain will assist in planning with client.

Goal

The client will relate improvement of pain and, when possible, increase daily activities.

Indicators

- Receive validation that pain exists.
- Practice selected noninvasive pain relief measures to manage pain.
- Relate improvement of pain and, when possible, increase daily activities.

Interventions	Rationales
1. Teach to differentiate between joint pain and stiffness.	1. When joint pain exists, techniques for joint protection are instituted. When flares are diminished, active ROM exercises are indicated (Holmes, 1998).
2. If joints are inflamed, rest and avoid activities that stress joints. Gentle ROM may be tried.	2. ROM can prevent contractures. Inflamed joints are at risk for injury.
3. Apply local heat or cold to affected joints for approximately 20 to 30 minutes three to four times a day. Avoid temperatures likely to cause skin or tissue damage by checking the temperature of warm soaks or covering a cold/ice pack with a towel.	3,4. Treatment of inflammatory joint pain focuses on the reduction of discomfort and inflammation by the use of local comfort measures, joint rest, and the use of anti-inflammatory or disease-modifying medications.

(continues on page 507)

Interventions continued	Rationales continued
4. Encourage a warm bath or shower the first thing in the morning to reduce morning stiffness.	
5. Encourage measures to protect affected joints: a. Perform gentle active ROM exercises once daily during periods of active inflammation. b. Use larger, stronger joints (e.g., forearm, not fingers). c. Rest 5–10 minutes periodically when trying to complete a task. d. Avoid stooping, bending, or overreaching. e. Change positions frequently; avoid positions of stress on joints. f. Use splints. g. Obtain assistance with ADLs if necessary. h. Maintain proper body alignment. i. Avoid pillows under the knees to prevent knee and hip flexion deformities. j. Use assistive devices as necessary.	5. Frequent rest periods take the weight off joints and relieve fatigue. Proper positioning is needed to minimize stress on joints (Holmes, 1998).
6. Encourage the use of adjunctive pain control measures: a. Progressive relaxation b. Transcutaneous electrical nerve stimulation (TENS) c. Biofeedback d. Imagery/music/acupuncture	6. Pain is a subjective, multifactorial experience that can be modified by the use of cognitive and physical techniques to reduce the intensity or perception of pain (Holmes, 1998).

Documentation

Progress notes
In affected joints: pain, swelling, warmth, erythema
Pain relief measures
Response to pain relief measures

High Risk for Ineffective Therapeutic Regimen Management Related to Insufficient Knowledge of Condition, Pharmacologic Therapy, Home Care, Stress Management, and Quackery

Focus Assessment Criteria	Clinical Significance
1. Knowing of or experience with arthritic conditions either personal or from relatives or friends; feelings, concerns, and questions	1. This assessment guides nurse in developing teaching strategies.
2. Readiness and ability to learn and retain information	2. A client or family failing to achieve learning goals requires a referral for assistance postdischarge.

Goals

The goals for this diagnosis represent those associated with discharge planning. Refer to the discharge criteria.

Interventions	Rationales

1. Explain inflammatory arthritis using teaching aids appropriate to client's and family member's levels of understanding. Explain the following:
a. Inflammatory process
b. Joint function and structure
c. Effects of inflammation on joints and juxtaarticular structures
d. Extra-articular manifestations of the disease process
e. Chronic nature of disease
f. Disease course (remission/exacerbation)
g. Low incidence of significant or total disability
h. Components of the standard treatment program:
  • Medications (e.g., aspirin, non-steroidal anti-inflammatory drugs, disease-modifying agents, cytotoxic agents, corticosteroids)
  • Local comfort measures
  • Exercise/rest
  • Joint protection/assistive devices
  • Consultation with other disciplines
	1. Inflammatory joint disease is a chronic illness. Education should emphasize a good understanding of the inflammatory process and actions the client can take to manage symptoms and minimize their impact on his or her life.

2. Allow significant others opportunities to share feelings and frustrations.
  • Adequate nutrition
  • Regular follow-up care
	2. Persons with RA may be difficult to live with, demanding, or manipulative (Holmes, 1998).

3. Teach client and family to identify characteristics of quackery: a. "Secret" formulas or devices for curing arthritis b. Advertisements using "case histories" and "testimonials" c. Rejection of standard components of treatment program d. Claims of persecution by the "medical establishment"	3. An accurate and full understanding of inflammatory joint disease and its treatment decreases the client's susceptibility to quackery.
4. Teach client to take prescribed medications properly and to report symptoms of side effects promptly.	4. Adhering to the schedule may help to prevent fluctuating drug blood levels and can reduce side effects. Prompt reporting of side effects enables intervention to prevent serious problems.

(continues on page 509)

Interventions continued	Rationales continued

5. Explain the proper use of other treatment modalities:
  a. Local heat or cold application
  b. Assistive devices
  c. Exercises
	5. Injury can further decrease mobility and motivation to continue therapies.

6. Explain the relationship of stress to inflammatory diseases. Discuss stress management techniques:
  a. Progressive relaxation
  b. Guided imagery
  c. Regular exercise
	6. Stressful events may be associated with an increase in disease activity. Effective use of stress management techniques can help to minimize the effects of stress on the disease process.

7. Reinforce the importance of routine follow-up care.	7. Follow-up care can identify complications early and help to reduce disabilities from disuse.
8. Refer to appropriate community resources such as The Arthritis Foundation, 1314 Spring St N.W., Atlanta, GA 30309.	8. Such resources can provide specific additional information to enhance self-care.

 Documentation

Discharge summary record
  Client and family teaching
  Outcome achievement or status
  Referrals if indicated

OSTEOMYELITIS

Osteomyelitis is a disease in which the bone and surrounding tissues are infected. The infection may result from a blood-borne infection from other sites (e.g., infected tonsils, pressure ulcer, an inner ear infection) or because of direct bone contamination as with an open fracture, trauma, or surgery. Osteomyelitis also may develop from vascular insufficiency, such as diabetes mellitus or severe atherosclerosis, or from the presence of indwelling fixation devices. The limited blood supply in the bone makes healing more difficult. Chronic osteomyelitis may occur, necessitating amputation of the extremity.

Time Frame
Initial or secondary diagnosis

DIAGNOSTIC CLUSTER*

Collaborative Problems	Refer to
PC: Bone Abscess	
PC: Sepsis	Fractured Hip and Femur

Nursing Diagnoses	Refer to
Pain related to soft-tissue edema secondary to infection	Fractured Hip and Femur
Impaired Physical Mobility related to limited range of motion of affected bone	Fractured Hip and Femur
High Risk for Ineffective Therapeutic Regimen Management related to insufficient knowledge of condition, etiology, course, pharmacologic therapy, nutritional requirements, pain management, and signs and symptoms of complications	

Related Care Plans

Long-Term Venous Access Devices

---

* This medical condition was not included in the validation study.

Discharge Criteria

Before discharge, the client or family will do the following:

1. Identify factors that contribute to osteomyelitis.
2. Relate the signs and symptoms that must be reported to a health care professional.
3. Verbalize an intent to implement life-style changes needed for healing.

510

Collaborative Problem

Potential Complication: Bone Abscess

Nursing Goal
The nurse will monitor for early signs/symptoms of bone abscesses and sepsis and collaboratively intervene to stabilize client.

Indicators
- Temperature 98–99.5°F
- Heart rate 60–100 beats/min
- Respiratory rate 16–20 breaths/min
- White blood count >12,000 cells/mm³, <4000 cells/mm³

Interventions	Rationales

1. Monitor:
  a. Fever and chills
  b. Bone pain
  c. Increasing tenderness
  d. Warmth
	1. As pus accumulates the pressure increases, causing ischemia in the bone compartment.

2. Assure that antibiotics are given round the clock.	2. Sustained high therapeutic blood levels of the antibiotic are necessary (Pons, 1991). Teach client the importance of taking the antibiotics for the entire course as ordered.

 Related Physician-Prescribed Interventions

Medications. Intravenous antibiotic therapy, analgesics

Diagnostic Studies. Cultures (blood/wound/stool, urine); sedimentation rate; CBC; urinalysis; prealbumin, total protein; C-reactive protein; radio nuclide bone scan; MRI

Therapies. Incision and drainage of abscesses; surgical debridement; casting or immobilization of affected bone; hyperbaric oxygen; appropriate physical therapy

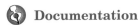 Documentation
Flow records
  Vital signs
  Pulses, color, warmth, sensation, and movement of distal areas
Progress notes
  Unusual complaints

Nursing Diagnoses

High Risk for Ineffective Therapeutic Regimen Management Related to Insufficient Knowledge of Condition, Etiology, Course, Pharmacologic Therapy, Nutritional Requirements, Pain Management, and Signs and Symptoms of Complications

Focus Assessment Criteria	Clinical Significance
1. Knowledge of condition	1. Assessment of knowledge of the possible chronicity of this condition determines the level of teaching needed.

Goals

The goals for this diagnosis represent those associated with discharge planning. Refer to the discharge criteria.

Interventions	Rationales

1. Determine knowledge of condition, prognosis, and treatment.
  a. Review proper handling techniques of pin sites or external fixation (if applicable).
  b. Instruct client to avoid tenting of skin around pin and to avoid application of thick ointment and occlusive dressing at pin site.
	1. The client's understanding contributes to improved compliance and reduced risk.
	  a. Stress on sites should be avoided.
	
	  b. Occlusion at pin site can encourage microorganism growth.

2. Teach infection control for drains and wounds:
  a. Use proper aseptic techniques for dressing changes, care of pins/external fixates.
  b. Strict handwashing before and after wound care.
  c. Use proper techniques for disposal of soiled dressing.
	2. These measures help to prevent introduction of additional microorganisms into the wound; they also reduce the risk of transmitting infection to others.

3. Discuss the nutritional requirements and dietary sources.
 	
  a. Calories per day: 2500–3000
 	
  b. Protein: 100 to 125 g; sources: dairy, meat, poultry, fish, and legumes
  c. B-complex vitamins; sources: meat, nuts, and fortified cereals
 	
  d. Vitamin C: 75–300 mg; sources: green vegetables and citrus fruits
  e. Phosphorus, magnesium, and vitamin D; sources: multivitamins
	3. Major complications of trauma and sepsis increase the metabolic rate from 10% to 50%. In the presence of insufficient protein, the body breaks down its own endogenous protein stores (Salmond, 1998).
	a,b. Increased caloric and protein intake is needed to enhance the body's protein-sparing capacity.
	
	  c. B-complex vitamins are required for metabolism of carbohydrates, fat, and protein.
	  d. Vitamin C is essential for collagen formation and wound healing (Salmond, 1998).
	  e. These nutrients are required for healing (Salmond, 1998).

4. Explain the need for supplements (e.g., milkshakes and puddings).	4. Supplements may be needed to ensure the daily caloric requirement.
5. Discuss techniques to manage pain. Refer to index under acute or chronic pain.	
6. Teach client to take prescribed antibiotic diligently.	6. A variety of microorganisms may cause osteomyelitis. More than one organism may be involved. More and more patients

(continues on page 513)

Interventions continued	Rationales continued
	may become immunocompromised, thus increasing the number of unusual pathogens such as fungi and mycobacteria.
7. Teach client to monitor and report complications: a. Fever b. Increasing pain c. Visible bone deformity d. Swelling e. Exudate	7. Fever and increasing pain can be indicative of sepsis. Sudden pain in affected limb can indicate a pathologic fracture.
8. Prepare client and family of the possibility of exacerbations.	8. Chronic osteomyelitis can occur if bacterial growth occurs in vascular scar tissue, which is impenetrable to antibiotics (Pons, 1991). Chronic osteomyelitis is most common following open fracture with direct contamination of the wound.
9. Stress the importance of balancing rest, activity, constructive stress management, and optimal nutrition.	9. Clients can be empowered by giving them choices in managing their health (Lamm, Dungan & Hiromoto, 1991).

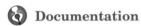 Documentation

Discharge summary record
   Client teaching
   Outcome achievement or status

OSTEOPOROSIS

In osteoporosis, the rate of bone resorption exceeds the rate of bone formation. As a result, the bones become progressively porous and brittle and are prone to fracture from minimal trauma and even normal stress. Small-framed, non-obese Caucasian women are at greatest risk.

 Time Frame
Secondary diagnosis

 DIAGNOSTIC CLUSTER*

Collaborative Problems

• Potential Complications:

Fractures
Kyphosis
Paralytic Ileus

Nursing Diagnoses

• High Risk for Ineffective Therapeutic Regimen Management related to insufficient knowledge of condition, risk factors, nutritional therapy, and prevention

---

*This medical condition was not included in the validation study.

Discharge Criteria

Before discharge, the client or family will

1. Relate those risk factors that can be modified or eliminated.
2. Describe dietary modifications.
3. Relate signs and symptoms that must be reported to a health care professional.

Collaborative Problems

Potential Complication: Fractures

Potential Complication: Kyphosis

Potential Complication: Paralytic Ileus

Nursing Goal

The nurse will monitor for signs/symptoms of (a) fractures, (b) kyphosis, and (c) paralytic ileus and collaboratively intervene to stabilize client.

Indicators

• No new onset of pain (a, b)
• No changes in height (a, b)
• Bowel sound present (c)

Interventions	Rationales
1. Monitor for signs and symptoms of fractures (vertebral, hip, or wrist): a. Pain in lower back or neck b. Localized tenderness c. Pain radiating to abdomen and flank d. Spasm of paravertebral muscles	1. Bones with high amounts of trabecular tissue (e.g., hip, vertebrae, wrist) are more affected by progressive osteoporosis.
2. Monitor for kyphosis of dorsal spine, marked by loss of height. Kyphosis is indicated when the distance between the foot and the symphysis pubis exceeds the distance between the head and the symphysis pubis by more than 1 cm.	2. This spinal change can cause height loss of 2.5 to 15 cm.
3. Monitor for signs and symptoms of paralytic ileus: a. Absent bowel sounds b. Abdominal discomfort and distention	3. Vertebral collapse involving the tenth to twelfth thoracic vertebrae (T10–T12) can interfere with bowel innervation, resulting in ileus.

Related Physician-Prescribed Interventions

Medications. Calcium, vitamin D supplements; salmon calcitonin; fluoride; estrogen replacement therapy in conjunction with progesterone; bisphosphonates; selective estrogen-receptor modulators

Laboratory Studies. Serum calcium and phosphate; alkaline phosphatase; hydroxyproline; urine calcium excretion; serum osteocalcin; hematocrit

Diagnostic Studies. X-ray examinations (bone density), dual-photon absorptiometry, single-photon absorptiometry, quantitative computed tomography (Mitlak & Nussbaum, 1993), dual-energy x-ray absorptiometry

Therapies. Braces (vertebral), surgery to repair fractures, kyphoplasty, casting

Documentation

Progress notes
    Complaints of pain or discomfort
Flow records
    Bowel sounds
    Height

Nursing Diagnoses

High Risk for Ineffective Therapeutic Regimen Management Related to Insufficient Knowledge of Condition, Risk Factors, Nutritional Therapy, and Prevention

Focus Assessment Criteria	Clinical Significance
1. Knowledge of or experience with osteoporosis	1. This assessment helps the nurse to plan teaching strategies.

(continues on page 516)

Focus Assessment Criteria continued	Clinical Significance continued
2. Readiness and ability to learn and retain information	2. A client or family failing to meet learning goals requires a referral for assistance postdischarge.

Goal

The goals for this diagnosis represent those associated with discharge planning. Refer to the discharge criteria.

Interventions	Rationales
1. Discuss osteoporosis using teaching aids appropriate to the client's or family's level of understanding (e.g., pictures, slides, models). Explain the following: a. Loss of bone density b. Increased incidence of vertebral, hip, and wrist fractures	1. Various teaching strategies may be necessary to maximize understanding and retention of information. a. Bone mass decreases as a result of decreased bone formation or increased bone resorption. Age 34 is the median age for initial bone loss in women (Freund, 1995). Genetics, estrogen, and risk factors strongly influence rate of bone loss. Risk factors include endocrine disorders, immobilization, nutritional abnormalities, chronic disease (e.g., malignant tumors), and collagen diseases (Core Curriculum, 2001). b. These bones contain large amounts of porous trabecular tissue, which makes them more susceptible to the effects of osteoporosis. About one half of women experience vertebral fracture due to osteoporosis before age 75. The incidence of osteoporosis-related hip fracture in women doubles every 5 years after age 50. Of individuals with hip fractures, 12% to 20% die within 1 year of the fracture. By age 90, more than one third of women have hip fractures (Freund, 1995).
2. Explain risk factors and which ones can be eliminated or modified (Hunt, 1998). a. Sedentary life style b. Thinness, small body frame	2. Focusing on those factors that can be modified can help to decrease feelings of helplessness (Hunt, 1998). a. Inactivity leads to increased rate of bone resorption. b. Thin women typically have less bone mass than obese women. Caucasian women with small skeletal frames are at greatest risk. African-American and Oriental women tend to have more bone mass and thus are at less risk.

(continues on page 517)

Interventions continued	**Rationales** continued
c. Diet low in calcium and vitamin D and high in phosphorus	c. Insufficient dietary calcium and vitamin D can contribute to decreased bone reformation. High phosphate intake associated with high-protein diets stimulates parathyroid activity and thus increases bone resorption.
d. Menopause or oophorectomy	d. Decreased plasma estrogen level increases bone sensitivity to the resorptive action of parathyroid hormone.
e. Medications	e. Various medications have been linked to progression of osteoporosis (e.g., some anti-convulsants, aluminum-containing antacids, thyroid supplements, isoniazid, prolonged heparin therapy, tetracycline, furosemide, and corticosteroids [particularly if dosage exceeds 15 mg/day for more than 2 years]). Corticosteroids affect calcium absorption by interfering with vitamin D metabolism. Discontinuation of therapy does not result in restoration of lost bone mass; however, it does prevent further disease progress.
f. Alcohol ingestion	f. Alcohol impairs calcium absorption in the intestines, increases urinary loss of calcium, and has a possible effect on liver activation of vitamin D.
g. Caffeine	g. Early research results provide some evidence that caffeine increases calcium loss in kidneys and intestines.
h. Low sodium fluoride levels	h. Sodium fluoride stimulates osteoblastic activity.
i. Cigarette smoking	i. On average, smokers are thinner than nonsmokers; moreover, female smokers usually experience menopause earlier than nonsmokers.
3. Refer to community resources such as smoking cessation workshops, Alcoholics Anonymous, and the Arthritis Foundation.	3. These resources can provide needed assistance after discharge.
4. Teach to monitor for and report signs and symptoms of fracture: a. Sudden severe pain in the lower back, particularly after lifting or bending b. Painful paravertebral muscle spasms c. Gradual vertebral collapse (assessed by changes in height or measurements indicating kyphosis) d. Chronic back pain e. Fatigue f. Constipation	4. Early detection and treatment of fractures can prevent serious tissue damage and disabilities. One quarter of older individuals with hip fractures die within a year. Only 25% of those with hip fractures regain full functional ability. Hip fractures have a high mortality, morbidity, and cost for both individuals and society (Anders & Ornellas, 1997).

(continues on page 518)

Interventions continued	**Rationales** continued

5. Reinforce explanations for nutritional therapy and consult with dietitian when indicated:
  a. Encourage calcium intake of 1000 to 1500 mg/day.
	5. Nutritional therapy is a critical component of treatment.
	
	  a. The National Osteoporosis Foundation recommends 1200 mg of calcium per day for individuals up to age 24, 1000 mg for adults, and 1500 mg in postmenopausal women not receiving estrogen replacement (Core Curriculum, 2001; Mitlak & Nussbaum, 1993; National Institutes of Health [NIH], 2000). Older women need increased intake to compensate for decreased absorption, and premenopausal women should prepare for expected bone resorption by increasing intake.

b. Identity foods high in calcium (e.g., sardines, salmon, tofu, dairy products, and dark green leafy vegetables).
  c. Monitor for signs and symptoms of lactose intolerance such as diarrhea, flatulence, and bloating.
  d. Recommended multivitamin containing 400 to 800 IU of vitamin D daily (Fujita, 1992).
  e. Identify food sources of vitamin D (e.g., fortified milk, cereals, egg yolks, liver, and saltwater fish).
 	
  f. Encourage adequate (not excessive) protein intake of approximately 44 g/day in most clients.
	b. Dietary sources provide a good means of increasing calcium intake.
	
	  c. Increased intake of dairy products may lead to development of lactose intolerance, particularly in older clients.
	  d,e. Vitamin D is necessary for the use and absorption of available calcium and phosphorus. However, excessive vitamin D intake can result in bone loss. Side effects, such as hypercalcemia, hypercalciuria, and kidney stones, can occur. (NIH, 2000)
	  f. Protein intake should not exceed normal recommended requirements because excessive protein can enhance bone loss by causing increased urinary acid and resulting increased calcium excretion.

6. Explain the need for increased physical activity and certain restrictions:
  a. Encourage exercise that results in movement, pull, and stress on the long bones (e.g., walking, stationary bicycling, and rowing).
 	
  b. Instruct the client to exercise at least three times a week for 30 to 60 minutes each session as ability allows.
	6. Immobilization results in bone resorption exceeding bone formation (Burckhardt, 1992).
	  a. Weightbearing exercise increases bone mass. Compressive forces of muscle contraction and stress, tension, and bending provide mechanical stimulation and bone growth and retention. A larger muscle mass provides greater protection against osteoporosis (Stacey, 1989). Caution should be used in choosing activities that do not carry a high risk of fractures. Activities such as jogging and bicycling over rough roads may increase pressure on weightbearing vertebrae.
	  b. A consistent exercise program stimulates bone formation and slows bone loss. It also provides a secondary benefit of improved neuromuscular conditioning, agility, and decreased likelihood of falls.

(continues on page 519)

Interventions continued	**Rationales** continued
c. Discourage flexion exercises of the spine and sudden bending, jarring, and strenuous lifting. Avoid activities that rotate the vertebral spine.	c. These maneuvers increase vertical compression force, increasing the risk of vertebral fractures. Extension or isometric exercises are more appropriate; there is less risk of fractures to fragile vertebrae as stress is decreased on the anterior portion of the vertebral body.
d. Plan adequate rest periods; lay in supine position for at least 15 minutes when chronic pain increases or at certain intervals during day.	d. Fatigue decreases the motivation to exercise.
e. Instruct the client in the use of a back brace, corset, or splint if necessary.	e. This intervention minimizes the possibility of spontaneous fractures.
f. Encourage family members or other caregivers to provide passive range-of-motion exercises for a client immobilized in bed.	f. Many studies have demonstrated that prolonged immobilization causes even young persons to experience bone loss (approximately 1% of bone mass per week).
7. Explain the importance of safety precautions such as the following: a. Supporting the back with a firm mattress, body supports, and good body mechanics b. Protecting against accidental falls by wearing walking shoes with low heels; removing environmental hazards such as throw rugs, slippery floors, electrical cords in pathways, and poor lighting; and avoiding alcohol, hypnotics, and tranquilizers c. Using assistive devices as necessary (e.g., a cane or crutches) d. Avoiding any flexion movement such as stooping, bending, and lifting. Explain that vertebral compression fractures can result from minimal trauma resulting from opening a window, lifting a child, coughing, or stooping.	7. Osteoporosis increases the risk of spontaneous fractures. a. Spontaneous fractures occur most often in the mid to lower thoracic and lumbar spine. b. Often a fall is caused by a spontaneous fracture of the hip. Falling from a standing position can result in a fracture of the proximal femur; falling on an outstretched hand can cause Colles' fracture. Even though wrist fractures heal easily, they are significant because they are predictors of hip fractures. c. Assistive devices can decrease the risk of falling. d. Any flexion movement should be eliminated to decrease the risk of fracture.
8. Explain any prescribed medication therapy; stress the importance of adhering to the plan and understanding possible side effects. As appropriate, reinforce the following (Kessenich, 1996): a. Calcium supplement: 1000 to 1500 mg/day; 1500 mg/day after menopause accompanied by increased fluid intake b. Vitamin D supplement: 100 to 500 IU/day. (*Note:* If vitamin D is used in conjunction with calcitriol, plasma calcium	8. Compliance with the medication regimen can slow the progression of osteoporosis. Awareness of possible side effects allows prompt reporting and intervention to minimize adverse effects. a. Risk of renal calculi can be diminished with increased fluid intake. b. Vitamin D supplements increase utilization of phosphorus and calcium in clients with no exposure to sunlight and

(continues on page 520)

Interventions continued	Rationales continued
levels should be monitored weekly for 4 to 6 weeks and then less frequently.)	with inadequate dietary vitamin intake. Hypercalcemia can result.
c. Parenteral Salmon Calcitonin: FDA-approved dose is 100 IU daily. Frequently 100 IU/day, three times a week is used initially; then after X-ray films and evaluation of serum calcium, dosage may decrease to 50 IU/day q 1–3 days.	c. Serum calcium levels should be monitored closely because of an increased risk of hypercalcemia with induced hyperparathyroidism. Calcitonin decreases further bone loss at vertebrae and femoral sites. There seems to be some protection from postmenopausal bone loss for women who are not able or willing to take estrogen replacement therapy. This is an expensive therapy that may reduce pain associated with fractures. Initial therapy sometimes produces flushing and nausea. An intranasal calcitonin preparation is being evaluated in clinical trials in the United States. This preparation seems to prevent bone loss for at least 2 years in postmenopausal women (Kessenich, 1996).
d. Sodium fluoride: usually 60 mg/day at separate time from calcium administration	d. Taking calcium with fluoride may interfere with fluoride absorption. Fluoride acts as a stimulator for osteoblasts and increases cancellous bone mass. The dosage seems to be an important factor in preventing fractures, with nonvertebral fractures increasing at higher doses. Lower doses, <50 mg, have a beneficial effect on vertebral fractures; however, the trabecular bone mass of the spine is not increased as it is at higher doses. This indicates a narrow window for the most therapeutic dose (Arcangelo & Peterson, 2001).
e. Alendronate (Fosamax) orally 10 mg/day	e. Bisphosphonates decrease bone resorption and prevent bone loss (Kessenich, 1996; NAON, 2001).
9. Provide information regarding the National Osteoporosis Foundation, 1232 22nd Street, N.W., Washington DC, 20037-1292, (202) 223-2226, website: http://www.nof.org.	

 Documentation

Discharge summary record
   Client teaching
   Outcome achievement or status
   Referrals if indicated

Infectious and Immunodeficient Disorders

HUMAN IMMUNODEFICIENCY VIRUS/ ACQUIRED IMMUNODEFICIENCY SYNDROME

An infection caused by the human immunodeficiency virus (HIV), acquired immunodeficiency syndrome (AIDS) was first reported in the United States in 1981. AIDS represents the end stage of a continuum of HIV infection and its sequelae. Major modes of infection transmission include sexual activity with an infected person and exposure to infected needles, blood, or blood products. A fetus can contract HIV infection from an infected mother perinatally. HIV infects primarily the T4-cell lymphocytes; this interferes with cell-mediated immunity. The clinical consequences of this progressive, immune deficit are opportunistic infections and malignancies. Beginning in the 1990s, the increased number of available medications has slowed the course of HIV dramatically.

 Time Frame
Initial diagnosis
Recurrent acute episodes

⊕ DIAGNOSTIC CLUSTER

Collaborative Problems	**Refer to**
▲ PC: Opportunistic Infections	
△ PC: Malignancies	
▲ PC: Septicemia	Thermal Injury
△ PC: Myelosuppression	Leukemia

Nursing Diagnoses	**Refer to**
▲ Risk for Infection Transmission related to the infectious nature of the client's blood and body fluids	
* High Risk for Imbalanced Nutrition: Less Than Body Requirements related to HIV infection, opportunistic infections/malignancies associated with AIDS	
* High Risk for Ineffective Coping related to situational crisis (i.e., new HIV or AIDS diagnosis, first hospitalization)	
* High Risk for Caregiver Role Strain related to AIDS-associated shame/stigma, and uncertainty about course of illness and demands on caregiver	

(continues on page 524)

Nursing Diagnoses continued	**Refer to** continued
▲ High Risk for Ineffective Therapeutic Regimen Management related to functional and/or cognitive deficits associated with advanced HIV infection and/or opportunistic events	
▲ High Risk for Ineffective Therapeutic Regimen Management related to insufficient knowledge of HIV, its transmission, prevention, treatment, and community resources	
△ Powerlessness related to unpredictable nature of condition	Chronic Obstructive Pulmonary Disease
△ Anxiety related to perceived effects of illness on life style and unknown future	Cancer: Initial Diagnosis
△ Grieving related to loss of body function and its effects on life style	Cancer: Initial Diagnosis
△ Powerlessness related to change from curative to palliative status	Cancer: Initial Diagnosis
▲ High Risk for Infection related to increased susceptibility secondary to compromised immune system	Leukemia
▲ Fatigue related to effects of disease, stress, chronic infections, and nutritional deficiency	Inflammatory Joint Disease
▲ High Risk for Impaired Oral Mucous Membrane related to compromised immune system	Chemotherapy
Related Care Plans Cancer (End-Stage)	

▲ This diagnosis was reported to be monitored for or managed frequently (75%–100%).
△ This diagnosis was reported to be monitored for or managed often (50%–74%).
*This diagnosis was not included in the validation study.

Discharge Criteria

Before discharge, the client or family will

1. Relate the implications of diagnosis.
2. Describe the prescribed medication regimen.

3. Identify modes of HIV transmission.
4. Identify infection control measures.
5. Describe signs and symptoms that must be reported to a health care professional.
6. Identify available community resources.

Collaborative Problems

Potential Complication: Opportunistic Infections

Potential Complication: Malignancies

Potential Complication: Septicemia

Potential Complication: Avascular Necrosis

Nursing Goal

The nurse will detect early signs and symptoms of (a) opportunistic infections (pneumonia, encephalitis, enteritis, cytomegalovirus, herpes simplex, herpes zoster, stomatitis, esophagitis, meningitis) and (b) malignancies, and collaboratively intervene to stabilize client.

Indicators

- Temperature 98–99.5°F (a)
- Respirations 16–20 breaths/min (a)
- No cough (a)
- Alert, oriented (a)
- No seizures, no headaches (a)
- Regular, formed stools (a)
- No herpetic or zoster lesions (a)
- Swallows with no difficulty (a)
- No change in vision (a)
- No weight loss (b)
- No new lesions (b)
- No lymphadenopathy (b)

Interventions	Rationales
1. Monitor for opportunistic infections:	1. Severe immune deficiencies with CD4 <200 cause opportunistic infections (OI) and malignancies. Antiretroviral therapy has dramatically reduced OIs.
a. Protozoal: • *Pneumocystis carinii* pneumonia (dry, nonproductive cough, fever, dyspnea) • *Toxoplasma gondii* encephalitis (headache, lethargy, seizures) • *Cryptosporidium* enteritis (watery diarrhea, malaise, nausea, abdominal cramps)	a. The most common and serious infection is *Pneumocystis carinii* pneumonia.
b. Viral (CD4 count <50): • Genital herpes simplex, herpes simplex perirectal abscesses (severe pain, bleeding, rectal discharge)	b. Herpes simplex is common and painful. The CMV infections are responsible for significant morbidity (e.g., blindness).

(continues on page 526)

Interventions continued	**Rationales** continued
• Cytomegalovirus (CMV) retinitis, colitis, pneumonitis, encephalitis, or other organ disease • Progressive multifocal leuko-encephalopathy (headache, decreased mentation) • Varicella zoster, disseminated (shingles) c. Fungal: • *Candida albicans* oral, stomatitis and esophagitis (exudate, complaints of unusual taste in mouth) • *Cryptococcus neoformans* meningitis (fever, headaches, blurred vision, stiff neck, confusion) d. Bacterial (CD4 count <50): • *Mycobacterium avium intracellulare* disseminated • *Mycobacterium tuberculosis* extrapulmonary and pulmonary	c. Fungal conditions are chronic with relapses. d. Bacterial infections frequently affect the pulmonary system.
2. Emphasize the need to report symptoms early. Advise that if client is severely compromised, some symptoms will not be present (e.g., increased temperature).	2. Early treatment can often prevent serious complications (e.g., septicemia) and increases the chance of a favorable response to treatment.
3. Administer medications for opportunistic infections. Consult a pharmacological reference for specific information (Arcangelo & Peterson, 2001). a. *Pneumocystis carinii* pneumonia (PCP) * Bactrim * Dapsone • Atovaquone • Clindamycin and primoaquine b. *Mycobacterium avium intracellulare* complex infection (MAC) * Azithromycin • Clarithromycin • Ethambutol • Rifabutin • Ciprofloxacin • Amikacin c. Cytomegalovirus disease (CMU) • Ganciclovir (oral, IV, intraocular) • Foscarnet • Cidofovir • Fomivirsen d. Candidiasis (oral/pharyngeal, esophageal, vulvo/vaginal) • Clotrimazole (topical, oral) • Amphotericin B (oral suspension, IV)	3. Rest and a nutritious diet provide the person with energy to heal and to increase defense systems. Stress management techniques help to decrease anxiety, which is fatiguing.

(continues on page 527)

Interventions continued	**Rationales** continued
• Fluconazole • Itraconazole • Ketoconazole	
4. Explain the need to balance activity and rest, consume a nutritious diet, and practice stress management techniques.	4. The malignancies that affect AIDS clients are related to immunosuppression: a. Kaposi's sarcoma is cancer of the lymphatic vessel (endothelial wall). It is not skin cancer. b. Non-Hodgkin's lymphomas can progress into the bone marrow, liver, spleen, and gastrointestinal and nervous systems.
5. Monitor for malignancies: a. Kaposi's sarcoma: • Painless, palpable lesions (purplish, pinkish, or red) frequently on trunk, neck, arms, and head • Extracutaneous lesions in GI tract, lymph nodes, buccal mucosa, and lungs b. Lymphoma (non-Hodgkin's, Burkitt's): • Painless lymphadenopathy (early site neck, axilla, inguinal area) • Pruritus, weight loss	5. Gram-positive and gram-negative organisms can invade open wounds, causing septicemia. A debilitated client is at increased risk. Sepsis produces massive vasodilation, resulting in hypovolemia and subsequent tissue hypoxia. Hypoxia leads to decreased renal function and cardiac output, triggering a compensatory response of increased respirations and heart rate in an attempt to correct hypoxia and acidosis. Bacteria in urine or blood indicate infection.
6. Monitor for signs and symptoms of septicemia: a. Temperature >101°F or <98.6°F b. Decreased urine output c. Tachycardia and tachypnea d. Pale, cool skin e. White blood cells (WBCs) and bacteria in urine f. Positive blood culture	
7. Monitor and support use of prescribed prophylactic medication (Dolin, Masur, & Saag, 2003). a. If CD4 <200, Bactrim DS 3× week (Monday, Wednesday, Friday) prophylaxis for *P. carinii* pneumonia b. If CD4 <50 Zithromax 1200 mg every week, prophylaxis for cytomegalovirus (CMV).	

◥ Related Physician-Prescribed Interventions

Medications. Antibiotics, antiretrovirals, antiemetics, antifungals, chemotherapy, antipyretics, nucleoside reverse transcriptase inhibitors (NRTI), antiviral agents, protease inhibitors (PI), antidiarrheals, non-nucleoside reverse transcriptase inhibitors (NNRTI)

Intravenous Therapy. Creatinine, hyperalimentation, BUN

Laboratory Studies. Liver function tests viral load, enzyme-linked immunosorbent assay (ELISA), complete blood count, cultures, T-lymphocyte cells, hepatitis panel, CD4 count, Western blot test, CD8 count, serum protein, genotype, phenotype

Diagnostic Studies. Magnetic resonance imaging (MRI), endoscopy, biopsies, thallium scan, chest x-ray film

Therapies. Nasogastric feeding

 Documentation

Flow records
Lesions (number, size, locations)
Respiratory assessment
Neurologic assessment (mentation, orientation, affect)
Mouth assessment
Progress notes
Complaints

Risk for Infection Transmission Related to the Infectious Nature of the Client's Blood and Body Fluids (This diagnosis is not currently on the NANDA list but has been included for clarity and usefulness.)

Focus Assessment Criteria	Clinical Significance
1. Client/caregiver/partner knowledge of modes of HIV transmission 2. Client/caregiver/partner knowledge and use of universal precautions as indicated 3. Client/partner knowledge and use of safer sex precautions	1–3. Knowledge of modes of transmission and prevention strategies can reduce the risk of transmission and the fears associated with it.
4. Institutional/agency policies that direct the management of exposures to client blood or infectious body fluids	4. Policies guiding exposures should be comprehensive, current, and supportive of both the client and the involved employee.

Goal

The client will take necessary steps to prevent infection transmission.

Interventions	Rationales
	1–6. Universal precautions are to prevent the transmission of blood-borne pathogens from client to caregiver. They are utilized with all clients regardless of diagnosis, age, or sexual orientation of the client. The particular precautions taken with each individual client are dependent on the potential of transmission related to the care to be rendered and not to the client's diagnosis.

(continues on page 529)

Interventions continued	Rationales continued
1. Wash hands before and after contact with client in care situation.	1. Handwashing is one of the most important means of preventing the spread of infection.
2. Wear latex gloves when performing procedures involving the client's body fluids including: blood, semen, vaginal fluids, cerebrospinal fluids, peritoneal fluids, amniotic fluids, synovial fluids, pleural fluids, pericardial fluids, or other body fluids with visible blood (e.g., urine, menses, stool, saliva, etc.). Do not reuse gloves (CDC, 2000).	2. Gloves provide a barrier from contact with infectious secretions and excretions.
3. Wear mask, goggles, or eye shield and gown when there is the potential for splash of body fluids during care of the client (e.g., suctioning, a tracheotomy, or caregiving for a client with explosive vomiting or diarrhea) (CDC, 2000).	3. Masks prevent transmission by air isolation of infectious agents if oral mucosal lesions are present. Gowns prevent soiling of clothes if contact with secretions/excretions is likely.
4. Handle needles, scalpels, and other sharp objects carefully to prevent injury to self or others after use with client. Never recap a needle, make sure to bend or break it, and carefully dispose of used needles and other sharps into a puncture-proof sharps container immediately after use (CDC, 2000).	4. Needle sticks and sharp injuries carry by far the highest risk of transmission of blood-borne pathogens to health care personnel.
5. Immediately and thoroughly wash hands or other skin surfaces that may have been contaminated with blood or other potentially infectious body fluids.	
6. Ensure easy access to an adequate supply of gloves, masks, gowns, and eye shields in all patient care areas. Nonlatex gloves and disposable resuscitation equipment should also be available.	6. Allergy to latex among the general population is on the rise.
7. Ensure comprehensive and current institutional or agency policies that direct the management of employee exposure to client blood and infectious body fluids.	7–8. Policies guiding exposure should be comprehensive, current, and supportive of both the client and the involved employee.

(continues on page 530)

Interventions continued	**Rationales** continued
8. Be supportive of colleagues, nursing and otherwise, who have sustained exposure to a client's blood or infectious body fluids. Support includes emotional support and protecting the person's confidentiality as much as possible.	
9. Instruct and provide written material on safer sex guidelines that include: a. Correct and consistent use of a latex condom with every act of vaginal, anal, and/or oral intercourse b. Provision for adequate lubrication during intercourse by use of a water-based lubricant c. Maintenance of a faithful monogamous sexual relationship with partner d. No sex or use of sex toys involving any exchange of blood or body fluids e. Avoidance of high-risk behavior conducive to transmission of blood-borne or sexually transmitted diseases including: • Sex with multiple partners • Sex or behavior that involves the exchange of blood or body fluids • Needle sharing during drug use, tattooing, acupuncture, or other activities • Rough sexual practices that can lead to breaks in the mucosal lining of the rectum, mouth, or vagina	9. Correct and consistent use of a latex condom with every act of intercourse has been shown to significantly reduce the risk of transmission of sexually transmitted diseases including HIV. Oil-based lubricants (e.g., Vaseline) can degrade latex condoms.
10. Instruct and provide written material on transmission precautions for the home setting including: a. No sharing of toothbrushes, razors, enema or douche equipment or other sharp objects b. Prompt and adequate disposal of needles and other sharps into a puncture proof "locked" container c. Proper handwashing after any contact with clients' blood or infectious body fluids d. Use of gloves for provision of client care involving contact with his or her blood or body fluids e. Cleaning up blood and body fluid spills by using gloves and paper towel to get up the majority of the spill before	10. Fear of HIV transmission is a common concern of caregivers of persons with HIV. HIV is rapidly inactivated by exposure to disinfecting agents. Household bleach solution (dilute 1:10 with water) is an inexpensive choice.

(continues on page 531)

Interventions continued	Rationales continued
disinfecting area with a 1:10 solution of bleach	
11. Provide facts to dispel myths regarding transmission of HIV including: a. HIV is **not** transmitted by skin-to-skin contact, mosquito bites, swimming pools, clothes, eating utensils, telephones, or toilet seats. b. Closed mouth kissing, sweat, tears, urine, and feces do not transmit HIV. c. HIV cannot be contracted while giving blood.	11. Dispelling myths and correcting misinformation can reduce anxiety and allow others to interact more normally with the client.
12. Provide client and caregiver with the National CDC AIDS hotline number (1-800-342-AIDS).	12. The hotline provides rapid access to accurate information.

High Risk for Imbalanced Nutrition: Less Than Body Requirements Related to HIV Infection, Opportunistic Infections/Malignancies Associated with AIDS

Focus Assessment Criteria	Clinical Significance
1. Diet history past and present 2. Calculation of nutrient intake	1,2. Changes in eating patterns, measurement of sufficiency of nutrient intake, and so on assist the health professional in evaluating factors related to the client's nutritional status.
3. Anthropometric measurements such as weight, height, skinfold thickness, and midarm circumference 4. Laboratory tests for anemia (blood count) and long-term protein calorie malnutrition (serum albumin) 5. Functional measurements of muscle power (e.g., hand-grip strength) and short-term visceral protein deficits (serum retinol-binding protein and prealbumin) when protein calorie malnutrition is suspected	3–5. Protein-calorie malnutrition (PCM) is a potential condition with any chronic disease affecting oral intake and gastrointestinal absorption of nutrients. PCM should be assessed for regularly in HIV + clients. Nutritional plans should be constructed in consultation with a dietitian in the face of evidence supporting the presence of PCM.

Goal

The client will ingest daily nutritional requirements in accordance with activity level and metabolic needs.

Indicators
- Relate importance of good nutrition.
- Identify deficiencies in daily intake.
- Relate methods to increase appetite.

Interventions	**Rationales**
1. Assess client for weight loss/malnutrition at regular intervals. 2. Consult with dietitian for nutritional assessment, calorie count, meal planning, and nutritional instruction as indicated.	1,2. The Task Force on Nutritional Support in AIDS recommends that all clients, including HIV asymptomatic, have a complete nutritional assessment on initial contact and then regularly with a health professional. The three goals for good nutritional management are as follows: a. Preserve lean body mass. b. Provide adequate levels of all nutrients. c. Minimize symptoms of malabsorption (Task Force on Nutrition Support in AIDS, 1989).
3. Instruct client on importance of and methods to increase calorie/protein in diet: a. Eat cheese, nuts, peanut butter, milk shakes, and so on between meals and at bedtime. b. Enrich soups, vegetables, or starchy foods with milk or cheese. c. Sweeten toast, cereals, and fruits with sugar, jelly, or honey. d. Use sour cream and heavy cream when possible. e. Eat hard-boiled eggs for snack.	3. Significant weight loss is a common finding among clients with HIV. Early nutritional assessment and institution of corrective measures may slow weight loss and avoid the nutritional complications often seen in the later stage of HIV infection (Task Force on Nutrition Support in AIDS, 1989).
4. Assist client with referrals and necessary coordination to assure consistent supply of nutritional supplements as indicated.	4. Some states cover the cost of nutritional supplements when a dietitian documents the need. Nutritional supplements are drinks containing several micronutrients and macronutrients. They are usually recommended when the client is experiencing difficulty gaining or maintaining weight or when food intake declines for whatever reason. Instant breakfast mixed with whole milk is a reasonable cost-effective alternative to commercially made supplements in some instances (Physicians Association for AIDS Care [PAAC], 1993).
5. Regularly assess for client anorexia and institute measures to increase client appetite as appropriate: a. Rule out psychological etiology (e.g., depression, anxiety).	5. Anorexia is a loss or change in appetite with a relative decrease in food intake that, left untreated, will result in a loss of body weight and cell mass. Anorexia can be a direct result of advanced HIV infection,

(continues on page 533)

Interventions continued	**Rationales** continued
b. Suggest small, more frequent meals throughout the day.	AIDS-associated opportunistic infections or malignancies, or any number of medications used to treat them (Task Force on Nutrition Support in AIDS, 1989).
c. Drink liquids 30 minutes before rather than during meals.	
d. Offer foods in a pleasant atmosphere, and encourage the presence of family/friends during meals as possible.	
e. Consult physician regarding the use of appetite stimulants when indicated.	
f. Avoid serving large food quantity by providing nutritionally dense foods (e.g., nutritional supplements).	

6. Instruct client on interventions to manage any contributing factors to weight loss/wasting.
   Contributing factors:
   • Mouth soreness:
     A. Avoid hot and cold foods.
     B. Avoid acid-containing drinks and spicy foods.
   • Difficulty swallowing:
     A. Avoid hard-to-swallow, sticky foods (e.g., peanut butter).
     B. Choose soft, moist foods (e.g., oatmeal, pudding).
     C. Dunk toast, crackers, and so on in soup, milk, and so forth to moisten them.

   • Changes in taste:
     A. Add spices to food (e.g., lemon juice, garlic).

   • Nausea and vomiting:
     A. Eat smaller, more frequent meals.
     B. Eat foods low in fat and sugar.
     C. Consult with physician regarding antiemetic medication.

   • Diarrhea:
     A. Avoid caffeine and fatty foods.
     B. Drink fruit juices to replace fluid and minerals.
     C. Eat foods low in lactose.
     D. Consult with physician regarding antidiarrheal medication.

6.

   • Oral and esophageal candidiasis and pharyngeal and esophageal ulcers are relatively common among those with advanced HIV infection. Candidiasis especially is easily recognizable and treatable (Task Force on Nutrition Support in AIDS, 1989).

   • Changes in taste are not uncommon with medications used to treat HIV infection and opportunistic infections (e.g., AZT and Pentamidine)
   • Nausea and vomiting may be present secondary to medication or an organic cause requiring treatment. Persistent vomiting may lead to dehydration, fluid and electrolyte imbalance, and weight loss (Task Force on Nutrition Support in AIDS, 1989).
   • Diarrhea is seen frequently in HIV infection and the opportunistic infection within the AIDS spectrum (e.g., cryptosporidium, CMV). Depending on the etiology, malabsorption, fever, or anorexia may accompany the diarrhea, increasing the likelihood of nutritional deficit (Task Force on Nutrition Support in AIDS, 1989).

7. Teach client the potential gastrointestinal side effects of his or her medications.

7. Many medications used in treating HIV infection and the opportunistic infections seen in AIDS have possible gastrointestinal

(continues on page 534)

Interventions continued	Rationales continued
	side effects. These side effects can potentially limit the client's nutritional intake and nutrient absorption (e.g., *AZT:* nausea and vomiting, altered sense of taste; *DDI:* nausea and vomiting, diarrhea; *TMP-SMX:* anorexia, glucose intolerance, stomatitis)
8. Instruct client/caregiver on methods to avoid food-borne illness: a. Thoroughly cook meat, fish, and eggs. b. Wash hands before handling foods. c. Maintain foods at a safe temperature. d. Wash fruits and vegetables before consumption. e. Use separate cutting boards for raw and cooked foods. f. Monitor the proper serving of foods in summer (e.g. hot foods are hot, cold are cold).	8. Persons with HIV infection are thought to be especially at risk of food-borne disease because of immunosuppression (Campbell & Cope, 1990; Hoyt & Stacts, 1991; PAAC, 1993).
9. Consult social worker to evaluate client for referral to agencies supportive of the nutritional needs of the HIV infected.	9. Fatigue and weakness seen in advanced HIV disease can prohibit client from adequate meal preparation. Home-delivered meals and food basket delivery are examples of services for HIV + clients seen in some areas (Campbell & Cope, 1990).

Documentation

High Risk for Ineffective Coping Related to Situational Crisis (i.e., New HIV or AIDS Diagnosis, First Hospitalization)

Focus Assessment Criteria	Clinical Significance
1. Psychosocial history	1. History of interpersonal relationships/education, career, and so on provides insight into client's potential for various psychological dysfunction.
2. Current distress and crisis	2. Client's levels of anxiety and fear are often directly related to the extent of the crisis he or she is experiencing.
3. Social support	3. The amount and accessibility of social support must be known to adequately plan strategies to strengthen present supports and garner additional assistance as needed.

(continues on page 535)

Focus Assessment Criteria continued	Clinical Significance continued
4. Life-cycle phase	4. Age-related goals, values, and so on contribute to the client's ability to cope with crisis.
5. Illness phase	5. Where the clients are on the continuum of HIV infection will affect their perceptions and way of coping.
6. Individual identity	6. Who the client is and his or her values, goals, and so on will greatly affect how he or she perceives and copes with the crisis associated with HIV infection.
7. Loss and grief	7. Besides personal loss of function, goals, and so on, HIV-infected clients often experience the death of friends and loved ones to AIDS. The degree of loss will affect their coping ability.

Goal

The client will make decisions and follow through with appropriate actions to change provocative situations in personal environment.

Indicators

- Verbalize feelings related to emotional state.
- Focus on the present.
- Identify response patterns and the consequences of resulting behavior.
- Identify personal strengths and accept support through the nursing relationship.

Interventions	Rationales
1. Encourage client's expression of anxiety, anger, and fear. Listen attentively and nonjudgmentally.	1. Listening is credited as a helpful strategy to assist clients coping with AIDS. Anger at AIDS-associated prejudice or lack of understanding of others occurs commonly among the HIV infected.
2. Determine client's past coping strategies, and assist them to develop coping strategies based on their previous successful outcomes and personal strengths.	2. Interventions constructed using the client's personal style and character are likely to be of lasting use to client. Previous successes should be built on when possible.
3. Discourage coping mechanisms that are maladaptive or self-defeating (i.e., alcohol, drugs, denial, compulsive behavior).	3. Substance abuse and "destructive" denial are behaviors often perceived to provide subjective relief. This relief, however, is usually temporary and ultimately self-defeating.

(continues on page 536)

Interventions continued	Rationales continued
4. Assist client with finding meaning in illness and not assuming the victim role.	4. "Focus should be on living with AIDS, not dying of it. Nurses can rekindle the spark that is needed to discover the meaning and purpose in suffering and even death" (Carson & Green, 1992, p. 217).
5. Encourage and reinforce client's hopes as appropriate.	5. "All life is based on hope and when hope is low or absent, people see their lives as finished . . . when professional caretakers see hope in the terminally ill as unrealistic and label it as denial, they lower the quality of the years remaining to the person, or force him or her to turn elsewhere for help" (Hall, 1990, p. 183).
6. Assist client to identify appropriate support systems (i.e., support group, community resources) and encourage their use.	6. Feelings of alienation and social isolation are common among the HIV infected. Support groups potentially are able to educate, support, and assist the client to anticipate and deal with the crises inevitable to the client's illness (Mallinson, 1999).
7. Encourage/provide exercise, recreation, diversional activities, and independent activities-of-daily-living performance.	7. Diversional activities can provide opportunities of rest from mental and emotional distress. Maximal independence and participation in activities can increase self-confidence and self-esteem.
8. Instruct client on stress-management techniques (i.e., distraction, relaxation imagery) as appropriate.	8. Stress reduction techniques can assist the client in dealing with personal fears and anxieties.
9. Assist client with coordination of care using advocacy as necessary.	9. The physical demands of chronic infection and the frequent complexity of care arrangements can prohibit consistent compliance and follow-up with medical care and counseling. Nurses, by making appropriate referrals for the client, decrease demands on the client and are able to advocate for the client as indicated.

High Risk for Caregiver Role Strain Related to AIDS-associated Shame/Stigma, and Uncertainty About Course of Illness and Demands on Caregiver

Focus Assessment Criteria	Clinical Significance
1. Who have clients shared their HIV status with? Is there any conflict between clients and caregivers concerning who knows or who "should" know?	1. To maintain client confidentiality, it must be ascertained who knows and who does not know client's HIV status. No one should be told client's HIV status without the client's approval.

(continues on page 537)

Focus Assessment Criteria *continued*	Clinical Significance *continued*
2. Who else is HIV + (e.g., partner, caregiver, child, spouse, etc.)?	2. Caregivers themselves may be HIV +, which could impact on caregiving ability, or caregivers might be caring for or have cared for others who are HIV +.
3. Health and functional level of caregivers (i.e., infected partners, elderly parent).	3. If caregivers are HIV + or elderly, will they be able to tolerate the demands their caregiving places on them?
4. Level of support for AIDS caregiving by others (i.e., emotional and practical support).	4. Are caregivers getting any support for their caregiving role? If so, is it adequate to assist them with the caregiving demands?
5. Status of durable power of attorney (DPOA) and Living Will.	5. Who has the legal ability or who do clients wish to handle their affairs and oversee their health care decisions, should they be unable to do so? Having persons of clients' choice having their DPOA is especially important when there is lack of communication or conflict between patient's biologic family and caregiver.

Goals

The person will relate a plan on how to continue social activities despite caregiving responsibilities.

Indicators
- Identify activities that are important for self.
- Relate intent to enlist the help of at least two people.

Interventions	Rationales
1. Explore the meanings and beliefs that caregivers hold regarding the client's HIV infection. 2. Explore the caregivers' prior knowledge of and current feelings about the client's sexual behavior or drug use.	1,2. Caregivers' feelings of shame or guilt regarding client's HIV infection or life style may prohibit optimal caregiving. They may need help expressing their feelings regarding these traditionally taboo topics (Brown & Powell-Cope, 1991; Flaskerud & Ungrarski, 1999; Powell-Cope & Brown, 1992).
3. Consistent acknowledgment and support of caregiving role.	3. AIDS caregivers often receive little to no support for their caregiving role. Their fear of discrimination and hatred toward themselves or the client stops them from disclosing their situation. This leads to feelings of isolation (Brown & Powell-Cope, 1991; Flaskerud & Ungrarski, 1999; Powell-Cope & Brown, 1992).

(continues on page 538)

Interventions continued	Rationales continued
4. Assist caregivers with anticipating the uncertainty, role changes and unpredictability of their caregiving role, and course of the HIV infection itself.	4. Uncertainty is a common concern of caregivers of persons with life-threatening illnesses. The ability to anticipate certain events or changes can allay some anxiety for caregivers (Brown & Powell-Cope, 1991).
5. Assist caregivers with their decision making regarding whom to tell about their AIDS caregiving role.	5. Fear of rejection and isolation can make the decision of who to tell anxiety provoking and overpowering to AIDS caregivers (Powell-Cope & Brown, 1992).
6. Assist caregivers with the "staging" method of disclosure of the AIDS caregiving role as appropriate.	6. Disclosure by "staging" of the information is less anxiety provoking than full disclosure (e.g., *Stage I* = "My son is sick." *Stage II* = "My son is under a doctor's care and needs to stay with me until he is back on his feet." *Stage III* = "My son has AIDS and needs my help.") (Powell-Cope & Brown, 1992).
7. Provide anticipatory guidance and counseling to AIDS caregivers as they prepare to go public with their caregiving role.	7. The process of "going public" with their AIDS caregiving role is complex and stressful for caregivers planning to do so. Rehearsal of how and when to disclose and how to handle potential responses can minimize the stress on the caregiver (Powell-Cope & Brown, 1992).
8. Reinforce caregivers' knowledge of HIV transmission, infection control precautions for the home, and so on. Provide written information on same and remain available for questions.	8. Fear of HIV transmission to self and other members of household is a major concern of AIDS caregivers (Brown & Powell-Cope, 1991).
9. Teach signs and symptoms of burnout and stress-reduction techniques.	9. AIDS caregivers are subject to burnout and need help to avoid it if possible. If burnout is inevitable, caregivers need to be able to identify it early in its onset so as to be able to plan for respite care.
10. Identify and assist with use of community resources supportive of AIDS caregiver such as community case management services, AIDS caregivers' support groups, day care, respite care, and so on.	10. AIDS caregivers need support that recognizes their unique needs and support should be used to reinforce their caregiving.

(continues on page 539)

Interventions continued	Rationales continued
11. Encourage caregivers to pursue personal goals during their AIDS caregiving.	11. Pursuing personal goals during their caregiving assists caregivers to be able to focus on their own interests and lives. These goals carry on and provide their lives with meaning after the death of the client (Ferrell & Boyle, 1992).
12. Allow caregivers to express frustration/anger at health care system and health care professionals as appropriate.	12. Expressing anger and frustration at health professionals or the health care systems after perceived situations involving insensitivity or a lack of understanding is a way for caregivers to express their feelings (Ferrell & Boyle, 1992).

High Risk for Ineffective Therapeutic Regimen Management Related to Functional and/or Cognitive Deficits Associated with Advanced HIV Infection and/or Opportunistic Events

Focus Assessment Criteria	Clinical Significance
1. *Bio/psycho/social/spiritual status* of the client with emphasis on care, treatment, functional needs, quality of life definition, and short- and long-term goals	1. A holistic client assessment including his or her health-related goals and quality of life definition is the foundation of any plan to attain these goals.
2. *Family/caregiver support ability* (family as defined by the client)	2. Adequate caregiver support, emotionally and practically, is crucial in an optimal care situation for a client with deficits associated with HIV infection.
3. *Care environment adequacy* with emphasis on safety, accessibility, and basic need provision.	3. The setting in which the client lives must contain the resources to safely and adequately meet care needs over time.
4. *Community resources:* HIV-specific and service-specific agencies and programs. The question that needs to be considered in relation to these four assessment areas is: Can the client's care, safety, and treatment needs be met by the client and their family/caregivers with the resources available in the care environment and community?	4. What are the services and programs accessible to the client to assist in optimally maintaining their therapeutic regimen?

Goals

The goals for this diagnosis represent those associated with discharge planning. Refer to the discharge criteria.

Interventions	Rationales
I. *Client-Specific Interventions* 1. Assist the client in clarifying his or her wishes regarding medical treatment issues and short- and long-term goals in relation to his or her quality of life definition.	1. Effective interventions can be planned and implemented only with the client's full understanding and agreement.
2. Collaborate with client's primary care provider to simplify the medical regimen as possible and to maximize the client's comfort and symptom management.	2. Medications with limited or questionable efficacy can sometimes be discontinued without loss of clinical benefit to the client. Other medications are able to be taken less often in certain circumstances, thus simplifying the overall regimen.
3. Assist client to find health care providers who are accessible, experienced at HIV management, and sensitive to the client's gender, cultural, and life style issues.	3. Clients with HIV-experienced providers live longer and suffer less morbidity overall than do those HIV-infected individuals who receive their care from HIV-inexperienced providers.
4. Educate the client about HIV and opportunistic illness management and the importance of adherence for maximum clinical benefit.	4. Ongoing client-specific education related to the expected benefits of therapy is basic to any effort to assist their long-term adherence.
5. Arrange for a comprehensive system of ongoing client assessment of the ability to manage the therapeutic regimen by utilizing an HIV-specific or health care system case management program.	5. A plan for formal ongoing assessment of the client's ability to manage his or her regimen and evaluation of the adequacy to the interventions to support their management is crucial to the regimen's success in the long term.
6. Assist client's understanding of the actual or potential effects of the use of denial or substance abuse on his or her ability to maintain therapeutic regimen. Refer motivated clients for mental health or substance abuse assistance as indicated.	6. Depression, anxiety, and substance abuse can all interfere with the client's ability to attain his or her health-related goals.
7. Advocate for the client to the insurance carrier for uncovered benefits, using cost-effective rationale as indicated.	7. A well-reasoned argument using clinical benefit and cost-effectiveness can sometimes convince an insurance carrier to reimburse for a normally uncovered benefit.
8. Consult with the dietitian, social worker, or case manager to evaluate client eligibility for special programs or service according to need (e.g., pharmacy providing overnight drug delivery or state Medicaid program coverage of nutritional supplements).	8. HIV-specific programs and services vary from state to state. A variety of health care professionals may be needed to arrange for a specific service.

(continues on page 541)

Interventions continued	**Rationales** continued
9. Refer the client to a social worker or attorney for assistance with power of attorney, living will or last will, and testament arrangements as indicated.	9. Creating a living will or giving a trusted friend, partner, or family member power of attorney for health care allows the client some confidence that his or her wishes and quality of life definition will be respected in the event that he or she is unable to make decisions related to care.
10. Consult physical therapy, occupational therapy, or a rehabilitation specialist for client functional determination as indicated.	10. Physical medicine and rehabilitation physicians specialize in determining the functional potential of clients. With the input of physical and occupational therapists, they develop plans to maximize that potential.
II. *Family/caregiver specific* (with the consent of the client) 11. Facilitate family or caregivers' meeting to communicate the client's wishes, evaluate the adequacy of client supports, and delegate care tasks.	11. Clear communication of the client's needs and wishes related to their care to those persons directly involved in their care is of the utmost importance.
12. Educate family/caregivers on HIV transmission precautions in the home setting and specific care tasks required (e.g., medication administration, proper body mechanics for client transfer assistance).	12. Fear of HIV transmission is common among caregivers of clients with HIV infection.
13. Counsel caregiver on anticipating the client's care requirements and integrating these activities into his or her life.	13. Uncertainty is a common concern of caregivers of persons with life-threatening illnesses. The ability to anticipate certain events or changes can allay some anxiety for caregivers
14. Refer for personal care services, chore provision grant, or "buddy" services when indicated and available.	14. A variety of caregiving support services is available depending on locale and client eligibility.
15. Arrange for client "day care" services when the primary caregiver is employed and other supports are lacking.	15. Balancing caregiving responsibilities with employment can be difficult to impossible for persons caring for someone with cognitive and/or functional deficits. Day care arrangements for the client, if eligible, are available in some areas.
16. Refer caregivers to a respite program when indicated and available.	16. AIDS caregivers need support that recognizes their unique needs and support should be used to reinforce their caregiving.

(continues on page 542)

Interventions continued	Rationales continued
III. *Care environment specific* 17. Arrange for home nursing services for client.	17. Most insurance carrier policies cover home nursing services when the client is home bound and requires skilled care.
18. Consult with social worker or care manager to arrange for client placement at a skilled nursing facility, hospice facility, residential living program, or other program or facility commensurate with client's wishes or short- and long-term goals.	18. The client's care needs and wishes regarding living situation adequacy in relation to those needs are two essential factors affecting the decision for or against an alternative care setting.

Documentation

Discharge summary record
   Client teaching
   Outcome achievement or status
   Referrals if indicated

High Risk for Ineffective Therapeutic Regimen Management Related to Insufficient Knowledge of HIV, Its Transmission, Prevention, Treatment, and Community Resources

Focus Assessment Criteria	Clinical Significance
1. Client's current knowledge of HIV, HIV transmission, prevention, treatment, and community resources	1. Assessing client's understanding of HIV disease and its treatment allows the nurse to plan constant and optimal teaching strategies. Accurate knowledge is built on and reinforced, and misconceptions are clarified.
2. Client's readiness to learn	2. The strategies and time committed necessary to teach someone motivated to learn are very different from those for the person not accepting of the need to learn about the condition and its treatment.
3. Client's ability to learn and return information	3. If client is unable to learn or remember information presented, alternative or additional interventions must be considered (e.g., incorporation of family/caregivers into teaching).
4. Client's cultural beliefs about HIV disease	4. The client's cultural beliefs regarding HIV and its treatment will affect every aspect of his or her learning. The nurse should be able to anticipate these beliefs and incorporate them into teaching strategies as necessary.

(continues on page 543)

Focus Assessment Criteria continued	Clinical Significance continued
5. Client's educational level attained	5. Years of formal education completed by the client will help in the planning of optimal teaching strategies and educational aids to enhance client learning.
6. Client's primary language	6. Will the client learn better in English or another language? Should the use of an interpreter be considered (with client consent only)?
7. Client's visual and hearing acuity	7. The client's visual and hearing acuities obviously will affect the teaching strategies and aides chosen to enhance client learning.

Goals

The goals for this diagnosis represent those associated with discharge planning. Refer to the discharge criteria.

Interventions	Rationales
1. Teach the basic pathophysiology of HIV infection and concepts of the immune system.	1. The client's understanding of HIV and its effect on the body is the basis of all further learning.
2. Explain HIV infection treatment including those decisions related to the CD4 level and viral load. These include the initiation of antiretroviral therapy and prophylaxis against certain opportunistic infections (e.g., PCP, MAC).	2. Besides symptoms the client may experience as a result of their HIV infection progression, their CD4 and viral load levels are essential to the initiation of antiretroviral therapy and prophylaxis against such opportunistic infections as *Pneumocystis carinii* pneumonia (Agency for Health Care Policy and Research, 1994; Melroe, Stawarz, Simpsons, & Henry, 1997).
3. Teach HIV routes of transmission and preventive measures/risk reduction activities.	3. The importance of efforts to prevent HIV transmission to infected persons as well as prevention of reinfection by a resistant strain of HIV or with other STDs if person is already infected cannot be overstated!
4. Explain the rationale and intended effects of the treatment program: a. Enhanced immune function b. Limitation of HIV infection c. Prevention of opportunistic events	4. Client agreement with commitment to treatment is tied to his or her understanding of treatment goals.

(continues on page 544)

Interventions continued	Rationales continued
5. Teach name, action, dose, safe use, and potential side effects and interactions of medications.	5. Many individuals will better adhere to therapy if they understand the intended effect of the individual medications on their bodies.
6. Stress the importance of close adherence to combination antiretroviral therapy to prevent viral resistance to therapy.	6. Combination antiretroviral therapy, taken as directed, offers more effective long-term suppression of HIV infection and prevents the emergence of resistant HIV strains by maintenance of a constant effective level in the bloodstream (Sanford, Sonde, & Gilbert, 1996).
7. Explain the risks of missing doses of antiretroviral medications.	7. Poor adherence to antiretroviral drugs can result in development of resistant virus to multiple medications—even entire classes, such as protease inhibitors (Murphy, Lu, Martin, Hoffman & Marelich, 2002).
8. Assist client to identify techniques to take pills on schedule (Bartlett & Finkbeiner, 2000). a. When brushing teeth (twice a day) b. Alarm watch c. Sectioned pill containers d. When watching favorite television shows e. If you miss a dose, take it when you remember; do not "double up."	8. A decrease of 10% of the total pills taken weekly caused a doubling of HIV (Bangsberg et al., 2000).
9. Encourage person to share condition with persons in same household.	9. Keeping a secret and hiding pills increase the risk of missing doses.
10. Teach health promotion/illness prevention practices: a. Safer sex b. Nutrition c. Avoidance of food-/water-borne illnesses	10. a. Safer sex reduces the risk of HIV transmission to uninfected persons and reduces the risk of the client's reinfection by HIV or other STDs. b. The link between nutrition and immunologic function is well established (Casey, 1997). c. Persons with HIV infection are thought to be especially at risk of water- and food-borne illnesses because of immunosuppression (Campbell & Cope, 1990; Hoyt & Stacts, 1991; PAAC, 1993).

(continues on page 545)

Interventions continued	**Rationales** continued
d. Effective coping	d,e. Stress has been associated with reactivation of herpes simplex infection and malignancy because of its negative effect on the immune system (Flaskerud & Ungrarski, 1999).
e. Stress reduction	
f. Immunizations	f. Those immunizations that prevent disease and are safe for use with the HIV-infected individual include pneumococcal, influenza, and HBV. Live attenuated vaccines are contraindicated in persons with advanced HIV infection (Dolin et al., 2003).
g. Adequate rest	g. Adequate and consistent periods of rest and sleep can lessen the effects of stress on the body (Flaskerud & Ungrarski , 1999).
11. Explain factors impinging on the attainment of the client's health-related goals: a. Unsafe sexual practices b. Poor nutrition c. Substance abuse	11. c. Heroin, cocaine, ETOH, marijuana, and amphetamines are all possible factors in immune suppression. Substance abuse also interferes with adherence to medication regimen (Dolin et al., 2003).
d. Tobacco use	d. The detrimental effects of nicotine addiction are well known.
e. Depression/stress f. Lack of adherence to therapy	f. Strict adherence to combination antiretroviral therapy is necessary to prevent subtherapeutic levels of medication conducive to the emergence of viral resistance and consequent disease progression.
12. Provide information and encourage appropriate utilization of community resources supportive of persons living with HIV.	12. There are numerous organizations available locally and nationally for a variety of services and support to persons living with HIV and their caregivers.
13. Include significant other/family participation in all phases of client education (only with client's consent).	13. Ideally, the involvement of supportive others in the client's education regarding HIV and its treatment reinforces the client's learning and supports the caregiver and caregiver's commitment to the client.
14. Instruct client on signs and symptoms to report to health care provider: a. Visual changes	14. a. Blurred vision, "floaters," and other visual complaints can signify CMV retinitis of HIV retinopathy. CMV retinitis causes blindness if not treated.

(continues on page 546)

Interventions continued	**Rationales** continued
b. Anorexia / weight loss	b. Anorexia or weight loss can be a sign of disease progression, opportunistic disease, or HIV wasting syndrome.
c. Difficult or painful swallowing	c. Dysphagia or odynophagia are symptomatic of esophageal candidiasis or other GI tract infection or ulceration requiring treatment.
d. Persistent or severe diarrhea	d. Besides causing dehydration and electrolyte imbalances, diarrhea in the HIV-infected individual can be symptomatic of anything from a food intolerance or medication side effect to an opportunistic pathogen.
e. Dyspnea or resistant cough	e. Cough or dyspnea in the HIV-infected person can be a sign of TB, PCP, or other bacterial or opportunistic infection.
f. Headache / stiff neck	f. A headache with a stiff neck can be a sign of meningitis, bacterial or otherwise. Persistent headache can indicate a central nervous system malignancy or infection or sinusitis.
g. Fever / chills / night sweats	g. This combination of signs and symptoms can signify HIV progression or a local systemic infection.
h. Fatigue	h. Fatigue can be the first sign of infection or generalized sepsis even in the absence of other signs and symptoms.

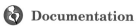 **Documentation**

Discharge summary record
   Client teaching
   Outcome achievement or status
   Referrals if indicated

SYSTEMIC LUPUS ERYTHEMATOSUS

Systemic lupus erythematosus (SLE) is a chronic, inflammatory, autoimmune disease of connective tissues. SLE can involve every organ system and can range in severity from very mild to severe. It can affect pleural and pericardial membranes, joints, skin, blood cells, and nervous and glomerular tissue. The etiology has not been confirmed, but latent viruses, genetic factors, hormones, and medications have been linked to onset. The female preponderance of lupus clients is 10 to 1 with more occurrences in blacks and Hispanics. The triggering of abnormal immune function results in the formation of antibodies directed against various components of the body (autoantibodies) (Holmes, 1998; Ruiz-Irastorza et al., 2001).

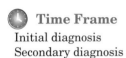 **Time Frame**

Initial diagnosis
Secondary diagnosis

⊙⊙ DIAGNOSTIC CLUSTER*

Collaborative Problems	Refer to
PC: Polymyositis, Serositis, Pericarditis	
PC: Vasculitis	
PC: Hematologic Abnormalities	
PC: Raynaud's Disease	
PC: Neuropsychiatric Disorders	

Nursing Diagnoses	Refer to
High Risk for Injury related to increased dermal vulnerability secondary to disease process	
High Risk for Ineffective Therapeutic Regimen Management related to insufficient knowledge of condition, rest versus activity requirements, pharmacologic therapy, signs and symptoms of complications, risk factors, and community resources	
Powerlessness related to unpredictable course of disease	Diabetes Mellitus
Fatigue related to decreased mobility joint pain and effects of chronic inflammation	Inflammatory Joint Disease

(continues on page 548)

Nursing Diagnoses continued	**Refer to** continued
High Risk for Disturbed Self-Concept related to inability to achieve developmental tasks secondary to disabling condition and changes in appearance	Multiple Sclerosis
Related Care Plan Corticosteroid Therapy	

* This medical condition was not included in the validation study.

Discharge Criteria

Before discharge, the client or family will

1. State the intent to share concerns with a trusted friend.
2. Identify components of a standard treatment program.
3. Relate proper use of medications.
4. Describe actions to reduce the risk of exacerbation.
5. Identify signs and symptoms that must be reported to a health care professional.

Collaborative Problems

Potential Complication: Polymyositis, Serositis, Pericarditis

Potential Complication: Vasculitis

Potential Complication: Hematologic Abnormalities

Potential Complication: Raynaud's Syndrome

Potential Complication: Neuropsychiatric Disorders

Nursing Goal

The nurse will detect early signs and symptoms of: (a) polymyositis, serositis; (b) pericarditis; (c) vasculitis; (d) hematologic abnormalities; (e) Raynaud's disease; and (f) neurologic disorders, and collaboratively intervene to stabilize client.

Indicators
- No new complaints of pain (a, b, c, f)
- Blood pressure >90/60 HH mg (c)
- Pulse 60–100 beats/min (c)
- Respirations 16–20 breaths/min (c)
- Temperature 98–99.5°F (c)
- Capillary refill <3 seconds (e)
- Liver function tests
  ○ Alanine aminotransferase (ALT) (c)
  ○ Aspartate aminotransferase (AST) (c)
  ○ Bilirubin total D.1–1.2mg/dL (c)
  ○ Prothrombin time 9.5–12 seconds (c, d)
  ○ Partial prothrombin time 20–45 seconds (c, d)
  ○ Bleeding time 1–9 minutes (c, d)
- Stool for occult blood: negative (c)
- Arterial blood gases
  ○ Oxygen saturation (SaO_2) 94–100% (c)
  ○ Carbon dioxide ($PaCO_2$) 35–45 mm Hg (c)
  ○ Serum pH 7.35–7.45 (c)

- Renal function
  - Creatinine 0.7–1.4 mg/dL (c)
  - Blood urea nitrogen 10–20 mg/dL (c)
  - Prealbumin (c)
  - Urine creatinine clearance (c)
  - Complement C4 70–150 mg/dL (c)
  - Complement C3 16–45 mg/dL (c)
- Complete blood count
  - Hemoglobin (d)
    - Male 13–18 gm/dL
    - Female 12–16 gm/dL
  - Hematocrit (d)
    - Male 42–50%
    - Female 40–48%
  - Red blood cells (d)
    - Male 4.6–5.9 million/mm^2
    - Female 4.2–5.4 million/mm^2
  - White blood cells 5,000–10,800/cu mm (d)
  - Platelets 100,000–400,000/cu mm (d)
- No c/o cyanosis, membranes tingling, or pain in fingers/hands (c, e)
- No seizures (c, f)
- Intact sensation and motor function (c, f)
- Clear, oriented (c, f)

Interventions	Rationales

1. Monitor for polymyositis, serositis, and pericarditis:
  a. Tendinitis (pain radiating down an extremity)
  b. Bursitis (pain in shoulder, knee, elbow, or hip)
  c. Pericarditis (pain beneath left clavicle and in the neck and left scapular region; aggravated by movement)
	1. Antibodies are produced that damage the cell membrane constituents, DNA, nucleoprotein, and histones. The resulting inflammation stimulates antigens that in turn stimulate autoantibodies, and the cycle begins anew (Holmes, 1998).

2. Monitor for the effects of vasculitis:
  a. Hypertension
  b. Peripheral vascular disease
  c. Pericarditis
  d. Hepatomegaly
  e. Splenomegaly
  f. Gastritis
  g. Pneumonitis
  h. Seizures
  i. Renal disease
	2. Excessive autoantibodies combine with antigens to form immune complexes. These complexes are deposited in vascular and tissue surfaces, triggering an inflammatory response and eventually local tissue injury. Thus SLE can affect any organ system (Porth, 2002).

3. Monitor for hematologic disorders:
  a. Hemolytic anemia
  b. Leukopenia
  c. Lymphopenia
  d. Thrombocytopenia
	3. Antibodies against red blood cells result in hemolytic anemia. Antibodies against platelets result in thrombocytopenia. B-lymphocyte production is regulated by a balance of CD4 + and CD8 + lymphocytes. (T cells). This balance is disrupted by SLE (Porth, 2002).

(continues on page 550)

Interventions continued	**Rationales** continued

4. Monitor laboratory findings for early signs of vasculitis and hematological disorders:
  a. Liver function tests
  b. PT, PPT
  c. Bleeding time
  d. Stool for occult blood
  e. Arterial blood gases
  f. BUN, creatinine, prealbumin
  g. Serum pH
  h. Urine creatinine clearance
  i. Complement C3, complement C4
	4. Inflammation of vessel walls decreases blood supply to major organs, causing necrosis, sclerosis, and dysfunction.

5. Teach client to report purpura and ecchymosis.	5. They are manifestations of platelet deficiencies.

6. Monitor for Raynaud's syndrome:
  a. Vasospasm of arteries in fingers resulting in pallor changing to cyanosis and ending in rubor
  b. Numbness, tingling, and pain in affected digits
	6. In Raynaud's syndrome, inflammation and subsequent damage to connective tissue produces vasospasm of arteries and arterioles of the fingers and hands (Porth, 2002).

7. Monitor for neurological disorders:
  a. Seizures
  b. Headaches
  c. Myasthenia gravis
  d. Guillain-Barré syndrome
  e. Polyneuropathy
  f. Cranial neuropathy
  g. Acute confusion
	7. The pathological cause of CNS symptoms is unclear. They are thought to result from acute vasculitis that impedes blood flow causing clots, hemorrhage, or both. Seizures are usually related to renal failure (McCowan, 1998).

8. Monitor for psychiatric disorders:
  a. Anxiety disorder
  b. Cognitive dysfunction
  c. Mood disorder
  d. Psychosis
	8. The cause of psychiatric disorders in clients with SLE is unknown. They have been associated with triggering the onset of SLE (McCowan, 1998).

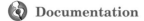 ### Related Physician-Prescribed Interventions

Medications. Cyclophosphamide, cyclosporine, thalidomide, mycophenolate mofetil methotrexate, nonsteroidal anti-inflammatory agents, antimalarials, cytotoxic agents, corticosteroids

Laboratory Studies. Complete blood count with differential, complement human C4, antiphospholipid antibodies, complement human C3, anticardiolipin (IgM, IgG), BUN, lupus anticoagulant, serum creatinine, urinalysis, 24-hour urine, creatinine clearance, ANA, anti-DNA

Therapies. Plasmapheresis, stem-cell transplantation, immunoablative therapy, joint replacement

Diagnostic Studies. EEG, chest x-ray, EKG, renal biopsy

Documentation
Flow records
  Vital signs
  Peripheral pulses
Progress notes
  Complaints

Nursing Diagnoses

High Risk for Injury Related to Increased Dermal Vulnerability Secondary to Disease Process

Focus Assessment Criteria	Clinical Significance
1. Knowledge of need to avoid sun exposure	1. In SLE, the skin is extremely sensitive to sun exposure.
2. Presence of skin manifestations of SLE	2. Common skin manifestations of SLE include the characteristic "butterfly" facial rash, discoid skin lesions, and patchy alopecia. Other SLE skin manifestations, such as digital or leg ulcers, result from immune complex deposition vasculitis and generally signal active systemic disease.

Goal

The client will identify causative factors that may increase disease activity (e.g., sun exposure).

Indicators

- Identify measures to reduce damage to skin by the sun.
- Identify strategies to manage skin damage should it occur.
- Identify signs and symptoms of cellulitis.

Interventions	Rationales
1. Explain the relationship between sun exposure and disease activity.	1. Through an unknown mechanism, exposure to ultraviolet light can precipitate an exacerbation of both skin and systemic diseases. The client's understanding of this relationship should encourage him or her to limit sun exposure.
2. Identify strategies to limit sun exposure: a. Avoid sun exposure between 10 am and 2 pm. b. Use sunscreen (15 SPF); reapply after swimming or exercise. c. Select lightweight long-sleeved clothing and wide-brimmed hats.	2. A client with SLE should make every attempt to minimize sun exposure.
3. Explain the need to avoid fluorescent lighting or a too-hot stove.	3. Like sunlight, fluorescent lighting produces ultraviolet rays.
4. Teach the client to keep skin ulcers clean and the skin moist.	4. Skin changes associated with SLE increase the vulnerability to injury. Reducing

(continues on page ◦ 552)

Interventions continued	Rationales continued
	bacteria on the skin reduces risk of infection. Dry skin is more susceptible to breakdown.
5. Teach to recognize signs and symptoms of vasculitis and to report them promptly to a health care professional: a. Tenderness b. Swelling c. Warmth d. Redness	5. Vascular inflammation of the smallest blood vessels, capillaries, and venules can cause occlusion.

 Documentation

Flow record
　Skin assessment
Discharge summary record
　Client teaching
　Response to teaching

High Risk for Ineffective Therapeutic Regimen Management Related to Insufficient Knowledge of Condition, Rest Versus Activity Requirements, Pharmacologic Therapy, Signs and Symptoms of Complications, Risk Factors, and Community Resources

Focus Assessment Criteria	Clinical Significance
1. Readiness and ability to learn and retain information	1. A client or family failing to achieve learning goals requires a referral for assistance postdischarge.
2. Knowledge of or experience with SLE	2. This assessment helps the nurse to plan effective teaching strategies.

Goals

The goals for this diagnosis represent those associated with discharge planning. See the discharge criteria.

Interventions	Rationales
1. Explain SLE using teaching aids appropriate to client's and family's levels of understanding. Discuss the following:	1. Understanding may help to improve compliance and reduce exacerbations.

(continues on page 553)

Interventions continued	**Rationales** continued

a. The inflammatory process
   b. Organ systems at risk of involvement
      (see Potential Complications in this care
      plan for more information)
   c. Chronic nature of disease (remission/
      exacerbation)
   d. Components of standard treatment
      program
   e. Medications
   f. Exercise and rest
   g. Regular follow-up care	

2. Teach client to take medications properly and to report symptoms of side effects. Drugs prescribed for SLE may include the following:
   a. Nonsteroidal anti-inflammatory drugs
   b. Corticosteroids (refer to the Cortico-steroid care plan for more information)
   c. Immunosuppressive agents such as azathioprine (Imuran) and cyclophos-phamide (Cytoxan)
   d. Antimalarial agents such as hydroxy-chloroquine (Plaquenil)
	2. Knowledge of and proper adherence to the medication regimen can help to reduce complications and detect side effects early.

3. Teach the need to balance activity and rest. (Refer to the Inflammatory Joint Dis-ease care plan for specific strategies.)	3. The chronic fatigue associated with SLE necessitates strategies to prevent exhaus-tion and maintain the highest level of independent functioning (Albano & Wallace, 2001).
4. Teach the need for meticulous, gentle mouth care.	4. Vasculitis can increase the risk of mouth lesions and injury.

5. Teach client to report signs and symptoms of complications:
 	
   a. Chest pain and dyspnea
 	
   b. Fever
   c. Ecchymoses
 	
   d. Edema
 	
   e. Decreased urine output, concentrated urine
   f. Nausea and vomiting
 	
   g. Leg cramps
	5. Early detection of complications enables prompt interventions to prevent serious tis-sue damage or dysfunction (Holmes, 1998).
	   a. Chest pain and dyspnea may indicate pericarditis or pleural effusion.
	   b. Fever may point to infection.
	   c. Ecchymoses may indicate a clotting disorder.
	   d. Edema may signal renal or hepatic insufficiency.
	   e. These urine changes may indicate renal insufficiency.
	   f. Nausea and vomiting can indicate GI dysfunction.
	   g. Leg cramps may result from peripheral vascular insufficiency.

(continues on page 554)

Interventions continued	Rationales continued
6. Explain the relationship of stress and autoimmune disorders. Discuss stress management techniques: a. Progressive relaxation b. Guided imagery c. Regular exercise (e.g., walking, swimming) d. Refer to counselor and psychiatrist as appropriate.	6. Stress may be associated with an increase in disease activity. Stress management techniques can reduce the stress and fatigue associated with unmanaged conflicts (Albano & Wallace, 2001).
7. Refer to appropriate community resources: a. Arthritis Foundation, (800) 283-7800, www.arthritis.org b. Lupus Foundation of America, (800) 558-0121, www.lupus.org c. National Arthritis, Musculoskeletal and Skin Disease Information Clearinghouse, (301) 495-4484	7. Additional self-help information may be very useful for self-care. Provide excellent support and education for patient and family (Albano & Wallace, 2001).

 Documentation

Discharge summary record
  Client teaching
  Outcome achievement or status
  Referrals if indicated

Neoplastic Disorders

CANCER: INITIAL DIAGNOSIS

Cancer involves a disturbance in normal cell growth in which abnormal cells arise from normal cells, reproduce rapidly, and infiltrate tissues, lymph, and blood vessels. The destruction caused by cancer depends on its site, whether or not it metastasizes, its obstructive effects, and its effects on the body's defense system (e.g., nutrition, hematopoiesis). Cancer is classified according to the cell of origin: malignant tumors from epithelial tissue are called carcinomas and those from connective tissue are known as sarcomas. Treatment varies depending on classification, cancer stage, and other factors.

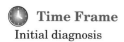 **Time Frame**
Initial diagnosis

DIAGNOSTIC CLUSTER	
Nursing Diagnoses	**Refer to**
▲ Anxiety related to unfamiliar hospital environment, uncertainty about outcomes, feelings of helplessness and hopelessness, and insufficient knowledge about cancer and treatment	
△ High Risk for Disturbed Self-Concept related to changes in life style, role responsibilities, and appearance	
▲ Interrupted Family Processes related to fears associated with recent cancer diagnosis, disruptions associated with treatments, financial problems, and uncertain future	
△ Decisional Conflict related to treatment modality choices	
▲ Grieving related to potential loss of body function and the perceived effects of cancer on life style	
△ High Risk for Spiritual Distress related to conflicts centering on the meaning of life, cancer, spiritual beliefs, and death	Cancer: End-Stage

(continues on page 558)

Nursing Diagnoses continued	Refer to continued
Related Care Plans Chemotherapy Radiation Therapy	

▲ This diagnosis was reported to be monitored for or managed frequently (75%–100%).
△ This diagnosis was reported to be monitored for or managed often (50%–74%).

Discharge Criteria

Before discharge, the client or family will

1. Relate the intent to share concerns with a trusted confidante.
2. Describe early signs of family dysfunction.
3. Identify signs and symptoms that must be reported to a health care professional.
4. Identify available community resources.

Collaborative Problems

The collaborative problems caused by cancer depend on its site, whether it metastasizes, its obstructive effects, and its effects on the body's defense system (e.g., white blood count, renal insufficiency). For example, cancer of the breast can metastasize to the brain, lung, liver, and bone. In this case, the collaborative problems PC: Increased Intracranial Pressure, PC: Hepatic Insufficiency, PC: Respiratory Insufficiency, and PC: Pathological Fractures would be appropriate. Refer to the index of collaborative problems for specific care plans where those collaborative problems are detailed.

 Related Physician-Prescribed Interventions

Medications. Vary depending on stage of disease

Intravenous Therapy. None

Laboratory Studies. CBC with differential, liver function tests, renal function tests, blood chemistry, T-helper/T-suppressor ratio, lysozyme, complement C4, complement human C3, total acid, urine inorganic phosphorus, urine catecholamines, urine alpha amino nitrogen, serum electrolytes

Selected Markers. (Griffin-Brown, 2000):

Enzyme	Associated Malignancy
Test Lactic dehydrogenase (LDH)	Lymphoma, seminoma, leukemia, metastatic carcinoma
Prostatic acid phosphatase (PAP)	Metastatic cancer of the prostate, myeloma, lung cancer, osteogenic sarcoma
Placental alkaline phosphatase (PLAP)	Seminoma, lung, ovary, uterus
Neuron-specific enolase (NSE)	Small-cell lung cancer, neuroendocrine tumors, neuroblastoma, medullary thyroid cancer

(continues on page 559)

Enzyme continued	**Associated Malignancy** continued
Creatine kinase-BB (CK-BB)	Breast, colon, ovary, prostate cancers; small-cell lung cancer
Terminal deoxynucleotidal transferase (TdT)	Lymphoblastic malignancy
Hormones Parathyroid hormone (PTH)	Ectopic hyperparathyroidism from cancer of the kidney, lung (squamous cell), pancreas, ovary, myeloma
Calcitonin	Medullary thyroid, small cell lung, breast cancer, and carcinoid
Adrenocorticotropic hormone (ACTH)	Lung, prostate, gastrointestinal cancers, neuroendocrine tumors
Antidiuretic hormone (ADH)	Small lung cancer, adenocarcinomas
Human-chorionic gonadotropin, beta subunit (B-HCG)	Germ cell tumors of testicle and ovary; ectopic production in cancer of stomach, pancreas, lung, colon, liver
Metabolic Products 5-Hydroxyindoleacetic acid (5-HIAA)	Carcinoid, lung
Vanillylmandelic acid (VMA)	Neuroblastoma

Proteins
Protein electrophoresis (urine-Bence Jones)
  IgG
  IgA
  IgM
  IgD
  IgD
Beta-2 microglobulin
	Myeloma, lymphoma (serum-immunoglobulins)

Antigens Alpha-fetoprotein (AFP)	Nonseminomatous germ cell testicular cancer, choriocarcinoma, gonadal teratoblastoma in children, cancer of the pancreas, colon, lung, stomach, biliary system, liver
Carcinoembryonic antigen (CEA)	Cancer of the colon-rectum, stomach, pancreas, prostate, lungs, breast

(continues on page 560)

Enzyme continued	Associated Malignancy continued
Prostrate-specific antigen (PSA)	Prostrate cancer
Tissue polypeptide antigen (TPA)	Breast, colon, lung, pancreas cancer
CA-125	Ovary (epithelial), pancreas, breast, colon, lung, liver cancer
CA-a9-9	Pancreas, colon, gastric cancer
CA-15-3	Breast cancer
CA-27-29	Breast cancer
CA-72-4	Gastric cancer
Others Lipid-associated sialic acid (LSA)	Leukemia, lymphoma, melanoma, most solid tumors
Chromosome rearrangements (deletion, translocation)	Melanoma, small cell lung, renal, testicular cancers, liposarcoma, neuroblastoma, lymphoma, leukemia, and others
Amplified oncogenes (MYC)	Neuroblastoma, small cell lung cancer, lymphoma, breast cancer
EP1B-B	Glioblastoma, squamous cell carcinomas, breast, gastric, esophagus cancers
C-ERB-B2 (HER-2)	Breast and ovarian cancers, adenocarcinomas

Diagnostic Studies. Magnetic resonance imaging (MRI); varied sites; bone marrow aspiration; bone scan; x-rays (chest, abdomen); liver-spleen scan; bone scan; positron emission tomography (PET); computerized axillomography (CT) (chest, abdomen, musculoskeletal, bladder, lung, head, neck); GI barium studies; ultrasound (liver, abdomen, ovary, esophagus, transrectal, transvaginal)

Nursing Diagnoses

Anxiety Related to Unfamiliar Hospital Environment, Uncertainty about Outcomes, Feelings of Helplessness and Hopelessness, and Insufficient Knowledge about Cancer and Treatment

Focus Assessment Criteria	Clinical Significance
1. Level of understanding of condition, past experiences with cancer	1–3. This assessment helps the nurse to identify learning needs and plan appropriate teaching strategies. Health professionals recognize that cancer is a chronic disease that can be cured or controlled with treatment. In the general public, however, the term *cancer* conjures thoughts of death. Lack of knowledge and negative attitudes about cancer, coupled with the unfamiliarity of medical treatments and the hospital environment, cause most newly diagnosed clients to respond with anxiety and fear even when the prognosis is good. The physiologic and psychological effects of treatments produce changes in body image, life style, and function that also can contribute to fear and anxiety (Barsevick, Much, & Sweeney, 2000).
2. Familiarity with hospital environment, diagnostic tests, and treatment plan	
3. Life style, strengths, coping mechanisms, and available support systems	

Goal

The client will report increased psychological comfort.

Indicators
- Share concerns regarding the cancer diagnosis.
- Identify one strategy that reduces anxiety.

Interventions	Rationales

1. Provide opportunities for client and family members to share feelings (anger, guilt, loss, and pain).
  a. Initiate frequent contacts and provide an atmosphere that promotes calm and relaxation.
  b. Convey a nonjudgmental attitude and listen attentively.
  c. Explore own feelings and behaviors.
	1. Frequent contact by caregiver indicates acceptance and may facilitate trust. Client may be hesitant to approach the staff because of negative self-concept. The nurse should not make assumptions about a client's or family member's reaction; validating the person's particular fears and concerns helps to increase awareness. The nurse should be aware of how the client and family are reacting and how their reactions are influencing the nurse's feeling and behavior (Barsevick, Much, & Sweeney, 2000).

2. Encourage an open discussion of cancer including experiences of others and potential for cancer's cure or control.	2. The nurse who can talk openly about life after a cancer diagnosis offers encouragement and hope (Poncar, 1994).
3. Explain hospital routines and reinforce the physician's explanations of scheduled tests and proposed treatment plan. Focus on what the client can expect.	3. Accurate descriptions of sensations and procedures help to ease anxiety and fear associated with the unknown. (Christman & Kirchoff, 1992).

(continues on page 562)

Interventions continued	Rationales continued

4. Identify those at risk for unsuccessful adjustment:
  a. Poor ego strength
  b. Ineffective problem-solving ability
  c. Poor motivation
  d. External focus of control
  e. Poor overall health
  f. Lack of positive support systems
  g. Unstable economic status
  h. Rejection of counseling (Shipes, 1987)
	4. A client identified as high-risk may need referrals for counseling. Successful adjustment is influenced by factors such as previous coping success, achievement of developmental tasks, extent to which the disorder and treatment interfere with goal-directed activity, sense of self-determination and control, and realistic perception of the disorder (Bushkin, 1993).

5. Convey a sense of hope.	5. Clients who are reacting to a new cancer diagnosis must begin with hope. Hope is necessary to cope with the rigors of treatment (Barsevick, Much, & Sweeney, 2000).
6. Promote physical activity and exercise. Assist to determine level of activity advisable.	6. Physical activity provides diversion and a sense of normalcy. Clients who exercise may improve their quality of life (Smith, 1996).

 Documentation

Progress notes
  Present emotional status
  Interventions utilized
  Response to interventions

High Risk for Disturbed Self-Concept Related to Changes in Life Style, Role Responsibilities, and Appearance

Focus Assessment Criteria	Clinical Significance
1. Previous exposure to persons with cancer 2. Ability to express feelings about condition 3. Ability to share feelings with family members and significant others 4. Self-concept and others' perceptions of client's self-concept	1–4. This information helps nurse to detect patterns of response due to adaptation. It may be helpful to note how the client's support persons view the client's self-concept; they can provide insight into factors that may have had a negative impact on self-concept, and they tend to be sensitive to subtle changes.
5. Sense of well-being 6. Participation in self-care 7. Evidence of adapting life style to accommodate disabilities	5,6. Participation in self-care and adapting goals to disability indicates attempts to cope with the changes (Hamburg and Adams, 1953).

Goal

The client will relate the intent to continue previous life style as much as possible.

Indicators

- Communicate feelings about possible changes.
- Participate in self-care.

Interventions	Rationales
1. Contact client frequently and treat him or her with warm, positive regard.	1. Frequent contact by the caregiver indicates acceptance and may facilitate trust. Client may be hesitant to approach the staff because of negative self-concept.
2. Encourage client to express feelings and thoughts about the following: a. Condition b. Progress c. Prognosis d. Effects on life style e. Support system f. Treatments	2. Encouraging client to share feelings can provide a safe outlet for fears and frustration and can increase self-awareness.
3. Provide reliable information and clarify any misconceptions.	3. Misconceptions can needlessly increase anxiety and damage self-concept.
4. Help client to identify positive attributes and possible new opportunities.	4. Client may tend to focus only on the change in self-image and not on the positive characteristics that contribute to the whole concept of self. The nurse must reinforce these positive aspects and encourage the client to reincorporate them into his or her new self-concept.
5. Assist with hygiene and grooming as needed.	5. Participation in self-care and planning can aid positive coping.
6. Encourage visitors.	6. Frequent visits by support persons can help the client feel that he or she is still a worthwhile, acceptable person; this should promote a positive self-concept.
7. Help client to identify strategies to increase independence and maintain role responsibilities: a. Prioritizing activities b. Getting assistance with less valued or most fatiguing activities, e.g., shopping, housekeeping	7. A strong component of self-concept is the ability to perform functions expected of one's role, thus decreasing dependency and reducing the need for others' involvement.

(continues on page 564)

Interventions continued	**Rationales** continued
c. Using energy conservation techniques (Refer to the nursing diagnosis Fatigue in the Inflammatory Joint Disease care plan for specific strategies.) d. Using mobility aids and assistive devices as needed	
8. Discuss ways that the client can provide support to support persons: a. Actively listening to their problems b. Attempting to decrease the focus on disabilities (Refer to Chapter 3, The Ill Adult: Issues and Responses, for more information.) c. Help client to identify ways of integrating the cancer experience into her or his life rather than allowing cancer to take over life.	8. The nurse can help the client learn how to balance relationships and preserve the family system. The experience of cancer is different for everyone. What is vitally important to one person may be inconsequential to another (Stevens, 1992).
9. Help client to identify potential opportunities for self-growth through living with cancer: a. Living and getting the most out of each day b. Value of relationships c. Increase in knowledge, personal strength, and understanding d. Spiritual and moral development	9. Experiences with cancer can provide the client with opportunities to reevaluate his or her life and to focus on personal priorities.
10. Allow client's support persons to share their feelings regarding the diagnosis and actual or anticipated effects (anger, rage, depression, or guilt).	10. Cancer can have a negative impact on the client's family financially, socially, and emotionally.
11. Assess for signs of negative response to changes in appearance: a. Refusal to discuss loss b. Denial of changes c. Decreased self-care ability d. Social isolation e. Refusal to discuss future	11. A client at high risk for unsuccessful adjustment should be identified for additional interventions or referrals.
12. Assist with management of alopecia as necessary: a. Explain when hair loss occurs (usually within 2 to 3 weeks of initiation of therapy) and when regrowth will begin (usually 4 to 6 weeks after discontinuation of therapy).	12. Embarrassment from alopecia can contribute to isolation and negative self-concept.

(continues on page 565)

Interventions continued	Rationales continued

b. Suggest cutting long hair to minimize fallout.
   c. Suggest resources for wigs and hairpieces.
   d. Discuss measures to reduce hair loss in low-dose therapy (e.g., wash hair only twice a week, use a mild shampoo, or avoid brushing).
   e. Encourage good grooming, hygiene, and other measures to enhance appearance (e.g., makeup, manicures, and new clothes).	

13. Discuss possible emotional reactions—sadness, depression, and displaced anger. Encourage verbalization of feelings.	13. Changes in appearance often initiate the grieving process.
14. Discuss the advantages and disadvantages of scalp tourniquets and ice caps to prevent hair loss. The advantages are that they provide some control over hair loss and may reduce hair loss, especially in low-dose chemotherapy or radiation therapy. The disadvantages include possible micrometastasis to scalp not protected by chemotherapy, discomfort, and high cost.	14. Understanding advantages and disadvantages allows the client to make an informed decision regarding these treatments.
15. Refer an at-risk client for professional counseling.	15. Some clients may need follow-up therapy to aid with effective adjustment.

 Documentation

Progress notes
   Present emotional status
   Interventions
   Response to interventions

Interrupted Family Processes Related to Fears Associated with Recent Cancer Diagnosis, Disruptions Associated with Treatments, Financial Problems, and Uncertain Future

Focus Assessment Criteria	Clinical Significance
1. Understanding condition	1–7. The family unit is a system based on interdependence between members and patterns that provides structure and support. Chronic illness in one family member disrupts these relationships and patterns.
2. Family coping patterns	
3. Current response	

(continues on page 566)

Focus Assessment Criteria continued	Clinical Significance continued
4. Intrafamilial stresses 5. Problem behavior in children 6. Stressful behavior (Cooper, 1984): • Nervousness • Sleeplessness • Loss of appetite • Inability to concentrate • Irritability 7. Available resources	Cancer and its treatment may be as threatening to the family as to the client. Common sources of fear and disruption include the following: a. The mistaken belief that cancer is contagious and can be "caught." b. Concerns about the hereditary nature of cancer c. Guilt d. Anger/depression e. Revulsion at client's appearance f. Concerns about caregiving ability g. Worry about death h. Financial problems i. Feeling alone; lack of family support j. Concerns k. Shock These feelings and concerns can affect family communication, function, and support, and can alter family processes.

Goal

The family will maintain a functional system of mutual support for each other.

Indicators
• Verbalize feelings regarding the diagnosis and prognosis.
• Identify signs of family dysfunction.
• Identify appropriate resources to seek when needed.

Interventions	Rationales
1. Convey an understanding of the situation and its impact on the family.	1. Communicating understanding and a sense of caring and concern facilitates trust and strengthens the nurse's relationship with client and family.
2. Explore family members' perceptions of the situation. Encourage verbalization of feelings such as guilt, anger, blame and grief.	2. Verbalization can provide an opportunity for clarification and validation of feelings and concerns; this contributes to family unity. Spouses report increased anxiety prior to discharge from hospital and anger at client for egocentricity during home-care period.
3. Determine if present coping mechanisms are effective.	3.

(continues on page 567)

Interventions continued	**Rationales** continued

4. Take steps to promote family strengths:
  a. Acknowledge assistance of family members.
  b. Involve family in client care.
  c. Encourage time away from caregiving to prevent burnout.
  d. Encourage humor.
  e. Encourage communication.
  (Refer to Chapter 3, The Ill Adult: Issues and Responses for more information.)
	4. This can help to maintain the existing family structure and its function as a supportive unit. Cancer challenges one's values and beliefs; this can result in changed cognitive, affective, and behavioral responses.

5. Assist to reorganize roles at home, set new priorities, and redistribute responsibilities.	5. Planning and prioritizing can help to maintain family integrity and reduce stress.
6. Prepare family for signs of stress, depression, anxiety, anger, and dependency in client and other family members.	6. Anticipatory guidance can alert members to potential problems before they occur, enabling prompt intervention at early signs.
7. Encourage family to call on its social network (e.g., friends, relatives, church members) for emotional and other support.	7. Outside assistance may help to reduce the perception that the family must "go it alone."
8. Encourage open communication between significant others.	8. Family members are reluctant to discuss distressing information or their feelings with the person.

9. Identify dysfunctional coping mechanisms:
  a. Substance abuse
  b. Continued denial
  c. Exploitation of one or more family members
  d. Separation or avoidance. Refer for counseling as necessary.
	9. A family with a history of unsuccessful coping may need additional resources. A family with unresolved conflicts before diagnosis is at high risk.

10. Direct to community agencies and other sources of assistance (e.g., financial, housekeeping, direct care, and childcare) as needed.	10. Family may need assistance to help with management at home.

 Documentation

Progress notes
  Present family functioning
  Interventions
  Response to interventions
  Discharge summary record
  Referrals if indicated

Decisional Conflict Related to Treatment Modality Choices

Focus Assessment Criteria	Clinical Significance
1. Knowledge of cancer diagnosis, treatment options, and treatment plan	1–4. These assessments provide the nurse with needed information to assist the client and family with informed decision making.
2. Decision-making pattern	
3. Other involved parties (e.g., relatives, friends, and physician)	
4. Possible conflicts (e.g., religion, culture, and family)	

Goal

The client and family members will

1. Relate the advantages and disadvantages of choices.
2. Share their fears and concerns regarding a decision.
3. Make an informed choice.

Interventions	Rationales
1. Provide, reinforce, and clarify information about the diagnosis, treatment options, and alternative therapies.	1. Client and family need specific, accurate information to make an informed decision. Cancer gives a sense of being out of control. Exploration of all options may help client to regain a sense of control (Fryback & Reinert, 1997).
2. Allow client and family members opportunities to share feelings and concerns regarding the decision.	2. Conflict is more intense when the decision has potentially negative impacts or conflicting opinions exist. Anxiety and fear have a negative impact on decision-making ability. Providing opportunities to share feelings and concerns can help to reduce anxiety.
3. Ensure that client and family clearly understand what is involved in each treatment alternative.	3. Informed decisions support a person's right to self-determination. Clients must be prepared for the emotional and physical problems they will face.
4. As appropriate, assure client that he or she does not have to abide by decisions that others make but can choose for himself or herself. Discourage family members and others from undermining the client's confidence in decision-making ability.	4. Each person has the right to make his or her own decisions and to expect respect from others.

(continues on page 569)

Interventions continued	Rationales continued
5. Provide as much time as possible for decision making.	5. Effective and informed decision-making requires time to consider all alternatives thoroughly.
6. If indicated, encourage client to seek a second professional opinion.	6. A second opinion can confirm information and validate options.

🌐 Documentation

Progress notes
   Dialogues

Grieving Related to Potential Loss of Body Function and the Perceived Effects of Cancer on Life Style

Focus Assessment Criteria	Clinical Significance
1. Signs and symptoms of grief reaction (e.g., crying, anger, withdrawal) 2. Significance of loss, coping mechanisms 3. Personal strengths, support systems	1–3. At diagnosis, most clients with cancer experience losses secondary to the disease and its treatment; major losses may include the following: a. Loss of functional ability b. Change in role c. Social isolation d. Loss of intimacy e. Anticipatory loss of life These losses, like any, are accompanied by grief feelings. Evaluation of the losses, the client's response, coping mechanisms, personal strengths, and support systems guides the nurse in planning appropriate interventions.

Goal

The client and family members will

1. Express grief.
2. Describe the personal meaning of the loss.
3. Report an intent to discuss his or her feelings with significant others.

Interventions	Rationales
1. Provide opportunities for client and family members to ventilate feelings, discuss the loss openly, and explore the personal meaning of the loss. Explain that grief is a common and healthy reaction.	1. A cancer diagnosis typically gives rise to feelings of powerlessness, anger, profound sadness, and other grief responses. Open, honest discussions can help the client and family members accept and cope with the situation and their responses to it.

(continues on page 570)

Interventions continued	**Rationales** continued
2. Encourage use of positive coping strategies that have proved successful in the past.	2. Positive coping strategies aid acceptance and problem solving.
3. Encourage client to express positive self-attributes.	3. Focusing on positive attributes increases self-acceptance and acceptance of the diagnosis.

4. Implement measures to support the family and promote cohesiveness:
  a. Help family members acknowledge losses.
  b. Explain the grieving process.
  c. Encourage client to verbalize feelings.
  d. Allow participation in care to promote comfort.
  e. Encourage discussing the relationship's significance.
	4. Family cohesiveness is important to client support.

5. Promote grief work with each response:
  a. Denial:
   • Encourage acceptance of the situation; do not reinforce denial by giving false reassurance.
   • Promote hope through assurances of care, comfort, and support.
   • Explain the use of denial by one family member to other members.
   • Do not push a person to move past denial until he or she is emotionally ready.
  b. Isolation:
   • Convey acceptance by encouraging expressions of grief.
   • Promote open, honest communication to encourage sharing.
   • Reinforce the client's self-worth by providing privacy when desired.
   • Encourage socialization as feasible (e.g., support groups, church activities).
  c. Depression:
   • Reinforce the client's self-esteem.
   • Employ empathetic sharing and acknowledge grief.
   • Identify the degree of depression and develop appropriate strategies.
  d. Anger:
   • Explain to other family members that anger represents an attempt to control the environment; it stems from frustration at the inability to control the disease.
   • Encourage verbalization of anger.
	5. Grieving involves profound emotional responses; interventions depend on the particular response.

(continues on page 571)

Interventions continued	**Rationales** continued
e. Guilt: • Acknowledge the person's expressed self-image. • Encourage identification of the relationship's positive aspects. • Avoid arguing and participating in the person's system of "I should have . . ." and "I shouldn't have. . . ." f. Fear: • Focus on the present and maintain a safe and secure environment. • Help person explore reasons for and meanings of the fears. g. Rejection: • Provide reassurance by explaining what is happening. • Explain this response to other family members. h. Hysteria: • Reduce environmental stressors (e.g., limit personnel). • Provide a safe, private area in which to express grief.	
6. Act as a guide to the client through the grief experience by understanding needs and providing help where needed (Bushkin, 1993).	
7. Validate and reflect impressions with client.	7. It is important to realize that clients with cancer often have their own realities that may differ from the nurse's view (Yates, 1993).

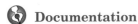 **Documentation**

Progress notes
  Present emotional status
  Interventions
  Response to nursing interventions

CANCER: END-STAGE

Approximately 400,000 people in the United States die of cancer each year. Cancer that treatment cannot control metastasizes to adjacent organs and structures or spreads through the blood and lymphatics to a distant site such as the liver, brain, or bones. For example, a client with end-stage colon cancer may have a tumor in the colon causing bowel obstruction. Metastasis to the liver causes ascites, edema, and clotting problems; metastasis to the lung promotes respiratory alterations.

End-stage cancer with metastasis can result in many structural and functional problems, depending on the body area(s) or system(s) affected. Potential complications also depend on the affected site; only those specific to end-stage cancer are discussed in this care plan. In addition, the client and his or her significant others face multiple challenges of pain, loss, and decreased functioning.

Time Frame
Terminal stage (care in home, hospital, long-term care facility, or hospice)

DIAGNOSTIC CLUSTER*

Collaborative Problems	Refer to
PC: Hypercalcemia	
PC: Cachexia	
PC: Malignant Effusions	
PC: Narcotic Toxicity	
PC: Pathologic Fractures	
PC: Spinal Cord Compression	
PC: Superior Vena Cava Syndrome	
PC: Intracerebral Metastasis	Cerebrovascular Accident (Stroke)
PC: Myelosuppression	Chemotherapy

Nursing Diagnoses	Refer to
Acute and/or Chronic Pain related to direct tumor involvement and/or associated with cancer therapy (surgery, radiation, chemotherapy)	
Grieving related to terminal illness, impending death, functional losses, and withdrawal of or from others	
Powerlessness related to change from curative status to palliative status	
Hopelessness related to overwhelming functional losses or impending death	

(continues on page 573)

Nursing Diagnoses continued	Refer to continued
High Risk for Spiritual Distress related to fear of death, overwhelming grief, belief system conflicts, and unresolved relationship conflicts	
High Risk for Ineffective Therapeutic Regimen Management related to insufficient knowledge of home care, pain management, signs and symptoms of complications, and community resources available	
Imbalanced Nutrition: Less Than Body Requirements related to decreased oral intake, increased metabolic demands of tumor, and altered lipid metabolism	Chemotherapy
Constipation related to decreased dietary fiber intake, decreased intestinal mobility secondary to narcotic medications and inactivity	Immobility or Unconsciousness
Pruritus related to dry skin secondary to dehydration or accumulation of bile salts secondary to biliary duct obstruction	Hepatitis (Viral)
Ineffective Airway Clearance related to decreased ability to expectorate secretions secondary to weakness, increased viscosity, and pain	Pneumonia
Disuse Syndrome related to pain, weakness, fatigue, and edema	Immobility or Unconsciousness
High Risk for Injury related to weakness, fatigue secondary to anemia, electrolyte imbalances, or somnolence secondary to medications or disease process	Cerebrovascular Accident (Stroke)
Self-Care Deficit related to fatigue, weakness, sedation, pain, and decreased sensory-perceptual capacity	Immobility or Unconsciousness
Disturbed Self-Concept related to dependence on others to meet basic needs	Multiple Sclerosis
Interrupted Family Processes related to change to terminal status, unresolved relationship conflicts, and concerns regarding coping and managing home care	Multiple Sclerosis

(continues on page 574)

Nursing Diagnoses continued

Related Care Plans

Specific Surgical Care Plan
Radiation Therapy
Chemotherapy

---

*This medical condition was not included in the validation study.

Discharge Criteria

Before discharge, the client or family will

1. Relate the intent to share feelings with a trusted friend.
2. Relate strategies to manage discomfort.
3. Identify personal strengths.
4. Identify community resources available for assistance.
5. Describe signs and symptoms of complication that must be reported to a health care professional.
6. Identify two sources of spiritual comfort.

Collaborative Problems

Potential Complication: Hypercalcemia

Potential Complication: Cachexia

Potential Complication: Malignant Effusions

Potential Complication: Narcotic Toxicity

Potential Complication: Pathologic Fractures

Potential Complication: Spinal Cord Compression

Potential Complication: Superior Vena Cava Syndrome

Nursing Goal

The nurse will detect early signs and symptoms of (a) hypercalcemia, (b) cachexia, (c) malignant effusions (plural ascites pericardial), (d) narcotic toxicity, (e) pathologic fractures, (f) spinal cord compression, and (g) superior vena cava syndrome and collaboratively intervene to stabilize client.

Indicators
- Alert, oriented (a, d, g)
- EKG: normal sinus rhythm (a)
- No seizures (a)
- No nausea or vomiting (a)
- No significant weight gain or loss (b)
- No edema (b, c, e, g)
- No anorexia or early satiety (b, c)
- Pulse 60–100 beats/min (b, d)
- Respirations 16–20 breaths/min (b, d)
- Easy, rhythmic breathing (b, c, d)
- No pleuritic pain (b)
- Full breath sounds in all quadrants (b, c)
- No increase in abdominal girth (c)
- No visual changes (g)
- No hoarseness or stridor (g)
- No bone pain (e)

- Full range of motion (e)
- No visible bone deformity (e)
- No sensory or motor losses (f)
- No neck or back pain (f)
- Normal bowel movements (f)
- No venous distention (c, g)
- Serum magnesium 1.3–2.4 mEq/L (c)
- Serum sodium 135–145 mEq/L (c)
- Serum potassium 3.8–5 mEq/L (c)
- Serum calcium 8.5–10.5 mg/dL (a,c)
- Serum albumin 3.5–5 g/dL (c)
- Serum prealbumin 20 50 g/dL (c)
- Serum protein 6–8 g/dL (c)
- Partial prothrombin time (PTT) 20–45 sec (c)
- Hemoglobin (c)
  - Male: 13–18 g/dL
  - Female: 12–16 g/dL
- Hematocrit (c)
  - Male: 42%–50%
  - Female: 40%–48%
- Platelets 100,000–400,000/cu mm (c)
- Blood urea nitrogen (BUN) 10–20 mg/dL (c)
- Alanine aminotransferase (ALT) 7–40 U/mL (c)
- Aspartate aminotransferase (AST) 10–40 U/mL (c)

Interventions	Rationales

1. Monitor for signs and symptoms of hypercalcemia:
  a. Altered mental status
  b. Dysrhythmias
  c. Numbness or tingling in fingers and toes
  d. Muscle cramps
  e. Seizures
  f. Nausea/vomiting
	1. Hypercalcemia (serum calcium >11 mg/dL) is a common complication of end-stage cancer. It occurs most often in multiple myeloma, lung cancer, head and neck cancer, breast cancer, and metastatic bone cancer, owing to disturbed calcium reabsorption (Wickham, 2000).

2. Monitor for signs/symptoms of cachexia:
  a. Weight loss
  b. Early satiety
  c. Edema
  d. Anorexia
	2. A client with advanced cancer has an abnormal sugar tolerance with resistance or decreased sensitivity to insulin; this inhibits cell nourishment. Cachexia results from the increased metabolic demands of the tumor, altered lipid metabolism, and anorexia. Impaired carbohydrate meta-bolism causes increased metabolism of fats and protein, which—especially in the presence of metabolic acidosis—can lead to negative nitrogen balance. Nutritional deficiencies are associated with development of pressure sores, impaired cellular and hormonal immunity, higher risk for infection, apathy, and depression (Foltz, 2000).

(continues on page 576)

Interventions continued	**Rationales** continued
3. Monitor laboratory values: a. Serum calcium, ionized calcium b. CBC with differential c. Serum albumin, transferrin, prealbumin d. Blood urea nitrogen (BUN) e. Creatinine f. Electrolytes and magnesium g. Liver function tests	3. Selected laboratory studies are done to monitor nutritional status and to detect early changes in renal function. Potassium and magnesium losses can occur with hydration and diuretic treatment. Hydration depends on extent of dehydration, renal excretory capacity, and cardiovascular condition (DeVita, Hellman, & Rosenberg, 2001; Wickham, 2000).

4. Monitor for malignant effusions (excessive accumulation of fluid in the pleural space, peritoneal cavity [ascites], or pericardial space):
a. Pleural effusion:
  • Cough (dry)
  • Variable dyspnea
  • Pleuritic pain
  • Diminished and delayed chest movement on the involved side
  • Bulging of intercostal spaces (in a large effusion)
  • Decreased breath sounds auscultated over the effusion
  • Decreased vocal and tactile fremitus
  • Increased respiratory rate and depth
b. Ascites:
  • Abdominal distention
  • Increased abdominal girth
  • Shortness of breath
  • Fatigue
  • Fluid wave
  • Generalized edema
  • Reduced bladder capacity
  • Ankle edema
  • Indigestion
  • Early satiety
  • Decreased serum albumin and protein values
  • Abnormal clotting factors and electrolyte values
c. Pericardial effusion:
  • Dyspnea, dry cough, chest pain
  • Weakness and dizziness
  • Upright, forward-leaning posture
  • Muffled heart/breath sounds
  • Friction rub
  • Orthopnea
  • Neck vein distention
  • Increased central venous pressure
	4. Effusions cause pain and discomfort and inhibit function.
	
	a. Collections of fluid (either transudates or exudates) in the pleural cavity, pleural effusions are common with cancer. Fluid pressure dynamics are affected by direct pressure by tumor or lymphatic or venous obstruction of severe hypoproteinemia (Wickham, 2000).
	
	b. Accumulation of serous fluid in the peritoneal cavity is caused by obstruction in portal circulation. Tumors also can involve lymphatic channels that interfere with drainage of peritoneal cavity, and humoral factors may cause capillary leakage (DeVita et al., 2001).
	
	c. Tumors of the lung and breast, leukemia, lymphomas, melanomas, and sarcomas metastasize to the pericardium and promote pericardial effusions. These effusions interfere with cardiac function, reducing cardiac volume during diastole and decreasing cardiac output and venous return.

(continues on page 577)

Interventions continued	**Rationales** continued
5. Monitor abdominal girth and weight daily.	5. These measurements help to detect fluid retention and ascites.

6. Monitor for signs of narcotic toxicity:
  a. Increased sedation
  b. Drowsiness
  c. Depressed respiratory rate
	6. Many health professionals are overly concerned about narcotic toxicity and may needlessly withhold narcotics from a terminally ill client. A client in severe pain can tolerate very high doses of narcotics without developing excessive sedation and respiratory depression.

7. As necessary, intervene for narcotic toxicity:
  a. Monitor sedation level frequently. Expect peak effects from narcotics 5 to 10 minutes after intravenous rejection, 30 minutes after intramuscular (IM) injection; and 90 minutes after subcutaneous (SC) injection.
  b. Withhold narcotic dose if sedation level increases; assess results.
  c. If respirations fall below 12, monitor patient carefully; below 10, notify physician.
  d. If respirations continue to fall, consult with physician for a narcotic antagonist (e.g., Naloxone).
	7. Narcotic toxicity can occur if excretion is impaired (e.g., in liver dysfunction). Sedation usually precedes respiratory depression; withholding drugs when sedation occurs usually heads off respiratory depression. Narcotic antagonists reduce opioid effects by competing for the same receptor sites.

8. Monitor for signs and symptoms of pathologic fracture:
  a. Localized pain that becomes continuous and unrelenting
  b. Visible bone deformity
  c. Crepitation on movement
  d. Loss of movement or use
  e. Localized soft tissue edema
  f. Skin discoloration
  g. Tenderness to percussion over involved spine
	8. Pathologic fractures occur in about 9% of clients with metastatic disease. Bones most susceptible to tumor invasion are those with the greatest bone marrow activity and blood flow—the vertebrae, pelvis, ribs, skull, and sternum. The most common sites for long bone metastasis are the femur and humerus (DeVita et al., 2001).

9. Maintain alignment and immobilize the site if fracture is suspected.	9. Immobilization helps to reduce soft tissue damage from dislocations.
10. If a stabilization device is necessary, refer to the Casts care plan for specific interventions.	10. Devices may be necessary to stabilize bones.

(continues on page 578)

Interventions continued	**Rationales** continued
11. Monitor for signs and symptoms of spinal cord compression Flaherty, 2000): a. Early signs: • Neck or back pain—gradual onset relieved by sitting, increased by lying or movements • Motor weakness • Sensory loss b. Late signs: • Motor loss • Urinary retention, overflow, incontinence • Constipation, incontinence, difficulty expelling stool. • Poor sphincter control	11. Spinal cord compression results from tumor invasion into the epidural space or from bony erosion and altered vertebral alignment secondary to fracture. Symptoms vary depending on the extent and location of compression. Treatments include radiation therapy and corticosteroids for compression resulting from an extradural mass and a decompression laminectomy for compression owing to bony erosion.
12. Maintain bed rest.	12. Immobility reduces the risk of injury to the spinal cord.
13. Monitor respiratory, bowel, and bladder function.	13. The level of the cord compression influences respiratory (cervical), bowel (lumbar), and bladder (lumbar) functioning.
14. Monitor for signs and symptoms of superior vena cava syndrome (SVCS) (Sitton, 2000): a. Early signs: • Facial, trunk, upper extremity edema • Pronounced venous pattern on trunk • Neck vein distention • Cough b. Late signs: • Hoarseness • Stridor • Engorged conjunctiva • Headache • Dizziness • Visual disturbances • Change in mental status • Respiratory distress	14. SVCS occurs when the superior vena cava becomes occluded by a tumor or thrombus. Commonly associated with lung cancer, breast cancer, and lymphomas, SVCS causes impaired venous return from the head and upper extremities, resulting in upper body edema and prominent collateral circulation (Sitton, 2000).

❦ Related Physician-Prescribed Interventions

Medications. Dependent on symptomatology, chemotherapy, analgesics, antiemetics

Intravenous Therapy. Replacement (fluid, electrolytes); transfusions; albumin

Laboratory Studies. Dependent on history, clinical symptomatology; serum protein; complete blood count; carcinogenic antigens; blood chemistry; electrolytes

Diagnostic Studies. Varies according to site, clinical symptomatology

Therapies. Refer to Cancer: Initial Diagnosis

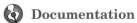 **Documentation**

Flow records
   Daily weights
   Vital signs
   Auscultation findings (lung, heart)
   Abdominal girth
   Intake and output
Progress notes
   New complaints

Nursing Diagnoses

Acute and/or Chronic Pain Related to Direct Tumor Involvement and/or Associated with Cancer Therapy (Surgery, Radiation, Chemotherapy)

Focus Assessment Criteria	Clinical Significance

1. Description of pain
  a. Onset, location, duration
  b. Intensity, quality, time of day
  c. Factors that increase pain
  d. Factors that decrease pain
  e. Associated factors (nausea, vomiting, pruritus)
	1. A thorough assessment is needed for successful management of cancer pain (Yeager, McGuire, & Sheidler, 2000).

2. Client's perception of pain severity based on a scale of 0 to 10 (0 = no pain, 10 = worst pain) rated as follows:
  a. At its worst
  b. At its best
  c. After each pain relief intervention
	2. This scale provides a good method of evaluating the subjective experience of pain.

3. Physical signs of pain (e.g., increased pulse rate and respirations, elevated blood pressure, restlessness, facial grimacing, guarding).	3. In some clients with acute pain, objective signs may be more reliable indicators of pain; for whatever reason, some clients are reluctant to express pain or request pain relief medications. Objective symptoms of pain may be absent in a patient with chronic pain because of damage to afferent pain fibers.
4. Activity pattern, emotional response/anxiety, depression, suffering, sleep/rest patterns, and fatigue	4. This assessment evaluates the effects of pain on functioning. Suffering is a state of severe distress commonly associated with pain.
5. Medications (type, dosage, interval)	5. A medication history can help to evaluate effectiveness of pharmacologic pain relief.
6. Sedation level, respiratory rate	6. These data establish a baseline for subsequent assessments.
7. Use of noninvasive pain relief techniques	7. Noninvasive measures that promote comfort and relaxation can reduce pain.

Goals

The client will report relief after pain measures and an increase in activity.

Indicators

• Participate in pain management decisions.
• Relate that others validate that their pain exists.
• Practice one non-invasive pain relief measure.

Interventions	Rationales

1. Assist in identifying the source of pain:
  a. Obstruction
  b. Effusions
  c. Invasive lines
  d. Immobility
  e. Skeletal source
  f. Muscular source
	1. Do not assume that all pain is related to tissue destruction. Pain of different origins requires different interventions for relief.

2. Convey that you acknowledge and accept his or her pain.	2. A client who believes that he or she must convince skeptical caregivers of the seriousness of his or her pain experiences increased anxiety, which can increase pain.

3. Review pharmacological options.
  a. NSAIDs
 	
  b. Steroids
 	
  c. Opioids
 	
  d. Adjuvant analgesics
 	
    • Tricyclic antidepressants
 	
    • Anticonvulsants
 	
    • NMDA-receptor antagonist
 	
    • Psychostimulants
	3.
	  a. They can be useful for metastatic bone pain from compression of tendons, muscles, pleura, and peritoneum; soft tissue pain; and nonobstructive visceral pain (Polomano, McGuire, & Sheidler, 2000). NSAIDS are also effective against mild pain.
	  b. Indirectly or directly, steroids reduce swelling, inflammation, and compression resulting from tumor growth. They also are an appetite stimulant and antiemetic (Polomano et al., 2000).
	  c. Opioids interfere with pain perception in the brain; they are useful for moderate to severe pain (Polomano et al., 2000).
	  d. These medications enhance the action of pain-modulating symptoms especially in treatment of neuropathic pain (Polomano et al., 2000).
	    • They have been found useful in relieving pain from infiltration as a result of treatment-related injury (e.g., postmastectomy pain syndrome).
	    • They have been found useful in relieving neuropathic pain.
	    • Ketamine has been found to reduce neuropathic pain.
	    • These agents counteract the sedation seen with opioid analgesics.

(continues on page 581)

Interventions continued	**Rationales** continued

4. Provide selected interventions with type of medication
  a. NSAIDs
    • Provide medicine with food or milk.
    • Monitor for GI bleeding and ulcers (e.g., hemoccult, c/o pain, nausea).
    • Monitor liver and renal function laboratory test results.
  b. Steroids
    Refer to Corticosteroid Care Plan.
  c. Opioids
    • Start with low dose and increase until adequate analgesic is achieved.
    • Aggressively manage nausea and vomiting with antiemetics. Use "round the clock" medications for 1–2 weeks.
    • Provide laxatives for constipation (e.g., Metamucil, senna lactulose, docusate).
  For dry mouth, rinse mouth often, suck on sugarless candies, and drink liquids often.
	4.
	  a. Prostaglandins cause loss of protective epithelial lining in GI tract and kidney. Elimination of drug is primarily through hepatic metabolism. The goal is to balance the incidence of side effects with effective pain management.
	
	  c. The chemoreceptor trigger zone in the brain is sensitive to chemical stimuli of opioids (Polomano, 2000). Opioids reduce peristalsis and decrease saliva production.

5. Treat break-through pain with immediate-release formulations.	5. Pain can vary through the day and night

6. Differentiate pain from other symptoms (Panke, 2000):
  a. Delirium
  b. Increased agitation
  c. Restlessness
	6. A terminally ill person may moan and grimace in response to pain as well as delirium.

7. If increased pain is suspected, upwardly titrate the pain medication.	7. If the symptoms decrease, then pain is probably the cause (Panke, 2002).

8. Provide accurate information:
  a. Explain the cause of the pain, if known.
  b. Explain how long the pain should last.
  c. Reassure that narcotic addiction is not likely to develop from the pain relief regimen. Physical dependency may occur.
	8. A client who understands and is prepared for pain by detailed explanations tends to experience less stress—and, consequently, less pain—than a client who receives vague or no explanations. Physical dependency is easily resolved by slowly reducing the amount of pain medication when the patient is free of pain (Miaskowski & Donovan, 1992).

9. Provide privacy for the client during acute pain episodes.	9. Privacy reduces embarrassment and anxiety and enables more effective coping.

(continues on page 582)

Interventions continued	**Rationales** continued

10. Recognize and treat pain promptly with prescribed analgesics.
   a. Determine the preferred route of administration; consult with physician.
 	
   b. Assess vital signs, especially respiratory rate, before and after administration.
   c. Consult with pharmacist for possible adverse interactions with other medications the client is taking, such as muscle relaxants and tranquilizers.
   d. Consult with physician for a regular narcotic administration schedule.
 	
   e. If necessary, use the PRN approach to pain medication; administer before treatment procedures or activity, and instruct client to request pain medications as needed before pain becomes severe.
   f. About ½ hour after administration, assess pain relief and patient satisfaction with pain relief plan.
	10.
	
	   a. If frequent injections are necessary, the intravenous route is preferred because it is not painful and absorption is guaranteed.
	   b. Narcotics depress the brain's respiratory center.
	
	   c. Some medications potentiate the effects of narcotics.
	
	   d. The scheduled approach may reduce the total 24-hour drug dose as compared to the PRN approach and may reduce the client's anxiety associated with having to ask for and wait for PRN medications.
	   e. The PRN approach is effective for breakthrough pain or to manage additional pain from treatments and procedures.
	
	   f. Response to analgesics can vary with stress levels, fatigue, and pain intensity.

11. Consult with physician for co-analgesic medications, as necessary:
   a. Bone pain—aspirin or ibuprofen
   b. Increased intracranial pressure—dexamethasone
   c. Postherpetic neuralgia—amitriptyline
   d. Nerve pressure—prednisone
   e. Gastric distention—metoclopramide
   f. Muscle spasm—diazepam
   g. Lymphodermia—diuretics
   h. Infection—antibiotics
   i. Neuropathic pain—Tegretol and amitriptyline
	11. In addition to narcotics, other medications can help to relieve pain and discomfort.

12. Explain and assist with noninvasive pain relief measures:
   a. Splinting
   b. Positioning
   c. Distraction
   d. Massage
   e. Relaxation techniques
   f. Music therapy
	12. Certain measures can relieve pain by preventing painful stimuli from reaching higher brain centers. They also may improve the client's sense of control over pain.

(continues on page 583)

Interventions continued	Rationales continued
13. Consult with physician for other invasive pain relief measures: a. Radiation b. Nerve block c. Surgery d. Advanced analgesic technologies (patient-controlled analgesia and morphine drips)	13. Radiation can reduce the tumor size to decrease compression on structures and reduce obstructions. Nerve blocks cause an interruption in nerve function through injection of a local anesthetic (temporary) or a neurodestructive agent (permanent). Surgery can decrease tumor bulk to reduce pressure and obstruction.
14. Emphasize the need to report unsatisfactory pain relief.	14. Prompt reporting enables rapid adjustment to control pain.

🕮 Documentation

Medication administration record
Type, dose, time, route of all medications
Progress notes
Unsatisfactory relief from pain
Noninvasive relief measures

Grieving Related to Terminal Illness, Impending Death, Functional Losses, and Withdrawal of or from Others

Focus Assessment Criteria	Clinical Significance
1. Response to earlier losses, current losses, and feelings	1. End-stage cancer results in many losses; major losses include: a. Loss of functional ability b. Change in role and lifestyle c. Social isolation d. Loss of intimacy e. Anticipatory loss of life f. Financial losses
2. Impact of losses on self	2. These losses, like any, are accompanied by grief feelings.
3. Acknowledgment of impending death	3. A dying person needs to acknowledge impending death so that grief work can begin.
4. Grief feelings of family members 5. Distress level of client and family members 6. Client-family relationship and support 7. Family communication and methods of coping	4–7. a. Family affects patient adjustment to cancer (Hull, 1992). b. Family concerns and feelings may vary. c. Family members may need help and support to maintain an effective closure relationship with the client.

Goals

The client will acknowledge that death is expected.

Indicators
- Verbalize losses and changes.
- Verbalize feelings associated with losses and changes.

Family members will maintain an effective closure relationship as evidenced by:

- Spending time with the client
- Maintaining loving, open communication with the client
- Participating in care

Interventions	Rationales
1. Provide opportunities for client and family members to ventilate feelings, discuss the loss openly, and explore the personal meaning of the loss. Explain that grief is a common and healthy reaction.	1. The knowledge that no further treatment is warranted and that death is imminent may give rise to feelings of powerlessness, anger, profound sadness, and other grief responses. Open, honest discussions can help client and family members accept and cope with the situation and their responses to it.
2. Encourage use of positive coping strategies that have proved successful in the past.	2. Positive coping strategies aid acceptance and problem solving.
3. Encourage client to express positive self-attributes.	3. Focusing on positive attributes increases self-acceptance and acceptance of imminent death.
4. Help client acknowledge and accept impending death; answer all questions honestly.	4. Grief work, the adaptive process of mourning, cannot begin until the impending death is acknowledged.
5. Promote grief work with each response: a. Denial: • Encourage acceptance of the situation; do not reinforce denial by giving false reassurance. • Promote hope through assurances of care, comfort, and support. • Explain the use of denial by one family member to other members. • Do not push a person to move past denial until he or she is emotionally ready. b. Isolation: • Convey acceptance by encouraging expressions of grief. • Promote open, honest communication to encourage sharing.	5. Grieving involves profound emotional responses; interventions depend on the particular response. • Anger is often perceived as negative. Anger, however, can energize behavior, facilitate expression of negative feelings, and function to help the client defend against a threat (Taylor, Baird, Malone, & McCorkle, 1993).

(continues on page 585)

Interventions continued	**Rationales** continued
<ul><li>Reinforce the client's self-worth by providing for privacy when desired.</li><li>Encourage socialization as feasible (e.g., support groups, church activities).</li></ul>c. Depression:<ul><li>Reinforce client's self-esteem.</li><li>Employ empathetic sharing and acknowledge grief.</li><li>Identify degree of depression and develop appropriate strategies.</li></ul>d. Anger:<ul><li>Explain to other family members that anger represents an attempt to control the environment and stems from frustration at the inability to control the disease.</li><li>Encourage verbalization of anger.</li></ul>e. Guilt:<ul><li>Acknowledge the person's expressed self-image.</li><li>Encourage identification of the relationship's positive aspects.</li><li>Avoid arguing and participating in the person's system of "I should have . . ." and "I shouldn't have . . . ."</li></ul>f. Fear:<ul><li>Focus on the present and maintain a safe and secure environment.</li><li>Help the person explore reasons for and meanings of the fears.</li></ul>g. Rejection:<ul><li>Provide reassurance by explaining what is happening.</li><li>Explain this response to other family members.</li></ul>h. Hysteria:<ul><li>Reduce environmental stressors (e.g., limit personnel).</li><li>Provide a safe, private area in which to express grief.</li></ul>	
6. Encourage client to engage in a life review by focusing on accomplishments and disappointments. Assist in attempts to resolve unresolved conflicts.	6. Life review provides an opportunity to prepare for life closure.
7. Implement measures to support the family and promote cohesiveness (Jassak, 1992): a. Seek family perceptions of what is happening. b. Help them to acknowledge losses and impending death.	7. Family cohesiveness is important to client support.

(continues on page 586)

Interventions continued	Rationales continued
c. Explain the grief process. d. Explain expected behaviors during terminal stages (denial, anger, depression, and withdrawal). e. Allow participation in care to promote comfort. f. Encourage discussing the relationship's significance. g. Promote adequate rest and nutrition. h. Assist with funeral home arrangements if needed. i. Refer to a bereavement support group. j. Identify resources for helping family and children cope with cancer (booklets, social service, hospice).	
8. Promote hope by assurances of attentive care, relief of discomfort, and support.	8. Terminally ill clients most appreciate the following nursing care measures: assisting with grooming, supporting independent functioning, providing pain medications when needed, and enhancing physical comfort.

 Documentation

Progress notes
Present emotional status
Interventions
Response to nursing interventions

Powerlessness Related to Change from Curative Status to Palliative Status

Focus Assessment Criteria	Clinical Significance
1. Perception of loss of control 2. Feelings of powerlessness and grief 3. Threat of death 4. Inability to make decisions and solve problems 5. Patient strengths and capabilities, available support	1–5. A client's response to loss of control depends on the personal meaning of the loss, individual coping patterns, personal characteristics, and responses of others.

Goal

The client will participate in decisions regarding care and activities.

Indicators

• Identify factors that can be controlled.
• Share feelings.

Interventions	Rationales

1.
  a. Determine client's usual response to problems.
 	
  b. Decrease ambiguity by identifying choices and options.
	1.
	  a. It is important to determine whether the client usually seeks to change own behaviors to control problems or expects others or external factors to control problems.
	  b. Understanding anticipated trajectory of disease and treatment plan promotes a sense of control (Bushkin, 1993).

2. Help client to identify personal strengths and assets.	2. Discouraging client from focusing only on limitations can promote self-esteem.
3. Assist in identifying energy patterns and scheduling activities to accommodate these patterns.	3. A review of the client's daily schedule helps in planning appropriate rest periods.
4. Help client to prioritize activities and schedule them during usual periods of high energy.	4. Scheduling can help client to participate in activities that promote feelings of self-worth and dignity.

5. Help client to identify components of the situation that can be controlled or maintained:
  a. Comfort
  b. Care schedule
  c. Family interaction and communication
  d. Home care decisions
  e. Death with dignity
  f. Funeral arrangements
	5. Loss of power in one area may be counter-balanced by the introduction of other sources of power or control.

6. Promote effective problem solving by breaking activities down into parts:
  a. Things to be resolved now
  b. Things that require time to resolve
  c. Things that cannot be changed (e.g., impending death)
	6. A sense of control may be established by breaking the situation down into some components that can be controlled.

7. As appropriate, provide client with opportunities to make decisions about certain aspects of the care plan.	7. Allowing client to make decisions reinforces respect for his or her right of self-determination.
8. Promote communication of feelings and concerns among family members and significant others.	8. Open communication can help to enlist the support of others.

(continues on page 588)

Interventions continued	Rationales continued
9. If family support is not available, do the following: a. Identify possible community resources for home support. b. Explain long-term care placement. c. Refer to social services or to a clergyman if appropriate. d. Provide social support using volunteer and professional services.	9. Although end-stage cancer cannot be cured and death will occur, clients and support persons need a sense of hope. Client should believe that he or she will be comfortable, that care needs will be met, that he or she can maintain relationships with others, and that he or she will die with dignity.

 Documentation

Progress notes
   Participation in self-care decisions
   Emotional status
   Interactions

Hopelessness Related to Overwhelming Functional Losses or Impending Death

Focus Assessment Criteria	Clinical Significance
1. Response to impending death 2. Available support	1,2. Hopelessness is a subjective emotional state that must be validated through assessment.
3. Spiritual beliefs	3. For some clients, spiritual beliefs can sustain hope for eternal peace when life on earth ends.

Goal

The client will die with dignity and peace.

Indicators

- Express confidence that he or she will receive the needed care and be comfortable.
- Share his or her suffering openly.

Interventions	Rationales
1. Discuss the medical situation honestly.	1. Promoting hope for a cure sets up the client and support persons for false hope and despair.
2. Redirect client to identify alternative sources of hope: a. Relationships b. Faith c. Things to accomplish	2. Recognizing positive aspects of one's life may facilitate coping with an aspect of one's life that is uncontrollable. Authentic relationships, self-representation, and feelings of belonging have been identified as a client's emotional needs in the living and dying phase.

(continues on page 589)

Interventions continued	**Rationales** continued

3. Help client to identify realistic hope in his or her situation:
  a. Client will be comfortable.
  b. Client will receive needed care.
  c. Client will maintain significant relationships.
  d. Client will die with dignity.
	3. Others can promote hope. Their support can help the client to gain confidence and autonomy.

4. Encourage client to appreciate the fullness of each moment, each day.	4. Redirecting thoughts can produce growth and strength even in a time of conflict.

5. Promote a positive psychosocial environment through measures such as the following:
  a. Providing favorite foods
  b. Encouraging personalization of the room
  c. Keeping the room clean and comfortable
	5. These techniques show that the client is respected and valued.

6. Help client to identify purpose in his life such as these ways:
  a. Model for others
  b. Love
  c. Advice
	6. The dying person can provide others with a gift—an example of how to live with imminent death and how to control one's death.

7. Provide client with a sense of confidence and assurance that he or she can deal with cancer. Explain that the nurse can be relied on to guide the client along the way.	7. A guide provides support and direction (Bushkin, 1993).

 Documentation

Progress notes
  Dialogues
  Emotional, spiritual status

High Risk for Spiritual Distress Related to Fear of Death, Overwhelming Grief, Belief System Crisis

Focus Assessment Criteria	**Clinical Significance**
1. Doubting or loss of faith	1–3. The stresses of terminal illness may threaten a client's relationship with a higher being, his beliefs, or others.
2. Religious practices, religious leader (access, visits)	
3. Present response (anger, guilt, self-hate, sadness)	

Goal

The client will express desire to perform religious or spiritual practice.

Indicators
* Express feelings regarding beliefs.
* Discuss the meaning and purpose of illness and death.

Interventions	Rationales
1. Communicate willingness to listen to the client's feelings regarding spiritual distress.	1. Client may view anger at God and a religious leader as a "forbidden" topic and may be reluctant to initiate discussions of spiritual conflicts.
2. Suggest contact with another spiritual support person, such as the hospital chaplain, if client is reluctant to share feelings with his or her usual spiritual advisor.	2. Other contacts may help client to move toward a new spiritual understanding.
3. Explore if client desires to engage in a religious practice or ritual and accommodate his or her request to the extent possible.	3. The client may value prayer and spiritual rituals highly.
4. Offer to pray with him or her or to read from a religious text.	4. This can help to meet client's spiritual needs.

🖐 Documentation

Progress notes
    Dialogues
    Interventions
    Spiritual status
    Referrals

High Risk for Ineffective Therapeutic Regimen Management Related to Insufficient Knowledge of Home Care, Pain Management, Signs and Symptoms of Complications, and Community Resources Available

Focus Assessment Criteria	Clinical Significance
1. Willingness and ability of caregiver(s) to learn treatment measures, manage equipment, and perform needed care	1,2. The wide-ranging aspects and consequences of end-stage cancer require that caregivers be well versed in all aspects of care.
2. Understanding home care needs	

Goals

The goals for this diagnosis represent those associated with discharge planning. Refer to the discharge criteria.

Interventions	Rationales

1. Discuss home care needs:
  a. Treatments:
    • Pressure ulcer care
    • Feeding tubes
    • Wound care
    • Tube care
    • Injections
    • Tracheostomy care
    • Ostomy care
    • Denver shunt management
  b. Equipment:
    • Supplemental oxygen
    • Suction equipment
    • IV equipment
    • Assistive devices (e.g., walker, wheelchair)
  c. Care needs:
    • Positioning
    • Feeding and bathing techniques
    • Transfer techniques
    • Injury prevention strategies
	1. Each client has specific individual care needs. Understanding can maximize treatment effectiveness.

2. Teach home care measures and evaluate ability.
  a. Provide written teaching materials for treatments and equipment when feasible.
  b. Demonstrate procedures, equipment, and care measures.
  c. Have the caregiver return demonstration under supervision until skill is evident.
  d. Provide for practice to increase caregiver's skill.
  e. Encourage verbalization of questions and concerns.
  f. Provide positive reinforcement.
	2. Specific instructions can reduce fear related to lack of knowledge and help the nurse determine what follow-up teaching is needed.

3. If renal insufficiency is present, use opioids with short-half lives such as oxycodone, fentanyl, or hydromorphone.	3. Renal insufficiency allows opioid metabolites, especially morphine, to accumulate and cause opioid toxicity.

4. Monitor for signs/symptoms of opioid toxicity:
  • Hallucinations
  • Myoclonus (muscle spasms)
  • Hyperirritability
	4. Excess metabolites cause opioid toxicity, which requires lowering the dose or changing the type of opioid.

5. Consider changing type of opioid because it is ineffective or has adverse effects.	5. Changing opioids may be required until there is a balance between pain relief and side effects (Panke, 2002).

(continues on page 592)

Interventions continued	**Rationales** continued
6. Consider sedation with clients who have advanced disease when intractable pain continues (Quill & Byock, 2000).	6. The primary goal is no longer prolongation of life but achieving optimal comfort for people with a do-not-resuscitate (DNR) status.
7. Consult with person and family for sedation use. Advise that sedation can be reduced and can be resumed anytime (Quill & Byock, 2000).	7. Consultation is needed to provide clear explanations and to acquire informed consent (Panke, 2002).
8. Clearly communicate the client's and family's decisions to the staff in the plan of care.	8. Controversies regarding the use of sedation at end of life are distinguishable from euthanasia (Panke, 2002).
9. Explain how and where to obtain needed equipment and supplies.	9. Knowledge of access postdischarge can reduce some apprehension and facilitate care.
10. Teach signs and symptoms that must be reported to a health care professional: a. Change in mental status, visual changes, or muscle coordination b. Muscle cramps, numbness c. Increasing dyspnea, edema, abdominal distention d. Increasing sedation, decreasing respirations e. Skeletal pain, loss of movement f. Neck or back pain, motor deficits, sensory deficits (e.g., paresthesias) g. Change in bowel or bladder function h. Facial edema, dyspnea, distended neck veins	10. Early reporting may enable prompt interventions to reduce or eliminate certain complications. a. Neurological changes may indicate cerebral metastasis, which can be sudden or insidious. Cancers of the lung, breast, testicles, thyroid, kidney, prostate, melanoma, and leukemia are associated with cerebral metastasis. b. Muscle cramps and numbness may point to calcium imbalance. c. These symptoms may indicate malignant effusions (pleural, ascites, pericardial). d. Sedation and respiratory depression may indicate narcotic toxicity. e. Pain and limited movement may indicate pathological fracture. f. These signs and symptoms may point to cord compression. g. Bladder or bowel changes may result from cord compression or ascites. h. These effects may indicate superior vena cava syndrome (SVCS), which is associated with lung cancer, breast cancer, and lymphoma.
11. If skeletal pain, loss of movement, or neck or back pain occurs, teach client to maintain bed rest and to immobilize the area until a health professional can examine it.	11. Immobilization helps to prevent further tissue damage.

(continues on page 593)

Interventions continued	Rationales continued
12. Discuss possible cancer- and death-related stressors, such as financial burdens, role responsibility changes, and dependency, with the family.	12. Terminal illness entails a wide range of stressors. Preparing the family for possible problems enables planning to prevent or minimize them.
13. Provide information about or initiate referrals to community resources (e.g., hospice, counselors, home health agencies, American Cancer Society).	13. Assistance may be needed with home management and with minimizing the potential destructive effects on the client and family.

 Documentation

Discharge summary record
Client teaching
Outcome achievement or status
Referrals if indicated

LEUKEMIA

In normal bone marrow, efficient regulatory mechanisms ensure a balance between cell proliferation and maturation and the needs of the individual. This control is missing or abnormal in leukemia, which results in arrest of the cell during maturation. This produces an abnormal proliferation of these immature cells, which crowd other marrow elements. The end results are inhibited growth and function of these elements, and gradual replacement of the marrow by leukemia cells.

Leukemia is classified according to the cell line involved. Acute myelogenous leukemia involves a malignant clone that arises in the myeloid, monocyte, erythroid, or megakaryocyte cells. Acute lymphocytic leukemia involves abnormal lymphoblast clones in the marrow, thymus, and lymph nodes. Chronic lymphocytic leukemia involves proliferation of long-lived incompetent lymphocytes. Chronic myelogenous leukemia involves proliferation of mature granulocytes in the bone marrow (Wujcik, 2000).

Hairy cell leukemia involves a proliferation of cytoplasmic projections on circulating mononuclear cells (Wujcik, 2000). The exact cause of leukemia is unknown, but the key event is damage to the DNA of the hematopoietic stem cells. Some presumed causes are chemicals (e.g., pesticides), medications (e.g., actinomycin), smoking, ionizing radiation, genetic factors, and viruses (e.g., Epstein-Barr).

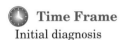 **Time Frame**

Initial diagnosis

 ⦾⦾ **DIAGNOSTIC CLUSTER*** **Collaborative Problems** PC: Bone Marrow Depression PC: Leukostasis PC: CNS Involvement PC: Massive Splenomegaly	
Nursing Diagnoses	**Refer to**
High Risk for Infection related to increased susceptibility secondary to leukemic process and side effects of chemotherapy	
High Risk for Ineffective Therapeutic Regimen Management related to insufficient knowledge of disease process, treatment, signs and symptoms of complications, reduction of risk factors, and community resources.	
High Risk for Impaired Social Interactions related to fear of rejection or actual rejection of others after diagnosis	Cancer (Initial Diagnosis)

(continues on page 595)

Nursing Diagnoses continued	Refer to continued
Powerlessness related to inability to control situation	Cancer (Initial Diagnosis)
High Risk for Ineffective Sexual Patterns related to fear secondary to potential for infection and injury	Cancer (Initial Diagnosis)
Related Care Plans Chemotherapy Cancer (Initial Diagnosis)	

* This medical condition was not included in the validation study.

Discharge Criteria

Before discharge, the client or family will

1. Describe the home care regimen including restrictions.
2. Identify the signs and symptoms of complications that must be reported to a health care professional.
3. Describe the necessary follow-up care.
4. Verbalize an awareness of available community resources.
5. Identify function of bone marrow including cell lines.

Collaborative Problems

Potential Complication: Bone Marrow Depression

Potential Complication: Leukostasis

Potential Complication: CNS Involvement

Potential Complication: Massive Splenomegaly

Nursing Goal

The nurse will detect early signs and symptoms of (a) bone marrow depression, (b) leukostasis, (c) CNS toxicity, and (d) massive splenomegaly, and collaboratively intervene to stabilize client.

Indicators
- Alert, oriented (c)
- Neutrophils 60% to 70% (a, b, d)
- Red blood cells (a, b, d)
    ○ Male: 4.6–5.9 million/mm^3
    ○ Female: 4.2–5.4 million/mm^3
- Platelets 150,000–400,000/mm^3 (a, b, d)
- No petechiae or purpura (a, b, d)
- No gum or nasal bleeding (a, b, d)
- Regular menses (a, b, d)
- No headache (c)
- Clear vision (c)
- Intact coordination, facial symmetry, and muscle strength (c)
- No splenomegaly (d)

Interventions	Rationales

1. Monitor for bone marrow depression:
  a. Decreased neutrophils
  b. Decreased red blood cells
  c. Decreased platelets
	1. Each day bone marrow produces and releases into the circulation red cells, platelets, and granulocytes to maintain hemostasis and oxygen requirements. In addition, the bone marrow participates in the defense against foreign invasion with antibody synthesis, initiating phagocytosis and antigen processing (Hays, 1990; Wujcik, 2000). Leukemia cells proliferate and infiltrate the bone marrow, decreasing red blood cells, platelets, and granulocytes.

2. Monitor for disseminated intravascular coagulation (DIC):
  a. Easy bruising
  b. Epistaxis
  c. Menorrhagia
  d. Gingival bleeding
  e. Central nervous system (CNS) hemorrhage
  f. Thrombosis (chronic DIC)
	2. DIC may occur with any acute leukemia but more often with acute promyelocytic. The cause is extensive triggering of the coagulation system. Excessive circulating thromboses may be the triggering cause in leukemia. At some point, the extensive hypercoagulation consumes available clotting factors, resulting in the body's inability to form stable clots (Gobel, 2000; Wujcik, 2000).

3. Report WBC counts over 50,000 to the physician; prepare to administer high doses of cytotoxic drugs.	3. Individuals with many circulating blasts are at risk for leukostasis. Leukostasis occurs when vessel walls rupture as the result of excessive numbers of blast cells (Wujcik, 2000).

4. Monitor for CNS leukemia:
  a. Altered level of consciousness
  b. Headaches
  c. Blurred vision
  d. Change in coordination, facial symmetry, or muscle strength
	4. CNS involvement can result from infiltration of leukemic cells into the cerebrospinal fluid, which increases intracerebral pressure and compresses cerebral tissue.

5. Complete a neurologic assessment before administering high-dose cytosine arabinoside (HDCA).	5. Cerebellar toxicity is a CNS toxic effect of high-dose HDCA (Wujcik, 2000).

6. Monitor for massive splenomegaly:
  • Enlarged spleen
  • Thrombocytopenia (decreased platelets)
  • Petechiae (pin point purplish-red spots)
  • Purpura (purple areas of bruising)
	6. Leukemia cells proliferate and infiltrate the spleen. Replacement of bone marrow by leukemia cells results in decreased platelet production (Porth, 2002).

(continues on page 597)

Interventions continued	**Rationales** continued
7. Teach client to assess for signs of bleeding every day to every shift as necessary (Gobel, 2000):	7. Regular total body assessment is necessary to detect early signs of bleeding, which is the second leading cause of death in leukemia. As platelet count decreases, the risk of bleeding increases as follows (Gobel, 2000):
a. Integumentary system: • Petechiae • Ecchymoses • Hematomas • Oozing from venipuncture sites • Cyanotic patches on arms/legs	a. >100,000: no risk
b. Eyes and ears: • Visual disturbances • Periorbital edema • Subconjunctival hemorrhage • Ear pain	b. 100,000–50,000: minimal risk
c. Nose, mouth, and throat: • Petechiae • Epistaxis • Tender or bleeding gums	c. 50,000–20,000: moderate risk
d. Cardiopulmonary system: • Crackles and wheezes • Stridor and dyspnea • Tachypnea and cyanosis • Hemoptysis	d. <20,000: severe risk
e. Gastrointestinal system: • Pain • Bleeding around rectum • Occult blood in stools	
f. Genitourinary system: • Bleeding • Increased menses • Decreased urine output	
g. Musculoskeletal system: • Painful joints	
h. Central nervous system: • Mental status changes • Vertigo • Seizures • Restlessness	
8. Transfuse blood components as ordered.	8. Potential transplant candidates should receive leuco-depleted blood products. Most clients need a specific blood component (e.g., platelets, plasma) (Gobel, 2000).
9. Minimize invasive procedures; avoid the following: a. Rectal temperatures b. Suppositories c. IM and SC injections d. Vaginal douches e. Bladder catheterization	9. Invasive procedures can cause tissue trauma and sources of infection (Gobel, 2000).

(continues on page 598)

Interventions continued	Rationales continued
10. Apply pressure to puncture sites for 3 to 5 minutes.	10. This prevents prolonged bleeding from puncture sites, which can cause damage to underlying structures such as nerves.

◤ Related Physician-Prescribed Interventions

Medications. Prednisone, antineoplastics, stool softeners, anthracycline, antiemetics, cyclophosphamide, analgesics, methotrexate, antineoplastics, teniposide, 6-mercaptopurine, cytarabine, am sarcine, idarubicin, interferon-alfa, vitamin D_3, all-trans-retinoic acid

Intravenous Therapy. Granulocyte transfusion, platelet transfusion, blood transfusion, electrolyte support, medication administration

Laboratory Studies. Reverse-transcriptase, polymerase chain reaction, complete blood count with differential, urinalysis, liver enzyme levels, BUN level, chemistry, prothrombin time, blood cultures, partial thromboplastin time, uric acid level, polymerase chain reaction, serum markers (see Cancer: Initial Diagnosis)

Diagnostic Studies. Bone marrow aspiration, tomography scan, chest X-ray film, liver-spleen scan, lumbar puncture, flow cytometric typing, electron microscopy, intracranial radiation, cytochemistry, immunophenotype

Therapies. Nutritional supplements, splenectomy, bone marrow transplant

Documentation
Flow records
   Intake and output
   Vital signs
   Weight
   Physical assessment
   Neurologic checks
Progress notes
   Abnormal assessment findings
   Interventions
   Response to interventions

Nursing Diagnoses

High Risk for Infection Related to Increased Susceptibility Secondary to Leukemic Process and Side Effects of Chemotherapy

Focus Assessment Criteria	Clinical Significance
1. History of infections	1. Infections in clients with leukemia result from the combined effects of bone marrow depression, treatment, invasive procedures, and hospitalization.
2. Vital signs	2. People with leukemia tend not to produce an inflammatory response; therefore, typical response to pathogens will not be present. A single elevation above 101.2°F with neutropenia should be reported.

(continues on page 599)

Focus Assessment Criteria continued	Clinical Significance continued
3. Biopsy, puncture, and catheterization sites	3–6. Most infections in clients with neutropenia are from the sinuses, skin, respiratory system, and gastrointestinal tract.
4. Respiratory system: cough, sputum, lung fields	
5. Gastrointestinal system: nausea, vomiting, diarrhea, perianal area	
6. Genitourinary system: intake and output, urine characteristics, frequency, burning, perineal area	
7. Laboratory values: WBCs, in particular granulocytes, cultures	7. WBCs, particularly granulocytes, are the first line of defense against infection. As levels decrease, susceptibility to infection increases as follows: a. 2,500–2,000/mm³: no risk b. 2,000–1,000/mm³: minimal risk c. 1,000–500/mm³: moderate risk d. <500/mm³: severe risk
8. Medication use (e.g., corticosteroids, antipyretics)	8. Corticosteroids and antipyretics mask signs and symptoms of infection, particularly fever (electron microscopy).

Goal

The client will report risk factors and precautions needed.

Indicators
- Identify risk factors that can be reduced.
- Relate early signs and symptoms of infection.

Interventions	Rationales
1. Institute measures to prevent exposure to known or potential sources of infection: a. Maintain protective isolation in accordance with institutional policy. b. Maintain meticulous handwashing. c. Provide scrupulous hygiene. d. Restrict visitors with colds, flu, or infections. e. Provide good perianal hygiene twice daily and after each bowel movement (e.g., sitz baths). f. Restrict fresh flowers and plants. g. Restrict fresh fruits and vegetables. h. Use mouth care protocol. i. Care for neutropenic clients first.	1. These precautions minimize client's exposure to bacterial, viral, and fungal pathogens, both exogenous and endogenous.

(continues on page 600)

Interventions continued	Rationales continued
2. Notify physician of any changes in vital signs.	2. Subtle changes in vital signs, particularly fever, may be only early signs of sepsis.
3. Obtain cultures of sputum, urine, diarrhea, blood, and abnormal body secretions as ordered.	3. Cultures can confirm infection and identify the causative organism.
4. Explain reasons for precautions and restrictions.	4. Client's understanding may improve compliance and reduce risk factors.
5. Reassure client and family that the increased susceptibility to infection is only temporary.	5. Granulocytopenia can persist for 6 to 12 weeks. Understanding the temporary nature of granulocytopenia may help to prevent client and family from becoming discouraged.
6. Minimize invasive procedures (e.g., rectal and vaginal examinations, indwelling [Foley] catheter insertion, and IM injections).	6. Certain procedures cause tissue trauma, increasing the susceptibility to infection.
7. Optimal nutrition supports protein synthesis and phagocytosis.	7. Explain the importance of good nutrition and vitamin and mineral supplementation.

🖐 Documentation

Flow records
    Vital signs
    Intake and output
    Assessments
    WBC/granulocyte count
Progress notes
    Abnormal findings or complaints
Discharge summary record
    Client teaching

High Risk for Ineffective Therapeutic Regimen Management Related to Insufficient Knowledge of Disease Process, Treatment, Signs and Symptoms of Complications, Reduction of Risk Factors, and Community Resources

Focus Assessment Criteria	Clinical Significance
1. Understanding of condition, past experiences with cancer	1. This assessment helps nurse to identify learning needs and plan appropriate teaching strategies.

(continues on page 601)

Focus Assessment Criteria continued	Clinical Significance continued
2. Life style, personal strengths, coping mechanisms, available support systems	2. Health professionals recognize that cancer is a chronic disease that can be cured or controlled with treatment. In the general public, however, the term *cancer* conjures thoughts of death. Lack of knowledge and negative attitudes about cancer coupled with the unfamiliarity of medical treatments and the hospital environment cause most newly diagnosed clients to respond with anxiety and fear, even when the prognosis is good. The physiologic and psychological effects of treatments produce changes in body image, life style, and function that also can contribute to fear and anxiety.

Goals

The goals for this diagnosis represent those associated with discharge planning. Refer to the discharge criteria.

Interventions	Rationales
1. Explain leukemia to client and family including the following aspects: a. Pathophysiology b. Function of bone marrow and its specific components c. Potential complications (e.g., infection, anemia, and bleeding)	1. Providing specific information about leukemia may improve compliance by helping client and family to understand the need for treatments and precautions (Wujcik, 2000).
2. Explain that anemia causes fatigue; stress the need for energy conservation. (Refer to the nursing diagnosis Fatigue in the Inflammatory Joint Disease care plan for specific strategies.)	2. Anemia results from inadequate red blood cell production secondary to increased WBC production. Energy conservation reduces fatigue (Wujcik, 2000).
3. Teach the importance of optimal nutrition.	3. Adequate intake of protein, carbohydrates, vitamins, and minerals is required for tissue rebuilding and increased resistance to infection.
4. Provide written information about and applications for registration to the Leukemia Society of America and local leukemia foundations.	4. These resources can provide emotional support and possibly financial assistance.

(continues on page 602)

Interventions continued	**Rationales** continued
5. Teach client the importance of good oral care and to inspect oral mucous membranes daily.	5. Inadequate defense mechanisms (e.g., abnormal WBC count, bone marrow suppression) increase the risk for infection.
6. Teach client the importance of good peri-anal hygiene and avoiding constipation and rectal trauma (e.g., enemas, thermometers).	6. Rectal abscesses can occur from trauma and constipation, increasing the susceptibility to infection.
7. Teach to avoid all immunizations.	7. An immunosuppressed client must avoid immunization because he or she lacks the ability to build antibodies and can contract the disease from the immunization.
8. Consult with pharmacist or physician before using over-the-counter (OTC) drugs.	8. Many OTC medications inhibit platelet functioning.
9. Teach measures to avoid bacteria in the diet: a. Avoid raw fruits and vegetables. b. Avoid fried foods in restaurants.	9. These foods are a potential source of bacteria pathogens.
10. Teach client to report the following signs of (Wujcik, 1996): a. Infection: • Fever • Excess cough and sputum production • Burning with urination b. Anemia: • Dyspnea • Increasing weakness c. Bleeding: • Nosebleeds • Blood in stools • Cloudy urine • Bruises	10. These signs and symptoms may indicate need for additional treatment (e.g., NSAIDS, aspirin).
11. Provide soft toothbrushes or sponges for oral hygiene. Explain the following to client and family: a. Rationales for precautions b. Signs and symptoms they must report to a health care professional c. The need to avoid medications that interfere with platelet function; provide a list.	11. This can help to prevent damage to oral mucosa, which is susceptible to bleeding and flossing. The client's and family's understanding can encourage compliance and reduce anxiety. Include function of platelets (Gobel, 2000).

(continues on page 603)

Interventions continued	**Rationales** continued

12. Teach client to avoid:
   a. Forceful coughing, sneezing, or nose blowing
 	
   b. Constipation and bowel straining
	12.
	   a. Epistaxis can be life threatening in a person with decreased platelets (Gobel, 2000).
	   b. Rectal bleeding can result from straining (Gobel, 2000).

13. Teach the importance of informing all health care providers about diagnosis:
   a. Dentist and hygienist
   b. Phlebotomist
	13. Precautions may be needed to prevent bleeding.

14. Encourage client to continue usual social activities as tolerated.	14. Long-term survivors report personal relationships to be the most important indicator for a positive quality of life (Zebrack, 2000).
15. Provide opportunities to discuss how the experience of leukemia has affected client's and family members' lives.	15. Some persons living with leukemia report a high ability to cope with stressors (Zebrack, 2000).
16. Consider referrals to counselors and therapists as needed.	16. Individuals facing a life-threatening condition may need assistance with adaption.

🕑 Documentation

Discharge summary record
   Client teaching
   Outcome achievement or status
   Referrals if indicated

Clinical Situations

ALCOHOL WITHDRAWAL

Clinically, only one of every ten alcoholics is diagnosed and clinicians do not ask about alcohol use unless it is obvious. It is critical to identify people who abuse alcohol to prevent potentially fatal withdrawal symptoms. The focus of medical and nursing care is to prevent, not to observe for, the complications of alcohol withdrawal (Babel, 1997). Prevention includes aggressive management of early withdrawal and close monitoring of the client's response.

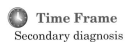 **Time Frame**

Secondary diagnosis

◯◯ DIAGNOSTIC CLUSTER*

Collaborative Problems   **Refer to**

PC: Delirium Tremens
PC: Autonomic Hyperactivity
PC: Seizures
PC: Alcohol Hallucinosis
PC: Hypovolemia   Thermal Injuries
PC: Hypoglycemia   Diabetes Mellitus

Nursing Diagnoses

- Imbalanced Nutrition: Less Than Body Requirements related to inadequate intake of balanced diet and water-soluble vitamins (thiamine, folic acid, and pyridoxine)
- High Risk for Deficient Fluid Volume related to abnormal fluid loss secondary to vomiting, diarrhea, dehydration, and diaphoresis
- High Risk for Violence related to (examples) impulsive behavior, disorientation, tremors, or impaired judgment
- Anxiety related to loss of control, memory losses, and fear of withdrawal
- Ineffective Coping: anger, dependence, or denial related to inability to constructively manage stressor without alcohol
- High Risk for Ineffective Therapeutic Regimen Management related to insufficient knowledge of condition, treatments available, high-risk situations, and community resources

---

* This clinical situation was not included in the validation study.

Discharge Criteria

The client will

1. Recognize that alcohol is a disease.
2. Acknowledge that alcoholism is not a healthy choice.
3. Identify treatments available for alcoholism.
4. Identify community resources available for skill building.

Collaborative Problems

Potential Complication: Delirium Tremens

Potential Complication: Autonomic Hyperactivity

Potential Complication: Seizures

Potential Complication: Alcohol Hallucinosis

Potential Complication: Hypovolemia

Potential Complication: Hypoglycemia

Nursing Goal

The nurse will detect early signs and symptoms of (a) delirium tremens, (b) autonomic hyperactivity, (c) seizures, (d) alcohol hallucinosis, (e) hypovolemia, and (f) hypoglycemia and will collaboratively intervene to stabilize the client.

Indicators

- No seizure activity (a, b, c)
- Calm, oriented (a, b, d)
- Temperature 98–99.5°F (d)
- Pulse, 60–100 beats/min (a, b, d)
- BP >90/60, <140/90 mm Hg (a, b, d)
- No reports of hallucinations (a, d)

Interventions	Rationales
1. Carefully attempt to determine if client abuses alcohol. Consult with family regarding perception of alcohol consumption. Explain why accurate information is necessary.	1. It is critical to identify high-risk clients so potentially fatal withdrawal symptoms can be prevented.
2. Obtain history of drinking pattern from client or significant others (Kappas-Larson & Lathrop, 1993). a. What was the day of last drink? b. How much was consumed on that day? c. On how many days of the last 30 did the client consume alcohol? d. What was the average intake? e. What was the most drank?	2. Alcoholics tend to underestimate alcohol consumed; therefore, multiply the amount a man tells you by two to three drinks and for a woman by four to five drinks (Smith-DiJulio, 2001).
3. Determine attitude toward drinking by asking CAGE questions. a. Have you ever thought you should *C*ut down your drinking? b. Have you ever been *A*nnoyed by criticism of your drinking? c. Have you ever felt *G*uilty about your drinking? d. Do you drink in the morning (i.e., *E*ye-opener) (Ewing, 1984)?	3. These questions can be used to identify possible defensiveness, pervasiveness, and attitudes about drinking.
4. Obtain history of previous withdrawals: a. Delirium tremens: • Time of onset • Manifestation	4. Withdrawal occurs between 6 to 96 hours after cessation of drinking. Withdrawal can occur in individuals who are considered "social drinkers" (6 oz of alcohol daily

(continues on page 609)

Interventions continued	**Rationales** continued
b. Seizures: • Time of onset • Type	for a period of 3 to 4 weeks). Withdrawal patterns may resemble those of previous episodes. Seizure patterns unlike previous episodes may indicate another underlying pathology (Babel, 1997).
5. Obtain complete history of prescription and nonprescription drugs taken.	5. Benzodiazepine or barbiturate withdrawal may mimic alcohol withdrawal and will complicate the picture. Substance abusers tend to cross-abuse substances (Babel, 1997).
6. Perform a physical examination to determine effects of alcohol-related conditions such as the following: a. Nutritional deficiencies b. Liver damage c. Hypertension d. Gastritis/ulcers e. Heart disease f. Emphysema g. Diabetes/hypoglycemia h. Acute pancreatitis i. Infections	6. The presence of any of these conditions will affect the medical regimen. Subjective histories are not always reliable with alcoholics. Alcoholics may not complain of symptoms.
7. Consult with primary provider regarding the client's risk and initiation of benzodiazepine therapy with dosage determined by assessment findings.	7. Benzodiazepine requirements in alcohol withdrawal are highly variable and client specific. Fixed schedules may oversedate or undersedate (Babel, 1997).
8. Observe for desired effects of benzodiazepine therapy: a. Relief from withdrawal symptoms b. Peaceful sleep but rousable	8. Benzodiazepine is the drug of choice in controlling withdrawal symptoms. Neuroleptics cause hypotension and lower seizure threshold. Barbiturates may effectively control symptoms of withdrawal but have no advantages over benzodiazepines (Babel, 1997).
9. Monitor for autonomic hyperactivity: a. Anxiety b. Insomnia c. Mild tachycardia d. Tremors e. Sensory hyperacuity f. Low-grade fever g. Disorientation h. Dehydration	9. Once a level drops ≤ 100 mg/dL below the person's normal level, he or she will typically manifest withdrawal. These symptoms can last up to 5 days. Withdrawal results in a hyper-metabolic state due to adrenergic excess and possible alteration of prostaglandin E_1 levels (Babel, 1997).
10. Monitor for withdrawal seizures: a. Determine time of onset.	10. Withdrawal seizures can occur between 6 to 96 hours after cessation of drinking.

(continues on page 610)

Interventions continued	**Rationales** continued
b. Refer to care plan for Seizure Disorders in index.	Seizures are usually nonfocal and grand mal, last for minutes or less, and occur singularly or in clusters of two to six (Babel, 1997).
11. Monitor for and intervene promptly in cases of status epilepticus: a. Follow institution's emergency protocol.	11. Status epilepticus is life threatening if not controlled immediately with IV diazepam.
12. Monitor for delirium tremens: a. Delirium component (vivid hallucinations, confusion, extreme disorientation, and fluctuating levels of awareness) b. Extreme hyperadrenergic stimulation (tachycardia, hypertension or hypotension, extreme tremor, agitation, diaphoresis, and fever)	12. Delirium tremens appears on either the 4th or 5th day after cessation of drinking and resolves within 5 days (Babel, 1997).
13. Monitor and determine onset of alcohol hallucinosis: • Visual, auditory, and tactile hallucinations, but the person senses that the hallucinations are not real and they are aware of their surroundings.	13. Alcohol hallucinosis occurs between 6 to 96 hours after abstinence and can last up to 3 days (Babel, 1997).
14. Monitor and restore fluid and electrolyte balances: a. Urine output b. Serum potassium c. Serum sodium d. Serum magnesium	14. Fluid and electrolyte losses from vomiting, profuse perspiration, and decreased antidiuretic hormone (from alcohol ingestion) cause dehydration. Increased neuromuscular activity can deplete magnesium/enil: IV glucose administration can cause intracellular shift of magnesium (Porth, 2002).
15. Monitor for hypoglycemia: a. Blood glucose	15. Alcohol depletes liver glycogen stores and impairs gluconeogenesis. Alcoholics also are malnourished (Nayduch, 2000).
16. Monitor vital signs every 30 minutes initially: a. Temperature, pulse, and respiration b. Blood pressure (BP)	16. Clients in withdrawal will have elevated heart rate, respirations, and fever. Those experiencing delirium tremens can be expected to have a low-grade fever. A rectal temperature greater than 99.9°F, however, is a clue to possible infection. Hypotension may be associated with pneumonia and a clue to infection (Porth, 2002).

(continues on page 611)

Interventions continued	Rationales continued

17. Monitor laboratory values:
   a. White blood cell count (WBC)
   b. Liver function studies
   c. Serum glucose
   d. Occult blood
   e. Albumin, prealbumin
   f. Serum alcohol level
   g. Electrolytes
	17. Laboratory values may indicate alcohol-related conditions as mentioned in 6. Alcohol abuse causes a range of immunopathologic events. In alcoholic liver disease, albumin is lowered because of decreased synthesis by liver and malnutrition (Porth, 2002).

18. Observe for side effects or overmedication of benzodiazepine therapy:
   a. Oversedation
   b. Slurred speech
   c. Ataxia
   d. Nystagmus
	18. All medications have a therapeutic window and are not without their side effects.

19. Maintain client IV running continuously.	19. Necessary for fluid replacement, dextrose, thiamine bolus, benzodiazepine, and magnesium sulfate administrations. Chlordiazepoxide and diazepam should not be given intramuscularly because of unpredictable absorption (Babel, 1997).
20. Control fever nonpharmacologically through use of cooling blankets, ice, and so forth.	20. Client may also have alcohol-related conditions such as varices, ulcers, gastritis, and cirrhosis that contraindicate the use of acetaminophen or ASA.

 Related Physician-Prescribed Interventions

Medications. Benzodiazepines, Dilantin, thiamine, multivitamins, folic acid, magnesium

Intravenous Therapy. Fluid replacement, dextrose 1 g/kg

Laboratory Studies. Complete blood cell count (CBC), serum prealbumin, liver function studies, serum potassium, serum glucose, serum sodium, serum alcohol level, serum magnesium, occult blood (stool), serum albumin

Diagnostic Studies. Electroencephalogram, if first occurrence of seizure or pattern changes

Therapies. Well-balanced diet with multivitamin supplement

 Documentation

Nursing history
Flow records
  Daily weight
  Vital signs
  Laboratory values
  Alcohol withdrawal symptoms
Progress notes
  Change in status
  Interventions
  Response to interventions

Nursing Diagnoses

Imbalanced Nutrition: Less Than Body Requirements Related to Inadequate Intake of Balanced Diet and Water-soluble Vitamins (Thiamine, Folic Acid, and Pyridoxine)

Focus Assessment Criteria	Clinical Significance
1. Intake (type of food, vitamin supplements)	1. Intake must be evaluated even if person appears well nourished because he or she has obtained calories from alcohol, not a well-balanced diet.
2. Weight (weekly)	2. Measurement is an indicator for evaluating results of change in diet.
3. Laboratory values: serum albumin, prealbumin	3. A lower serum albumin level is an indicator of malnutrition or decreased synthesis by liver (Dudek, 2001).

Goal

The client will relate what constitutes a well-balanced diet.

Indicators
- Describe the reasons for nutritional problems.
- Gain weight (specify amount).
- Relate need for vitamin supplements.

Interventions	Rationales
1. Discuss the importance of a well-balanced diet; the rationale for thiamine replacement; development and symptoms of Wernicke-Korsakoff syndrome (ophthalmoplegia, ptosis, palsy, disconjugate gaze, and altered consciousness). Effects of alcohol and thiamine depletion (Dudek, 2001).	1. Helping client to understand the benefits of well-balanced diet can improve compliance.
2. Provide three to four meals a day with multivitamins.	2. They will help restore nutritional status.
3. Maintain good oral hygiene (brush teeth and rinse mouth) before and after ingestion of food.	3. Accumulation of food particles in mouth can contribute to foul odors and taste that diminish appetite.

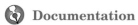 **Documentation**

Flow record
   Weight
   Intake (type and supplements)

High Risk for Deficient Fluid Volume Related to Abnormal Fluid Loss Secondary to Vomiting, Diarrhea, Dehydration, and Diaphoresis

Focus Assessment Criteria	Clinical Significance
1. Vital signs: blood pressure, temperature, pulse, and respirations	1–3. These assessments provide baseline data for comparison with subsequent assessment findings.
2. Skin turgor, mucous membranes, and urine output	
3. Consistency and frequency of stools	

Goal

The client will have moist mucous membranes and pale yellow urine with a specific gravity within normal limits.

Indicators

- Describe how alcohol causes dehydration.
- Maintain weight.

Interventions	Rationales

1. Monitor for early signs and symptoms of fluid volume deficit:
  a. Dry mucous membranes
  b. Amber urine
	1. Decreased circulating volume causes drying tissues and concentrated urine. Early detection enables prompt fluid replacement therapy to correct deficits.

2. Do not administer antiemetic medication.	2. Antiemetics lower seizure threshold.
3. Maintain patient IV running continuously.	3. This will replace fluid loss.
4. Monitor intake and output, making sure that intake compensates for output.	4. Dehydration may increase glomerular filtration rate, making output inadequate to clear wastes properly.
5. Weigh daily.	5. Accurate daily weights can detect fluid loss.

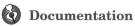 **Documentation**

Flow records
  Vital signs
  Intake and output
  Daily weights
  Medications
  Vomiting episodes

High Risk for Violence Related to (Examples) Impulsive Behavior, Disorientation, Tremors, or Impaired Judgment

Focus Assessment Criteria	Clinical Significance
1. Body language including affect and motor activity	1. Body language is an important indicator of impending violence especially when a person is unable to communicate emotions.
2. History of violence	2. History is also a strong predictor of violence

Goal

The client will have fewer violent responses.

Indicators

- Demonstrate control of behavior with assistance from others.
- Relate causative factors.

Interventions	Rationales
1. Promote interactions that increase client's sense of trust and value of self.	1. In agitated state, client may not be able to verbally express feelings but may act out these feelings in aggressive manner.
2. Establish an environment that decreases stimuli. a. Decrease noise level b. Soft lighting c. Personal possessions d. Single/semiprivate room e. Control number of people entering room	2. Client is already in an agitated/mentally compromised state, and environmental stimuli will unnecessarily increase this state and send client "over the edge."
3. Assess situations that have contributed to past violent episodes and attempt to modify the circumstances to prevent similar circumstances.	3. There can be a pattern to violence. Detecting and changing the pattern can eliminate the violence.
4. Assist individual in maintaining control over his or her behavior.	4. Losing control is a very frightening experience, more so than the violence.
5. If violence is imminent, systematically approach the individual with a group of four to five individuals. a. One nurse speaks to client and is in charge. b. One nurse for each limb.	5. This decreases the nurse's risk of danger, and the presence of four to five staff members reassures individual that the nursing staff will not let the client lose control.

(continues on page 615)

Interventions continued	Rationales continued
6. Use least resistive method of restraint for the shortest duration possible. a. Follow agency policy when using restraint.	6. This is in keeping with ethical and legal guidelines for restraint.
7. Make verbal contact with client as soon as possible after the aggressive incident.	7. This maintains client's sense of worth despite the aggressive behavior.
8. Initiate debriefing strategies among nursing staff involved in incident.	8. This allows nursing staff members to center themselves after critical and often unpleasant incidents.

🔖 Documentation

Progress notes
   Aggressive incident
   Actions taken
   Evaluation/outcome
Flow record
Restraint

Anxiety Related to Loss of Control, Memory Losses, and Fear of Withdrawal

Focus Assessment Criteria	Clinical Significance
1. Anxiety level: mild, moderate, severe, or panic	1. Extreme anxiety impairs learning and coping abilities. Assessment will provide indicator of the effectiveness of benzodiazepine therapy.
2. Past experience with withdrawals	2. Expectations and perceptions of withdrawal are influenced by past experiences. Withdrawals are extremely uncomfortable, and alcoholics try to avoid withdrawals.
3. Support system: availability and quality	3. Adequate support from family, friends, and other sources can provide comfort and help client to maintain self-esteem. Poor support can increase stress and impair coping ability.
4. Explain the effects of alcohol withdrawal on anxiety levels.	4. Helping client understand what is happening can decrease anxiety.

5. Teach and practice relaxation techniques when anxiety levels are lower.
   a. Deep breathing
   b. Progressive relaxation
   c. Imagery
   d. Music/Walkman
	5. Relaxation techniques can be transferred to other situations that cause anxiety to promote coping skills. Some theories in the field of addiction attribute alcoholism to uncontrolled or "free-floating" anxiety. Teaching can only be effective when anxiety levels are lower.

Goal

The client will report increased emotional comfort.

Indicators

- Relate cause of confusion and anxiety.
- Communicate feeling regarding present situation.

Interventions	Rationales
1. Create a quiet, calm environment. 2. Frequently orient client to time and place.	1,2. People experiencing withdrawal are anxious, hyperalert, terrified, and confused.
3. Encourage family or close friends (one at a time) to stay with person.	3. This may help to increase orientation.
4. Support efforts at recovery.	4. The person may be hostile, argumentative, and demanding with feelings of guilt and shame (Smith-DiJulio, 2001).
5. If person has illusions, hallucinations, or vivid nightmares, correct the misperception with a verbal explanation (e.g., "See they are not bugs, they are dots on the wallpaper").	5. Illusions and hallucinations are vivid and frightening; they result from severe disturbances in sensorium.

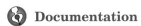 **Documentation**

Flow record
  Levels of anxiety and behavior response
Progress notes
  Unusual responses or situations

Ineffective Coping: Anger, Dependence, or Denial Related to Inability to Constructively Manage Stressors Without Alcohol

Focus Assessment Criteria	Clinical Significance

1. Emotional status and defense mechanisms:
   a. Anger
   b. Denial
   c. Self-esteem
   d. Perceived coping status
	1. Alcoholics use the denial defense mechanism to support their primary urge of drinking. Denial takes many and various forms such as excuse making, blaming, lying, minimizing, vagueness, power plays, and intellectualizing. These forms of denial impair the nurse–client relationship.

2. Family and social supports	2. Family and social supports are often severed and damaged as the alcoholism progresses. Family and social supports assist in the process of recovery.

Goal
The client will relate the intent to seek assistance after discharge.

Indicators
- Express painful emotions.
- Identify social supports.
- Practice self-esteem-building exercises.
- Label unsatisfactory protective behaviors.

Interventions	Rationales
1. Furnish a structured and supportive environment.	1. Structure is needed to control alcohol abuse. Support is needed to assist in the difficult task of withdrawing.
2. Increase client's awareness of unsatisfactory protective behaviors.	2. Alcohol abuse is an ineffective method of promoting self-care (Compton, 1989).
3. Empathically assist client to investigate thoughts and feelings so as to understand the source of pain.	3. Pain is the outcome of childhood experience when significant persons did not meet the child's unique needs and experiences (Nighorn, 1988).
4. Encourage clients to journal their thoughts, feelings, and behaviors.	4. Increases their awareness of the inter-relationship between thoughts, feelings, and behaviors (Carscadden, 1993).
5. Provide alternative ways to tolerate or handle painful emotions.	5. The alcoholic has difficulty tolerating painful emotions as a result of ego dysfunction and self-care deficits. They abuse alcohol to calm intense affects (Compton, 1989).

6. Encourage productive thinking patterns through the following:
  a. Positive self-talk
  b. Examining faulty assumptions about self/others
  c. Imagery
	6. Faulty or negative thinking is prevalent among alcoholics and stems from belief systems that started in their childhoods (Smith-DiJulio, 2001).

7. Reinforce positive coping behavior.	7. Reinforcement provides the feedback needed when new behaviors are tried.
8. Provide self-esteem–building exercises.	8. Self-esteem dysfunctions are critically involved with alcoholism (Nighorn, 1988).

(continues on page 618)

Interventions continued	Rationales continued
9. Encourage client to build social support networks through peer support groups and mobilization of friendship networks.	9. Chemicals lead addicts to develop a skewed sense of themselves and their relationships to the world. Peers can point out unrealistic views of self and world and also provide the needed emotional growth that was stunted by alcohol.
10. Access community program (e.g., individual counseling, AA).	10. Sobriety is a lifelong process.

Documentation

Progress notes
  Teaching
  Response to teaching

High Risk for Ineffective Therapeutic Regimen Management Related to Insufficient Knowledge of Condition, Treatments Available, High-risk Situations, and Community Resources.

Focus Assessment Criteria	Clinical Significance

1. Loss of control
  a. Drink more than planned
  b. Rules about use
  c. Break/dismiss rules
	1. Loss of control is an essential factor in making an accurate assessment of dependency along with withdrawal symptoms.

2. Social problems
  a. Change in friends
  b. Sexual acting out when drinking
  c. Friends complaining of alcohol use
	2. Social problems can be an early indicator of an alcohol problem.

3. Legal problems
  a. Driving infractions
  b. Assault
  c. Solicitation
  d. Burglary
  e. Drug trafficking
	3. The disease of alcoholism finds many substance abusers in a host of legal problems.

4. Family problems
  a. Family conflict
  b. Sexual problems with spouse
  c. Acting out of other family members
	4. The alcoholic's lack of emotional availability and hostility causes friction with loved ones, which builds into conflict and family squabbles.

5. Employment difficulties
  a. Coworker disputes
  b. Tardiness
  c. Absenteeism
  d. Inconsistent performance
  e. Labile, moody behavior
	5. For the gainfully employed, the job is often the last area to be affected by alcohol abuse. They hold the job as an example of how drinking is not a problem as well as because that income is needed to provide funds for alcohol.

Goals

The goals for this diagnosis represent those associated with discharge planning. Refer to discharge criteria.

Interventions	Rationales
1. Educate regarding the disease of alcoholism and its effects on self, family, job, and finances.	1. Learning alcoholism's effects can motivate a client to change behavior. It may be especially useful to do this while client experiences the discomforts of withdrawal.
2. Teach client to recognize and respond to the various alcohol-related medical conditions.	2. Continued alcohol abuse will lead to varying alcohol-related medical conditions as described in the collaborative problems.
3. Refer to community skill-building activities: a. Assertiveness training b. Stress management c. ADLs d. Anger management	3. The disease of addiction prevents individuals from learning adaptive social and other coping skills.
4. Improve family functioning through referral to community programs. a. Communication skills b. Boundaries and roles c. Education d. ALANON	4. Family functioning and individuals have suffered from the disease of alcoholism.

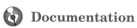 **Documentation**

Progress notes
  Teaching
  Response to teaching

IMMOBILITY OR UNCONSCIOUSNESS

This care plan addresses the needs of clients who are immobile and either unconscious or conscious. In addition to the following diagnostic cluster, refer to the specific coexisting medical disease or condition (e.g., renal failure and cancer).

⊗ DIAGNOSTIC CLUSTER

Collaborative Problems	Refer to
▲ PC: Pneumonia, Atelectasis	Cerebrovascular Accident (Stroke)
▲ PC: Fluid/Electrolyte Imbalance	General Surgery
▲ PC: Negative Nitrogen Balance	Chronic Renal Failure
△ PC: Sepsis	Urolithiasis
▲ PC: Thrombophlebitis	General Surgery
△ Renal Calculi	Chronic Renal Failure
△ PC: Urinary Tract Infection	Chronic Renal Failure
* PC: Osteoporosis	Corticosteroid Therapy

Nursing Diagnoses	Refer to
△ Disuse Syndrome related to effects of immobility on body systems	
▲ (Specify) Self-Care Deficit related to immobility	
△ Powerlessness related to feelings of loss of control and the restrictions placed on life style	
▲ High Risk for Ineffective Airway Clearance related to stasis of secretions secondary to inadequate cough and decreased mobility	COPD
▲ Total Incontinence related to unconscious state	Neurogenic Bladder
△ High Risk for Impaired Oral Mucous Membrane related to immobility to perform own mouth care and pooling of secretions	Pneumonia

▲ This diagnosis was reported to be monitored for or managed frequently (75%–100%).
△ This diagnosis was reported to be monitored for or managed often (50%–74%).
* This diagnosis was not included in the validation study.

Nursing Diagnoses

Disuse Syndrome Related to Effects of Immobility on Body Systems

Focus Assessment Criteria	Clinical Significance
1. Level of consciousness 2. Motor function in arms and legs 3. Mobility: ability to turn self, sit, stand, transfer, ambulate 4. Restrictive devices (e.g., casts, ventilator, Foley catheter, IV lines) 5. Range of motion: full or limited 6. Elimination pattern 7. Respiratory status 8. Circulatory status, skin condition 9. Intake and output	1–9. Musculoskeletal inactivity has adverse effects on all body systems. The nurse must assess the client's functional ability to determine the type and frequency of interventions required (Bullock, 1996; Milde, 1988).

Goal

The client will not experience complications of immobility.

Indicators
• Demonstrate intact skin and tissue integrity.
• Demonstrate maximum pulmonary function.
• Demonstrate maximum peripheral blood flow.
• Demonstrate full range of motion.
• Demonstrate adequate bowel, bladder, and renal functions.
• Explain rationale for treatments.
• Make decisions regarding care when possible.
• Share feelings regarding immobile state.

Interventions	Rationales
1. Explain the effects of immobility on body systems and the reason for interventions as indicated.	1. Understanding may help to elicit cooperation in reducing immobility.

2. Take steps to promote optimal respiratory function.
  a. Vary bed position, unless contra-indicated, to change the horizontal and vertical positions of the thorax gradually.
  b. Assist with repositioning, turning from side to side every hour if possible.
  c. Encourage deep breathing and controlled coughing exercises five times an hour.
	2. Immobility contributes to stasis of secretions and possible pneumonia or atelectasis. These measures help to increase lung expansion and the ability to expel secretions (Hickey, 2002).

(continues on page 622)

Interventions continued	**Rationales** continued
d. Teach to use a blow bottle or incentive spirometer every hour when awake. (A client with severe neuromuscular impairment may have to be awakened during the night as well.) e. For a child, try using colored water in the blow bottle; also have client blow up balloons, blow soap bubbles, blow cotton balls with a straw, and other "fun" breathing exercises. f. Auscultate lung fields every 8 hours or less if altered breath sounds occur. g. Encourage small, frequent feedings.	
3. Encourage increased oral fluid intake as indicated.	3. Optimal hydration liquefies secretions for easier expectoration and prevents stasis of secretions that provide a medium for microorganism growth.
4. Explain the effects of daily activity on elimination. Assist with ambulation when possible.	4. Activity influences bowel elimination by improving muscle tone and stimulating appetite and peristalsis.

5. Promote factors that contribute to optimal elimination.
  a. Balanced diet:
    • Review a list of foods high in bulk (e.g., fresh fruits with skins, bran, nuts and seeds, whole-grain breads and cereals, cooked fruits and vegetables, and fruit juices).
    • Discuss dietary preferences.
    • Encourage intake of approximately 800 g of fruits and vegetables (about four pieces of fresh fruit and a large salad) for normal daily bowel movement.
  b. Adequate fluid intake:
    • Encourage intake of at least 8 to 10 glasses (about 2,000 mL) daily unless contraindicated.
    • Discuss fluid preferences.
    • Set up a regular schedule for fluid intake.
  c. Regular time for defecation:
    • Identify normal defecation pattern before onset of constipation.
    • Review daily routine.
    • Include time for defecation as part of the regular daily routine.
    • Discuss a suitable time based on responsibilities, availability of facilities, etc.
	5.
	
	  a. A well-balanced diet high in fiber content stimulates peristalsis (McLane & McShane, 1992).
	
	  b. Sufficient fluid intake is necessary to maintain bowel patterns and promote proper stool consistency (McLane & McShane, 1992).
	
	  c. Taking advantage of circadian rhythms may aid in establishing a regular defecation schedule (McLane & McShane, 1992).

(continues on page 623)

Interventions continued	**Rationales** continued
• Suggest that client attempt defecation about an hour after a meal and remain in the bathroom a suitable length of time. d. Simulation of the home environment: • Have client use the bathroom instead of a bedpan if possible; offer a bedpan or a bedside commode if client cannot use the bathroom. • Assist client into position on the toilet, commode, or bedpan if necessary. • Provide privacy (e.g., close the door, draw curtains around the bed, play a television or radio to mask sounds, and make room deodorizer available). • Provide for comfort (e.g., provide reading materials as a diversion) and safety (e.g., make a call bell readily available). e. Proper positioning: • Assist client to a normal semisquatting position on toilet or commode if possible. • Assist onto a bedpan if necessary, elevating the head of the bed to high Fowler's position or to the elevation permitted. • Stress the need to avoid straining during defecation efforts.	d. Privacy and a sense of normalcy can promote relaxation, which can enhance defecation (McLane & McShane, 1992). e. Proper positioning uses the abdominal muscles and the force of gravity to aid defecation (McLane & McShane, 1992).
6. Institute measures to prevent pressure ulcers. (Refer to the Pressure Ulcers care plan for specific interventions.)	6. The immobile client is at risk for pressure ulcers—localized areas of cellular necrosis that tend to occur when soft tissue is compressed between a bony prominence and a firm surface for a prolonged period. Avoiding prolonged pressure can prevent pressure ulcer formation (Maklebust, Sieggreen, 2001).
7. Promote optimum circulation when the client is sitting. a. Limit sitting time for a client at high risk for ulcer development. b. Instruct client to lift self every 10 minutes using the chair arms if possible or assist client with this maneuver.	7. Capillary flow is increased if pressure is relieved and redistributed. Prolonged compromised capillary flow leads to tissue hypoxia and necrosis (Maklebust & Sieggreen, 2001).
8. With each position change, inspect areas at risk for developing ulcers: a. Ears b. Elbows c. Occiput	8. Certain areas over bony prominences are more prone to cellular compression (Maklebust & Sieggreen, 2001).

(continues on page 624)

Interventions continued	**Rationales** continued
d. Trochanter e. Heels f. Ischia g. Sacrum h. Scapula i. Scrotum	
9. Observe for erythema and blanching, palpate for warmth and tissue sponginess, and massage vulnerable areas lightly with each position change.	9. Erythema and blanching are early signs of tissue hypoxia. Deep massage can injure capillaries, but light massage stimulates local circulation (Maklebust & Sieggreen, 2001).

10. Teach the client to do the following:
  a. Elevate legs above level of the heart. (*Note:* This may be contraindicated if severe cardiac or respiratory disease is present.)
  b. Avoid standing or sitting with legs dependent for long periods.
  c. Consider using Ace bandages or below-knee elastic stockings.
 	
  d. Avoid using pillows behind the knees or a gatch on the bed elevated at the knees.
  e. Avoid leg crossing.
  f. Change positions, move extremities, or wiggle fingers and toes every hour.
  g. Avoid garters and tight elastic stockings above the knees.
  h. Perform leg exercises every hour when advisable.
	10.
	a,b. Immobility reduces venous return and increases intravascular pressure that contribute to venous stasis and thrombophlebitis (Caswell, 1993).
	
	c. Elastic stockings reduce venous pooling by exerting even pressure over the leg; they increase flow to deeper veins by reducing the caliber of the superficial vein (Caswell, 1993).
	d–g. External venous compression impedes venous flow (Caswell, 1993).
	
	h. Leg exercises promote the muscle pumping effect on the deep veins (Caswell, 1993).

11. Measure baseline circumference of calves and thighs daily if the client is at risk for deep venous thrombosis or if it is suspected.	11. Thrombophlebitis causes edema, which increases leg measurements (Caswell, 1993).

12. Institute measures to increase limb mobility.
  a. Perform range-of-motion (ROM) exercises as frequently as the client's condition warrants.
  b. Support limbs with pillows to prevent or reduce swelling.
  c. Encourage client to perform exercise regimens for specific joints as prescribed by physician or physical therapist.
	12. Joints without range of motion exercise develop contractures in 3 to 7 days because flexor muscles are stronger than extensor muscles (Maas, 1992).

(continues on page 625)

Interventions continued	**Rationales** continued
13. Take steps to maintain proper body alignment.	13. Prolonged immobility and impaired neurosensory function can cause permanent contractures (Hickey, 2002).
a. Use a footboard.	a. This measure prevents foot drop.
b. Avoid prolonged periods of sitting or lying in the same position.	b. This measure prevents hip flexion contractures.
c. Change position of the shoulder joints every 2 to 4 hours.	c. This measure can help to prevent shoulder contractures.
d. Use a small pillow or no pillow when client is in Fowler's position.	d. This measure prevents flexion contracture of the neck.
e. Support the hand and wrist in natural alignment.	e. This measure can help to prevent dependent edema and flexion contracture of wrist.
f. If client is supine or prone, place a rolled towel or small pillow under the lumbar curvature or under the end of the rib cage.	f. This measure prevents flexion or hyperflexion of lumbar curvature.
g. Place a trochanter roll or sandbags alongside hips and upper thighs.	g. This prevents external rotation of the femurs and hips.
h. If client is in the lateral position, place pillow(s) to support the leg from groin to foot and a pillow to flex the shoulder and elbow slightly; if needed, support the lower foot in dorsal flexion with a sandbag.	h. These measures prevent internal rotation and adduction of the femur and shoulder and prevent foot drop.
i. Use hand-wrist splints.	i. Splints prevent flexion or extension contractures of fingers and abduction of the thumbs.
14. Monitor for and take steps to reduce bone demineralization:	14. Lack of motion and weightbearing results in bone destruction that releases calcium into the bloodstream and results in hypercalcemia (Bullock & Henze, 2000).
a. Monitor for signs and symptoms of hypercalcemia (e.g., elevated serum calcium level, nausea and vomiting, polydipsia, polyuria, lethargy).	
b. Provide weightbearing whenever possible; use a tilt table if indicated.	
15. Take measures to prevent urinary stasis and calculi formation (Maas, 1992).	15. Peristaltic contractions of the ureters are insufficient in a reclining position and result in urine stasis in the renal pelvis.
a. Provide daily intake of fluid of 2,000 mL or greater (unless contraindicated).	a. Stones form more readily in concentrated urine.
b. Maintain urine pH below 6.0 (acidic) with acid ash foods (e.g., cereals, meats, poultry, fish, cranberry juice, and apple juice).	b. These measures reduce the formation of calcium calculi.
c. Teach client to avoid these foods: • Milk, milk products, and cheese • Bran cereals • Cranberries, plums, raspberries, gooseberries, olives	c. These foods are high in calcium and oxalate and can contribute to stone formation.

(continues on page 626)

Interventions continued	Rationales continued
• Asparagus, rhubarb, spinach, kale, Swiss chard, turnip greens, mustard greens, broccoli, beet greens • Legumes, whole grain rice • Sardines, shrimp, oysters • Chocolate • Peanut butter	

16. Maintain vigorous hydration unless contraindicated:
  a. Adult: 2,000 mL/day
  b. Adolescent: 3,000 to 4,000 mL/day
	16. Optimal hydration reduces the blood coagulability, liquefies secretions, inhibits stone formation, and promotes glomerular filtration of body wastes.

 Documentation

Flow records
  Exercise
  Turning
  Assessment results (circulatory, respiratory, skin)
Discharge summary record
  Client teaching

Self-Care Deficit (Specify) Related to Immobility

Focus Assessment Criteria	Clinical Significance
1. Self-feeding abilities 2. Self-bathing abilities 3. Self-dressing abilities 4. Self-toileting abilities 5. Motivation 6. Endurance	1–6. A baseline is needed to assess improvement in self-care activities.

Goal

The client will perform self-care activities (specify feeding, toileting, dressing, grooming, or bathing).

Indicators
• Demonstrate use of adaptive devices (specify) if necessary.
• Demonstrate optimal hygiene after care is provided.

Interventions	Rationales
1. Promote client's maximum involvement in feeding activities. a. Ascertain from client or family members what foods client likes and dislikes.	1. Eating has physiological, psychological, social, and cultural implications. Providing control over meals promotes overall well-being.

(continues on page 627)

Interventions continued	**Rationales** continued
b. Have client eat all meals in the same setting—pleasant surroundings that are not too distracting.	
c. Provide good oral hygiene before and after meals.	
d. Encourage client to wear dentures and eyeglasses as necessary.	
e. Place client in the most normal eating position suited to the physical disability (best is sitting in a chair at a table).	
f. Provide social contact during meals.	
g. Encourage eating of "finger foods" (e.g., bread, bacon, fruit, and hot dogs) to promote independence.	
h. To enhance independence, provide necessary adaptive devices (e.g., plate guard to avoid pushing food off plate, suction device under plate or bowl for stabilization, padded handles on utensils for a more secure grip, wrist or hand splints with clamp to hold eating utensils, special drinking cup, and rocker knife for cutting).	
i. Assist with setup if needed (e.g., opening containers, napkins, and condiment packages; cutting meat; and buttering bread).	
j. Arrange food so client has adequate amount of space to perform the task of eating.	
2. Promote client's maximum involvement in bathing activities:	2. Inability for self-care produces feelings of dependency and poor self-concept. With increased ability for self-care, self-esteem increases.
a. Bathing time and routine should be consistent to encourage greatest amount of independence.	
b. Encourage client to wear prescribed corrective lenses or hearing aid.	
c. Keep bathroom temperature warm; ascertain client's preferred water temperature.	
d. Provide for privacy during the bathing routine.	
e. Provide for adaptive equipment as needed (e.g., bath board for transferring to tub chair or stool, washing mitts with pocket for soap, adapted toothbrushes, shaver holders, and hand-held shower spray).	
f. Place bathing equipment in the location most suitable to client.	
g. Keep a call bell within reach if client is to bathe alone.	

(continues on page 628)

Interventions continued	Rationales continued

3. Promote client's maximum involvement in toileting activities:
  a. Observe client's ability to obtain equipment or get to the toilet unassisted.
  b. Provide only the amount of supervision and assistance necessary.
  c. Provide necessary adaptive devices to enhance independence and safety (e.g., commode chairs, spill-proof urinals, fracture bedpans, raised toilet seats, and support side rails for toilets).
  d. Avoid use of bedpans and urinals whenever possible; provide a normal atmosphere of elimination in the bathroom; use the same toilet to promote familiarity.
	3. These measures can reduce the embarrassment associated with assistance with toileting (Tracey, 1992).

4. Promote or provide assistance with grooming and dressing:
  a. Deodorant application daily
  b. Cosmetics of choice
  c. Hair care (shampoo and styling)
  d. Facial hair
  e. Nail and foot care
	4. Optimal personal grooming promotes psychological well-being (Tracey, 1992).

 Documentation

Progress notes
  Involvement in self-care

Powerlessness Related to Feelings of Loss of Control and the Restrictions Placed on Life Style

Focus Assessment Criteria	Clinical Significance
1. Understanding of activity restrictions 2. Perception of control 3. Effects on life style	1–3. A client's response to loss of control depends on the personal meaning of the loss, individual coping patterns, personal characteristics, and responses of others.

Goal

The client will verbalize the ability to influence selected situations.

Indicators
- Identify what factors can be controlled.
- Make decisions regarding his or her care.

Interventions	Rationales
1. Encourage client to share feelings and fears regarding restricted movement.	1. Open dialogue promotes sharing and well-being.

(continues on page 629)

Interventions continued	**Rationales** continued
2. Determine client's usual response to problems.	2. To plan effective care, nurse must determine whether the client usually seeks to change his or her own behaviors to control problems or expects others or external factors to control problems.
3. Encourage client to wear desired personal adornments (e.g., baseball cap, colorful socks) and clothes rather than pajamas.	3. Street clothes allow client to express his or her individuality, which promotes self-esteem and reduces feelings of powerlessness.

4. Plan strategies to reduce the monotony of immobility.
  a. Vary daily routine when possible.
  b. Have client participate in daily planning when possible.
  c. Try to make the routine as normal as possible (e.g., have client dress in street clothes during the day if feasible).
  d. Encourage visitors.
  e. Alter physical environment when possible (e.g., update bulletin boards, change pictures on the walls, rearrange furniture).
  f. Maintain a pleasant, cheerful environment. Position client near a window if possible. If appropriate, provide a goldfish bowl for visual variety.
  g. Provide various reading materials (or "books on tape" if impairment hinders reading ability), a television, and radio.
  h. Discourage excessive television watching.
  i. Plan some "special" activity daily to give client something to look forward to each day.
  j. Consider enlisting a volunteer to read to the client or help with activities if necessary.
  k. Encourage client to devise his or her own strategies to combat boredom.
	4. These measures may help to reduce the monotony of immobility and compensate for psychological effects of immobility (e.g., decreased attention span, decreased motivation).

5. Provide opportunities for client to make decisions regarding surroundings, activities, and routines, and short- and long-term goals as appropriate.	5. Mobility enables client to actualize decisions (e.g., when to eat, where to go, what to do). Loss of mobility can affect autonomy and control (Lubkin, 1995).
6. Encourage family members to request the client's opinions when making family decisions.	6. The family can provide opportunities for client to maintain role responsibilities; this can help to minimize feelings of powerlessness (Lubkin, 1995).

 Documentation

Progress notes
  Interactions
  Response

SEXUAL ASSAULT

Sexual assault is forced and violent oral, vaginal, or anal penetration of a person without his or her consent. This care plan focuses on nursing for a client who has been sexually assaulted and is hospitalized for injuries.

 Time Frame

Coexisting with (trauma requiring hospitalization)

DIAGNOSTIC CLUSTER*

Collaborative Problems   **Refer to**

PC: Sexually Transmitted Infection (STI)
PC: Unwanted Pregnancy
PC: Compartmental Syndrome

Nursing Diagnoses

- Rape Trauma Syndrome

Collaborative Problems associated with physical injuries sometimes caused by sexual assault include fractures, head injuries, abdominal injuries, and burns. Refer to the collaborative problem index for specific problems.
* This situation was not included in the validation study.

Discharge Criteria

The person will

1. Share feelings.
2. Describe rationales and treatment procedures.
3. Identify what needs to be done now and take steps toward the goals.
4. Relate the intent to seek professional help after discharge.
5. Identify members of support system and use them appropriately.

Collaborative Problems

Potential Complication: Sexually Transmitted Infection

Potential Complication: Unwanted Pregnancy

Nursing Goal

The nurse collaboratively intervenes to prevent (a) STIs and (b) unwanted pregnancy.

Indicators
- Continued negative results on pregnancy test (b)
- Continued negative results on chlamydia test (a)
- Continued negative results on gonorrhea test
- Continued negative results on microscopic examination of vaginal fluids (*Trichomonas vaginalis*)
- Continued negative results on rapid plasma reagin test (RPR)
- Continued negative HIV test

Interventions	Rationales
1. Explain the risks of STIs and pregnancy.	1. Both are possible results of sexual assault.
2. Screen individual cultures (cervical, urethra, rectal, oral) and blood specimens (syphilis, HIV).	2. Selected medications can eliminate pathogens that cause STIs.

3. Provide treatment 1 prophylaxis for:
  a. Chlamydia: Zithromax 1 gm
  b. Gonorrhea: Rocephin 250 mg IM (with 1% lidocaine as dilutant)
  c. Trichomonas: Flagyl 2 gm in two divided doses over 24 hours
  d. Syphilis: doxycycline 100 mg twice a day for 10 days
	3. The U.S. Centers for Disease Control recommends screening of all sexual assault victims (Feldhaus, 2002).

4. Explain risks of HIV transmission and prophylaxis (if within 48 hours of assault) (Moe & Grau, 2001).
  a. If desired, start medications immediately.
  b. If desired, provide 3 to 5 days of
   • Lamivudine 150 mg (one tablet every 12 hours)
   • Zidovudine 300 mg (one tablet every 12 hours).
  c. If assailant is known to be HIV positive, provide 5 days of
   • Zidovudine 300 mg (one tablet every 12 hours)
   • Indinavir 400 mg (2 tablets every 8 hours) or nelfinavir 250 mg (9 tablets every 12 hours).
	4. The seriousness of HIV infection has prompted HIV postexposure prophylaxis for sexually assaulted persons (Moe & Ledray, 2001).

5. Explain side effects of medications.	5. The client must understand side effects versus signs of diseases.

6. Determine if client is at risk for pregnancy.
  a. No contraceptive use
  b. No surgical sterilization
  c. History of infertility
  d. Premenopausal or postmenopausal
	6. At-risk clients should be identified (Feldhaus, 2002).

(continues on page 632)

Interventions continued	Rationales continued
7. Explain how emergency contraception (ECP) prevents implantation of fertilized egg.	7. ECP delays ovulation and interferes with tubal transport of egg or sperm (Arcangelo & Peterson, 2001).
8. If desired and within 72 hours of assault, provide ECP medication. Explain when to take the second dose.	8. ECP can cause nausea and vomiting from high estrogen content.
9. Provide antiemetic medication if needed.	

 Related Physician-Prescribed Interventions

Medications (refer to collaborative problems for specific medications). STD prophylaxis, ECP, HIV prophylaxis, antiemetics, analgesics, sedatives

Laboratory Studies. Vaginal, urethra, rectal cultures; HIV testing; RPR test; serum/urine drug screens

Diagnostic Studies. Microscopic examination of vaginal fluid smear (wet mount)

Documentation
Progress notes
  Present emotional status
  Interventions
  Responses in nursing interventions, police and counselor interviews, examination for evidence
  Subjective, objective, and general reactions
  Availability of significant others for support.
  Medications given and collection of specimens

Nursing Diagnoses

Rape Trauma Syndrome

Focus Assessment Criteria	Clinical Significance
1. Perception of event	1–4. Reaction depends on many variables:
2. Level of anxiety	• How frightening was the trauma?
3. Coping mechanisms	• How intense was the event?
4. Available support system	• How long did it last?
	• How was the victim coping before the event?

Goals
Refer to discharge criteria.

Interventions	Rationales
1. Provide interventions to decrease anxiety. 　a. Limit people to whom the victim must describe assault. 　b. Do not leave person alone. 　c. Maintain a nonjudgmental attitude. 　d. Show concern for person. 　e. Ensure confidentiality. 　f. Encourage talking. 　g. Allow person self-blame. 　h. Encourage problem solving. 　i. Enlist support system. 　j. Create a plan to increase sense of safety.	1. 　a. Repeatedly relating the incident increases shame and anxiety. 　b. Isolation can increase anxiety. 　c. This will lessen shame. 　d. Empathy will validate worth. 　e. This will encourage sharing. 　f. This helps person to sort feelings. 　g. This validates humanity. 　h. It increases client's sense of control. 　i. Support system provides some stability and safety. 　j. This will reduce fear and anxiety.
2. Assess for psychological responses: 　a. Subjective: 　　• Phobias, nightmares, and flashbacks 　　• Disbelief 　　• Denial and emotional shock 　　• Anger, fear, and anxiety 　　• Depression and guilt 　　• Expressions of numbness, shame, and self-blame 　　• Suicidal ideation 　　• With older adults, fear of losing independence 　　• Concerns about going mad, losing control, and having intrusive thoughts 　　• Difficulty with decision making 　b. Objective: 　　• Crying 　　• Silence, calm, composed 　　• Trembling hands 　　• Excessive bathing (seen particularly with child or adolescent) 　　• Avoiding interaction with others (staff and family) 　　• Wearing excessive clothing (two or three pairs of pants or panties) 　　• Pacing and excessive talking 　　• Mood swings and inappropriate laughing 　　• Self-abusive behaviors (head banging or scratching) 　　• Increased startle response	2. Careful recording of psychological responses assists in recording progress in therapy, planning treatment, or identifying those at greatest risk. Behavior can differ from individual to individual. Feelings can be fast and furious or slow, trance-like, mixed, or clear. 　Victims may experience a wide range of feelings; either expressed or controlled. Previous coping skills often dissipate.
3. Assist client to identify major concerns (psychological, medical, and legal) and his or her perception of needed help.	3. Sexual assault is always associated with coercion and threatened or actual violence. It is by this means the assailant takes control from the victim. Involving the victim in decision-making begins reestablishing a sense of control (Smith-DiJulio, 2001).

(continues on page 634)

Interventions continued	Rationales continued

4. Whenever possible, provide crisis counseling within 1 hour of rape trauma event (Kilpatrick, 1983).
  a. Ask permission to contact the rape crisis counselor.
  b. Be flexible and individualize approach according to person's needs.
	4. a,b. Victim empowerment is the primary antidote to the trauma of sexual assault (Smith-DiJulio, 2001).

5. Promote a trusting relationship by providing emotional support with unconditional positive regard and acceptance.
 	
  a. Stay with person during acute stage or arrange for other support.
  b. Brief person on police and hospital procedures during acute stage.
  c. Assist during medical examination and explain all procedures in advance.
  d. Help person to meet personal needs (bathing after examination and evidence has been acquired).
  e. Listen attentively to person's requests.
  f. Maintain unhurried attitude toward person and family.
  g. Avoid rescue feelings toward person.
  h. Maintain nonjudgmental attitude.
  i. Support person's beliefs and value system; avoid labeling.
  j. Reassure that symptoms are normal responses that will lessen and improve with time.
	5. Providing immediate and ongoing empathy and support prepares victims for referral to more in-depth psychological counseling (Tyra, 1993). Main issues in the acute stage are being in control, fearing being left alone, and having someone to listen (Smith-DiJulio, 2001).
	a–i. Helping and other deep interpersonal transactions demand a certain intensity of presence. Being with a client is attending in its deepest sense.
	    Victims are vulnerable to any statement that can be construed as blaming. Their normal defenses are weakened. When asked too many questions, clients can feel "grilled." This interferes with the rapport between helper and client. Statements are gentler forms of probes than questions (e.g., "I can see fear in your eyes; tell me about it" versus "Are you afraid?").
	
	j. The victim needs to understand that a wide range of behavior and emotional responses is normal.

6. Explain the care and examination she or he will experience (D'Epiro, 1986).
 	
  a. Maintaining eye contact, conduct the examinations in an unhurried manner.
 	
  b. Explain every detail before action.
 	
  c. During pelvic examination, explain the position and the instruments.
	6. Because the victim's right to deny or consent has been violently violated, it is important to seek permission for subsequent care (Heinrich, 1987). It is important to tell the patient as much as is practical or possible about what is happening and why. Even in life-threatening situations, any sense of control given to the victim is helpful.
	a. Unhurried and confident actions, eye contact, and affirming the victim is safe help to calm and assure that he or she is alive and worthy.
	b. Cognitive dysfunction impairs short-term memory (see Anxiety).
	c. The victim of rape needs to understand the common reactions to this experience. The evidentiary examination is

(continues on page 635)

Interventions continued	**Rationales** continued
	especially distressing because it can be reminiscent of the assault (Ledray, 1992).
7. Explain the legal issues and police investigation (Heinrich, 1987).	7. According to Backman (1990), reporting the crime to authorities is clearly associated with improved emotional outcomes for victims. This is an important step in helping the victim recognize the reality of the crime.

7. Explain the legal issues and police investigation (Heinrich, 1987).
   a. Explain the need to collect specimens for future possible court use.
   b. Explain that the choice to report the rape is the victim's.
   c. If the police interview is permitted:
      • Negotiate with victim and police for an advantageous time.
      • Explain to victim what kind of questions will be asked.
      • Remain with the victim during the interview; do not ask questions or offer answers.
      • If the officer is insensitive, intimidating, offensive in manner, or asks improper questions, discuss this with the officer in private. If the behavior continues, use proper channels and make a complaint.

7. According to Backman (1990), reporting the crime to authorities is clearly associated with improved emotional outcomes for victims. This is an important step in helping the victim recognize the reality of the crime.

8. Fulfill medical and legal responsibilities by documentation ([AALNC], 2001; Heinrich, 1987)
   a. History of rape (date, time, and place)
   b. Nature of injuries, use of force, weapons used, threats of violence or retribution, and restraints used
   c. Nature of assault (fondling, oral, anal, vaginal penetration, ejaculation, use of condom)
   d. Postassault activities (douching, bathing, showering, gargling, urinating, defecating, changing clothes, eating or drinking)
   e. Present state (use of drugs or alcohol)
   f. Medical history, tetanus immunization status, gynecologic history (last menstrual period), and last voluntary intercourse
   g. Emotional state and mental status
   h. Examination findings, smears/cultures taken, blood tests, evidence collected, and photographs (if appropriate)
   i. Document to whom, when, and what evidence is delivered
   j. Label all evidence with name, identification number, date, time collected, collector's name, and source

8. Strict adherence to procedures and policies can enhance the future legal case. When possible, a sexual assault nurse examiner (SANE) should manage the victim's care.

(continues on page 636)

Interventions continued	**Rationales** continued
9. If the attack was a drug-facilitated sexual assault (DFSA): a. Assess for possible involuntary drug ingestion: • Reports exist that victim appeared intoxicated within 15 minutes after drinking a beverage. • Victim remembers very little after drinking the beverage. • Victim awakens hours later undressed or partially dressed, or with vaginal or rectal soreness. • Victim reports nausea and vomiting upon awakening. b. If suspicious of DFSA (and within 72 hours of ingestion), collect blood and urine specimens while maintaining proper chain of custody. c. Document if victim has taken or used drugs recreationally or by prescription.	9. a. These signs and symptoms increase the probability of DFSA (Ledray, 2001). b. If the samples are to be used as evidence, proper handling must be strictly followed (Ledray, 2001). c. If this is not known ahead of time, the victim's credibility can be questioned (Ledray, 2001).
10. Provide interventions to assist with regaining control (Smith-DiJulio, 2001): a. Listen, listen, listen. b. Encourage verbalizing of thoughts and feelings. c. Empower survivors by involving them in decision making and in their treatment plan. Explore their identified needs.	10. a. Probably the best response is simply for the nurse to listen without judgment and ask more then once what to do to support the client's recovery (Carosella, 1995). b. Many traumatized people repeat their stories over and over. This is part of the healing and diminishes with time. c. Victims should not be forced to talk until they are ready. Having the name and number of a person to call helps when the client is ready.
11. Reassure that feelings and reactions are normal responses and accept where clients are in the recovery process: a. Crying or silence • Sit quietly with them. • Offer to listen when they are ready to talk. • Affirm and validate their feelings. • Reassure of normalcy: "You have a lot to be sad about." "I am here for you when you're ready to talk."	11. Expert nursing care can minimize victims' emotional trauma, prevent further victimization, and promote recovery. Whatever help the nurse offers, honest empathy and nonjudgmental listening are crucial. a. Emotional care must aim to convey respect and understanding; communicate empathy, reassurance, and support; encourage ventilation of feelings; preserve dignity; empower the victim; provide anticipatory guidance; and ensure adequate follow-up.

(continues on page 637)

Interventions continued	**Rationales** continued

b. Anger
  - Understand that anger can be displaced onto caregivers or significant others.
  - Redirect and acknowledge its validity: "You're very angry." "You have every right to be." "You were assaulted." "Who wouldn't be angry?"
  - Allow the anger.
  - Try not to personalize or be offended. It's not you they are angry with.
  - Later when clients are calmer, help to restore their dignity by calmly exploring the basis for their feelings.

b. Intense anger may cause feelings of being out of control or out of touch.

c. Self-blame, self-abuse, feeling repulsive
  - Avoid using "should," "ought to," "must," "never." These words can be interpreted as blaming.

  - Assure the victim that "rape exists because there are rapists, not because there are victims" (Carosella, 1995).
  - Reassure: "You made the right decisions. You survived."
  - Provide comfort measures.
  - Provide scented soaps, bubble bath, etc.

c.
  - Victims of rape feel vulnerable and repulsive to others. Feeling comfortable can increase the client's sense of security.
  - Comfort creates a sense of healing and eases feelings of dirtiness.

d. Flashbacks, dreams, night terrors.
  - Reassure clients that they are safe.
  - If possible do not leave them alone; phone support people.
  - Identify if there were triggers prompting the reaction.
  - Encourage rest and avoiding stress.

d. Dreams are an attempt to make sense of what happened. The most positive way to view dreams is as an attempt to reclaim power. Identifying triggers helps to link them to a past experience, rather than only the present. This differentiation begins to make the present feel safe.
  - Incidence of flashbacks increases with fatigue or stress.
  - Feeling empowerment means you can do something to avert or minimize future trauma.
  - We need order to feel safe: "Everyone said what helped most was routine, routine, routine."

e. Fear
  - Problem-solve ways to feel safer.
  - Turn to support system.
  - Plan days and engage in diversional activities.
  - Avoid stressful situations.
  - Be available.
  - Don't leave client alone.
  - Have victim change residence and telephone number.

(continues on page 638)

Interventions continued	Rationales continued
• Encourage use of objects that symbolize safety (nightlight). • Help victim to use coping methods that have previously proved effective. • Suggest that victim change locks. • Encourage victim to maintain routine. • Suggest self-defense classes.	

12. Explore available support systems. Involve significant others.
   a. Share with family and friends the victim's immediate needs for love and support.
   b. Encourage family to express feelings and to ask questions.
   c. Reassure the victim that his or her reactions are normal.
   d. Refer to counseling services.
 	
   e. Respect the victim's right to restrict unwanted visitors.
   f. Discuss fears of rejection.
   g. Explore sexual, intimate concerns.
   h. Encourage survivor to recognize positive responses or support from others.
   i. Expect many of the same reactions as the victim/survivor.
	a. Isolation can lead to withdrawal.
	
	d. Postponing professional help lengthens the time reactions persist and lengthens recovery.

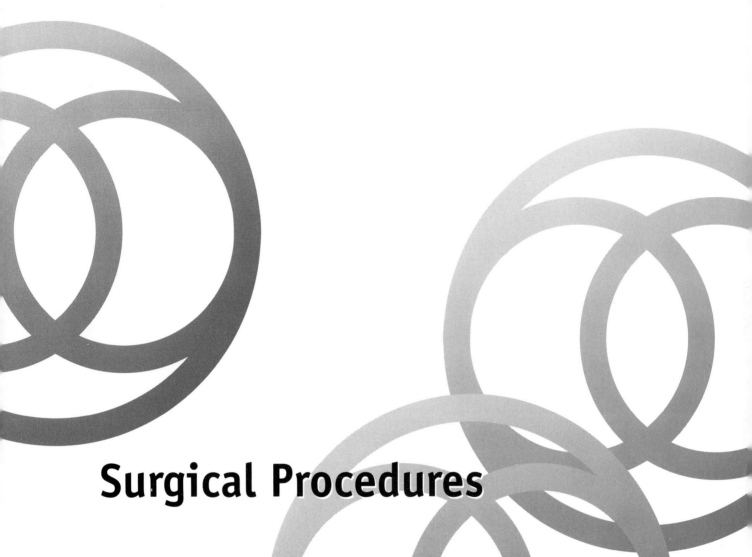

Surgical Procedures

GENERIC CARE PLAN
FOR THE SURGICAL CLIENT

Kathleen M. Killman, RN, C, MS

This care plan (Level I) presents nursing diagnoses and collaborative problems that commonly apply to clients (and their significant others) experiencing all types of surgery. Nursing diagnoses and collaborative problems specific to a surgical procedure are presented in the care plan (Level II) for that procedure.

 Time Frame

Preoperative and postoperative periods

 DIAGNOSTIC CLUSTER

Preoperative

Nursing Diagnosis

- Anxiety/Fear related to surgical experience, loss of control, unpredictable outcome, and insufficient knowledge of preoperative routines, postoperative exercises and activities, and postoperative changes and sensations

Postoperative

Collaborative Problems

PC: Hemorrhage
PC: Hypovolemia/Shock
PC: Evisceration/Dehiscence
PC: Paralytic Ileus
PC: Infection (Peritonitis)
PC: Urinary Retention
PC: Thrombophlebitis

Nursing Diagnoses

- Risk for Ineffective Respiratory Function related to immobility secondary to postanesthesia state and pain
- Risk for Infection related to a site for organism invasion secondary to surgery
- Acute Pain related to surgical interruption of body structures, flatus, and immobility
- Risk for Imbalanced Nutrition: Less Than Body Requirements related to increased protein and vitamin requirements for wound healing and decreased intake secondary to pain, nausea, vomiting, and diet restrictions
- Risk for Constipation related to decreased peristalsis secondary to immobility and the effects of anesthesia and narcotics
- Activity Intolerance related to pain and weakness secondary to anesthesia, tissue hypoxia, and insufficient fluid and nutrient intake
- Risk for Ineffective Therapeutic Regimen Management related to insufficient knowledge of care of operative site, restrictions (diet, activity), medications, signs and symptoms of complications, and follow-up care

---

Discharge Criteria

Before discharge, the client and/or family will

1. Describe any at-home activity restrictions.
2. Describe at-home wound and pain management.

3. Discuss fluid and nutritional requirements for proper wound healing.
4. List the signs and symptoms that must be reported to a health care professional.
5. Describe necessary follow-up care.

Preoperative: Nursing Diagnosis

Anxiety/Fear Related to Surgical Experience, Loss of Control, Unpredictable Outcome, and Insufficient Knowledge of Preoperative Routines, Postoperative Exercises and Activities, and Postoperative Changes and Sensations

Focus Assessment Criteria	Clinical Significance
1. Specific stressors and nature of concerns	1. Every client experiences some emotional reaction to surgery; the nature and degree of reaction depend on how client perceives the surgery and its anticipated effects—physical, psychological, financial, social, occupational, spiritual.
2. Past experiences or knowledge regarding surgery 3. Understanding planned surgical procedure	2,3. Accurate knowledge of planned procedure and care routines can help to reduce anxiety and fear related to the unknown.
4. Available support system	4. Adequate support from family, friends, and other sources can help client to cope with surgery and recovery.

5. Anxiety level:
   a. Mild (alert and aware of situation; learning and coping abilities intact)
   b. Moderate (physical signs present [e.g., increased pulse rate, muscle tremors; concentration difficult])
   c. Severe (more overt signs present, e.g., hyperventilation, tachycardia; perception altered greatly; learning and coping severely impaired)
   d. Panic (hyperactivity and other overt physical signs present; perception completely distorted; learning and coping impossible)
	5. Extreme anxiety impairs client's learning and coping abilities.

6. Readiness and ability to learn and retain information	6. A client or family failing to achieve learning goals requires a referral for assistance post-discharge.

Goal
The client will communicate feelings regarding the surgical experience.

Indicators
- Verbalize, if asked, what to expect regarding routines, environment, and sensations.
- Demonstrate postoperative exercises, splinting, and respiratory regimen.

Interventions	Rationales
1. Provide reassurance and comfort: stay with client, encourage her or him to share his feelings and concerns, listen attentively, and convey a sense of empathy and understanding.	1. Providing emotional support and encouraging client to share allows her or him to clarify fears and provides opportunities for nurse to provide realistic feedback and reassurance.
2. Correct any misconceptions and inaccurate information that the client has about the procedure.	2. Modifiable contributing factors to anxiety include incomplete and inaccurate information. Providing accurate information and correcting misconceptions may help to eliminate fears and reduce anxiety.
3. Determine if client desires spiritual support (e.g., visit from clergy or other spiritual leader, religious article, or ritual). Arrange for this support if necessary.	3. Many clients need spiritual support to enhance coping ability.
4. Allow and encourage family members and significant others to share their fears and concerns. Enlist their support for the client, but only if it is meaningful and productive.	4. Effective support from family members, other relatives, and friends can help client to cope with surgery and recovery.
5. Notify physician if client exhibits severe or panic anxiety.	5. Immediate notification enables prompt assessment and possible pharmacologic intervention.
6. Notify physician if client needs any further explanations about the procedure; beforehand, the physician should explain the following: a. Nature of the surgery b. Reason for and expected outcome of surgery c. Any risks involved d. Type of anesthetic to be used e. Expected length of recovery and any postoperative restrictions and instructions	6. The physician is responsible for explaining the surgery to the client and family; the nurse, for determining their level of understanding and then notifying the physician of the need to provide more information.
7. Involve family members or significant others in client teaching whenever possible.	7. Knowledgeable family members or significant others can serve as "coaches" to remind client of postoperative instructions and restrictions.
8. Provide instruction (bedside or group) on general information pertaining to the need for active participation, preoperative routines, environment, personnel, and postoperative exercises.	8. Preoperative teaching provides client with information; this can help to decrease anxiety and fear associated with the unknown and enhance client's sense of control over the situation.

(continues on page 644)

Interventions continued	**Rationales** continued
9. Present information or reinforce learning using written materials (e.g., books, pamphlets, instruction sheets) or audiovisual aids (e.g., videotapes, slides, posters).	9. Simultaneous stimulation of multiple senses augments the learning process. Written materials can be retained and used as a reference after discharge. These materials may be especially useful for caregivers who did not participate in client teaching sessions.
10. Explain the importance and purpose of all preoperative procedures:	10. This information can help to relieve anxiety and fear associated with lack of knowledge of necessary preoperative activities and routines.
a. Enemas	a. Enemas are sometimes given to empty the bowel of fecal material; this can help to reduce risk of postoperative bowel obstruction as peristalsis resumes.
b. Nothing-by-mouth (NPO) status	b. Eliminating oral fluids preoperatively reduces risk of aspiration postoperatively.
c. Skin preparation	c. Tests and studies establish baseline values and help to detect any abnormalities before surgery.
d. Laboratory studies	d. Preoperative sedatives reduce anxiety and promote relaxation that increase the effectiveness of anesthesia and decrease secretions in response to intubation.
11. Discuss expected intraoperative procedures and sensations: a. Appearance of operating room and equipment b. Presence of surgical staff c. Administration of anesthesia d. Appearance of postanesthesia recovery room e. Recovery from anesthesia	11. Client's understanding of expected procedures and sensations can help to ameliorate fears.
12. Explain all expected postoperative routines and sensations:	12. Explaining what the client can expect, why the procedures are done, and why certain sensations may occur can help to reduce fears associated with the unknown and unexpected.
a. Parenteral fluid administration	a. Parenteral fluids replace fluids lost from NPO state and blood loss.
b. Vital sign monitoring	b. Careful monitoring is needed to determine status and track any changes.

(continues on page 645)

Interventions continued	**Rationales** continued
c. Dressing checks and changes	c. Until wound edges heal, wound must be protected from contaminants.
d. Nasogastric (NG) tube insertion and care	d. An NG tube promotes drainage and reduces abdominal distention and tension on the suture line.
e. Indwelling (Foley) catheter insertion and care	e. A Foley catheter drains the bladder until muscle tone returns as anesthesia is excreted.
f. Other devices such as intravenous (IV) lines, pumps, and drains	
g. Symptoms including nausea, vomiting, and pain	g. Nausea and vomiting are common side effects of preoperative medications and anesthesia; other contributing factors include certain types of surgery, obesity, electrolyte imbalance, rapid position changes, and psychological and environmental factors. Pain commonly occurs as medications lose their effectiveness.
h. The availability of analgesics and antiemetics if needed	
13. As applicable, teach client (using return demonstration to ensure understanding and ability) how to do the following: a. Turn, cough, and deep-breathe. b. Support the incision site while coughing. c. Change position in bed every 1 to 2 hours. d. Sit up, get out of bed, and ambulate as soon as possible after surgery (prolonged sitting should be avoided).	13. Client's understanding of postoperative care measures can help to reduce anxiety associated with the unknown and promote compliance. Teaching the client about postoperative routines before surgery ensures that her or his understanding is not impaired postoperatively by the continuing effects of sedation.
14. Explain the importance of progressive activities postoperatively including early ambulation and self-care as soon as client is able.	14. Activity improves circulation and helps to prevent pooling of respiratory secretions. Self-care promotes self-esteem and can help to enhance recovery.
15. Explain important hospital policies to family members or significant others (e.g., visiting hours, number of visitors allowed at one time, location of waiting rooms, how physician will contact them after surgery).	15. Providing family members and significant others with this information can help to reduce their anxiety and allow them to better support the client.
16. Evaluate client's and family's or significant others' abilities to achieve preset, mutually planned learning goals.	16. This assessment identifies the need for any additional teaching and support.

Documentation

Flow records
  Progress notes
  Unusual interactions
Multidisciplinary client education record
  Preoperative teaching

Postoperative: Collaborative Problems

Potential Complication: Hemorrhage

Potential Complication: Hypovolemia/Shock

Potential Complication: Evisceration/Dehiscence

Potential Complication: Paralytic Ileus

Potential Complication: Infection (Peritonitis)

Potential Complication: Urinary Retention

Potential Complication: Thrombophlebitis

Nursing Goal

The nurse will monitor for early signs and symptoms of (a) hemorrhage; (b) hypovolemia/shock; (c) evisceration/dehiscence; (d) paralytic ileus; (e) infection; (f) urinary retention; and (g) thrombophlebitis and will intervene collaboratively to stabilize the client.

Indicators
- Calm, alert, oriented (a, b)
- Respirations 16–20 beats/min (a, b)
- Respirations relaxed and rhythmic (a, b)
- Breath sound present all lobes (a, b)
- No rales or wheezing (a, b)
- Pulse 60–100 breaths/min (a, b)
- BP > 90/60, < 140/90 mm Hg (a, b)
- Capillary refill < 3 sec (a, b)
- Peripheral pulses full, equal (a, b)
- Skin warm and dry (a, b)
- Temperature 98.5–99°F (a, b, e)
- Urine output > 30 mL/hr (a, b)
- Usual skin color (a, b)
- Surgical wound intact (c, e)
- Minimal drainage serosanguinous (e)
- Bowel sounds present (b, d)
- No nausea and vomiting (b, d)
- No abdominal distention (b, d)
- Decreasing abdominal tenderness (c, e)
- Decreasing wound tenderness (c, e)
- No bladder distension (f)
- No difficulty voiding (f)
- Negative Homans' sign (no pain with dorsiflexion of foot) (g)
- No calf tenderness, warmth, edema (g)
- White blood cells 4,000–10,000 mm^3 (e)
- Hemoglobin (a)
  - Male 14–18 g/dL
  - Female 12–16 g/dL
- Hematocrit (a)
  - Male 42%–52%
  - Female 37%–47%
- Oxygen saturation (SaO_2) > 94% (a, b)

Interventions	Rationales

1. Monitor for signs and symptoms of hemorrhage/shock and promptly report changes to surgeon:
  a. Increased pulse rate with normal or slightly decreased blood pressure
  b. Urine output <30 mL/hr
  c. Restlessness, agitation, decreased mentation
  d. Increased capillary refill over 3 seconds
  e. Decreased oxygen saturation < 94% (pulse oximetry)
  f. Increased respiratory rate
  g. Diminished peripheral pulses
  h. Cool, pale, or cyanotic skin
  i. Thirst
	1. The compensatory response to decreased circulatory volume aims to increase blood oxygen through increased heart and respiratory rates and decreased peripheral circulation (manifested by diminished peripheral pulses and cool skin). Decreased oxygen to the brain results in altered mentation.

2. Monitor fluid status; evaluate the following:
  a. Intake (parenteral and oral)
  b. Output and other losses (urine, drainage, and vomiting)
	2. Fluid loss during surgery and as a result of NPO status can disrupt fluid balance in a high-risk client. Stress can cause sodium and water retention.

3. Teach client to splint the surgical wound with a pillow when coughing, sneezing, or vomiting.	3. Splinting reduces stress on the suture line by equalizing pressure across the wound.
4. Monitor surgical site for bleeding, dehiscence, and evisceration.	4. Careful monitoring enables early detection of complications.

5. If dehiscence or evisceration occurs, contact surgeon immediately and do the following:
  a. Place client in low Fowler's position.
  b. Instruct client to lie still and quiet.
  c. Cover protruding viscera with a wet sterile dressing.
	5. Rapid interventions can reduce severity of complications.
	
	  a. Low Fowler's position uses gravity to minimize further tissue protrusion.
	  b. Lying still and quiet also minimizes tissue protrusion.
	  c. A wet sterile dressing helps to maintain tissue viability.

6. Do not initiate fluids until bowel sounds are present; begin with small amounts. Monitor client's response to resumption of fluids and foods and note the nature and amount of any emesis.
 	
7. Monitor for signs of paralytic ileus:
  a. Absent bowel sounds
  b. Nausea, vomiting
  c. Abdominal distention
	6,7. Intraoperative manipulation of abdominal organs and the depressive effects of narcotics and anesthetics on peristalsis can cause paralytic ileus usually between the third and fifth postoperative day. Pain typically is localized, sharp, and intermittent.

(continues on page 648)

Interventions continued	**Rationales** continued

8. Monitor for signs and symptoms of infection/sepsis (refer also to the nursing diagnosis High Risk for Infection):
  a. Increased temperature
  b. Chills
  c. Malaise
  d. Elevated white blood cell (WBC) count
  e. Increasing abdominal tenderness
  f. Wound tenderness, redness, or edema
	8. Microorganisms can be introduced into the body during surgery or through the incision. Circulating pathogens trigger the body's defense mechanisms: WBCs are released to destroy some pathogens, and the hypothalamus raises the body temperature to kill others. Wound redness, tenderness, and edema result from lymphocyte migration to the area.

9. Monitor for signs of urinary retention:
  a. Bladder distention
  b. Urine overflows (30 to 60 mL or urine every 15 to 30 minutes)
	9. Anesthesia produces muscle relaxation, affecting the bladder. As muscle tone returns, spasms of the bladder sphincter prevent urine outflow, causing bladder distention. When urine retention increases the intravesical pressure, the sphincter releases urine and control of flow is regained.

10. Instruct client to report bladder discomfort or inability to void.	10. Bladder discomfort and failure to void may be early signs of urinary retention.

11. If client does not void within 8 to 10 hours after surgery or complains of bladder discomfort, do the following:
  a. Warm the bedpan.
  b. Encourage client to get out of bed to use the bathroom if possible.
  c. Instruct a male client to stand when urinating if possible.
  d. Run water in the sink as client attempts to void.
  e. Pour warm water over client's perineum.
	11. These measures may help to promote relaxation of the urinary sphincter and facilitate voiding.

12. If client still cannot void, follow protocols for straight catheterization as ordered.	12. Straight catheterization is preferable to indwelling catheterization because it carries less risk of urinary tract infection from ascending pathogens.

13. Monitor for signs and symptoms of thrombophlebitis:
  a. Positive Homans' sign (pain on dorsiflexion of the foot, due to insufficient circulation)
  b. Calf tenderness, unusual warmth, or redness
	13. Vasoconstriction due to hypothermia decreases peripheral circulation. Anesthesia and immobility reduce vasomotor tone, resulting in decreased venous return with peripheral blood pooling. In combination, these factors increase risk of thrombophlebitis.

14. Apply antiembolic hose as ordered.	14. They apply even compression, enhance venous return, and reduce venous pooling.

(continues on page 649)

Interventions continued	Rationales continued
15. Remind client to move and flex legs every hour.	15. This will increase circulation.
16. Encourage client to perform leg exercises. Discourage placing pillows under the knees, use of a knee gatch, crossing the legs, and prolonged sitting. Use TED hose/compression boots as appropriate.	16. These measures help to increase venous return and prevent venous stasis.

Related Physician-Prescribed Interventions

Medications.
Preoperative: Sedatives, narcotic analgesics, anticholinergics
Postoperative: Narcotic analgesics, antiemetics

Intravenous Therapy. Fluid and electrolyte replacement

Laboratory Studies. Complete blood count, urinalysis, chemistry profile

Diagnostic Studies. Chest x-ray film, electrocardiography

Therapies. Indwelling catheterization, incentive spirometry, wound care, liquid diet progressed to full diet as tolerated, preoperative NPO status, antiembolic hose, pulse oximetry

Documentation
Flow records
    Vital signs (pulses, respirations, blood pressure, temperature)
    Circulation (color, peripheral pulses)
    Intake (oral, parenteral)
    Output (urinary, tubes, specific gravity)
    Bowel function (bowel sounds, defecation, distension)
    Wound (color, drainage)
Progress notes
    Unusual complaints or assessment findings
    Interventions
Multidisciplinary client education record
    Post operative teaching

Postoperative: Nursing Diagnoses

Risk for Ineffective Respiratory Function Related to Immobility Secondary to Postanesthesia State and Pain

Focus Assessment Criteria	Clinical Significance

1. Respiratory status:
  a. Rate and rhythm
  b. Breath and lung sounds
  c. Effectiveness of coughing effort
	1. In the immediate postoperative period, hypoventilation and decreased sensorium, resulting from CNS depression by narcotics and anesthesia, increase risk of aspiration.

2. Risk factors for postoperative respiratory problems:	2. Even after recovery from anesthesia, respiratory effort is reduced owing to fatigue,

(continues on page 650)

Focus Assessment Criteria continued	Clinical Significance continued
a. Smoking b. Obesity c. Chronic respiratory disease d. Liver dysfunction e. Prolonged immobility f. Surgical incision near the diaphragm g. Debilitation h. Malnutrition or dehydration i. Elderly	pain, and immobility. These effects—particularly in combination with one or more of the listed risk factors—increase a client's risk of postoperative respiratory problems.

Goal

The client will exhibit clear lung fields.

Indicators

- Breath sounds present in all lobes
- Relaxed rhythmic respirations

Interventions	Rationales
1. Auscultate lung fields for diminished and abnormal breath sounds.	1. Presence of rales indicates retained secretions. Diminished breath sounds may indicate atelectasis.
2. Take measures to prevent aspiration. Position client on side with pillows supporting the back and with knees slightly flexed.	2. In the postoperative period, decreased sensorium and hypoventilation contribute to increased risk of aspiration.
3. Reinforce preoperative client teaching about the importance of turning, coughing, and deep breathing and leg exercises every 1 to 2 hours.	3. Postoperative pain may discourage compliance; reinforcing the importance of these measures may improve compliance.
4. Promote the following as soon as client returns to unit: a. Deep breaths b. Coughing (except if contraindicated) c. Frequent turning d. Incentive spirometry if indicated e. Early ambulation	4. Exercises and movement promote lung expansion and mobilization of secretions. Incentive spirometry promotes deep breathing by providing a visual indicator of the effectiveness of the breathing effort. Coughing assists to dislodge mucus plugs. Coughing is contraindicated in people who have had a head injury, intracranial surgery, eye surgery, or plastic surgery because it increases intracranial and intraocular pressure and tension on delicate tissues (plastic surgery)
5. Encourage adequate oral fluid intake as indicated.	5. Adequate hydration liquefies secretions, which enables easier expectoration and prevents stasis of secretions that provide a medium for microorganism growth. It also helps to decrease blood viscosity, which reduces risk of clot formation.

Documentation
Flow record
   Temperature
   Respiratory rate and rhythm
   Breath sounds
   Respiratory treatments and client's response
Progress notes
   Unsatisfactory response to respiratory treatments
Multidisciplinary client education record

Risk for Infection Related to a Site for Organism Invasion Secondary to Surgery

Focus Assessment Criteria	Clinical Significance
1. Surgical site and drains	1–3. Surgical interruption of skin integrity disrupts the body's first line of defense against infection and allows direct entry of microorganisms. In most cases, a surgical wound should close within 24 hours by primary intention.
2. Type and progression of wound healing	
3. Signs of infection or delayed healing	

Goal
The client will demonstrate healing of wound.

Indicators
• No abnormal drainage
• Intact, approximated wound edges

Interventions	Rationales

1. Monitor for signs and symptoms of wound infection:
  a. Increased swelling and redness
  b. Wound separation
  c. Increased or purulent drainage
  d. Prolonged subnormal temperature or significantly elevated temperature
	1. Tissue responds to pathogen infiltration with increased blood and lymph flow (manifested by edema, redness, and increased drainage) and reduced epithelialization (marked by wound separation). Circulating pathogens trigger the hypothalamus to elevate the body temperature; certain pathogens cannot survive at higher temperatures.

2. Monitor wound healing by noting the following:
  a. Evidence of intact, approximated wound edges (primary intention)
  b. Evidence of granulation tissue (secondary and tertiary intention)
	2. A surgical wound with edges approximated by sutures usually heals by primary intention. Granulation tissue is not visible and scar formation is minimal. In contrast, a surgical wound with a drain or an abscess heals by secondary intention or granulation and has more distinct scar formation. A restructured wound heals by third intention and results in a wider and deeper scar.

(continues on page 652)

Interventions continued	Rationales continued
3. Teach client about factors that can delay wound healing:	3.
a. Dehydrated wound tissue	a. Studies report that epithelial migration is impeded under dry crust; movement is three times faster over moist tissue.
b. Wound infection	b. The exudate in infected wounds impairs epithelialization and wound closure.
c. Inadequate nutrition and hydration	c. To repair tissue, the body needs increased protein and carbohydrate intake and adequate hydration for vascular transport of oxygen and wastes.
d. Compromised blood supply	d. Blood supply to injured tissue must be adequate to transport leukocytes and remove wastes.
e. Increased stress or excessive activity	e. Increased stress and activity result in higher levels of chalone, a mitotic inhibitor that depresses epidermal regeneration.
4. Take steps to prevent infection: a. Wash hands before and after dressing changes. b. Wear gloves until wound is sealed. c. Thoroughly clean area around drainage tubes. d. Keep tubing away from incision. e. Discard unused irrigation solutions after 24 hours.	4. These measures help to prevent introduction of microorganisms into the wound; they also reduce the risk of transmitting infection to others.
5. Explain when a dressing is indicated for wounds healing by primary intention and by secondary intention.	5. A wound healing by primary intention requires a dressing to protect it from contamination until the edges seal (usually by 24 hours). A wound healing by secondary intention requires a dressing to maintain adequate hydration; the dressing is not needed after wound edges seal.
6. Minimize skin irritation by the following means: a. Using a collection pouch, if indicated b. Changing saturated dressings often	6. Preventing skin irritation eliminates a potential source of microorganism entry.
7. Protect wound and surrounding skin from drainage by these methods: a. Using a collection pouch if indicated b. Applying a skin barrier	7. Protecting skin can help to minimize excoriation by acid drainage. A semi-permeable skin barrier provides a moist environment for healing and prevents bacteria entry.

(continues on page 653)

Interventions continued	Rationales continued

8. Teach and assist client in the following:
  a. Supporting the surgical site when moving
  b. Splinting the area when coughing, sneezing, or vomiting
  c. Reducing flatus accumulation
	8. A wound typically requires 3 weeks for strong scar formation. Stress on the suture line before this occurs can cause disruption.

9. Consult with an enterostomal or a clinical nurse specialist for specific skin care measures.	9. Management of a complex wound or impaired healing requires expert nursing consultation.

 Documentation

Progress notes
  Signs and symptoms of infection
Flow records
  Temperature
  Status of wound

Acute Pain Related to Surgical Interruption of Body Structures, Flatus, and Immobility

Focus Assessment Criteria	Clinical Significance

1. Source of pain such as
  a. Surgical site
  b. Chest tube site
  c. Invasive line
  d. Generalized discomfort
  e. Angina
  f. Flatus
	1. Postoperative surgical site pain results from destruction of nerves and tissue during surgery. When assessing a client's pain, to intervene appropriately try to differentiate between postoperative incision pain and the discomfort stemming from flatus or immobility.

2. Severity of pain, based on a scale of 0 to 10 (0 = no pain; 10 = the most severe pain) rated as follows:
  a. At its best
  b. At its worst
  c. After each pain relief measure
	2. Such a rating scale provides an objective means of evaluating the subjective experience of pain.

3. Physical signs of pain (e.g., increased heart and respiratory rates, elevated blood pressure, restlessness, facial grimacing, guarding)	3. Clients experience and express pain in different ways; some are reluctant to verbalize pain or request pain medications. Objective signs may alert the nurse to such a client's pain.

4. Factors that influence pain tolerance:
  a. Knowledge of pain and its cause
  b. Meaning of pain
  c. Ability to control pain
  d. Energy level
  e. Stress level
  f. Cultural background
  g. Response of others
	4. Pain tolerance refers to the duration and intensity of pain that a client is willing to endure. Pain tolerance differs greatly among clients and also may vary in an individual client in different situations.

Goal

A client will report progressive reduction of pain and an increase in activity.

Indicators

- Relate factors that increase pain.
- Report effective interventions.

Interventions	Rationales
1. Collaborate with client to determine effective pain relief interventions.	1. A client experiencing pain may feel a loss of control over his body and his life. Collaboration can help minimize this feeling.
2. Express your acceptance of client's pain. Acknowledge the pain's presence, listen attentively to client's complaints, and convey that you are assessing the pain because you want to understand it better, not because you are trying to determine if it really exists.	2. A client who feels the need to convince health care providers that she or he actually is experiencing pain is likely to have increased anxiety that can lead to increased pain.
3. Reduce client's fear and clear up any misinformation by doing the following: a. Teaching what to expect; describing the sensation as precisely as possible including how long it should last b. Explaining pain relief methods such as distraction, heat application, and progressive relaxation	3. A client who is prepared for a painful procedure with a detailed explanation of the sensations that he or she will feel usually experiences less stress and pain than a client who receives vague or no explanations.
4. Explain the differences between involuntary physiologic responses and voluntary behavioral responses regarding drug use. a. Involuntary physiologic responses: • Drug tolerance is a physiologic phenomenon in which, after repeated doses, the prescribed dose begins to lose its effectiveness. • Physical dependence is a physiologic state that results from repeated administration of a drug. Withdrawal is experienced if the drug is abruptly discontinued. Tapering the drug dosage helps to manage withdrawal symptoms. b. Voluntary behavioral responses: • Drug abuse is the use of a drug in any manner that deviates from culturally acceptable medical and social uses (McCafferty, 1989). Addiction is a behavioral pattern of drug use characterized by overwhelming involvement with use of the drug and	4. Many clients and families are misinformed regarding the nature and risks of drug addiction and consequently may be reluctant to request pain medication.

(continues on page 655)

Interventions continued	Rationales continued
securing its supply and the high tendency to relapse after withdrawal (Johnson, 2000).	
5. Provide client with privacy for his or her pain experience (e.g., close curtains and room door, ask others to leave the room).	5. Privacy allows client to express pain in his or her own manner, which can help to reduce anxiety and ease pain.
6. Provide optimal pain relief with prescribed analgesics: a. Determine preferred administration route—by mouth, intramuscular, intravenous, or rectal. Consult with physician or advanced practice nurse.	6. a. The proper administration route optimizes efficacy of pain medications. The oral route is preferred in most cases; for some drugs, the liquid dosage form may be given to a client who has difficulty swallowing. If frequent injections are necessary, the intravenous (IV) route is preferred to minimize pain and maximize absorption; however, IV administration may produce more profound side effects than other routes.
b. Assess vital signs—especially respiratory rate—before and after administering any narcotic agent.	b. Narcotics can depress the respiratory center of the brain.
c. Consult with a pharmacist regarding possible adverse interactions between the prescribed drug and other medications the client is taking (e.g., muscle relaxants, tranquilizers).	c. Some medications potentiate the effects of narcotics; identifying such medications before administration can prevent excessive sedation.
d. Take a preventive approach to pain medication, i.e., administer medication before activity (e.g., ambulation) to enhance participation (but be sure to evaluate the hazards of sedation); instruct client to request pain medication as needed before pain becomes severe.	d. The preventive approach may reduce the total 24-hour dose as compared with the PRN approach; it also provides a more constant blood drug level, reduces the client's craving for the drug, and eliminates the anxiety associated with having to ask for and wait for PRN relief.
e. After administering pain medication, return in ½ hour to evaluate its effectiveness.	e. Each client responds differently to pain medication; careful monitoring is needed to assess individual response. For example, too often every surgical client is expected to respond to 50 mg of meperidine (Demerol) every 3 to 4 hours regardless of body size, type of surgery, or previous experiences.
7. Explain and assist with noninvasive and nonpharmacologic pain relief measures: a. Splinting the incision site b. Proper positioning c. Distraction d. Breathing exercises	7. These measures can help to reduce pain by substituting another stimulus to prevent painful stimuli from reaching higher brain centers. In addition, relaxation reduces muscle tension and may help increase client's sense of control over pain.

(continues on page 656)

Interventions continued	Rationales continued
e. Massage f. Heat and cold application g. Relaxation techniques	

8. Assist client in coping with the aftermath of the pain experience:
  a. If indicated, inform client that the painful procedure is completed and that the pain should soon subside.
  b. Encourage client to discuss the experience.
  c. Clarify any misconceptions the client still may have.
  d. Praise the client for her or his endurance and behavior.
	8. These measures can help to reduce anxiety and help client to regain the sense of control altered by the painful experience.

9. Teach client to expel flatus by the following measures:
  a. Walking as soon as possible after surgery
  b. Changing positions regularly as possible (e.g., lying prone, assuming the knee–chest position)
	9. Postoperatively, sluggish peristalsis results in accumulation of nonabsorbable gas. Pain occurs when unaffected bowel segments contract in an attempt to expel gas. Activity speeds the return of peristalsis and the expulsion of flatus; proper positioning helps gas rise for expulsion.

Documentation

Medication administration record
  Type, route, and dosage schedule of all prescribed medications
Progress notes
  Unsatisfactory relief from pain-relief measures
Multidisciplinary client education record

Risk for Imbalanced Nutrition: Less Than Body Requirements Related to Increased Protein and Vitamin Requirements for Wound Healing and Decreased Intake Secondary to Pain, Nausea, Vomiting, and Diet Restrictions

Focus Assessment Criteria	Clinical Significance
1. Nutritional status (intake, weight)	1. Wound healing requires sufficient intake of protein, carbohydrates, vitamins, and minerals for fibroblast formation and granulation tissue and collagen production.

2. Presence of the following:
  a. Bowel sounds
  b. Nausea
  c. Vomiting
  d. Flatus
	2. Gastrointestinal (GI) function is impaired by many surgeries, anesthesia, oral intake restrictions, and immobility. The more rapidly a client resumes her or his normal diet postoperatively, the more quickly normal GI function will return.

Goal

The client will resume ingestion of the daily nutritional requirements.

Indicators

- Selections from the four basic food groups
- 2000 to 3000 mL of fluids
- Adequate fiber, vitamins, and minerals

Interventions	Rationales
1. Explain the need for an optimal daily nutritional intake including these items: a. Increased protein and carbohydrate intake b. Increased intake of vitamins A, B, B_{12}, C, D, and E, and niacin c. Adequate intake of minerals (zinc, magnesium, calcium, copper)	1. Understanding the importance of optimal nutrition may encourage client to comply with the dietary regimen.
2. Take measures to reduce pain: a. Plan care so that painful or unpleasant procedures are not scheduled before mealtimes. b. Administer pain medication as ordered. c. Position for optimal comfort.	2. Pain causes fatigue, which can reduce appetite.
3. Explain the possible causes of the client's nausea and vomiting: a. Side effect of preoperative medications and anesthesia b. Surgical procedure c. Obesity d. Electrolyte imbalance e. Gastric distention f. Too-rapid or strenuous movement Reassure client that these symptoms are normal.	3. Client's understanding of the source and normalcy of nausea and vomiting can reduce anxiety, which may help to reduce symptoms.
4. Take steps to reduce nausea and vomiting: a. Restrict fluids before meals and large amounts of fluids at any time; instead, encourage client to ingest small amounts of ice chips or cool clear liquids (e.g., dilute tea, Jell-O water, flat ginger ale, or cola) frequently, unless vomiting persists. b. Teach client to move slowly. c. Reduce or eliminate unpleasant sights and odors. d. Provide good mouth care after client vomits.	4. a. Gastric distention from fluid ingestion can trigger the vagal visceral afferent pathways that stimulate the medulla oblongata (vomiting center). b. Rapid movements stimulate the vomiting center by triggering vestibulo-cerebellar afferents. c. Noxious odors and sights can stimulate the vomiting center. d. Good oral care reduces the noxious taste.

(continues on page 658)

Interventions continued	Rationales continued
e. Teach deep breathing techniques.	e. Deep breaths can help to excrete anesthetic agents.
f. Instruct client to avoid lying down flat for at least 2 hours after eating. (A client who must rest should sit or recline with head at least 4 inches higher than feet.)	f. Pressure on the stomach can trigger vagal visceral afferent stimulation of the vomiting center in the brain.
g. Ensure patency of any nasogastric (NG) tube.	g. A malfunctioning NG tube can cause gastric distention.
h. Teach client to practice relaxation exercises during episodes of nausea.	h. Concentrating on relaxation activities may help to block stimulation of the vomiting center.
5. Maintain good oral hygiene at all times.	5. A clean, refreshed mouth can stimulate appetite.
6. Administer an antiemetic agent before meals if indicated.	6. Antiemetics prevent nausea and vomiting.

 Documentation

Flow record
  Intake (amount, type, time)
  Vomiting (amount, description)
Multidisciplinary client education record

Risk for Constipation Related to Decreased Peristalsis Secondary to Immobility and the Effects of Anesthesia and Narcotics

Focus Assessment Criteria	Clinical Significance

1. Preoperative and postoperative elimination patterns
 	
2. Abdominal status:
  a. Distention
  b. Bowel sounds
	1,2. Postoperatively, decreased GI motility can result from disruption of autonomic innervation due to stress, surgical manipulation of the intestine, immobility, and effects of medications. Preoperative elimination patterns and postoperative abdominal status serve as criteria for assessing bowel function.

Goal

The client will resume effective preoperative bowel function.

Indicators

- No bowel distention
- Bowel sounds in all quadrants

Interventions	Rationales
1. Assess bowel sounds to determine when to introduce liquids. Advance diet as ordered.	1. Presence of bowel sounds indicates return of peristalsis.
2. Explain the effects of daily activity on elimination. Assist with ambulation when possible.	2. Activity influences bowel elimination by improving abdominal muscle tone and stimulating appetite and peristalsis.
3. Promote factors that contribute to optimal elimination. a. Balanced diet: • Review a list of foods high in bulk (e.g., fresh fruits with skins, bran, nuts and seeds, whole grain breads and cereals, cooked fruits and vegetables, and fruit juices). • Discuss dietary preferences. • Encourage intake of approximately 800 g of fruits and vegetables (about four pieces of fresh fruit and a large salad) for normal daily bowel movement. b. Adequate fluid intake: • Encourage intake of at least 8 to 10 glasses (about 2000 mL) daily unless contraindicated. • Discuss fluid preferences. • Set up a regular schedule for fluid intake. c. Regular time for defecation: • Identify the normal defecation pattern before the onset of constipation. • Review daily routine. • Include time for defecation as part of the regular daily routine. • Discuss a suitable time based on responsibilities, availability of facilities, and so on. • Suggest that client attempt defecation about 1 hour following a meal and remain in the bathroom a suitable length of time. d. Simulation of the home environment: • Have client use the bathroom instead of a bedpan if possible; offer a bedpan or a bedside commode if the client cannot use the bathroom. • Assist into position on the toilet, commode, or bedpan if necessary.	3. a. A well-balanced diet high in fiber content stimulates peristalsis. b. Sufficient fluid intake is necessary to maintain bowel patterns and promote proper stool consistency. c. Taking advantage of circadian rhythms may aid in establishing a regular defecation schedule. d. Privacy and a sense of normalcy can promote relaxation, which can enhance defecation.

(continues on page 660)

Interventions continued	Rationales continued
• Provide privacy (e.g., close door, draw curtains around the bed, play a TV or radio to mask sounds, make room deodorizer available). • Provide for comfort (e.g., provide reading materials as a diversion) and safety (e.g., make a call bell readily available). e. Proper positioning: • Assist client to a normal semi-squatting position on the toilet or commode if possible. • Assist onto a bedpan if necessary, elevating the head of the bed to high Fowler's position or to the elevation permitted. • Stress the need to avoid straining during defecation efforts.	e. Proper positioning uses the abdominal muscles and the force of gravity to aid defecation. Straining can activate Valsalva's response, which may lead to reduced cardiac output.
4. Notify physician if bowel sounds do not return within 6 to 10 hours or if elimination does not return within 2 to 3 days postoperatively.	4. Absence of bowel sounds may indicate paralytic ileus; absence of bowel movements may indicate obstruction.

 Documentation

Flow record
  Bowel movements
  Bowel sounds

Activity Intolerance Related to Pain and Weakness Secondary to Anesthesia, Tissue Hypoxia, and Insufficient Fluid and Nutrient Intake

Focus Assessment Criteria	Clinical Significance
1. Degree of activity progression 2. Response to activity	1,2. Surgery, NPO status, and pain can compromise a client's energy and ability to participate in ADLs. The client should demonstrate steady activity progression.

Goal

The client will increase tolerance to activities of daily living (ADLs).

Indicators

• Progressive ambulation
• Ability to perform ADLs

Interventions	Rationales
1. Encourage progress in client's activity level during each shift as indicated: a. Allow client's legs to dangle first; support client from the side. b. Place the bed in high position and raise the head of the bed. c. Increase client's time out of bed by 15 minutes each time. Allow client to set a comfortable rate of ambulation and agree on a distance goal for each shift. d. Encourage client to increase activity when pain is at a minimum or after pain relief measures take effect.	1. A gradual increase in activity allows the client's cardiopulmonary system to return to its preoperative state without excessive strain. a. Dangling the legs helps to minimize orthostatic hypotension. b. Raising the head of the bed helps to reduce stress on suture lines. c. Gradual increases toward mutually established, realistic goals can promote compliance and prevent overexertion.
2. Increase client's self-care activities from partial to complete self-care as indicated.	2. Client's participation in self-care improves physiologic functioning, reduces fatigue from inactivity, and improves sense of self-esteem and well-being.
3. If client is not progressing at the expected or desired rate, do the following: a. Take vital signs prior to activity. b. Repeat vital sign assessment after activity. c. Repeat again after client has rested for 3 minutes. d. Assess for abnormal responses to increased activity: • Decreased pulse rate • Decreased or unchanged systolic blood pressure • Excessively increased or decreased respiratory rate • Failure of pulse to return to near the resting rate within 3 minutes after discontinuing activity • Complaints of confusion or vertigo • Uncoordinated movements	3. Activity tolerance depends on client's ability to adapt to the physiologic requirements of increased activity. The expected immediate physiologic responses to activity are increased blood pressure and increased respiratory rate and depth. After 3 minutes, pulse rate should decrease to within 10 beats/minute of client's usual resting rate. Abnormal findings represent the body's inability to meet the increased oxygen demands imposed by activity.
4. Plan regular rest periods according to client's daily schedule.	4. Regular rest periods allow the body to conserve and restore energy.
5. Identify and encourage client's progress. Keep a record of progress particularly for a client who is progressing slowly.	5. Encouragement and realization of progress can give client an incentive for continued progression.

Documentation

Flow record
  Vital signs
  Ambulation (time, amount)
Progress notes
  Abnormal or unexpected response to increased activity

Risk for Ineffective Therapeutic Regimen Management Related to Insufficient Knowledge of Care of Operative Site, Restrictions (Diet, Activity), Medications, Signs and Symptoms of Complications, and Follow-up Care

Focus Assessment Criteria	Clinical Significance
1. Readiness and ability to learn and retain information	1. A client or family failing to achieve learning goals requires a referral for assistance post-discharge.

Goals

The goals for this diagnosis represent those associated with discharge planning. Refer to the discharge criteria.

Interventions	Rationales

1. As appropriate, explain and demonstrate care of an uncomplicated surgical wound:
  a. Washing with soap and water
  b. Dressing changes using clean technique
	1. Uncomplicated wounds have sealed edges after 24 hours and therefore do not require aseptic technique or a dressing; however, a dressing may be applied if wound is at risk for injury.

2. As appropriate, explain and demonstrate care of a complicated surgical wound:
  a. Aseptic technique
  b. Handwashing before and after dressing changes
  c. Avoiding touching the inner surface of the soiled dressing and discarding it in a sealed plastic bag
  d. The use of sterile hemostats if indicated
  e. Wound assessment—condition and drainage
  f. Wound cleaning
  g. Drainage tubes if indicated
  h. Dressing reapplication
	2. Aseptic technique is necessary to prevent wound contamination during dressing changes. Handwashing helps to prevent contamination of the wound and the spread of infection. Proper handling and disposal of contaminated dressings helps to prevent infection transmission. Daily assessment is necessary to evaluate healing and detect complications.

3. Reinforce activity restrictions as indicated (e.g., bending, lifting).	3. Avoiding certain activities decreases the risk of wound dehiscence before scar formation occurs (usually after 3 weeks).

(continues on page 663)

Interventions continued	Rationales continued

4. Explain the importance of the following:
  a. Avoiding ill persons and crowds
  b. Drinking 8 to 10 glasses of fluid daily
  c. Maintaining a balanced diet
	4. Wound healing requires optimal nutrition, hydration, and rest as well as avoiding potential sources of infection.

5. Review with client and family the purpose, dosage, administration, and side effects of all prescribed medications.	5. Complete understanding can help to prevent drug administration errors.

6. Teach client and family to watch for and report signs and symptoms of possible complications:
  a. Persistent temperature elevation
  b. Difficulty breathing, chest pain
  c. Change in sputum characteristics
  d. Increasing weakness, fatigue, pain, or abdominal distention
  e. Wound changes (e.g., separation, unusual or increased drainage, increased redness or swelling)
  f. Voiding difficulties, burning on urination, urinary frequency, or cloudy, foul-smelling urine
  g. Pain, swelling, and warmth in calf
  h. Other signs and symptoms of complications specific to surgical procedure performed
	6. Early detection and reporting danger signs and symptoms enable prompt intervention to minimize severity of complications.

7. Whenever possible, provide written instructions.	7. Written instructions provide an information resource for use at home.
8. Evaluate client's and family's understanding of information provided.	8. Knowledge gaps may indicate need for a referral for assistance at home.

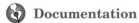 **Documentation**

Flow records
  Discharge instructions
  Follow-up instructions
Discharge summary record
  Status at discharge (pain, activity, wound healing)
  Achievement of goals (individual or family)
Multidisciplinary client education record

GENERIC CARE PLAN FOR THE AMBULATORY SURGICAL CLIENT

Kathleen M. Killman, RN, C, MS

This care plan (Level I) presents nursing diagnoses and collaborative problems that commonly apply to clients (and their significant others) experiencing all types of surgery in the ambulatory setting. Nursing diagnoses and collaborative problems specific to a surgical procedure are presented in the care plan (Level II) for that procedure.

 Time Frame

Preoperative and postoperative periods

 DIAGNOSTIC CLUSTER

Preoperative

Nursing Diagnosis

- Anxiety/Fear related to surgical experience, loss of control, unpredictable outcome, expected pain, and insufficient knowledge of preoperative routines, postoperative exercises and activities, and postoperative changes and sensations

Postoperative

Collaborative Problems

Potential Complications:

Hemorrhage
Hypovolemia/Shock
Evisceration/Dehiscence
Paralytic Ileus
Infection (Peritonitis)
Urinary Retention
Thrombophlebitis

Nursing Diagnoses

- Acute Pain related to surgical interruption of body structures
- Risk for Infection related to a site for organism invasion secondary to surgery
- Risk for Ineffective Therapeutic Regimen Management related to insufficient knowledge of care of operative site, restrictions (diet, activity), medications, signs and symptoms of complications, and follow-up care

---

Discharge Criteria

Before discharge, the client and/or family will

1. Describe any at-home activity restrictions.
2. Describe at-home wound and pain management.
3. Discuss fluid and nutritional requirements for proper wound healing.
4. List the signs and symptoms that must be reported to a health care professional.
5. Describe necessary follow-up care.

Preoperative: Nursing Diagnosis

Anxiety/Fear Related to Surgical Experience, Loss of Control, Unpredictable Outcome, Expected Pain, and Insufficient Knowledge of Preoperative Routines, Postoperative Exercises and Activities, and Postoperative Changes and Sensations

Focus Assessment Criteria	Clinical Significance
1. Specific stressors and nature of concerns	1. Every client experiences some emotional reaction to surgery; the nature and degree of this reaction depend on how the client perceives the surgery and its anticipated effects—physical, psychological, financial, social, occupational, spiritual.
2. Past experiences or knowledge regarding surgery 3. Understanding planned surgical procedure	2,3. Accurate knowledge of the planned procedure and care routines can help to reduce anxiety and fear related to the unknown.
4. Available support system	4. Adequate support from family, friends, and other sources can help client to cope with surgery and recovery.

5. Anxiety level:
  a. Mild (alert and aware of situation; learning and coping abilities intact)
  b. Moderate (physical signs present [e.g., increased pulse rate, muscle tremors; concentration difficult])
  c. Severe (more overt signs present [e.g., hyperventilation, tachycardia; perception altered greatly; learning and coping severely impaired])
  d. Panic (hyperactivity and other overt physical signs present; perception completely distorted; learning and coping impossible)
	5. Extreme anxiety impairs client's learning and coping abilities.

6. Readiness and ability to learn and retain information	6. A client or family failing to achieve learning goals requires a referral for assistance postdischarge.

Goal

The client will communicate feelings regarding the surgical experience.

Indicators
- Verbalize, if asked, what to expect regarding routines, environment, and sensations.
- Demonstrate postoperative exercises.

Interventions	Rationales
1. Provide reassurance and comfort; stay with client, encourage him or her to share feelings and concerns, listen attentively, and convey a sense of empathy and understanding.	1. Providing emotional support and encouraging client to share allows him or her to clarify fears and provides opportunities for nurse to provide realistic feedback and reassurance.
2. Correct any misconceptions and inaccurate information the client has about the procedure.	2. Modifiable contributing factors to anxiety include incomplete and inaccurate information. Providing accurate information and correcting misconceptions may help to eliminate fears and reduce anxiety.
3. Determine if the client desires spiritual support (e.g., visit from clergy or other spiritual leader, religious article, ritual). Arrange for this support if necessary.	3. Many clients need spiritual support to enhance coping ability.
4. Allow and encourage family members and significant others to share their fears and concerns. Enlist their support for client but only if its is meaningful and productive.	4. Effective support from family members, other relatives, and friends can help client to cope with surgery and recovery.
5. Notify physician if client exhibits severe or panic anxiety.	5. Immediate notification enables prompt assessment and possible pharmacologic intervention.
6. Notify physician if client needs any further explanations about the procedure; beforehand, the physician should explain the following: a. Nature of the surgery b. Reason for and expected outcome of surgery c. Any risks involved d. Type of anesthetic to be used e. Expected length of recovery and any postoperative restrictions and instructions	6. The physician is responsible for explaining the surgery to the client and family; the nurse, for determining their level of understanding then notifying the physician of the need to provide more information.
7. Involve family members or significant others in client teaching whenever possible.	7. Knowledgeable family members or significant others can serve as "coaches" to remind client of postoperative instructions and restrictions.

(continues on page 667)

Interventions continued	Rationales continued
8. Provide instruction (bedside or group) on general information pertaining to the need for active participation, preoperative routines, environment, personnel, and postoperative routine.	8. Preoperative teaching provides client with information that can help decrease anxiety and fear associated with the unknown and enhance his or her sense of control over the situation.
9. Present information or reinforce learning using written materials (e.g., books, pamphlets, instruction sheets) or audiovisual aids (e.g., videotapes, slides, posters).	9. Simultaneous stimulation of multiple senses augments the learning process. Written materials can be retained and used as a reference after discharge. These materials may be especially useful for caregivers who did not participate in client teaching sessions.
10. Explain the importance and purpose of all preoperative procedures (some of these explanations may occur preadmission): a. Enemas b. Nothing-by-mouth (NPO) status c. Skin preparation d. Laboratory studies	10. This information can help to relieve anxiety and fear associated with lack of knowledge of necessary preoperative activities and routines. a. Enemas are sometimes given to empty the bowel of fecal material; this can help to reduce risk of postoperative bowel obstruction as peristalsis resumes. b. Eliminating oral fluids preoperatively reduces risk of aspiration postoperatively. c. Tests and studies establish baseline values and help to detect any abnormalities before surgery. d. Preoperative sedatives reduce anxiety and promote relaxation, which increase the effectiveness of anesthesia and decrease secretions in response to intubation.
11. Discuss expected intraoperative procedures and sensations: a. Appearance of operating room and equipment b. Presence of surgical staff c. Administration of anesthesia d. Appearance of postanesthesia recovery room e. Recovery from anesthesia	11. The client understanding the expected procedures and sensations can help to ameliorate fears.
12. Explain all expected postoperative routines and sensations:	12. Explaining what the client can expect, why the procedures are done, and why certain sensations may occur can help to reduce fears associated with the unknown and unexpected.

(continues on page 668)

Interventions continued	**Rationales** continued
a. Parenteral fluid administration (if applicable)	a. Parenteral fluids replace fluids lost from NPO state and blood loss.
b. Vital sign monitoring	b. Careful monitoring is needed to determine status and track any changes.
c. Dressing checks and changes	c. Until wound edges heal, wound must be protected from contaminants.
d. Indwelling (Foley) catheter insertion and care (if applicable)	d. A Foley catheter drains the bladder until muscle tone returns as anesthesia is excreted.
e. Other devices such as IV lines, pumps, and drains as necessary	e–g. Nausea and vomiting are common side effects of preoperative medications and anesthesia; other contributing factors include certain types of surgery, obesity, electrolyte imbalance, rapid position changes, and psychological and environmental factors. Pain commonly occurs as medications lose their effectiveness.
f. Symptoms including nausea, vomiting, and pain	
g. Availability of analgesics and antiemetics if needed	
13. As applicable, teach client (using return demonstration to ensure understanding and ability) how to do the following: a. Cough and deep breathe. b. Support incision site while coughing. c. Sit up, get out of bed, and ambulate as soon as possible after surgery (prolonged sitting should be avoided).	13. Client's understanding of postoperative care measures can help to reduce anxiety associated with the unknown and promote compliance. Teaching client about postoperative routines before surgery ensures that the continuing effects of sedation postoperatively do not impair his or her understanding.
14. Explain the importance of progressive activities postoperatively, including early ambulation and self-care as soon as client is able.	14. Activity improves circulation and helps to prevent pooling of respiratory secretions. Self-care promotes self-esteem and can help to enhance recovery.
15. Explain important hospital policies (e.g., visiting hours, number of visitors allowed at one time, location of waiting rooms, how physician will contact them after surgery) to family members or significant others.	15. Providing family members and significant others with this information can help to reduce their anxiety and allow them to better support the client.
16. Evaluate client's and family's or significant others' abilities to achieve preset, mutually planned learning goals; if indicated, initiate a home health referral.	16. This assessment identifies the need for any additional teaching and support.

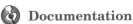 **Documentation**

Flow records
  Progress notes
  Unusual interactions
Multidisciplinary client education record
  Preoperative teaching

Postoperative: Collaborative Problems

Potential Complication: Hemorrhage

Potential Complication: Hypovolemia/Shock

Potential Complication: Evisceration/Dehiscence

Potential Complication: Paralytic Ileus

Potential Complication: Infection (Peritonitis)

Potential Complication: Urinary Retention

Potential Complication: Thrombophlebitis

Nursing Goal

The nurse will monitor for early signs and symptoms of (a) hemorrhage, (b) hypovolemia/shock, (c) evisceration/dehiscence, (d) paralytic ileus, (e) infection, (f) urinary retention, and (g) thrombophlebitis and will intervene collaboratively to stabilize the client.

Indicators
- Calm, alert, oriented (a, b)
- Respirations 16–20 breaths/min (a, b)
- Respirations relaxed and rhythmic (a, b)
- Breath sounds present all lobes (a, b)
- No rales or wheezing (a, b)
- Pulse 60–100 beats/min (a, b)
- BP > 90/60, < 140/90 mm Hg (a, b)
- Capillary refill < 3 sec (a, b)
- Peripheral pulses full, equal (a, b)
- Skin warm and dry (a, b)
- Temperature 98.5–99°F (a, b, e)
- Urine output > 30 mL/hr (a, b)
- Usual skin color (a, b)
- Surgical wound intact (c, e)
- Minimal drainage serosanguineous (e)
- Bowel sounds present (b, d)
- No nausea and vomiting (b, d)
- No abdominal distention (b, d)
- Decreasing abdominal tenderness (c, e)
- Decreasing wound tenderness (c, e)
- No bladder distension (f)
- No difficulty voiding (f)
- Negative Homans' sign (no pain with dorsiflexion of foot) (g)
- No calf tenderness, warmth, edema (g)
- White blood cells 4,000–10,000 mm^3 (e)
- Hemoglobin (a)
  - Male 14–18 g/dL
  - Female 12–16 g/dL
- Hematocrit (a)
  - Male 42%–52%
  - Female 37%–47%
- Oxygen saturation (SaO$_2$) > 94% (a, b)

Interventions	Rationales
1. Monitor for signs and symptoms of hemorrhage/shock: a. Increased pulse rate with normal or slightly decreased blood pressure b. Urine output < 30 mL/hr c. Restlessness, agitation, decreased mentation d. Increased respiratory rate e. Diminished peripheral pulses f. Cool, pale, or cyanotic skin g. Thirst	1. The compensatory response to decreased circulatory volume aims to increase blood oxygen through increased heart and respiratory rates and decreased peripheral circulation (manifested by diminished peripheral pulses and cool skin). Decreased oxygen to the brain results in altered mentation.
2. Monitor fluid status; evaluate the following: a. Intake (parenteral and oral) b. Output and other losses (urine, drainage, and vomiting)	2. Fluid loss during surgery and as a result of NPO status can disrupt fluid balance in a high-risk client. Stress can cause sodium and water retention.
3. Monitor surgical site for bleeding, dehiscence, and evisceration.	3. Careful monitoring enables early detection of complications.
4. Teach client to splint the surgical wound with a pillow when coughing, sneezing, or vomiting.	4. Splinting reduces stress on the suture line by equalizing pressure across the wound.
5. If dehiscence or evisceration occur, do the following: a. Place client in low Fowler's position. b. Instruct client to lie still and quiet. c. Cover protruding viscera with a wet sterile dressing.	5. Rapid interventions can reduce severity of complications. a. This position uses gravity to minimize further tissue protrusion. b. Doing so also minimizes tissue protrusion. c. A wet sterile dressing helps to maintain tissue viability.
6. Do not initiate fluids until bowel sounds are present; begin with small amounts. Monitor client's response to resumption of fluids and foods and note the nature and amount of any emesis. 7. Monitor for signs of paralytic ileus: a. Absent bowel sounds b. Nausea, vomiting c. Abdominal distention	6,7. Intraoperative manipulation of abdominal organs and the depressive effects of narcotics and anesthetics on peristalsis can cause paralytic ileus usually between the third and fifth postoperative days. Pain typically is localized, sharp, and intermittent.
8. Explain to client/family how to monitor for signs and symptoms of infection/sepsis (refer also to the nursing diagnosis Risk for Infection).	8. Microorganisms can be introduced into the body during surgery or through the incision. Circulating pathogens trigger the body's defense mechanisms:

(continues on page 671)

Interventions continued	**Rationales** continued

a. Increased temperature
   b. Chills
   c. Malaise
   d. Increasing abdominal tenderness
   e. Wound tenderness, redness, or
      edema
	WBCs are released to destroy some pathogens, and the hypothalamus raises the body temperature to kill others. Wound redness, tenderness, and edema result from lymphocyte migration to the area.

9. Monitor for signs of urinary retention:
   a. Bladder distention
   b. Urine overflow (30 to 60 mL or urine
      every 15 to 30 minutes)
	9. Anesthesia produces muscle relaxation, affecting the bladder. As muscle tone returns, spasms of the bladder sphincter prevent urine outflow, causing bladder distention. When urine retention increases the intravesical pressure, the sphincter releases urine and control of flow is regained.

10. Instruct client to report bladder discomfort or inability to void.	10. Bladder discomfort and failure to void may be early signs of urinary retention.

11. If client does not void within 8 to 10 hours after surgery or complains of bladder discomfort, do the following:
   a. Warm the bedpan.
   b. Encourage client to get out of bed to
      use the bathroom if possible.
   c. Instruct a male client to stand when
      urinating if possible.
   d. Run water in the sink as client attempts
      to void.
   e. Pour warm water over client's
      perineum.
	11. These measures may help to promote relaxation of the urinary sphincter and facilitate voiding.

12. If client still cannot void, follow protocols for straight catheterization as ordered.	12. Straight catheterization is preferable to indwelling catheterization because it carries less risk of urinary tract infection from ascending pathogens.

13. Explain to client/family how to monitor for signs and symptoms of thrombophlebitis:
   a. Calf tenderness, unusual warmth, or
      redness
	13. Vasoconstriction from hypothermia decreases peripheral circulation. Anesthesia and immobility reduce vasomotor tone resulting in decreased venous return with peripheral blood pooling. In combination, these factors increase the risk of thrombophlebitis.

14. Instruct client/family on use of TED hose if applicable.	14. They help to increase venous return and prevent venous stasis.

Related Physician-Prescribed Interventions

Medications
Preoperative. Sedatives, narcotic analgesics, anticholinergics
Postoperative. Narcotic analgesics, antiemetics

Intravenous Therapy. Fluid and electrolyte replacement

Laboratory Studies. Complete blood count, urinalysis, chemistry profile

Diagnostic Studies. Chest x-ray film, electrocardiography

Therapies. Indwelling catheterization, wound care, liquid diet progressed to full diet as tolerated, preoperative NPO status, antiembolic hose, pulse oximetry

 Documentation

Flow records
    Vital signs (pulses, respirations, blood pressure, temperature)
    Circulation (color, peripheral pulses)
    Intake (oral, parenteral)
    Output (urinary, tubes, specific gravity)
    Bowel function (bowel sounds, defecation, distension)
    Wound (color, drainage)
Discharge instructions
    Signs and symptoms of infection, thrombophlebitis
    Use of TED hose if indicated
    Splinting the wound
Progress notes
    Unusual complaints or assessment findings
    Interventions
Multidisciplinary client education record
    Postoperative teaching

Risk for Infection Related to a Site for Organism Invasion Secondary to Surgery

Focus Assessment Criteria	Clinical Significance
1. Surgical site and drains 2. Type and progression of wound healing 3. Signs of infection or delayed healing	1–3. Surgical interruption of skin integrity disrupts the body's first line of defense against infection and allows direct entry of microorganisms. In most cases, a surgical wound should close within 24 hours by primary intention.

Goal

The client will verbalize the signs and symptoms of infection and whom to contact if these occur.

Indicators
• No abnormal drainage
• Intact approximated wound edges

Interventions	Rationales

1. Teach client/family how to monitor for signs and symptoms of wound infection:
  a. Increased swelling and redness
  b. Wound separation
	1. Tissue responds to pathogen infiltration with increased blood and lymph flow (manifested by edema, redness, and increased drainage) and reduced epithelialization

(continues on page 673)

Interventions continued	**Rationales** continued
c. Increased or purulent drainage d. Significantly elevated temperature	(marked by wound separation). Circulating pathogens trigger the hypothalamus to elevate body temperature; certain pathogens cannot survive at higher temperatures.
2. Teach client/family how to monitor wound healing by noting evidence of intact, approximated wound edges (primary intention)	2. A surgical wound with edges approximated by sutures usually heals by primary intention. Granulation tissue is not visible; scar formation is minimal. In contrast, a surgical wound with a drain or an abscess heals by secondary intention or granulation and had more distinct scar formation.
3. Teach client and family about factors that can delay wound healing: a. Dehydrated wound tissue b. Wound infection c. Inadequate nutrition and hydration d. Compromised blood supply e. Increased stress or excessive activity	3. a. Studies report that epithelial migration is impeded under dry crust; movement is three times faster over moist tissue. b. The exudate in infected wounds impairs epithelialization and wound closure. c. To repair tissue, the body needs increased protein and carbohydrate intake and adequate hydration for vascular transport of oxygen and wastes. d. Blood supply to injured tissue must be adequate to transport leukocytes and remove wastes. e. Stress and activity result in higher levels of chalone, a mitotic inhibitor that depresses epidermal regeneration.
4. Take steps to prevent infection: a. Wash hands before and after dressing changes. b. Wear gloves until wound is sealed. c. Thoroughly clean area around drainage tubes. d. Keep tubing away from incision. e. Discard unused irrigation solutions after 24 hours.	4. These measures help to prevent introduction of microorganisms into the wound and also reduce risk of transmitting infection to others.
5. Explain when a dressing is indicated for wounds healing by primary intention and by secondary intention.	5. A wound healing by primary intention requires a dressing to protect it from contamination until the edges seal (usually 24 hours). A wound healing by secondary intention requires a dressing to maintain adequate hydration; the dressing is not needed after wound edges seal.

(continues on page 674)

Interventions continued	Rationales continued
6. Minimize skin irritation by the following means: a. Use a collection pouch if indicated. b. Change saturated dressings often.	6. Preventing skin irritation eliminates a potential source of microorganism entry.
7. Protect wound and surrounding skin from drainage by these methods: a. Use a collection pouch if indicated. b. Apply a skin barrier.	7. Protecting the skin can help to minimize excoriation by acid drainage. A semipermeable skin barrier provides a moist environment for healing and prevents entry of bacteria.
8. Teach and assist client with the following: a. Supporting surgical site when moving b. Splinting area when coughing, sneezing, or vomiting c. Reducing flatus accumulation	8. A wound typically requires 3 weeks for strong scar formation. Stress on the suture line before this occurs can cause disruption.
9. Consult with an enterostomal or a clinical nurse specialist for specific skin care measures.	9. Management of a complex wound or impaired healing requires expert nursing consultation.

 Documentation

Progress notes
   Signs and symptoms of infection
Flow records
   Temperature
   Status of wound

Acute Pain Related to Surgical Interruption of Body Structures

Focus Assessment Criteria	Clinical Significance
1. Source of pain such as a. Surgical site b. Invasive line c. Generalized discomfort d. Flatus	1. Postoperative surgical site pain results from destruction of nerves and tissue during surgery. When assessing a client's pain, to intervene appropriately the nurse must try to differentiate between postoperative incision pain and discomfort stemming from flatus or immobility.
2. Severity of pain, based on a scale of 0 to 10 (0 = no pain; 10 = the most severe pain) rated as follows: a. At its best b. At its worst c. After each pain-relief measure	2. Such a rating scale provides an objective means of evaluating the subjective experience of pain.

(continues on page 675)

Focus Assessment Criteria continued	Clinical Significance continued
3. Client's goal for pain relief (using 0 to 10 scale)	3. An awareness of client's goal for pain relief assists nurse in more accurately evaluating the effectiveness of pain-relief measures. Clients in pain (especially chronic pain) may expect pain only to be lessened, not relieved completely.
4. Physical signs of pain (e.g., increased heart and respiratory rates, elevated blood pressure, restlessness, facial grimacing, guarding)	4. Clients experience and express pain in different ways; some are reluctant to verbalize pain or request pain medications. Objective signs may alert nurse to such a client's pain.

5. Factors that influence pain tolerance:
  a. Knowledge of pain and its cause
  b. Meaning of pain
  c. Ability to control pain
  d. Energy level
  e. Stress level
  f. Cultural background
  g. Response of others
	5. Pain tolerance refers to the duration and intensity of pain that a client is willing to endure. Pain tolerance differs greatly among clients and also may vary in an individual client in different situations.

Goal

The client will report progressive reduction of pain and increased activity.

Indicators

- Relate factors that increase pain.
- Report effective interventions.

Interventions	Rationales
1. Collaborate with client to determine effective pain-relief interventions.	1. A client experiencing pain may feel a loss of control over his or her body and life. Collaboration can help to minimize this feeling.
2. Express your acceptance of client's pain. Acknowledge the pain's presence, listen attentively to complaints, and convey that you are assessing the pain because you want to understand it better, not because you are trying to determine if it really exists.	2. A client who feels the need to convince health care providers that he or she actually is experiencing pain is likely to have increased anxiety that can lead to increased pain.
3. Reduce client's fear and clear up any misinformation by doing the following: a. Teach what to expect; describe sensations as precisely as possible including how long they should last.	3. A client who is prepared for a painful procedure with a detailed explanation of the sensations that he or she will feel usually experiences less stress and pain than a client who receives vague or no explanations.

(continues on page 676)

Interventions continued	Rationales continued
b. Explain pain-relief methods such as distraction, heat application, ice application, progressive relaxation, visualization, and deep breathing.	
4. Explain the differences between involuntary physiologic responses and voluntary behavioral responses regarding drug use. a. Involuntary physiologic responses: • Drug tolerance is a physiologic phenomenon in which, after repeated doses, the prescribed dose begins to lose its effectiveness. • Physical dependence is a physiologic state that results from repeated administration of a drug. Withdrawal is experienced if the drug is abruptly discontinued. Tapering the drug dosage helps to manage withdrawal symptoms. b. Voluntary behavioral responses: • Drug abuse is the use of a drug in any manner that deviates from culturally acceptable medical and social uses (McCaffery & Beebe, 1989). Addiction is a behavioral pattern of drug use characterized by overwhelming involvement with use of the drug and securing its supply and the high tendency to relapse after withdrawal Johnson, 2000).	4. Many clients and families are misinformed regarding the nature and risks of drug addiction and consequently may be reluctant to request pain medication.
5. Provide client with privacy for his or her pain experience (e.g., close curtains and room door, ask others to leave the room).	5. Privacy allows client to express pain in his or her own manner, which can help reduce anxiety and ease pain.
6. Provide optimal pain relief with prescribed analgesics: a. Determine the preferred administration route—by mouth, IM, IV, or rectal. Consult with physician.	6. a. Proper administration route optimizes efficacy of pain medications. The oral route is preferred in most cases; for some drugs, the liquid dosage form may be given to a client who has difficulty swallowing. If frequent injections are necessary, the IV route is preferred to minimize pain and maximize absorption; however, IV administration may produce more profound side effects than other routes.
b. Assess vital signs—especially respiratory rate—before and after administering any narcotic agent.	b. Narcotics can depress the respiratory center of the brain.

(continues on page 677)

Interventions continued	**Rationales** continued
c. Consult with a pharmacist regarding possible adverse interactions between the prescribed drug and other medications (e.g., muscle relaxants, tranquilizers) the client is taking. d. Take a preventive approach to pain medication, i.e., administer medication before activity (e.g., ambulation) to enhance participation (but be sure to evaluate the hazards of sedation); instruct client to request pain medication as needed before pain becomes severe. e. After administering pain medication, return in 30 minutes to evaluate its effectiveness.	c. Some medications potentiate the effects of narcotics; identifying such medications before administration can prevent excessive sedation. d. The preventive approach may reduce the total 24-hour dose as compared with the PRN approach; it also provides a more constant blood drug level, reduces the client's craving for the drug, and eliminates the anxiety associated with having to ask for and wait for PRN relief. e. Each client responds differently to pain medication; careful monitoring is needed to assess individual response. For example, too often every surgical client is expected to respond to 50 mg of meperidine (Demerol) every 3 to 4 hours regardless of body size, type of surgery, or previous experiences.

7. Explain and assist with noninvasive and nonpharmacologic pain relief measures:
  a. Splinting incision site
  b. Proper positioning
  c. Distraction
  d. Breathing exercises
  e. Massage
  f. Heat and cold application
  g. Relaxation techniques
	7. These measures can help to reduce pain by substituting another stimulus to prevent painful stimuli from reaching higher brain centers. In addition, relaxation reduces muscle tension and may help increase client's sense of control over the pain.

8. Assist client in coping with the aftermath of the pain experience:
  a. If indicated, inform client that the painful procedure is completed and that the pain should soon subside.
  b. Encourage client to discuss the experience.
  c. Clarify any misconceptions the client still may have.
  d. Praise client for endurance and behavior.
	8. These measures can help to reduce anxiety and help client regain the sense of control that the painful experience altered.

9. Teach client to expel flatus by the following measures:
  a. Walk as soon as possible after surgery.
  b. Change positions regularly as possible (e.g., lie prone, assume the knee–chest position).
	9. Postoperatively, sluggish peristalsis results in accumulation of nonabsorbable gas. Pain occurs when unaffected bowel segments contract in an attempt to expel gas. Activity speeds the return of peristalsis and the expulsion of flatus; proper positioning helps gas rise for expulsion.

Documentation

Medication administration record
    Type, route, and dosage schedule of all prescribed medications
Progress notes
    Specific complaints of pain using 0 to 10 scale
    Response to pain relief measures
    Tolerance of oral pain medication
Multidisciplinary client education record
    Medications
    Pain relief measures

Risk for Ineffective Therapeutic Regimen Management Related to Insufficient Knowledge of Care of Operative Site, Restrictions (Diet, Activity), Medications, Signs and Symptoms of Complications, and Follow-up Care

Focus Assessment Criteria	Clinical Significance
1. Readiness and ability to learn and retain information	1. A client or family failing to achieve learning goals requires a referral for assistance postdischarge.

Goals

The goals for this diagnosis represent those associated with discharge planning. Refer to the discharge criteria.

Interventions	Rationales
1. As appropriate, explain and demonstrate care of an uncomplicated surgical wound: 　a. Washing with soap and water 　b. Dressing changes using clean technique	1. Uncomplicated wounds have sealed edges after 24 hours and therefore do not require aseptic technique or a dressing; however, a dressing may be applied if the wound is at risk for injury.
2. As appropriate, explain and demonstrate care of a complicated surgical wound: 　a. Aseptic technique 　b. Handwashing before and after dressing changes 　c. Avoiding touching the inner surface of the soiled dressing and discarding it in a sealed plastic bag 　d. Use of sterile hemostats if indicated 　e. Wound assessment—condition and drainage 　f. Wound cleaning 　g. T-tube care if indicated 　h. Dressing reapplication	2. Aseptic technique is necessary to prevent wound contamination during dressing changes. Handwashing helps to prevent contamination of the wound and the spread of infection. Proper handling and disposal of contaminated dressings helps to prevent infection transmission. Daily assessment is necessary to evaluate healing and detect complications.
3. Reinforce activity restrictions (e.g., bending, lifting) as indicated.	3. Avoiding certain activities decreases risk of wound dehiscence before scar formation occurs (usually after 3 weeks).

(continues on page 679)

Interventions continued	**Rationales** continued

4. Explain the importance of the following:
  a. Avoid ill people and crowds.
  b. Drink 8 to 10 glasses of fluid daily.
  c. Maintain a balanced diet.
	4. Wound healing requires optimal nutrition, hydration, and rest as well as avoiding potential sources of infection.

5. Review with client and family the purpose, dosage, administration, and side effects of all prescribed medications.	5. Complete understanding can help to prevent drug administration errors.

6. Teach client and family to watch for and report signs and symptoms of possible complications:
  a. Persistent temperature elevation
  b. Difficulty breathing, chest pain
  c. Change in sputum characteristics
  d. Increasing weakness, fatigue, pain, or abdominal distention
  e. Wound changes (e.g., separation, unusual or increased drainage, increased redness or swelling)
  f. Voiding difficulties: burning on urination; urinary frequency; or cloudy, foul-smelling urine
  g. Pain, swelling, and warmth in the calf
  h. Other signs and symptoms of complications specific to surgical procedure performed
	6. Early detection and reporting of danger signs and symptoms enable prompt intervention to minimize severity of complications.

7. Whenever possible, provide written instructions (in the client's first language).	7. Written instructions provide an information resource for use at home.
8. Evaluate client's and family's understanding of the information provided.	8. Knowledge gaps may indicate the need for a referral for assistance at home.

 Documentation

Flow records
  Discharge instructions
  Follow-up instructions
Discharge summary record
  Status at discharge (pain, activity, wound healing)
  Achievement of goals (individual or family)
Multidisciplinary client education record
  Wound care
  Pain management

ABDOMINAL AORTIC ANEURYSM RESECTION

This procedure involves surgical resection of an aneurysm—a localized or diffuse arterial outpouching of an artery—and a replacement graft of the aorta. Aneurysm can result from arteriosclerosis, trauma to the artery, congenital weakness, or previous infections. There are four types of aortic aneurysms: ascending aorta, aortic arch, descending thoracic aorta, and abdominal aortic. Repair of three types, excluding abdominal, requires cardiopulmonary bypass and hypothermia during surgery (Akers, 1989; Santilli & Santilli, 1997).

 Time Frame

Preoperative and postoperative periods

DIAGNOSTIC CLUSTER

Preoperative Period

Collaborative Problems	**Refer to**
▲ PC: Rupture of Aneurysm	

Postoperative Period

Collaborative Problems	**Refer to**
▲ PC: Distal Vessel Thrombosis or Emboli	
▲ PC: Renal Failure	
△ PC: Mesenteric Ischemia/Thrombosis	
△ PC: Spinal Cord Ischemia	

Nursing Diagnoses	**Refer to**
△ High Risk for Ineffective Therapeutic Regimen Management related to insufficient knowledge of home care, activity restrictions, signs and symptoms of complications, and follow-up care	
▲ High Risk for Infection related to location of surgical incision	Arterial Bypass Graft
High Risk for Sexual Dysfunction (male) related to possible loss of ejaculate and erections secondary to surgery or atherosclerosis	Colostomy

Related Care Plan

General Surgery Generic Care Plan
(Appendix II)

▲ This diagnosis was reported to be monitored for or managed frequently (75%–100%).
△ This diagnosis was reported to be monitored for or managed often (50%–74%).

Discharge Criteria

Before discharge, the client or family will

1. State wound care measures to perform at home.
2. Verbalize precautions regarding activities.
3. State signs and symptoms that must be reported to a health care professional.

Preoperative: Collaborative Problems

Potential Complication: Ruptured Aneurysm

Nursing Goal

The nurse will detect early signs and symptoms of (a) rupture of aneurysm, (b) distal vessel thrombosis/emboli, (c) renal failure, (d) mesenteric ischemia/thrombosis, and (e) spinal cord ischemia and will collaboratively intervene to stabilize the client.

Indicators
- Calm, oriented (a, d)
- All pulses palpable and strong (a, b, e)
- No abdominal pelvic chest pain (a, b)
- Non-tender abdomen (a, b, d)
- Capillary refill <3 seconds (b)
- No numbness of extremities (b, e)
- Urine output >30 ml/dL (c, e)
- Blood urea nitrogen 5–25 mg/dL (c)
- Serum creatinine
  - Male 0.6–1.5 gm/dL
  - Female 0.6–1.1 gm/dL
- White blood count 4,300–10,800 mm³ (d)
- Hematocrit (d)
  - Male 42%–52%
  - Female 37%–47%
- Sensory/motor intact (e)
- Bowel sounds present 5–30 times per min (d)
- Flatus present (d)
- Soft-formed bowel movements (d)

Interventions	Rationales
1. Monitor all pulses (carotid, brachial, radial, ulnar, femoral, popliteal, dorsalis pedis, and posterior tibial) and blood pressure.	1. A carotid bruit must be evaluated preoperatively to rule out risk of stroke during the operation. Assessing upper extremity pulses establishes a baseline for follow up after arterial lines are in place and arterial punctures are made for blood gas analysis. Assessing lower extremity pulses establishes a baseline for postoperative assessment. A potential complication of aneurysm repair is thrombosis or embolus of distal vessels. Also, clients with abdominal aneurysm have a higher incidence of popliteal aneurysm than the general population.
2. Monitor for signs and symptoms of aneurysm rupture:	2. The larger the aneurysm, the greater the risk of rupture. Aneurysms greater than

(continues on page 682)

Interventions continued	Rationales continued
	6 cm in diameter have a high risk of rupture within a year of discovery.
a. Acute abdominal pain with intense back or pelvic pain	a. Pain results from massive tissue hypoxia and profuse bleeding into the abdominal cavity.
b. Tender, pulsating abdomen	b. Abdominal pulsations and tenderness result from rhythmic pulsations of the artery and tissue hypoxia respectively.
c. Restlessness	c. Restlessness is a response to tissue hypoxia.
d. Shock	d. Shock may result from massive blood loss and tissue hypoxia.
3. Initiate emergency measures as necessary: • Oxygen • Intravenous line • Antihypertensive medications	3. Surgery for ruptured aneurysm carries a mortality rate of 30% to 50%; without immediate surgery, however, mortality rate is near 100%.

 Documentation

Flow records
  Vital signs
Progress notes
  Unusual events
  Interventions

Postoperative: Collaborative Problems

Potential Complication: Distal Vessel Thrombosis or Emboli

Potential Complication: Renal Failure

Potential Complication: Mesenteric Ischemia/Thrombosis

Potential Complication: Spinal Cord Ischemia

Nursing Goal
The nurse will identify and report vascular complications.

Interventions	Rationales

1. Monitor for signs of thrombosis in distal vessels:
  a. Diminished distal pulses, increased capillary refill time (>3 seconds)
  b. Pallor or darkened patches of skin
	1. Prolonged hypotension may result in thrombosis because of decreased blood flow.

(continues on page 683)

Interventions continued	Rationales continued
2. Instruct client to report numbness or tingling in the extremities.	2. Thrombosis of an artery supplying the leg results in a cool, pale, numb, or tingling extremity.
3. If client complains of pain, assess its location and characteristics.	3. It is important to differentiate pain of surgical manipulation from ischemic pain. Microembolization from the aneurysm to the distal skin causes skin infarctions manifested by point discomfort at the infarct and a dark pink-purple discoloration.

4. Monitor for signs of renal failure:
  a. Decreased urine output (<30 mL/hr)
  b. Elevated blood urea nitrogen (BUN), creatinine
  c. Occult blood in urine
	4. During abdominal aorta surgery, the renal arteries are at risk for thrombosis if they are involved in the aneurysm, are clamped for the operation, or are hypoperfused anytime during periods of hypotension. Impaired renal function can result. The endovascular technique reduces subclinical renal damage and colonic ischemia (Solomon, Yee, & Soulen, 2000).

5. Monitor for signs and symptoms of mesenteric thrombosis:
  a. Decreased bowel sounds
 	
  b. Constipation or diarrhea
 	
  c. Increasing abdominal pain
 	
  d. Elevated WBCs (20,000 to 30,000/mm³)
	5. The mesenteric artery, like the renal artery, is at risk for thrombosis.
	  a. Bowel sounds usually are not heard before the third postoperative day.
	  b. A liquid bowel movement before the third postoperative day may point to bowel ischemia.
	  c. Postoperative pain normally decreases each day.
	  d. Elevated WBC count indicates possible bowel necrosis.

6. Monitor for signs and symptoms of spinal cord ischemia:
 	
  a. Urinary retention or incontinence
	6. The spinal arteries are at risk for thrombosis for the same reasons as the renal arteries.
	  a. Inadequate perfusion above the second lumbar vertebra (L2) can result in bladder dysfunction.

7. Carefully monitor intake, output, and hydration and renal status (e.g., central venous pressure every hour for the first 24 hours postoperatively).	7. Hypovolemia can cause thrombosis of graft and decrease renal perfusion. Cross-clamping during surgery will disrupt blood flow to the renal arteries.
8. Monitor blood pressure and report elevations from baseline.	8. Hypertension can result from vasoconstrictor and can potentiate graft rupture.

9. Monitor for intra-abdominal bleeding:
  a. Increased abdominal girth
  b. Decreased hematocrit
	9. Intra-abdominal bleeding can occur during the first 24 hours postoperatively.

(continues on page 684)

Interventions continued	Rationales continued
c. Hypotension d. Tachycardia	
10. Palpate or Doppler peripheral pulses every hour for the first 24 hours.	10. Early detection of graft failure can prevent limb loss.
11. Monitor for ileus: a. Absence of bowel sounds b. Absence of flatus c. Abdominal distention	11. Manual manipulation and displacement of the bowel during surgery will cause bruising and resultant decreased peristalsis.
12. Monitor patency of gastrostomy or naso-gastric tube.	12. Nasogastric suctioning is used for 4 to 5 days postoperatively to decompress the bowel until peristalsis returns.

 Related Physician-Prescribed Interventions

Medications. Dependent on underlying etiology, antihypertensive (e.g., nitroprusside), beta blockers

Intravenous Therapy. Fluid and electrolyte replacement

Laboratory Studies. Refer to the General Surgery care plan, Appendix II.

Diagnostic Studies. Plain radiograph, CT scan, angiogram, MRI, B-mode ultrasound, computed tomographic angiography

Therapies. Oxygen, endovascular stents-graft; also refer to the General Surgery care plan.

 Documentation

Flow records
Vital signs
   Circulation (distal, pulses, color)
   Bowel sounds, presence of occult blood
   Lower extremities (sensation, motor function)
   Urine (output, occult blood)
Progress notes
   Characteristics of pain
   Unrelieved pain
   Interventions
   Response to interventions

Postoperative: Nursing Diagnoses

High Risk for Ineffective Therapeutic Regimen Management Related to Insufficient Knowledge of Home Care, Activity Restrictions, Signs and Symptoms of Complications, and Follow-up Care

Focus Assessment Criteria	Clinical Significance
1. Readiness and ability to learn and retain information	1. A client or family failing to achieve learning goals requires a referral for assistance post-discharge.

Goals

The goals for this diagnosis represent those associated with discharge planning. Refer to the discharge criteria.

Interventions	Rationales
1. For wound care measures and rationale, refer to the General Surgery care plan.	1.
2. If an aorto-bifemoral graft was performed, reinforce the need for a slouched position when sitting.	2. A slouched position helps to prevent graft kinking and possible occlusion.
3. Reinforce activity restrictions (e.g., car riding, stair climbing, lifting).	3. About 5 to 6 weeks after abdominal surgery for the client in good nutritional status, the collagen matrix of the wound becomes strong enough to withstand stress from activity. Surgeon may prefer to limit activity for a longer period because certain activities place tension on the surgical site (Nichols, 1991).
4. If client smokes, reinforce the health benefits of quitting and refer client to a smoking cessation program if available.	4. Tobacco acts as a potent vasoconstrictor that increases stress on the graft (Emma, 1992).
5. Instruct client to report any changes in color, temperature, or sensation in legs.	5. These signs and symptoms may indicate thrombosis or embolism that requires immediate evaluation.
6. Instruct client to report any GI bleeding immediately.	6. Duodenal bleeding may be a sign of erosion of the aortic graft into the duodenum.
7. Instruct client to inform all health care providers about the presence of a prosthetic graft before any invasive procedures.	7. Puncture or exposure of a prosthetic graft risks graft infection that may compromise the client's life.
8. Stress the importance of managing hypertension if indicated.	8. Hypertension can cause false aneurysms at the anastomosis site.

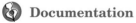 **Documentation**

Discharge summary record
  Client and family teaching
  Response to teaching

AMPUTATION

Amputation is the surgical severing and removal of a limb. Amputations are caused by accidents (23%), disease (74%), and congenital disorders (3%). The rate of lower extremity amputation is about 15 times greater in the person with diabetes. There are five categories of lower extremity amputations: hip disarticulation, above knee, knee disarticulation, below knee, and Syme (ankle and foot) (Williamson, 1998).

 Time Frame

Preoperative and postoperative periods

 DIAGNOSTIC CLUSTER

Preoperative Period

Nursing Diagnoses

▲ Anxiety related to insufficient knowledge of postoperative routines, postoperative sensations, and crutch-walking techniques

Related Care Plan

▲ General Surgery Generic Care Plan

Postoperative Period

Collaborative Problems

▲ PC: Edema of Stump
▲ PC: Wound Hematoma
▲ PC: Hemorrhage
Infection

Nursing Diagnoses

△ High Risk for Disturbed Body Image related to perceived negative effects of amputation and response of others to appearance
▲ High Risk for Impaired Physical Mobility related to limited movement secondary to amputation and pain
▲ Grieving related to loss of limb and its effects on life style
▲ Acute/Chronic Pain related to phantom limb sensations secondary to peripheral nerve stimulation and abnormal impulses to central nervous system
▲ High Risk for Injury related to altered gait and hazards of assistive devices
△ High Risk for Ineffective Therapeutic Regimen Management related to insufficient knowledge of activity of daily living (ADL) adaptations, stump care, prosthesis care, gait training, and follow-up care

---

▲ This diagnosis was reported to be monitored for or managed frequently (75%–100%).
△ This diagnosis was reported to be monitored for or managed often (50%–74%).

Discharge Criteria

Before discharge, the client and family will

1. Describe daily stump care.
2. Explain phantom sensations and interventions to reduce them.
3. Describe measures to protect the stump from injury.

4. Demonstrate prosthesis application and care if indicated.
5. Demonstrate ability to transfer from bed to chair safely.
6. Demonstrate ability to get to the bathroom safely.
7. Demonstrate ability to ascend and descend stairs safely.
8. Demonstrate exercises taught in physical therapy.

Preoperative: Nursing Diagnosis

Anxiety Related to Insufficient Knowledge of Postoperative Routines, Postoperative Sensations, and Crutch-walking Techniques

Focus Assessment Criteria	Clinical Significance
1. Understanding the following: a. Reason for amputation b. Surgical procedure c. Postoperative expectations (i.e., phantom limb sensation, adjustment to prosthetics)	1. Amputation poses a threat to body image and life style. The reason for the amputation influences the present response. Fear and anxiety are commonly related to loss of limb and adjustment to prosthetic.

Goal

The client will identify his or her expectations of the postoperative period.

Indicators
• Ask questions.
• Express concerns.

Interventions	Rationales
1. Explore client's feelings about the impending surgery. a. Allow person to direct discussion. b. Do not assume or project how the client feels.	1. Some may perceive amputation as a devastating event, whereas others will view the surgery as an opportunity to eliminate pain and improve quality of life.
2. Help to establish realistic expectations.	2. Successful prosthetic rehabilitation requires cooperation; coordination; tremendous physical energy; and a well-fitting, comfortable prosthesis (Piasecki, 2001; Yetzer, 1996).
3. Consult with other team members to see the client preoperatively (e.g., physical therapy, prosthetist, or discharge coordinator).	3. Preoperative instruction on postoperative activity helps client to focus on rehabilitation instead of on the surgery; this may help to reduce anxiety.
4. Discuss postoperative expectations, including the following:	4. These explanations help to reduce fears associated with unknown situations and to decrease anxiety.

(continues on page 688)

Interventions continued	Rationales continued
a. Appearance of the stump	a. See rationales 8 and 9.
b. Positioning	b. The stump will be elevated for 24 hours after surgery to prevent edema. Client will be assisted into the prone positions three to four times a day to prevent hip contractures (Piasecki, 2001).
c. Ambulation	c. Dangling and transfer to a chair may occur on first postoperative day. As soon as client is strong enough, use of crutches or a walker will be started (Piasecki, 2001).
d. Phantom pain	d. Research suggests that 85% of amputees have phantom limb pain ranging from daily to weekly to yearly (Hill, Nioen, Krussen, & McGreath, 1995).
5. Instruct on the following postoperatively: a. Active and active-resistive exercises b. Transfer maneuvers c. Use of crutches or walker	5. Training initiated preoperatively can increase mobility postoperatively (Piasecki, 2001).
6. Consult with physician regarding whether there will be immediate prosthetic fitting or a conventional delayed prosthetic fitting.	6. Postoperative care varies with each approach (Piasecki, 2001; Yetzer, 1996).
7. If immediate postsurgical prosthetic fitting is planned, explain that a rigid dressing and cast will be applied at the time of surgery.	7. A socket on the distal end of the cast provides an attachment for a pylon prosthetic unit (Piasecki, 2001).
8. If conventional delayed prosthesis fitting is planned, explain why the stump is covered with a dressing and an elastic bandage.	8. This method shrinks and shapes the stump. A temporary or intermediate prosthesis will be fitted in 3 to 6 weeks (Piasecki, 2001).
9. Explain that fitting for a permanent prosthesis will occur approximately 3 months after surgery.	9. With or without immediate postsurgical fitting, the stump needs this time for complete healing and shrinkage (Piasecki, 2001).
10. Explain that immediately after surgery, client will perceive the amputated limb as being the same shape and size as before surgery (Davis, 1993).	10. Immediately after surgery, all amputees feel the phantom limb as it was before surgery (Davis, 1993).

Documentation

Progress notes
   Assessment of learning readiness and ability
   Client teaching
   Response to teaching

Postoperative: Collaborative Problems

Potential Complication: Edema of Stump

Potential Complication: Wound Hematoma

Potential Complication: Hemorrhage

Potential Complication: Infection

Nursing Goal

The nurse will detect early signs and symptoms of (a) edema of stump, (b) hematoma, (c) hemorrhage, and (d) infection and will collaboratively intervene to stabilize the client.

Indicators

- Diminishing edema (a)
- No evidence of bleeding (c)
- Approximated suture line (a,b)
- No point tenderness (b)
- Temperature 98–99.5°F (d)
- Pulse 60–100 beats/min (c)
- BP >90/60, <140/90 (c)
- Hematocrit (c)
  - Male 42–52%
  - Female 37–47%
- White blood cells 4,300–10,800 mm³ (d)

Interventions	Rationales
1. Elevate stump the first 24 hours only.	1. Elevation the first 24 hours will reduce edema and promote venous return. Elevation of the limb after 24 hours can cause flexion contractions (Williamson, 1998).

2. Monitor incision for the following:
  a. Edema along suture line
  b. Areas of compression (if Ace wraps are used)
  c. Areas of pressure (if a cast is used)
  d. Bleeding
	2. Traumatized tissue responds with lymphedema. Excessive edema must be detected to prevent tension on the suture line that can cause bleeding. Tissue compression from edema can compromise circulation (Williamson, 1998).

3. Monitor for signs of hematoma:
  a. Unapproximated suture line
  b. Ruddy color changes of skin along suture line
  c. Oozing dark blood from suture line
  d. Point tenderness on palpation
	3. Amputation flaps may be pulled over large areas of "space," creating pockets that may contain old blood. Hematoma may compromise flap healing and delay rehabilitation (Ray, 2000).

4. Evaluate the fit of elastic bandages and reapply every 4 to 6 hours using figure-of-eight turns.	4. Proper bandaging provides wound protection, controls tissue edema, molds the limb for prosthetic fitting, and remains secure with movement (Williamson, 1998).

Related Physician-Prescribed Interventions

Medications. Analgesics

Laboratory Studies. Dependent on underlying condition and symptomatology

Diagnostic Studies. Dependent on symptomatology

Therapies. Physical therapy, occupational therapy, prosthesis

 Documentation

Flow records
   Appearance of suture line
   Appearance of skin around suture line
   Drainage
Progress notes
   Abnormal findings

Postoperative: Nursing Diagnoses

High Risk for Disturbed Body Image Related to Perceived Negative Effects of Amputation and Response of Others to Appearance

Focus Assessment Criteria	Clinical Significance
1. Ability to express feelings about appearance	1. Self-concept includes perceptions and feelings about self-worth, attractiveness, lovability, and capacity. The client's ability to express these perceptions and feelings allows the nurse to plan effective interventions to help enhance self-concept.
2. Perception of effects on life style	2. The client's emotional response to the loss is influenced in large part by the extent to which disability interferes with personal goals.
3. Ability to participate in self-care including dressing changes	3. A client's successful coping with physical loss is manifested by his or her involvement with self-care and care of the surgical site (Hamburg & Adams, 1953).
4. Present response (e.g., denial, mourning, awareness, or managing)	4. The grieving process in response to a recent disability involves denial or minimal thinking of loss, realization of loss and mourning, and eventually managing and incorporating the loss into one's life style.

Goal

The client will communicate feelings about his or her changed appearance.

Indicators
- Express an interest in dress and grooming.
- Discuss feelings with family.

Interventions	Rationales
1. Contact client frequently and treat him or her with warm, positive regard.	1. Frequent contact by the caregiver indicates acceptance and may facilitate trust. Client may be hesitant to approach the staff because of negative self-concept; nurse must reach out (Dudas, 1997).
2. Encourage client to verbalize feelings about appearance and perceptions of life style impacts. 3. Validate client's perceptions and assure client that they are normal and appropriate.	2,3. Expressing feelings and perceptions increases the client's self-awareness and helps nurse to plan effective interventions to address client's needs. Validating client's perceptions provides reassurance and can decrease anxiety (Dudas, 1997).
4. Assist client in identifying personal attributes and strengths. 5. Facilitate adjustment through active listening.	4,5. This can help client to focus on the positive characteristics that contribute to the whole concept of self rather than on only the change in body image. Nurse should reinforce these positive aspects and encourage client to reincorporate them into his or her new self-concept (Dudas, 1997).
6. Encourage optimal hygiene, grooming, and other self-care activities.	6. Participation in self-care and planning promotes positive coping with the change.
7. Encourage client to perform as many activities as possible unassisted.	7. Nonparticipation in self-care and overprotection by caregivers tends to promote feelings of helplessness and dependence.

8. When appropriate, do the following:
  a. Share your perceptions of the loss and the client's response to it.
  b. Explain the nature of the loss.
  c. Discuss the anticipated changes in life style.
	8. Open, honest discussions—expressing that changes will occur but that they are manageable—promote feelings of control.

9. Prepare significant others for physical and emotional changes.	9. Support can be given more freely and more realistically if others are prepared (Dudas, 1997).
10. Discuss with client's support system the importance of communicating client's value and importance.	10. This will enhance self-esteem and promote adjustment.
11. Facilitate use of prosthesis as soon as possible.	11. Restoration of mobility has a positive effect on self-concept (Williamson, 1992).
12. Refer a client at high risk for unsuccessful adjustment to counseling as appropriate.	12. Professional counseling is indicated for a client with poor ego strengths and inadequate coping resources.

Documentation

Progress notes
   Present emotional status
   Dialogues

High Risk for Impaired Physical Mobility Related to Limited Movement Secondary to Pain

Focus Assessment Criteria	Clinical Significance
1. ROM of all joints preoperatively	1. This baseline assessment provides data against which to compare postoperative assessment findings.
2. Postoperative ROM after client has received pain medication	2. ROM may be restricted by pain and improved after administration of pain medication.

Goal

The client will report increased use of affected limb.

Indicators

* Demonstrate safe use of adaptive devices.
* Use safety measures to prevent injury.

Interventions	Rationales
1. Elevate the limb for the first 24 hours only.	1. Elevation will reduce edema. Continued elevation can cause flexion contractures (Williamson, 1992).
2. Initiate transfer to chair and ambulation as soon as indicated.	2. These activities are usually initiated 12 to 24 hours after surgery (Williamson, 1992).
3. Consult with physical therapy to begin exercises.	3. Exercises are indicated for muscle strengthening and to prevent abduction and flexion contractures (Williamson, 1992).
4. Assist client into a prone position three to four times a day for at least 15 minutes. 5. Encourage client to sleep in this position.	4,5. Abdominal lying places the pelvic joints in an extended position that extends extensor muscles and prevents contractures (Williamson, 1992).
6. Teach client to perform active ROM exercises on unaffected limbs at least four times a day. (*Note:* Perform passive ROM only if client cannot do it actively.)	6. Active ROM increases muscle mass, tone, and strength and improves cardiac and respiratory functioning.

(continues on page 693)

Interventions continued	Rationales continued
7. Teach client to avoid prolonged sitting.	7. Prolonged sitting can cause hip flexion contractures.
8. Discuss the increased energy requirements needed to use a prosthesis.	8. Walking with a prosthesis requires more effort because of its weight and the loss of the usual muscle coordination. Clients who are successful see more advantages than disadvantages with prosthetic use (Williamson, 1992).
9. Explore with client activities that are important to resume (e.g., bowling or swimming). Discuss what client can do to resume activity.	9. Successful adaption to prosthesis use is dependent on the person's belief that one's behavior will improve one's situation (Bandura, 1992).
10. If appropriate, arrange for someone who has successfully adapted to a prosthesis to visit client.	10. Successful coping is promoted by witnessing others successfully coping (Bandura, 1992).
11. Emphasize progress, no matter how small. Convey that the client can successfully manage adaptation to the prosthesis.	11. Other people's belief that they can successfully cope increases one's own confidence (Bandura, 1992).

 Documentation

Flow records
   Exercises
Progress notes
   Range of motion

Nursing Diagnosis

Grieving Related to Loss of a Limb and Its Effects on Life Style

Focus Assessment Criteria	Clinical Significance
1. Signs and symptoms of grief reaction (e.g., crying, withdrawal, anxiety, restlessness, decreased appetite, or increased dependency)	1. Losses related to function and independence usually provoke a profound grief response. Persons experiencing amputation after long, painful, unsuccessful treatment may view this as a relief (Williamson, 1992).

Goal
The client will describe the meaning of the loss.

Indicators
- Express grief.
- Report an intent to discuss feelings with family members or significant others.

Interventions	Rationales
1. Provide opportunities for client and family members to ventilate feelings, discuss the loss openly, and explore the personal meaning of the loss. Explain that grief is a common and healthy reaction.	1. Amputation may give rise to feelings of powerlessness, anger, profound sadness, and other grief responses. Open, honest discussions can help the client and family members to accept and cope with the situation and their responses to it (Butler, Turkal & Seidl, 1992; Williamson, 1998).
2. Encourage use of positive coping strategies that have proved successful in the past.	2. Positive coping strategies aid acceptance and problem solving (Piasecki, 2001).
3. Encourage client to express positive self-attributes.	3. Focusing on positive attributes increases self-acceptance and acceptance of the loss (Piasecki, 2001).
4. Assess family's or significant others' responses to the situation by focusing on the following: a. Their perception of the short- and long-term affects of disability b. Past and present family dynamics	4. Successful adjustment depends on the client's and support persons' realistic perceptions of the situation (Piasecki, 2001).
5. Help family members and significant others to cope. a. Explore their perceptions of how the situation will progress. b. Identify behaviors that facilitate adaptation. c. Encourage them to maintain usual roles and behaviors. d. Encourage including the client in family decision-making. e. Discuss the reality of everyday emotions such as anger, guilt, and jealousy; relate the hazards of denying these feelings. f. Explain the dangers of trying to minimize grief and interfering with the normal grieving process.	5. A positive response by client's family or significant others is one of the most important factors in client's own acceptance of the loss (Butler, Turkal & Seidl, 1992).
6. Promote grief work with each response. a. Denial: • Encourage acceptance of the situation; do not reinforce denial by giving false reassurance. • Promote hope through assurances of care, comfort, and support. • Explain the use of denial by one family member to other members.	6. Grieving involves profound emotional responses; interventions depend on the particular response.

(continues on page 695)

Interventions continued	Rationales continued

• Do not push a person to move past denial until he or she is emotionally ready.
 b. Isolation:
   • Convey acceptance by encouraging expressions of grief.
   • Promote open, honest communication to encourage sharing.
   • Reinforce client's self-worth by providing for privacy when desired.
   • Encourage socialization as feasible (e.g., support groups or church activities).
 c. Depression:
   • Reinforce client's self-esteem.
   • Employ empathetic sharing and acknowledge grief.
   • Identify degree of depression and develop appropriate strategies.
 d. Anger:
   • Explain to other family members that anger represents an attempt to control the environment stemming from frustration at the inability to control the disease.
   • Encourage verbalization of anger.
 e. Guilt:
   • Acknowledge person's expressed self-image.
   • Encourage identification of the relationship's positive aspects.
   • Avoid arguing and participating in the person's system of "I should have . . ." and "I shouldn't have. . ."
 f. Fear:
   • Focus on the present and maintain a safe and secure environment.
   • Help person to explore reasons for and meanings of the fears.
 g. Rejection:
   • Provide reassurance by explaining what is happening.
   • Explain this response to other family members.
 h. Hysteria:
   • Reduce environmental stressors (e.g., limit personnel).
   • Provide a safe, private area in which to express grief.	

7. Refer client to Amputee Support group. • Have amputee visitor see patient.	7. This allows patient and family opportunity to ventilate and ask questions.

Documentation

Progress notes
  Present emotional status
  Interventions
  Response to interventions

* This diagnosis is not currently on the NANDA list but has been included for clarity or usefulness.

Acute/Chronic Pain Related to Phantom Limb Sensations Secondary to Peripheral Nerve Stimulation and Abnormal Impulses to Central Nervous System

Focus Assessment Criteria	Clinical Significance

1. Presence and character of phantom sensation (Katz, 1996):
  a. Feeling limb is present
  b. Limb is floating in midair
  c. Phantom limb "telescopes" into remaining stump
  d. Pain that resembles pain felt before surgery
  e. Tight band just below the level of amputation
  f. Pleasant, warm, and tingling feeling
	1. Eighty percent of amputees experience significant phantom limb sensations at intervals during the first year following surgery (Williamson, 1992).

Goal

The client will report decreased phantom pain.

Indicators

- State the reasons for phantom sensation.
- Demonstrate techniques for managing phantom sensation.

Interventions	Rationales
1. Explain that the sensations are normal and encourage client to report them.	1. Client may be hesitant to discuss phantom sensations for fear of appearing abnormal.
2. Explain that phantom sensations may manifest themselves as discomfort, pain, itching, tingling, warmth, or other sensations previously felt on that limb.	2. Phantom sensations are caused by stimulation of the nerve proximal to the amputation that previously extended to the limb. Client perceives the stimulation as originating from the absent limb. The exact cause of phantom limb pain is not agreed on. Stimulus of peripheral nerves proximal to the amputation is thought to be a cause. Another explanation is that severed nerves may send abnormal impulses that are perceived by the brain as abnormal (Davis, 1993; Katz, 1996).

(continues on page 697)

Interventions continued	Rationales continued
3. Explain that stress, anxiety, fatigue, depression, excitement, and weather changes may intensify phantom limb pain.	3. Psychological stressors do not cause phantom limb pain but can trigger or increase it (Katz, 1996).

4. Explain measures that have been effective in alleviating phantom limb pain.
  a. Applying heat to stump
  b. Applying pressure to stump (e.g., elastic bandages)
  c. Distraction, diversion techniques, and relaxation exercises
  d. Massage therapy (after 2 weeks postoperatively)
	4. Stimulation causing a second sensation may serve to override the phantom sensation (Williamson, 1992).

5. Avoid administering narcotics or analgesics for phantom pain. Check with physician about administration of other medications.	5. Narcotics are ineffective for phantom limb pain but are effective for surgical stump pain (Katz, 1996).
6. Advise client to consult with pain specialists if phantom limb pain is unmanageable.	6. Phantom limb pain causes disability and loss of employment (Hill, Nioen, Krussen, & McGreath, 1995).
7. Advise client that phantom pain may begin right after surgery or not until 2 to 3 months later.	7. This explanation will help to reduce fears associated with unknown situations.

 Documentation

Progress notes
  Reports of pain
  Interventions
  Response to interventions

High Risk for Injury Related to Altered Gait and Hazards of Assistive Devices

Focus Assessment Criteria	Clinical Significance
1. Knowledge of prosthesis use and assistive devices	1. Assessment guides nurse in planning appropriate teaching strategies.
2. Fit and comfort of prosthesis	2. Prosthetic devices should not be uncomfortable during use. Over time, weight change or muscle atrophy may necessitate adjustments in a device.

(continues on page 698)

Focus Assessment Criteria continued	Clinical Significance continued
3. Strength (arms, unaffected leg)	3. The upper body strength and the unaffected leg influence gait.
4. Ability to perform ADLs	4. Use of a leg prosthesis requires an additional 60% to 80% of energy expenditure. This may hinder client's ability to perform ADLs (Yetzer, 1996).

Goal

The client will not injure self.

Indicators

- Relate the potential safety problems associated with use of a prosthesis or an assistive device.
- Ask for assistance as needed.

Interventions	Rationales
1. Reinforce exercise and activities prescribed by physical therapist.	1. Exercises increase muscle strength needed for transfers and ambulation.
2. Provide an assistive device (such as walker or cane) to compensate for altered gait as necessary.	2. Client may need an assistive device to enable ambulation or reduce the risk of falling.
3. Teach client to eliminate environmental hazards from the home, such as the following: a. Throw rugs b. Clutter c. Dim lighting d. Uneven or slippery floors	3. Removing hazards can reduce risks of slipping and falling.
4. Encourage client to request assistance as needed when in an unfamiliar environment or situation.	4. Assistance may help to prevent injury.
5. Encourage client to report altered gait to physician or prosthetist.	5. Altered gait may be due to a poorly fitted prosthesis or other reasons; it requires further evaluation.

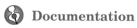 **Documentation**

Progress notes
    Assessment of learning readiness/ability
    Ability to perform ADLs

Discharge summary record
  Client teaching
  Response to teaching

High Risk for Ineffective Therapeutic Regimen Management Related to Insufficient Knowledge of Activity of Daily Living (ADL) Adaptations, Stump Care, Prosthesis Care, Gait Training, and Follow-up Care

Focus Assessment Criteria	Clinical Significance
1. Self-care limitations imposed by amputation 2. Knowledge of self-care activities 3. Support system	1–3. Assessment of self-care ability and support system determines whether or not client needs assistance at home.

Goals

The goals for this diagnosis represent those associated with discharge planning. Refer to the discharge criteria.

Interventions	Rationales

1. Teach foot care for the remaining foot including the following:
  a. Daily foot bath
  b. Thorough drying
  c. Daily inspection for corns, calluses, blisters, and signs of infection
  d. Professional nail cutting
  e. Wearing clean socks daily
  f. Wearing sturdy slippers or shoes
	1. Daily care is necessary to deflect or prevent injury, especially if a circulatory disorder was a contributing factor to amputation (Yetzer, Kauffman, & Sopp, 1994).

2. Instruct client to place a chair or other large object next to the bed at home to prevent him or her from getting out of bed at night and attempting to stand on the stump when not fully awake.	2. Phantom sensations include a kinesthetic awareness of the absent limb. A half-asleep client arising during the night may fall and damage the healing stump (Davis, 1993).
3. Instruct client to avoid tobacco; refer to a smoking cessation program if necessary.	3. Nicotine in tobacco constricts arterial vessels, which decreases blood flow to the healing stump. If amputation was related to atherosclerosis, tobacco use may threaten the stump's survival (Rudolph, 1992).

4. Explain the risks for infection and the need to report:
  a. Fever
  b. Increased pain
  c. Increased swelling
  d. Skin necrosis
	4. Hematomas of the wound contribute to infection. Coexisting diabetes mellitus reduces resistance to bacteria and causes diminished circulation. Tissue necrosis also can result from decreased circulation, chronic swelling, and infection.

(continues on page 700)

Interventions continued	Rationales continued

5. Teach the client to prepare the stump for a prosthesis as appropriate:
  a. Regularly examine the stump for expected changes (e.g., muscle and scar atrophy) and unexpected changes (e.g., skin breakdown, redness, tenderness, increased warmth or coolness, and numbness or tingling).
  b. When the incision is closed, perform daily stump care to include the following:
    • Washing with soap and water
    • Drying thoroughly
    • Avoiding creams and ointments
  c. Wrap the stump with Ace bandages using figure-of-eight turns.
	5.
	
	  a. Shrinkage occurs as scar tissue retracts. Increasing redness or tenderness may indicate infection.
	
	  b. Daily cleansing helps to prevent infection. Creams and ointments may soften the skin to the point at which it is easily broken down.
	
	  c. Elastic compression reduces edema in the stump. Edema interferes with wound healing and prolongs the rehabilitation time. Wrapping using figure-of-eight turns also helps to shape the stump for better fit into the prosthesis. Ace bandages wrapped horizontally can impede circulation.

6. Reinforce the need to continue exercises at home. (For more information, see the nursing diagnosis High Risk for Impaired Physical Mobility in this care plan).	6. Active ROM exercises increase muscle mass, tone, and strength pressure joint mobility and improve cardiac and respiratory function.
7. Evaluate client's ability to manage the home, shop, prepare food, and do other ADLs. If indicated, initiate referrals to community and social service agencies, i.e., Amputee Support Group.	7. Referrals may be indicated to provide additional assistance after discharge.
8. Refer client to rehabilitative facility.	8. The sooner the person engages in rehabilitation, the more successful is prosthetic ambulation (Munin et al., 2001).

 Documentation

Discharge summary record
  Client and family teaching
  Response to teaching
  Referrals if indicated

ARTERIAL BYPASS GRAFTING IN THE LOWER EXTREMITY

This procedure involves grafting an autogenous vein or an artificial graft to bypass an arterial occlusion and restore continuous blood flow. Depending on the extent of the occlusion, the bypass graft can reach from the top of the femoral artery to the proximal popliteal artery, to the tibioperoneal trunk, or to small arteries in the ankle (Folcarelli & Carleton, 1997).

 Time Frame

Preoperative and postoperative periods

 DIAGNOSTIC CLUSTER

Collaborative Problems

▲ PC: Thrombosis of Graft
△ PC: Compartment Syndrome
   Lymphocele
▲ PC: Disruption of Anastomosis

Nursing Diagnoses

▲ High Risk for Infection related to location of surgical incision
△ High Risk for Impaired Skin Integrity related to immobility and vulnerability of heels
▲ Acute Pain related to increased tissue perfusion to previous ischemic tissue
△ High Risk for Ineffective Therapeutic Regimen Management related to insufficient knowledge of wound care, signs and symptoms of complications, activity restrictions, and follow-up care

Related Care Plans

▲ General Surgery Generic Care Plan
▲ Abdominal Aortic Aneurysm Resection

▲ This diagnosis was reported to be monitored for or managed frequently (75%–100%).
△ This diagnosis was reported to be monitored for or managed often (50%–74%).

Discharge Criteria

Before discharge, the client and/or family will

1. Demonstrate proper wound care.
2. Demonstrate correct pulse palpation technique.
3. State the signs and symptoms that must be reported to a health care professional.

Collaborative Problems

Potential Complication: Thrombosis of Graft

Potential Complication: Compartment Syndrome

Potential Complication: Lymphocele

Potential Complication: Disruption of Anastomosis

Nursing Goal

The nurse will detect early signs and symptoms of (a) thrombosis of graft, (b) compartment syndrome, (c) lymphocele, and (d) disruption of anastomosis and will collaboratively intervene to stabilize client.

Indicators

- Capillary refill <3 seconds (a, b, d)
- Peripheral pulses: full, present (a)
- Warm, not mottled limbs (a, b)
- Intact sensation (a, b)
- Minimal limb edema (b)
- No pain with passive stretching (a, b)
- Intact muscle tension (a, b)
- Increasing wound drainage (c)
- Increasing local swelling (b, c)
- No bounding pulsation over graft (d)
- Can move toes (b)

Interventions	Rationales
1. Keep bed's side rails up.	1. Every practical measure should be taken to prevent graft trauma from injury.
2. Keep the limb warm but *do not* use electric heating pads or hot water bottles.	2. Peripheral nerve ischemia causes diminished sensation. High temperatures of heating devices may damage tissue without the client feeling discomfort.
3. Instruct client to sit in a "slouched" position and not to cross legs. If leg elevation is ordered, elevate the entire leg and the pelvis to heart level.	3. Sharp flexion and pressure on the graft must be avoided to prevent graft damage (Edwards, Abullarade, & Turnbull, 1996).
4. Monitor graft patency, palpate a graft patency, palpate a graft near the skin surface, and assess distal pulses for changes from baseline (e.g., Doppler pressure).	4. Graft patency is essential to arterial circulation.
5. Monitor circulatory status, color, temperature, sensation, and motor function in the affected leg every hour and as needed.	5. A sudden change in temperature, drop in pressure, or absence of pulses indicates graft thrombosis. Changes in sensation or motor function can indicate compartment syndrome (Edwards, Abullarade, & Turnbull, 1996).
6. Immediately report changes in color, temperature, sensation, pulses, or pressure to physician (e.g., pain in toes or foot).	6. Sudden decrease in arterial flow indicating thrombosed graft is an emergency requiring immediate surgical exploration of the graft (Edwards, Abullarade, & Turnbull, 1996).

(continues on page 703)

Interventions continued	**Rationales** continued

7. Monitor for signs and symptoms of compartment syndrome:
  a. Edema of revascularized limb
  b. Complaints of pain with passive stretching of the muscle
  c. Decreased sensation, motor function, or paresthesias of the distal limb
  d. Increased tension and firmness of muscle
	7. After a period of ischemia comes a period of increased capillary wall permeability. Restoration of arterial flow causes plasma and extracellular fluid to flow into the tissues, producing massive swelling in calf muscles. Pain and muscle tension result as the tissues are prevented from extending outward by the fascia and the inward pressure obliterates the circulation. The nerves become anoxic, causing paresthesias and motor deficits (Tumbarello, 2000).

8. Immediately report changes in status to the physician.	8. Postoperative edema is expected in the new vascularized limb. Careful assessment alerts the nurse to edema severe enough to cause compartment syndrome. Treatment must be initiated within 8 hours to preserve function of the extremity (Edwards, Abullarade, & Turnbull, 1996).

9. Monitor for signs and symptoms of lymphocele:
  a. Discomfort accompanied by local swelling
  b. Large amounts of clear or pink-tinged drainage
	9. A major lymphatic channel courses through the inner thigh area. If the lymphatic chain is lacerated during the operation, drainage may occur. The large amount of accumulated fluid seeks the path of least resistance and usually drains through the incision.

10. Support the affected leg and
  a. Discontinue elevation and ice.
  b. Loosen dressings.
	10. Support can reduce muscle spasms.

11. Apply compression dressings only if ordered by physician.	11. Although compression may possibly halt the flow of lymph long enough for the lymphatic vessel to seal, this usually is not the case; so surgical intervention may be required to repair the draining lymphatic chain. Compression should be used only on the physician's order; overly vigorous compression may damage the new graft.

12. Monitor for disruption of anastomosis:
  a. Decrease in perfusion of distal extremity
  b. Bounding aneurysmal pulsation over the anastomosis site. If bleeding occurs, apply firm constant pressure over site and notify physician.
	12. Hemorrhage from anastomotic disruption is an emergency requiring immediate surgical intervention.

Related Physician-Prescribed Interventions

Medications. Vasodilators, anticoagulant therapy, mannitol

Intravenous Therapy. Fluid/electrolyte replacement

Laboratory Studies. Prothrombin time, platelet count, serum creatinine phosphokinase, urine creatinine clearance

Diagnostic Studies. Doppler ultrasonography

Therapies. Hyperbaric oxygen therapy; also refer to the General Surgery care plan.

Documentation

Flow records
 Vital signs
 Distal pulses
 Circulatory status
Progress notes
 Presence and description of pain
 Unusual events, actions, responses
 Wound drainage and appearance

Nursing Diagnoses

High Risk for Infection Related to Location of Surgical Incision

Focus Assessment Criteria	Clinical Significance
1. Groin wound every shift	1. A superficial infection that would be benign in another surgical site can lead to graft failure.

Goal

The client will exhibit wound healing free of infection.

Indicators

- State early signs of infection.
- Demonstrate wound care.

Interventions	Rationales
1. If the wound does not have a polyurethane film dressing from the operating room, cover with a dry, sterile gauze dressing. Be certain that no skin surfaces come in contact with each other.	1. Minimizing moisture in the groin wound decreases the risk of infection (Maklebust & Sieggreen, 2001).
2. If client has a pendulous abdomen, teach her or him to position body so that the abdomen does not cover the groin wound.	2. Keeping the wound free of skin overlays decreases moisture, which is a medium for microorganism growth (Maklebust & Sieggreen, 2001).

(continues on page 705)

Interventions continued	Rationales continued
3. If tissue becomes macerated, increase the frequency of gauze dressing changes. Expose the groin to air for 15-minute periods during the day.	3. Air will help to dry the wound.
4. Teach client the importance of avoiding wound maceration and graft infection.	4. Graft failure can result from a wound infection.
5. Refer to Generic Surgical care plan for additional interventions.	

 Documentation

Flow records
   Interventions
   Response to interventions

High Risk for Impaired Skin Integrity Related to Immobility and Vulnerability of Heels

Goal

The client will maintain intact skin over heels.

Indicators
- Describe measures to protect heels.
- Relate why heels are at risk.

Interventions	Rationales
1. Observe for signs and symptoms of tissue ischemia (e.g., blanching or redness). Palpate for changes in tissue consistency beneath the skin.	1. Pressure ulcer formation may begin deep in the tissue. A client with peripheral vascular disease secondary to atherosclerosis is at high risk for pressure ulcer formation because of the ischemia already present in the tissue (Maklebust & Sieggreen, 2001).
2. Explain why heels are especially vulnerable to skin breakdown from excessive pressure.	2. A compromised arterial supply may be just enough to maintain viability of a leg but inadequate to heal an ulcer in the leg.
3. Take measures to alleviate pressure on heels (e.g., elevate heels from bed and avoid heel protectors).	3. Skin pressure triggers ulcer formation. Elevation reduces direct pressure; heel protectors are a direct pressure device (Maklebust & Sieggreen, 2001).

Documentation

Flow records
    Skin condition
    Interventions

Acute Pain Related to Increased Tissue Perfusion to Previous Ischemic Tissue

Focus Assessment Criteria	Clinical Significance
1. Comfort level, descriptions of sensations 2. Operative leg for evidence of ischemia	1,2. The nurse must investigate the underlying cause of pain to rule out an ischemic origin.

Goal

The client will report pain relief after interventions.

Indicators

• State the reason for the pain.
• Relate signs/symptoms of ischemia.

Interventions	Rationales
1. Explain the source of pain and reassure client that the sensation is temporary and will decrease each day.	1. Pain occurs as previously ischemic sensory nerve endings are being reperfused and less as reperfusion progresses.
2. Assess carefully to differentiate between the pain of reperfusion and pain of ischemia. (Ischemic tissue is cool; reperfused tissue is warm and edematous.) Notify physician immediately if you suspect ischemia.	2. Ischemic pain may indicate graft failure and warrants immediate evaluation.
3. Refer to the nursing diagnosis Acute Pain in the General Surgery care plan (Appendix II) for more information.	

 Documentation

Progress notes
    Unrelieved pain
    Interventions
    Response to interventions

High Risk for Ineffective Therapeutic Regimen Management Related to Insufficient Knowledge of Wound Care, Signs and Symptoms of Complications, Activity Restrictions, and Follow-up Care

Focus Assessment Criteria	Clinical Significance
1. Readiness and ability to learn and retain information	1. A client or family failing to achieve learning goals requires a referral for assistance postdischarge.

Goals

The goals for this diagnosis represent those associated with discharge planning. Refer to the discharge criteria.

Interventions	Rationales
1. Teach client and family the proper wound care techniques. (Refer to the nursing diagnosis High Risk for Ineffective Therapeutic Regimen Management in the General Surgery care plan, Appendix II, for specific measures.)	1. Proper wound care can prevent infection that delays healing (Edwards, Abullarade, & Turnbull, 1996).
2. Reinforce teaching regarding activity restrictions and mobility (Edwards, Abullarade, & Turnbull, 1996). a. Increase activity as prescribed. b. Avoid long periods (>20 minutes) of standing or sitting with legs bent at the groin and knee. c. Ambulate as advised; plan a walking program.	2. The client's understanding may encourage compliance with the therapeutic regimen. a. Activity should be increased gradually to promote circulation and reduce loss of strength. b. Dependent positioning of the legs increases postoperative swelling. Positions of hip–knee flexion impede venous return. c. Early ambulation is recommended to restore muscle activity and enhance venous blood return.
3. Teach client and support persons how to assess graft patency. a. Assess pulses and capillary refill. b. Palpate the graft for pulsations if near the surface.	3. Monitoring circulatory status must be continued at home.
4. Teach client and others to recognize signs and symptoms of problems and report them immediately. a. Absence of pulses b. Change in temperature of leg or foot c. Paresthesias and other changes in sensation d. Pain e. Wound or sore in affected leg f. Changes in incision (e.g., redness, drainage)	4. Reporting these signs of compromised circulation, infection, or possible graft failure promptly enables intervention to prevent serious complications. Diminished circulation impedes healing; infection can cause graft failure (Edwards, Abullarade & Turnbull, 1996).

(continues on page 708)

Interventions continued	Rationales continued
5. Reinforce teaching regarding foot care and prevention of injury to the leg. Refer to Peripheral Arterial care plan for specific teaching.	5. Continued care and precautions are necessary at home.
6. Discuss the options if impotence occurs (e.g., referral to urologist or counselor).	6. Operative disruption of internal iliac blood supply or sympathetic fibers may cause impotence (Rutherford, 1995).

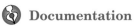 Documentation

Discharge summary record
  Client and family teaching
  Response to teaching

BREAST SURGERY (LUMPECTOMY, MASTECTOMY)

The treatment for breast cancer is removal of the tumor followed by radiation, chemotherapy, hormonal therapy, or combinations of these. The types of surgery differ in the amount of breast tissue removed, dissection of lymph nodes, and removal of pectoral muscles. *Lumpectomy* is the removal of the cancerous tissue and a small amount of adjacent tissue with overlying skin left in place. Axillary nodes may be dissected through a separate incision. *Quadrantectomy* is the removal of a quarter of the breast with the tumor including skin and most axillary lymph nodes. *Total mastectomy* is the removal of the entire breast and some lymph nodes. *Modified radical mastectomy* is the removal of the entire breast and all axillary lymph nodes. *Radical mastectomy* is the removal of the entire breast, skin, pectoral muscles, and all axillary lymph nodes. If the breast is removed, breast reconstruction with implants and nipple-areolar construction or autologous transplants are planned (Chapman & Goodman, 2000).

 Time Frame
Preoperative and postoperative periods

 DIAGNOSTIC CLUSTER

Preoperative Period

Nursing Diagnoses

▲ Anxiety/Fear related to perceived effects of mastectomy (immediate: pain, edema; postdischarge: relationships, work) and prognosis

Postoperative Period

Collaborative Problems

▲ PC: Neurovascular Compromise

Refer to General Surgery Care Plan for additional collaborative problems.

Nursing Diagnoses	Refer to
▲ High Risk for Impaired Physical Mobility (arm, shoulder) related to lymphedema, nerve/muscle damage, and pain	
▲ High Risk for Injury related to compromised lymph drainage, motor, and sensory function in affected arm	
▲ High Risk for Disturbed Self-Concept related to perceived negative effects of loss on functioning	Cancer: Initial Diagnosis

(continues on page 710)

Nursing Diagnoses continued	Refer to continued
▲ Grieving related to loss of breast and change in appearance	Cancer (Initial Diagnosis)
▲ High Risk for Ineffective Therapeutic Regimen Management related to insufficient knowledge of wound care, exercises, breast prosthesis, signs and symptoms of complications, hand/arm precautions, community resources, and follow-up care **Related Care Plan** General Surgery Generic Care Plan	

▲ This diagnosis was reported to be monitored for or managed frequently (75%–100%).

Discharge Criteria

Before discharge, the client and family will

1. Demonstrate hand and arm exercises.
2. Describe hand and arm precautions.
3. Demonstrate breast self-examination.
4. State care measures to perform at home.
5. Discuss strategies for performing ADLs.
6. State necessary precautions.
7. State the signs and symptoms that must be reported to a health care professional.
8. Verbalize an intent to share feelings and concerns with significant others.
9. Identify available community resources and self-help groups.

Preoperative: Nursing Diagnosis

Anxiety/Fear Related to Perceived Mastectomy and Prognosis

Focus Assessment Criteria	Clinical Significance
1. Nature of concerns and fears	1. Breast surgery poses a threat to body image; breast cancer may pose a threat to life. Client's emotional reaction to surgery depends in large part on her perception of its effects (e.g., physical, psychological, social, spiritual, and financial) on her life.
2. Understanding of mastectomy including past experience and information from others who have undergone the surgery	2. Many women have heard "horror stories" about mastectomy. Many of these stories involve older types of surgery that often did involve widespread tissue destruction. By comparison, today's procedures are much less destructive (Hoskins et al., 1996).

(continues on page 711)

Focus Assessment Criteria continued	Clinical Significance continued
3. Support systems, coping patterns	3. Women have cited family support as essential in helping them to cope (Hoskins et al., 1996).
4. Anxiety level (mild, moderate, severe, or panic)	4. High anxiety impairs learning.

Goal

The client will share concerns regarding the surgery and its outcome.

Indicators
- Describe actions that can help reduce postoperative edema and immobility.
- State an intent to share feelings with significant other or a friend.

Interventions	Rationales
1. Encourage client to verbalize her concerns and fears. Stay with client and family as much as possible and convey empathy and concern.	1. Both lumpectomy and mastectomy clients report anxiety and depression. The anxiety of lumpectomy clients was attributed to feelings of uncertainty regarding prognosis and possible reoccurrence. Mastectomy clients reported anxiety regarding the impact of surgery on relationships and appearance (Hoskins et al., 1996).
2. Initiate dialogue regarding concerns about the cancer diagnosis.	2. Open, honest dialogue can help to instill realistic hope. Avoiding the topic only promotes feelings of despair and isolation. A woman who loses a breast may feel self-conscious, inferior, and undesirable (Spencer, 1996).
3. If client is agreeable, arrange for a visitor from Reach for Recovery.	3. A person who has undergone mastectomy can give the client insights into the emotional aspects of the procedure and offer hope for a successful outcome.
4. Explain expected events simply, such as the following: a. Preoperative and postoperative routines b. Possible development of lymphedema and sensory changes after surgery c. Postoperative positioning and exercises d. Presence of drainage tubes	4. Explaining what to expect can help to reduce fear of the unknown and anxiety over unexpected events. Simple explanations will not overwhelm an already stressful situation.

(continues on page 712)

Interventions continued	Rationales continued
5. Explain that a temporary soft prosthesis can be worn immediately.	5. A temporary prosthesis enhances appearance and reduces the sense of imbalance that can result from breast removal. Understanding that a prosthesis can be worn immediately after recovery can help to allay anxiety associated with appearance.
6. Allow client's partner to share his or her concerns alone.	6. Research has shown that satisfaction with marital support and support from other adults positively affects the woman's adjustment (Hoskins et al., 1996).
7. Validate to client and partner that their concerns and fears are normal and expected.	7. Validation can help to reduce fear associated with such feelings as rejection, repulsion, abandonment, and loss of attractiveness.
8. Discuss with client and significant other that the greatest period of distress is 2 to 3 months postsurgery and that counseling may be helpful.	8. Research has shown that the initial emotional appraisal of threat gradually changes over time to a cognitive appraisal that leads to uncertainty and increased anxiety (Hoskins et al., 1996).
9. Discuss with client and significant other possible responses of others (e.g., minimization or avoidance).	9. Lumpectomy clients receive less psychological support from friends, family, and coworkers who minimize the seriousness of that surgery versus mastectomy (Hughes, 1993).
10. Encourage client to discuss options with physician regarding breast reconstruction or tissue expansion (Hinojosa & Layman, 1996).	10. Breast reconstruction can be done at the time of mastectomy or any time after.

 Documentation

Progress notes
  Dialogues
  Interventions
Response to interventions

Postoperative: Collaborative Problems

Potential Complication: Neurovascular Compromise

Nursing Goal

The nurse will detect early signs and symptoms of neurovascular compromise and collaboratively intervene to stabilize client.

Indicators
- Radial pulses full, bounding
- No numbness or tingling of hand
- Capillary refill <3 seconds
- Warm, not mottled extremity
- Intact finger flexion and extension

Interventions	Rationales

1. Monitor for signs and symptoms of neuro-vascular compromise by comparing findings between limbs.
   a. Diminished or absent radial pulse
   b. Numbness or tingling in hand
   c. Capillary refill time >3 seconds
   d. Pallor, blanching, or cyanosis, and coolness of extremity
   e. Inability to flex or extend fingers
	1. Removal of lymph nodes causes edema, leading to entrapment of peripheral nerves at the cervical outlet or wrist; edema is marked by decreased sensation, movement, and circulation. The degree of lymphedema is dependent on amount of collateral lymphatic avenues removed (Chapman & Goodman, 2000).

 Related Physician-Prescribed Interventions

Medications. Refer to the Cancer: Initial Diagnosis and General Surgery care plans.

Diagnostic Studies. Mammogram; thermography; ultrasound; computed tomography (CT) scan; xeroradiography; breast node biopsies (fine-needle core, wire localization); positron emission tomography (PET); scintimammography

Therapies. Back brace, physical therapy, temporary soft prosthesis, radiation, breast reconstruction, prosthesis, implants

 Documentation
Flow records
   Radial pulse assessment
   Affected arm: color, sensation, capillary refill time, movement

Postoperative: Nursing Diagnoses

High Risk for Impaired Physical Mobility (Arm, Shoulder) Related to Lymphedema, Nerve/Muscle Damage, and Pain

Focus Assessment Criteria	Clinical Significance
1. Motion in the affected arm and shoulder	1. Assessment is needed to determine the baseline and to gauge progress.
2. Level of pain and fatigue	2. Pain and fatigue can interfere with ability and motivation to participate in self-care.
3. Balance	3. Postoperative factors (e.g., large dressing and limited use of one arm) can impair balance and predispose to injury.

Goal

The client will demonstrate progressive mobility to the extent possible within limitations imposed by the surgery.

Interventions	Rationales
1. Explain the need to increase mobility to the maximum extent tolerated and specify the hazards of immobility.	1. Explanations can help to elicit cooperation despite discomfort or fear of falling.
2. Provide appropriate pain relief. (Refer to the General Surgery care plan in Appendix II for specific interventions.)	2. Pain reduces the ability and motivation to perform ROM and other exercises and to walk.
3. Explain the reasons for poor balance; accompany client while she walks.	3. A large compression bandage and impaired arm movement can interfere with balance and increase the risk of falling.
4. Instruct client to elevate the affected arm on a pillow when sitting or reclining.	4. Elevation facilitates lymphatic drainage and prevents pooling.
5. Provide client with written instructions for the following exercises to be performed 3 times a day (5–10 times each) (Chapman & Goodman, 2000): a. Postoperatively days 1 to 5: Rotate wrist in circular fashion, touch fingers to shoulder, and extend arm fully. b. After drains are removed: • Stand and hold a chair with other arm and bend over slightly. Swing your affected arm in small circles and gradually increase in size. Make 10 circles; then rest and repeat in the opposite direction. • Swing arm forward and back as far as you can without pulling on the incision. • Bend over slightly and swing arms across the chest in each direction. • Sit in a chair with both arms at your sides. Shrug both shoulders, then relax. • While sitting or standing, pull shoulders back, then bring shoulder blades together. c. After sutures are removed: • Lie in bed with arm extended, raise arm over your head, and extend backward.	5. a. These exercises increase circulation and help with preventing edema. b. These exercises promote muscle movement without stretching (Chapman & Goodman, 2000). c. These exercises will stretch and regain ROM in shoulders if done in all directions every day (Chapman & Goodman, 2000).

(continues on page 715)

Interventions continued	Rationales continued

• Lie in bed, grasp a cane or short pole with both hands across your lap. Extend arms straight up and over your head and return.
• Repeat, rotating the cane clockwise then counterclockwise while raised over your head.
• Stand and extend arm straight over your head and down.
• Extend your elbow out from your side at a 90-degree angle; hold it for 10 seconds then relax.
• Extend your arm straight out from your side even with your shoulder; extend arm straight up toward the ceiling.
• Stand sideways to the wall. Extend arm out so fingers touch the wall. Creep up the wall a little more each day. Repeat while facing wall.
d. After 6 weeks:
    • Water aerobics
    • Overall fitness program
	d. A regular exercise program three times a week will strengthen arm and shoulder and client to regain previous function (Chapman & Goodman, 2000).

6. Initiate passive ROM exercises on the affected arm as prescribed.	6. These exercises increase circulation and help to maintain function.
7. As activities are increased, encourage client to use the affected arm as much as possible.	7. Frequent arm movement prevents lymphedema and contractures.

 Documentation

Progress notes
  Level of function
  Exercises (type, frequency)

High Risk for Injury Related to Compromised Lymph Drainage, Motor, and Sensory Function in Affected Arm

Focus Assessment Criteria	Clinical Significance
1. Edema 2. Sensory and motor function in affected arm 3. Pain	1–3. Extensive mastectomy involving surgery to soft tissue, muscles, and nerves can create slight to profound changes in the lymphatic system. The resultant edema causes tissue compression, decreasing circulation, and impairing sensorimotor function. The overall incidence of lymphedema is 20% (Chapman & Goodman, 2000).

Goal

The client will report no injuries to affected arm.

Indicators

• Relate factors that contribute to lymphedema.
• Describe activities that are hazardous to the affected arm.

Interventions	Rationales
1. Monitor for signs and symptoms of sensori-motor impairment: a. Impaired joint movement b. Muscle weakness c. Numbness or tingling	1. These signs can indicate entrapment of nerves at the cervical outlet or wrist from lymphedema or damage to thoracodorsal nerve.
2. Monitor regular measurements of arm circumference for changes.	2. Regular measurements can detect increasing lymphedema.
3. Consult with physician for additional interventions as needed such as diuretics, elastic wraps, intermittent pneumatic compression.	3. If lymphedema increases, more aggressive therapy may be indicated.
4. Teach client to avoid the following: a. Vaccines, blood samples, injections, and blood pressure measurements in affected arm b. Constrictive jewelry and clothing c. Carrying a shoulder bag or heavy object with the affected arm d. Brassieres with thin shoulder straps (use ones with wide straps or no straps instead) e. Lifting objects weighing more than 5 to 10 lbs f. Strenuous exercise g. Leaning on arm	4. a,b. Constriction to the arm can exacerbate lymphedema. c. Shoulder bags and heavy objects increase pressure at the shoulder joint and increase blood flow to affected arm. d. Thin straps also produce constriction on the shoulder. e,f,g. Anything that increases blood flow to the affected area contributes to lymphedema (Chapman & Goodman, 2000).
5. Teach precautions to prevent trauma to the affected arm and hand: a. Using long glove potholders b. Avoiding cuts and scratches c. Avoiding injections and venipunctures of any kind d. Using a thimble when sewing e. Avoiding strong detergents or other chemical agents f. Wearing heavy gardening gloves and avoiding gardening in thorny plants g. Using electric razor under arms	5. Trauma to tissue with compromised lymphatic drainage exacerbates lymphedema (Chapman & Goodman, 2000).

(continues on page 717)

Interventions continued	Rationales continued
6. Teach client to cleanse wounds to the arm or hand promptly and to observe carefully for early signs of infection (e.g., redness, increased warmth). Stress the need to report any signs promptly.	6. Compromised lymph drainage compromises the body's defense against infection; this necessitates increased emphasis on infection prevention.
7. Teach client to keep wrist higher than elbow and elbow higher than heart whenever possible.	7. This will reduce edema.

Documentation
Discharge summary record
  Client teaching
  Outcome achievement or status

High Risk for Ineffective Therapeutic Regimen Management Related to Insufficient Knowledge of Wound Care, Exercises, Breast Prosthesis, Signs and Symptoms of Complications, Hand/Arm Precautions, Community Resources, and Follow-up Care

Focus Assessment Criteria	Clinical Significance
1. Readiness and ability to learn and retain information	1. A client or family failing to achieve learning goals requires a referral for assistance post-discharge.

Goals
The goals for this diagnosis represent those associated with discharge planning. Refer to the discharge criteria.

Interventions	Rationales
1. Teach breast self-examination techniques; instruct client to examine both breasts periodically.	1. Periodic, careful breast self-examination can detect problems early; this improves the likelihood of successful treatment.

2. Teach wound care measures. (Refer to the General Surgery care plan in Appendix II for details.)
  a. Avoid using strong deodorants and shaving of axilla for 2 weeks after surgery (Chapman and Goodman, 2000).
	2. Proper wound care is essential to reduce risk of infection.
	
	  a. Irritation to the axilla site should be avoided to decrease risk of infection (Chapman and Goodman, 2000).

(continues on page 718)

Interventions continued	**Rationales** continued
3. Provide information about breast prostheses. Emphasize the importance of a properly fitted prosthesis.	3. A prosthesis of optimal contour, size, and weight provides normal appearance, promotes good posture, and helps to prevent back and shoulder strain.
4. Explain the benefits of strengthening and aerobic exercises.	4. Strengthening exercises increase lymph flow with muscle-pumping action. Aerobic activity elevates the heart and respiratory rates; this stimulates the lymphatic transport (Chapman & Goodman, 2000).
5. Encourage client to maintain ideal body weight.	5. Adipose tissue compresses and reduces lymphatic transport (Chapman & Goodman, 2000).
6. Refer to specialist in lymphedema if needed.	6. Early interventions at the first sign of lymphedema can reduce long-term complications.
7. Explain use of compression sleeve if ordered.	7. Compression increases lymphatic return and reduces edema.
8. Explain to expect fatigue during next months (Badger, Braden, & Michel, 2001).	8. Fatigue has been found to be the most frequently reported side effect (Badger, Braden, & Michel, 2001).
9. Encourage client to seek professional counseling for assistance with coping and depression.	9. Depression is common and affects quality of life significantly (Badger, Braden, & Michel, 2001).
10. Provide written instructions for exercises to perform at home and reemphasize their importance.	10. Research has shown that after breast surgery women experience significant attentional deficits in post-surgical period regardless of extent of surgery (Cimprich, 1992).
11. Instruct client to inspect arm and hand daily and to report promptly any signs and symptoms of complications including these: a. Increasing edema or weakness b. Numbness or tingling c. Impaired hand or arm movement d. Warmth, redness, or rashes e. Pain	11. These signs and symptoms point to increasing lymphedema, which can lead to impaired sensorimotor function or infection.

(continues on page 719)

Interventions continued	Rationales continued
12. Discuss available community resources (e.g., Reach for Recovery, ENCORE). Encourage contact and initiate referrals if appropriate.	12. Personal sources of information are found to be more important than written materials (Bilodeau & Degner, 1996).
13. As appropriate, explore client's feelings concerning radiation therapy or chemotherapy, if planned.	13. Both radiation and chemotherapy carry side effects that necessitate client teaching to enhance self-care and coping.

 Documentation

Discharge summary record
   Client and family teaching
   Outcome achievement or status
   Referrals if indicated

CAROTID ENDARTERECTOMY

The surgical removal of atherosclerotic plaque or thrombus from the carotid artery, carotid endarterectomy is indicated to prevent cerebrovascular accident in clients who have experienced a transient ischemic attack. If the occlusion is severe, a bypass graft may be necessary (Hickey, 2001).

 Time Frame
Preoperative and postoperative periods

 DIAGNOSTIC CLUSTER

Preoperative Period

Nursing Diagnosis

▲ Anxiety related to anticipated surgery and unfamiliarity with preoperative and postoperative routines and postoperative sensations

Postoperative Period

Collaborative Problems

Circulatory
▲ PC: Thrombosis
▲ PC: Hypotension
▲ PC: Hypertension
▲ PC: Hemorrhage
▲ PC: Cerebral Infarction
Neurological
▲ PC: Cerebral Infarction
   Cranial Nerve Impairment
▲ PC: Facial
▲ PC: Hypoglossal
▲ PC: Glossopharyngeal
△ PC: Vagal
△ PC: Local Nerve Impairment
▲ PC: Respiratory Obstruction

Nursing Diagnoses

▲ High Risk for Injury related to syncope secondary to vascular insufficiency
△ High Risk for Ineffective Therapeutic Regimen Management related to insufficient knowledge of home care, signs and symptoms of complications, risk factors, activity restrictions, and follow-up care

Related Care Plan

General Surgery Generic Care Plan

▲ This diagnosis was reported to be monitored for or managed frequently (75%–100%).
△ This diagnosis was reported to be monitored for or managed often (50%–74%).

Discharge Criteria

Before discharge, the client and family will

1. Describe wound care techniques.
2. State activity restrictions for home care.
3. Demonstrate range-of-motion (ROM) exercises.
4. State the signs and symptoms that must be reported to a health care professional.
5. Identify risk factors and describe their relationship to arterial disease.

Preoperative: Nursing Diagnosis

Anxiety Related to Anticipated Surgery and Unfamiliarity with Preoperative and Postoperative Routines and Postoperative Sensations

Focus Assessment Criteria	Clinical Significance
1. Preoperative facial nerve function	1. This assessment establishes a baseline against which to compare postoperative assessment findings.
2. Anxiety level (mild, moderate, severe, or panic)	2. Assessing anxiety level guides the nurse in planning effective interventions (Redman & Thomas, 1996).

Goal

The client will relate postoperative expectations.

Interventions	Rationale
1. Discuss with client the possible effect of surgery on facial nerve function (i.e., numbness and asymmetry).	1. Alerting client of what to expect can reduce anxiety associated with fear of the unknown (Redman & Thomas, 1996).
2. Refer to the nursing diagnosis Anxiety in the General Surgery care plan, Appendix II, for specific interventions and rationales for preoperative anxiety.	

 Documentation

Progress notes
  Assessment results
  Client teaching
  Response to teaching

Postoperative: Collaborative Problems

Potential Complications: Circulatory Problems, Thrombosis, Hypotension, Hypertension, Hemorrhage, Cerebral Infarction

Potential Complications: Neurologic Problems, Cerebral Infarction, Cranial Nerve Impairment, Local Nerve Impairment

Potential Complication: Respiratory Obstruction

Nursing Goals

The nurse will detect early signs and symptoms of (a) vascular problems, (b) neurological deficits, (c) respiratory obstruction and collaboratively intervene to stabilize client.

Indicators

- Respirations—quiet, regular, unlabored (a, b, c)
- Respirations 16–20 per min (a, b, c)
- BP >90/60 <140/90 (a, b)
- Pulse 60–100 per min (a, b, c)
- Temperature 98-99.5°F (a)
- Alert, oriented (b)
- Pupils, equal, reactive to light (b)
- Intact motor function (b)
- Clear speech (b)
- Swallowing reflex intact (b)
- Facial symmetry (b)
- Full ROM upper/lower limbs (b)
- Urine output >30 ml/hour (a, b, c)
- Oxygen saturation (SaO_2) 94–100 mm Hg (a, b, c)
- Carbon dioxide ($PaCo_2$) 35–45 mm Hg (a, b, c)
- pH 7.35–7.45 (a, b, c)
- Hemoglobin males 13–15 gm/dL (a, b, c)
            females 12–10 gm/dL (a, b, c)
- Hematocrit males 42–50% (a, b, c)
            females 40–48% (a, b, c)
- Mean arterial pressure 60–160 mm Hg (a, b, c)
- White blood count 4,000–10,800 cu mm (a, b, c)

Interventions	Rationales

1. Monitor for the following:
   a. Respiratory obstruction (check trachea for deviation from midline, listen for respiratory stridor)
   b. Peri-incisional swelling or bleeding
	1. Edema or hematoma at the surgical site can cause mechanical obstruction.

2. Monitor for changes in neurological function.
   a. Level of consciousness
   b. Pupillary response
   c. Motor/sensory function of all four extremities (check hand grasps and ability to move legs).
	2. Stroke is a possible complication of carotid endarterectomy. Manifestations of cerebral infarction include neuromuscular impairment of the contralateral body side (Greenfield, 1997).

3. Monitor for cranial nerve dysfunction.
 	
   a. Hypoglossal nerve:
     • Difficulty with speech
     • Dysphagia
     • Upper airway obstruction
	3. The surgical procedure can temporarily or permanently disrupt cranial nerve functions (Hertzer, 1995).
	   a. The hypoglossal nerve controls intrinsic and extrinsic muscles for tongue movement.

(continues on page 723)

Interventions continued	Rationales continued

b. Facial nerve:
  • Upward protrusion of lower lip
c. Accessory nerves:
  • Sagging shoulder
  • Difficulty raising arm or shoulder
d. Vagus nerve:
  • Loss of gag reflex
  • Hoarseness
  • Asymmetrical movements of vocal cords
	b. The facial nerve controls facial motor function and taste.
	c. The accessory nerve controls the trapezius and sternocleidomastoid muscles.
	
	d. The vagus nerve regulates movements of swallowing and sensation to the pharynx and larynx.

4. Monitor for hypertension.	4. Hypertension can be anticipated in certain clients exhibiting predisposing factors such as preoperative hypertension or postoperative hypoxia and excessive fluid replacement.
5. As necessary, consult with the physician for IV pharmacologic management to prevent hypertensive episodes.	5. Hypertension can increase the risk of hemorrhage or disruption of arterial reconstruction.
6. Monitor for hypotension and bradycardia.	6. The removal of atherosclerotic plaque may cause increased pressure waves on the carotid sinus, leading to hypotension. Bradycardia may result from pressure on the carotid sinus during the operation or from postoperative edema. Postoperative cardiac complications are the leading cause of morbidity following carotid endarterectomy (Hickey, 1996).

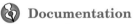 **Related Physician-Prescribed Interventions**

Refer to the Atherosclerosis care plan. Refer to the General Surgery care plan, Appendix II.

Documentation

Flow records
  Vital signs
  Patency of the temporal artery on the operative side
  Level of consciousness
  Pupillary response
  Motor function (hand grasp, leg movement)
  Cranial nerve function
  Wound assessment

Postoperative: Nursing Diagnoses

High Risk for Injury Related to Syncope Secondary to Vascular Insufficiency

Focus Assessment Criteria	Clinical Significance
1. Blood pressure, for postoperative orthostatic hypotension. (To assess, take readings with client lying down, then immediately on standing.)	1. Orthostatic hypotension causes episodes of cerebral hypoxia.

Goal

The client will

1. Relate methods of preventing sudden decreases in cerebral blood flow caused by orthostatic hypotension.
2. Demonstrate maneuvers to change position to avoid orthostatic hypotension.
3. Relate a decrease in episodes of dizziness or vertigo.

Interventions	Rationales
1. Remain with client during initial post-operative activity. 2. Instruct client to call for assistance when getting out of bed.	1,2. Syncope necessitates assistance to prevent injury.

3. Teach client to move slowly from the supine to the upright position to avoid orthostatic hypotension.
  a. Raise the head.
  b. Lower one leg at a time over the side of the bed.
  c. Sit for a few minutes before standing.
  d. Stand for a few minutes before walking.
	3. Slow movements minimize sudden decrease in cerebral blood flow by reducing the vascular rush to the large muscles.

4. Explain the relationship of dehydration, alcohol intake, and prolonged bed rest to orthostatic hypotension.	4. Dehydration and the vasodilating effects of alcohol decrease circulating volume. Prolonged bed rest increases venous pooling that contributes to orthostatic hypotension on arising. The client's understanding of these effects may encourage compliance with preventive measures.
5. Monitor use of antihypertensive medications.	5. Orthostatic hypotension can occur with certain antihypertensives (Malseed, Goldstein & Balkon, 1995).

 Documentation

Progress notes
  Complaints of vertigo
Discharge summary record
  Client teaching

High Risk for Ineffective Therapeutic Regimen Management Related to Insufficient Knowledge of Home Care, Signs and Symptoms of Complications, Risk Factors, Activity Restrictions, and Follow-up Care

Focus Assessment Criteria	Clinical Significance
1. Knowledge of arteriosclerotic disease, risk factors 2. Past experiences with risk factor modification	1,2. These assessments help to identify learning needs and guide the nurse in planning effective teaching strategies.
3. Readiness and ability to learn and retain information	3. A client or family failing to achieve learning goals requires a referral for assistance postdischarge.

Goals

The goals for this diagnosis represent those associated with discharge planning. Refer to the discharge criteria.

Interventions	Rationales
1. Teach client and family to watch for and report the following: a. Swelling or drainage from incision b. Numbness or weakness of opposite arm or leg c. Changes in speech or swallowing d. Changes in vision	1. These signs are indicative of progressive nerve or tissue compression.
2. Discuss the relationship of arterial disease and certain risk factors. a. Smoking b. Hyperlipidemia c. Obesity	2. a. Nicotine is a potent vasoconstrictor that reduces blood flow b. Lipoprotein abnormalities have been related to an increase in vascular diseases c. Obesity is usually associated with increased dietary intake of fats and cholesterol
3. Explore ways in which client can eliminate or reduce applicable risk factors. (Refer to the Atherosclerosis care plan for more information). 4. Explain the need for regular ROM exercises of head and neck.	3,4. Client's awareness that he or she can modify risk factors may encourage compliance with the treatment regimen.
5. Refer client to appropriate resources for assistance with risk factor modification: a. Dietitian for diet and weight loss counseling b. Smoking cessation program c. Exercise program (if approved by physician)	5. Client may need assistance for sustained management of risk factors after discharge.

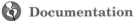 **Documentation**

Discharge summary record
  Client teaching
  Outcome achievement or status
Referrals if indicated

CATARACT EXTRACTION

Cataract extraction—surgical removal of the lens—can take several forms. The intracapsular procedure, which is performed less frequently, removes the capsule intact. The extracapsular procedure removes the anterior capsule, lens cortex, and nucleus. Removal is done with instruments or, more frequently, using the phacoemulsification procedure that uses ultrasound waves to disintegrate the lens which is then suctioned out. Regardless of the procedure, extraction allows insertion of an intraocular lens implant.

 Time Frame
Preoperative and postoperative periods

⊙⊙ DIAGNOSTIC CLUSTER

Preoperative Period

Nursing Diagnosis

▲ Fear related to upcoming surgery and potential failure to improve vision

Postoperative Period

Collaborative Problems

▲ PC: Hemorrhage
* PC: Increased intraocular pressure (IOP)
▲ PC: Endophthalmitis
  Dislocated intraocular lens

Nursing Diagnoses

△ Acute Pain related to increased intraocular pressure
▲ Risk for Infection related to increased susceptibility: surgical interruption of body surface
▲ Risk for Injury related to visual limitations and presence in unfamiliar environment
▲ High Risk for Ineffective Therapeutic Regimen Management related to insufficient knowledge of activities permitted, medications, complications, and follow-up care

---

▲ This diagnosis was reported to be monitored for or managed frequently (75%–100%).
△ This diagnosis was reported to be monitored for or managed often (50%–74%).
*This diagnosis was not included in the validation study.

Discharge Criteria

Before discharge, the client and family will

1. Discuss management of ADLs and activity restrictions if any.
2. Verbalize understanding of medication regimen.
3. State the signs and symptoms that must be reported to a health care professional.

Preoperative: Nursing Diagnosis

Fear Related to Upcoming Surgery and Potential Failure to Attain Improved Vision

Focus Assessment Criteria	Clinical Significance
1. Verbal and nonverbal indicators of anxiety	1. Risks associated with cataract surgery—e.g., potential failure to regain useful vision—may trigger anxiety and fear. Other factors, such as self-medication postoperatively and dependence on family as a result of surgery, also may contribute to anxiety. The nurse obtains this information by assessing sources of anxiety.
2. Understanding of cataract surgery including the following: a. Nature of procedure b. Risks and benefits c. Anesthetic: local, general d. Options for visual rehabilitation after surgery (e.g., intraocular lens implant [IOL], occasionally contact lenses)	2. Assessing client's knowledge level identifies learning needs and guides nurse in planning effective teaching strategies.
3. Amount of information the client seeks	3. Each client has different learning needs. One client may desire all the information possible about the procedure and its aftermath and may find that knowing details reduces anxiety; another may find too much detailed information overwhelming and anxiety-producing. Assessment allows the nurse to tailor client teaching to fit the client's desires.

Goal

The client will express any fears and concerns regarding the upcoming surgery.

Indicators

- Verbalize an understanding of perioperative routines and care measures.
- Ask questions regarding surgery.

Interventions	Rationales
1. Encourage verbalization and listen attentively.	1. Verbalizing feelings and concerns helps the nurse to identify sources of anxiety.
2. Reassure client that anxiety and fear are normal and expected responses to upcoming cataract surgery.	2. Validation and reassurance may help to reduce anxiety.

(continues on page 728)

Interventions continued	**Rationales** continued

3. Address any misconceptions the client expresses and provide accurate information, e.g.,
   a. Surgery removes the cataract, not the eye.
   b. A cataract is not film over the eye but a clouded lens in the eye.
   c. Most cataract surgeries are performed under local anesthesia.
	3. Misconceptions can contribute to anxiety and fear.

4. Present information using a variety of instructional methods and media:
   a. Print pamphlets
   b. Eye model
   c. Audiovisual programs
	4. Simultaneous stimulation of multiple senses enhances the teaching—learning process. Written materials also provide a source to refer to after discharge.

5. Explain required preadmission activities.
   a. Adherence to dietary instructions provided by anesthesia services
   b. Adjustments in medication regimen as ordered by the surgeon, anesthesiologist, or client's physician
   c. Use of antibiotic eyedrops the day before surgery
	5. Depending on the client's general health status, presence of concurrent medical problems, time of surgery, and physician's preferences, adjustments may be needed in diet (nothing by mouth for a specified period) and medications (e.g., withholding diuretics, decreasing insulin dose).

6. Discuss expected preoperative care measures:
   a. Dilating drops
   b. Intravenous (IV) access
   c. Bladder emptying
   d. Preoperative sedation prior to transport
 	
7. Provide information about activities, sights, and sounds associated with the intraoperative period.
   a. Presence and purpose of various personnel
   b. Noises of equipment
   c. Importance of lying still during the procedure
   d. Importance of communicating the need to move or cough before doing so during surgery
	6–7. Because cataract surgery is performed under local anesthesia and the client is awake, information about what to expect can help to reduce anxiety associated with fear of the unknown. It also enables client to participate better in care measures.

8. Reinforce physician's explanations of options for visual rehabilitation after surgery, as appropriate. a. IOL: These miniature plastic lenses are usually implanted during the surgery but can be implanted later. They provide the best visual correction when compared with other methods. One disadvantage is that they can dislocate occasionally.	8. Explaining options enables client to make an informed decision, when possible.

(continues on page 729)

Interventions continued	**Rationales** continued
b. Contact lenses: These create less than 5% of an image distortion and provide more focused central and peripheral vision than aphakic spectacles. Disadvantages include increased care and maintenance, high replacement costs, and intolerance in some clients. c. Aphakic spectacles: Hardly ever used in the United States because they cause distortion. They increase objects' image size by 25%–30% and cause objects to look barreled.	

 Documentation

Progress notes
   Client teaching
   Client's understanding of teaching and response

Postoperative: Collaborative Problems

Potential Complication: Hemorrhage

Potential Complication: Increased Intraocular Pressure (IOP)

Nursing Goal

The nurse will detect early signs and symptoms of (a) hemorrhage and (b) increased intraocular pressure.

Indicators

- No c/o of eye pain (a)
- No c/o of orbital pain (a)
- No sudden change in vision (a)
- No c/o of eyebrow pain (b)
- No c/o of nausea (b)
- No c/o halos around lights (b)

Interventions	**Rationales**

1. Monitor for signs and symptoms of hemorrhage.
  a. Pain in or around eyes
  b. Sudden onset of eye pain
  c. Changes in vision
	1. Ocular tissue is very vulnerable to bleeding because of its high vascularity and fragile vessels. Blood in anterior chambers (hyphemia) or in vitreous alters vision.

2. Monitor for signs and symptoms of increased intraocular pressure.
  a. Eyebrow pain
  b. Nausea
  c. Haloes around lights
	2. IOP may increase in response to surgery or medications such as steroid eye drops.

(continues on page 730)

Interventions continued	Rationales continued
3. Remind client to follow postoperative home eye care explained preoperatively, e.g., keeping eye shield on at night and glasses on during the day and sunglasses on when outside.	3. Eye shields or glasses are aimed at avoiding accidental bumping, scratching, or trauma.
4. Teach client to monitor for sign/symptoms of infection, IOP, and bleeding. Refer to Risk for Infection.	4. Because of the client's short hospitalization, the person/family will be instructed to monitor for postoperative complications.

 Related Physician-Prescribed Interventions

Medications. Antiemetics, analgesics, cycloplegics, antibodies (topical), antibiotic eye drops

Intravenous Therapy. Refer to the General Surgery care plan.

Laboratory Studies. Refer to the General Surgery care plan.

Diagnostic Studies. Snellen's eye chart, ophthalmoscopic examination, gonioscopy, B-scan ultrasonography, visual fields, potential acuity meter, brightness acuity testing, tonometry, slit-lamp examination

Therapies. Eye care

Documentation

Flow records
  Vital signs
  Eye assessment (suture lines, edema, pupils, vision)

Postoperative: Nursing Diagnoses

Acute Pain Related to Increased Intraocular Pressure

Focus Assessment Criteria	Clinical Significance

1. Location of pain; severity of pain based on a scale of 0 to 10 (0 = no pain, 10 = greatest pain), rated as follows:
  a. Before pain relief interventions
  b. One half hour after intervention
	1. This rating scale provides an objective method of evaluating the subjective experience of pain.

2. Associated signs and symptoms: a. Nausea	2. This assessment helps to differentiate normal postoperative pain from pain caused by increased intraocular pressure.
3. Usual response to pain	3. Assessing client's usual response to pain helps nurse to plan effective pain relief interventions.

Goal

The client will voice progressive pain reduction and pain relief after interventions.

Indicators
- Relate what increases pain.
- Relate what decreases pain.

Interventions	Rationales
1. Assist client in identifying effective pain relief measures.	1. Client has the most intimate knowledge of his or her pain and the effectiveness of relief measures.
2. Explain that pain may not occur until several hours after surgery.	2. Pain may not occur until the local anesthetic wears off; understanding this can help to reduce client's anxiety associated with the unexpected.
3. Support pain relief measures with prescribed analgesics.	3. Pharmacological therapy, such as mild analgesic, may be needed to provide adequate pain relief.

 Documentation

Progress notes
    Complaints of pain
    Interventions
    Response to interventions

Risk for Infection Related to Increased Susceptibility to Surgical Interruption of Body Surfaces

Focus Assessment Criteria	Clinical Significance

1. Signs of infection:
  a. Redness
  b. Acute eyelid edema
  c. Conjunctival injection (prominent conjunctival blood vessels)
  d. Crusting on eyelids or eyelashes
  e. Purulent matter between lids
  f. Elevated temperature
	1. Infection following ocular surgery can negatively affect visual acuity and successful surgical outcome. Postoperative care must focus on prevention, early detection, and prompt treatment of infection.

Goal

The client will exhibit healing of surgical site with no symptoms of infection.

Indicators
- Describe methods to protect eye.
- Demonstrate aseptic technique needed for medication administration.

Interventions	Rationales
1. Promote wound healing. 　a. Encourage a well-balanced diet and adequate fluid intake. 　b. Instruct client to keep a patch over the eye until the first eye drops are started 4–6 hours postoperative.	1. Optimal nutrition and hydration improve overall good health; this promotes healing of any surgical wound. Wearing an eye patch promotes healing by decreasing the irritative force of the eyelid against the suture line.
2. Use aseptic technique to instill eye drops. 　a. Wash hands before beginning. 　b. Hold dropper away from eye slightly so as not to touch eyelashes. 　c. When instilling, avoid contact between the eye, the drop, and the dropper. Teach the technique to client and family members.	2. Aseptic technique minimizes introduction of microorganisms and reduces risk of infection.
3. Assess for signs and symptoms of infection: 　a. Reddened, edematous eyelids 　b. Conjunctival injection (prominent blood vessels) 　c. Drainage on eyelids and lashes 　d. Purulent material in anterior chamber (between the cornea and iris) 　e. Elevated temperature 　f. Decreased visual acuity 　g. Abnormal laboratory values (e.g., elevated WBC count, abnormal culture, and sensitivity results)	3. Early detection of infection enables prompt treatment to minimize its seriousness.
4. Notify physician of any suspicious-looking drainage.	4. Abnormal drainage requires medical evaluation and possible initiation of pharmacological treatment.

 Documentation

Flow records
　Vital signs
　Condition of eye and suture line
Progress notes
　Abnormal findings

Risk for Injury Related to Visual Limitations and Presence in an Unfamiliar Environment

Focus Assessment Criteria	Clinical Significance
1. Visual acuity in each eye 2. Gait, previous history of falls	1–3. A client who has undergone ophthalmic surgery may not have immediate improve-

(continues on page 733)

Focus Assessment Criteria continued	Clinical Significance continued
3. Potential environment obstacles such as the following: a. Footstools and low furniture b. IV poles c. Wastebaskets d. Slippers	ment in vision. Preoperative assessment must include acuity of each eye; acuity of the unaffected eye indicates how the client views the environment, and acuity in the affected eye helps to guide the nurse in planning interventions to ensure safety.

Goal

The client will not experience injury or tissue trauma while on unit.

Indicators
- Identify risks factors present.
- Describe safety measures needed.

Interventions	Rationales
1. Orient client to the environment on arrival on surgical unit.	1. Client's familiarity with the environment may help to reduce accidents.
2. Place ambulation aids where client can see and reach them easily. Instruct client to request assistance before ambulating. Monitor use of ambulation aids.	2. These measures can help to reduce the risk of falls.
3. Teach client the importance of handwashing before eye care.	3. Handwashing is the most effective method of preventing infection.

 Documentation

Progress notes
  Visual acuity (preoperative)
Discharge summary record
  Client teaching

High Risk for Ineffective Therapeutic Regimen Management Related to Insufficient Knowledge of Activities Permitted Medications, Complications, and Follow-up Care

Focus Assessment Criteria	Clinical Significance
1. Knowledge of the therapeutic regimen	1. Assessing the client's and family's knowledge levels guides the nurse in planning teaching strategies.
2. Readiness and ability to learn and retain information	2. A client or family failing to achieve learning goals requires a referral for assistance postdischarge.

(continues on page 734)

Focus Assessment Criteria continued	Clinical Significance continued
3. Support systems, home environment	3. A client's ability to comply with the therapeutic regimen may be influenced (positively or negatively) by his or her home environment and available support systems.

Goals

The goals for this diagnosis represent those associated with discharge planning. Refer to the discharge criteria.

Interventions	Rationales

1. Discuss permitted activities after surgery:
  a. Reading
  b. Watching television
  c. Driving
  d. Cooking
  e. Light housekeeping
  f. Shower or tub bathing
	1. Beginning your discussions by outlining permitted activities rather than restrictions focuses the client on the positive rather than the negative aspects of recovery.

2. Reinforce activity restrictions specified by the physician; these may include avoiding the following activities:
  a. Lifting anything weighing over 20 lb
  b. Showering
  c. Straining during bowel movements
	2. Restrictions are needed to reduce eye movements and prevent increased intraocular pressure. Specific restrictions depend on various factors including the nature and extent of surgery, the physician's preference, and the client's age and overall health status. The client's understanding of the reasons for these restrictions can encourage compliance with them.

3. Reinforce the importance of avoiding rubbing or bumping the eye and of keeping the protective patch or shield in place throughout the first postoperative day. Glasses are worn during the day (with shield at night).	3. Rubbing or bumping the eye may interrupt suture line integrity and provide an entry point for microorganisms. Keeping the eye protected reduces risk of injury.

4. Explain the following information for each prescribed medication:
  a. Name, purpose, and action
  b. Dosage schedule (amount, times)
  c. Administration technique
  d. Special instructions or precautions
	4. Providing accurate information before discharge can promote compliance with the medication regimen and help prevent errors in administration.

5. Instruct client and family to report the following signs and symptoms:
  a. Persistent vision loss
  b. Eye pain not relieved by analgesics
	5. Early reporting of these signs and symptoms enables prompt intervention to prevent or minimize infection, increased intraocular pressure, hemorrhage, retinal detachment, or other complications.

(continues on page 735)

Interventions continued	**Rationales** continued
c. Vision abnormalities (e.g., light flashes or spots) d. Redness, increased drainage, or elevated temperature	
6. Instruct in ocular hygiene measures (i.e., removing crusty drainage by wiping the closed eyelid with a cotton ball moistened with ocular irrigating solution).	6. Secretions may adhere to eyelids and eyelashes. Removal promotes comfort and reduces the risk of infection by eliminating a source of microorganisms.
7. Stress the importance of adequate follow-up care with the schedule to be determined by the surgeon. The client should know the date and time of his or her first scheduled appointment before discharge.	7. Follow-up allows evaluation of healing and enables early detection of complications.
8. Provide written instructions on discharge.	8. Written instructions provide client and family with a source of information that they can consult as needed.

 Documentation
Discharge summary record
   Client and family teaching
   Outcome achievement or status

COLOSTOMY

Colostomy is the segmental resection of the transverse colon. Indications for colostomy include diverticulitis and cancer of the midtransverse colon. This procedure bypasses the rectum by diverting feces into an external appliance.

 Time Frame
Preoperative and postoperative periods

 DIAGNOSTIC CLUSTER

Preoperative Period

Nursing Diagnosis

▲ Anxiety related to lack of knowledge of colostomy care and perceived negative effects on life style

Postoperative Period

Collaborative Problems

• Potential Complications:

▲ Peristomal Ulceration/Herniation
▲ Stomal Necrosis, Retraction, Prolapse, Stenosis, Obstruction
Intra-abdominal sepsis
Large Bowel Obstruction
Perforation of Genitourinary Tract

Nursing Diagnoses

▲ High Risk for Disturbed Self-Concept related to effects of ostomy on body image and life style
△ High Risk for Ineffective Sexuality Patterns related to perceived negative impact of ostomy on sexual functioning and attractiveness
High Risk for Sexual Dysfunction related to physiological impotence secondary to damage to sympathetic nerves (male) or inadequate vaginal lubrication (female)
△ High Risk for Loneliness related to anxiety over possible odor and leakage from appliance
▲ High Risk for Ineffective Therapeutic Regimen Management related to insufficient knowledge of stoma pouching procedure, colostomy irrigation, peristomal skin care, perineal wound care, and incorporation of ostomy care into activities of daily living (ADLs)
△ Grieving related to implications of cancer diagnosis (*refer to:* Cancer: Initial Diagnosis)

Related Care Plan

General Surgery Generic Care Plan

▲ This diagnosis was reported to be monitored for or managed frequently (75%–100%).
△ This diagnosis was reported to be monitored for or managed often (50%–74%).
* This diagnosis was not included in the validation study.

Discharge Criteria

Before discharge, the client and family will

1. State conditions of ostomy care at home: stoma, pouching, irrigation, skin care.
2. Discuss strategies for incorporating ostomy management into ADLs.

3. Verbalize precautions for medication use and food intake.
4. State signs and symptoms that must be reported to a health care professional.
5. Verbalize an intent to share feelings and concerns related to ostomy with significant others.
6. Identify available community resources and self-help groups:
    a. Visiting nurse
    b. United Ostomy Association
    c. Recovery of Male Potency: Help for Impotent Male
    d. American Cancer Foundation
    e. Community supplier of ostomy equipment
    f. Financial reimbursement for ostomy equipment

Preoperative: Nursing Diagnosis

Anxiety Related to Lack of Knowledge of Colostomy Care and Perceived Negative Effects on Life Style

Focus Assessment Criteria	Clinical Significance
1. Understanding the underlying disorder necessitating colostomy (Society of Gastroenterology Nurses and Associates [SGNA], 1993) 2. Knowledge of structure and function of affected organs (SGNA, 1993) 3. Anticipated surgical procedure and stoma location 4. Previous exposure to person with an ostomy 5. Familiarity with stoma pouching equipment 6. Emotional status, cognitive ability, memory, vision, manual dexterity 7. Life style, strengths, coping mechanisms, available support systems	1–7. Assessing the client's knowledge of colostomy identifies learning needs and guides the nurse in planning effective teaching strategies. Assessing client's emotional status, mental and physical ability, and other related factors helps the nurse to evaluate the client's ability to accept, adjust to, and manage the ostomy and stoma (Righter, 1995).

Goal

The client will verbalize decreased anxiety related to fear of the unknown.

Indicators
- State reason for colostomy.
- Describe anatomic changes following colostomy surgery.
- Identify his or her own type of colostomy.

Interventions	Rationales
1. Identify and dispel any misinformation or misconceptions the client has regarding ostomy.	1. Replacing misinformation with facts can reduce anxiety.
2. Explain the normal anatomical structure and function of the gastrointestinal (GI) tract.	2. Knowledge increases confidence; confidence produces control and reduces anxiety.

(continues on page 738)

Interventions continued	**Rationales** continued
3. Explain the effects of the client's particular disorder on affected organs.	3. Understanding the disorder can help client accept the need for colostomy.
4. Use an anatomical diagram or model to show the resulting altered route of elimination.	4. Understanding how body waste elimination occurs after the rectum and anus are removed can help to allay anxiety related to altered body function.
5. Describe the stoma's appearance and anticipated location. Explain the following about the stoma: a. It will be the same color and moistness as oral mucous membrane. b. It will not hurt when touched because it has no sensory endings. c. It may bleed slightly when wiped; this is normal and not of concern. d. It will become smaller as the surgical area heals; color will remain the same. e. It may change in size depending on illness, hormone levels, and weight gain or loss.	5. Explaining expected events and sensations can help to reduce anxiety associated with the unknown and unexpected. Accurate descriptions of the stoma appearance help to ease shock at the first sight of it after ostomy surgery.
6. Discuss function of the stoma pouch. Explain that it serves as an external receptacle for storage of feces much as the colon acts as an internal storage receptacle.	6. Understanding the purpose and need for a pouch encourages client to accept it and participate in ostomy management.
7. Encourage client to handle the stoma pouching equipment.	7. Many clients are relieved to see the actual size and material of a stoma pouch. Often, uninformed clients have visions of large bags and complicated, difficult-to-manage equipment that can produce anxiety.
8. Plan a consult with ostomy nurse specialist.	8. This specialist can provide specific explanations.

 Documentation

Progress notes
   Present emotional status
   Client teaching

Postoperative: Collaborative Problems

Potential Complication
Peristomal Ulceration/Herniation

Potential Complication
Stomal Necrosis, Prolapse, Retraction, Stenosis, Obstruction

Potential Complication
Intraabdominal Sepsis

Potential Complication
Large Bowel Obstruction

Potential Complication
Perforation of Genitourinary Tract

Nursing Goal
The nurse will detect early signs and symptoms of (a) peristomal ulceration/herniation, (b) stomal complications, (c) intraabdominal sepsis, (d) large bowel obstruction, and (e) perforation of genitourinary tract and will collaboratively intervene to stabilize the client.

Indicators
- Intact bowel sounds all quadrants (d)
- Intact peristomal muscle tone (a, b)
- Free flowing ostomy fluid (a, b)
- No evidence of bleeding (a, b)
- No evidence of infection (c)
- No c/o nausea/vomiting/hiccups (c, d)
- Nondistended abdomen (d)
- Perineal wound intact (if sutured) (c)
- Temperature 98–99.5°F, no chills (c)
- BP >90/60, < 140/90 mm Hg (c)
- Pulse 60–100 beats/min (c)
- Respirations 16–20 breaths/min
- White blood cells 4,000–10,800/cu mm (c, e)
- Hemoglobin (e)
  - Males 13–19 gm/dL
  - Females 12–16 gm/dL
- Hematocrit (e)
  - Males 42–50%
  - Females 40–48%
- Urine output >30 ml/hr (e)

Interventions	Rationales

1. Monitor the peristomal area for the following:
  a. Decreased peristomal muscle tone
  b. Bulging beyond the normal skin surface and musculature
  c. Persistent ulceration
	1. Early detection of ulcerations and herniation can prevent serious tissue damage.

2. Monitor the following:
  a. Color, size, shape of stoma, and mucocutaneous separation
  b. Color, amount, and consistency of ostomy effluent
  c. Complaints of cramping abdominal pain, nausea and vomiting, and abdominal distention
  d. Ostomy appliance and appliance belt fit
	2.
	  a. Changes can indicate inflammation, retraction, prolapse, edema.
	  b. Changes can indicate bleeding or infection. Decreased output can indicate obstruction.
	  c. These complaints may indicate obstruction.
	  d. Improperly fitting appliance or belt can cause mechanical trauma to the stoma.

(continues on page 740)

Interventions continued	Rationales continued
3. If mucocutaneous separation occurs: • Fill separated area with absorptive powder or granules. • Cover with paste. • Reapply a new pouch.	3. Special techniques are needed to prevent fecal contamination.
4. Monitor perineal wound: a. Signs and symptoms of infection b. Bleeding c. Drainage	4. If perineal wound is closed, a drain will be in place.
5. If wound is open, follow wound care protocol.	5. If risk of infection is high, the wound will not be sutured closed and will need packing and irrigation.
6. Monitor for intraabdominal sepsis: a. c/o nausea, hiccups b. Spiking fevers, chills c. Tachycardia d. Elevated WBC	6. Leakage of GI fluid into peritoneal cavity (e.g., a leak at anastomotic site) can cause serious infections (e.g., staphylococcal).
7. Prepare for drainage procedure and/or surgical intervention.	7. Surgical intervention may be needed to drain abscess.
8. Monitor for large bowel obstruction. Notify physician if detected. a. Decreased bowel sounds b. Nausea, vomiting c. Abdominal distension	8. Intraoperative manipulation of abdominal organs and the depressive effects of anesthesia and narcotics can cause decreased peristalsis.
9. For additional collaborative problems (hemorrhage, hypovolemia, infection, urinary retention, thrombophlebitis), refer to General Surgery Care Plan.	

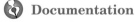 **Related Physician-Prescribed Interventions**

Refer also to the General Surgery care plan.

Medications. Antibiotics (e.g., kanamycin, erythromycin, neomycin); chemotherapy; immunotherapy; laxatives (preoperative)

Laboratory Studies. Carcinoembryonic antigen (CEA)

Diagnostic Studies. Flat plate of abdomen, computed tomography (CT) scan of abdomen

Therapies. Radiation therapy (preoperative, intraoperative, postoperative)

Documentation

Flow records
  Intake and output

Bowel sounds
  Wound status
Progress notes
  Stoma condition
Changes in physiologic status

Postoperative: Nursing Diagnoses

High Risk for Disturbed Self-Concept Related to Effects of Ostomy on Body Image and Life Style

Focus Assessment Criteria	Clinical Significance
1. Previous exposure to person(s) with an ostomy 2. Ability to visualize the stoma 3. Ability to express feelings about the stoma 4. Ability to share feelings about the ostomy with significant others 5. Ability to participate in the stoma pouching procedure 6. Ability to discuss plans to incorporate ostomy management into body image and life style 7. Evidence of negative self-concept	1–7. This assessment information helps the nurse evaluate present responses and progress. Participation in self-care and planning indicates positive attempts to cope with the changes.

Goal

The client will communicate feelings about the ostomy.

Indicators

• Acknowledge change in body structure and function.
• Participate in stoma care.

Interventions	Rationales
1. Contact client frequently and treat him or her with warm, positive regard.	1. Frequent contact by caregiver indicates acceptance and may facilitate trust. Client may be hesitant to approach staff because of negative self-concept.
2. Incorporate emotional support into technical ostomy self-care sessions.	2. This allows resolution of emotional issues during acquisition of technical skills. Shipes (1987) identified four stages of psychological adjustment that ostomy clients experience: a. *Narration.* Each client recounts his or her illness experience and reveals understanding of how and why he or she finds self in this situation. b. *Visualization and verbalization.* Client looks at and expresses feelings about his or her stoma.

(continues on page 742)

Interventions continued	**Rationales** continued
	c. *Participation.* Client progresses from observer to assistant then to independent performer of the mechanical aspects of ostomy care. d. *Exploration.* Client begins to explore methods of incorporating the ostomy into lifestyle. Use of this adjustment framework helps to establish guidelines for planning client's experiences in an organized manner.
3. Have client look at and touch stoma.	3. Nurse should not make assumptions about a client's reaction to ostomy surgery. Client may need help accepting the reality of the altered body appearance and function or dealing with an overwhelming situation.
4. Encourage client to verbalize feelings about the stoma and perceptions of its anticipated effects on his or her life style.	4. Sharing gives nurse an opportunity to identify and dispel misconceptions and allay anxiety and self-doubt.
5. Validate client's perceptions and reassure that such responses are normal and appropriate.	5. Validating client's perceptions promotes self-awareness and provides reassurance.
6. Have client practice using a pouch clamp on an empty pouch.	6. Beginning client teaching with a necessary skill that is separate from the body may be less threatening and may ease the fear of failure when performing on his or her own body.
7. Assist client with pouch emptying as necessary.	7. During ostomy care procedures, client will watch health care professionals for signs of revulsion. The nurse's attitude and support are of primary importance (Shipes, 1987).
8. Have client participate in pouch removal and pouch application. Provide feedback on progress; reinforce positive behavior and proper techniques.	8. Effective, thorough teaching helps client learn to master procedures.
9. Have client demonstrate the stoma pouching procedure independently in the presence of support persons.	9. Return demonstration lets nurse evaluate the need for any further teaching.

(continues on page 743)

Interventions continued	Rationales continued
10. Involve support persons in learning ostomy care principles. Assess client's interactions with support persons.	10. Others' response to the ostomy is one of the most important factors influencing client's acceptance of it.
11. Encourage client to discuss plans for incorporating ostomy care into his or her life style.	11. Evidence that client will pursue his or her goals and life style reflects positive adjustment.
12. Encourage client to verbalize positive self-attributes.	12. Identifying personal strengths promotes self-acceptance and positive self-concept.
13. Suggest that client meet with a person from the United Ostomy Association (UOA) who can share similar experiences.	13. In addition to the clinical expertise of the professional nurse, the ostomy client may choose to take advantage of a UOA visitor's actual experience with an ostomy (Maklebust, 1985).
14. Identify a client at risk for unsuccessful adjustment; look for these characteristics: a. Poor ego strength b. Ineffective problem-solving ability c. Difficulty learning new skills d. Lack of motivation e. External focus of control f. Poor health g. Unsatisfactory preoperative sex life h. Lack of positive support systems i. Unstable economic status j. Rejection of counseling (Shipes, 1987)	14. Successful adjustment to ostomies are influenced by factors such as the following: a. Previous coping success b. Achievement of developmental tasks presurgery c. Extent to which the disability interferes with goal-directed activity d. Sense of control e. Realistic perception of the event by the client and support persons
15. Refer an at-risk client for professional counseling.	15. In such a client, follow-up therapy is indicated to assist with effective adjustment.

 Documentation

Progress notes
  Present emotional status
  Interventions
  Response to interventions

High Risk for Ineffective Sexuality Patterns Related to Perceived Negative Impact of Ostomy on Sexual Functioning and Attractiveness

Focus Assessment Criteria	Clinical Significance
1. Importance of sex to the client 2. Availability of a partner	1–5. Assessment of current concerns and past sexual patterns provides direction

(continues on page 744)

Focus Assessment Criteria continued	Clinical Significance continued
3. Concerns about resuming intercourse 4. Preferred methods of sexual expression 5. Acceptability of alternative pleasuring activities to the client and partner	for planning effective nursing interventions.

Goal

The client will discuss own feelings and partner's concerns regarding the effect of ostomy surgery on sexual functioning.

Indicators

- Verbalize the intent to discuss concerns with partner before discharge.
- Relate resources available after discharge.

Interventions	Rationales
1. Reaffirm the need for frank discussion between sexual partners and the need for time for the partner to become accustomed to changes in the client's body.	1. Client may worry about his or her partner's acceptance; partner may be afraid of hurting the client and needs to know that the stoma is not harmed by sexual activity.
2. Role-play ways for client and partner to discuss concerns about sex.	2. Role-playing helps a person to gain insight by placing him or her in the position of another. It also may promote more spontaneous sharing of fears and concerns.
3. Discuss the possibility that client may project his or her own feelings onto the partner. Encourage frequent validation of feelings between partners.	3. The client may have erroneous assumptions about the partner (e.g., may erroneously assume that the partner is "turned off" by the ostomy).
4. Reaffirm the need for closeness and expressions of caring; involve client and partner in touching, stroking, massage, and so on.	4. Sexual pleasure and gratification are not limited to intercourse. Other expressions of caring may prove more meaningful.
5. Explore any fears client may express regarding mutilation, unacceptability, and other concerns that might limit his or her involvement in relationships.	5. These fears might limit involvement in relationships.
6. Discuss the possible availability of a penile prosthesis if the client is physiologically unable to maintain or sustain an erection sufficient for intercourse. Explain that penile implants provide the erection needed for intercourse and do not alter sensations or the ability to ejaculate.	6. Realizing that a prosthesis may be available may reassure client and reduce anxiety about performance; this actually could help to improve function.

(continues on page 745)

Interventions continued	Rationales continued
7. Refer client to a certified sex or mental health counselor if desired.	7. Certain sexual problems require continuing therapy and the advanced knowledge of therapists.

🎯 **Documentation**
Progress notes
    Assessment data
    Interventions
    Response to interventions
    Referrals if indicated

High Risk for Sexual Dysfunction Related to Physiologic Impotence Secondary to Damage to Sympathetic Nerve (Male) or Inadequate Vaginal Lubrication (Female)

Focus Assessment Criteria	Clinical Significance

1. Knowledge of the effects of surgery on sexual function.
  a. In men, abdominoperineal resection often damages sympathetic nerves in the presacral area that controls emission. This may result in retrograde ejaculation into the bladder and a "dry" orgasm. During abdominoperineal surgery, the parasympathetic nerves that control blood flow to the penis can be damaged, possibly resulting in erectile dysfunction.
  b. In women, there is little objective evidence of sexual dysfunction following abdominoperineal resection. The most common female sexual complaint is dyspareunia, which may result in "female impotence" (Galis, 1996).
	1. Assessing the client's knowledge of possible effects on sexual function guides the nurse in planning effective interventions.

Goal

The client will describe possible physiologic effects of surgery on sexual functioning.

Indicators
• Relate alternative methods of sexual expression.
• Relate intent to seek counseling if needed.

Interventions	Rationales

1. In men:
  a. Suggest that sexual activity need not always culminate in vaginal intercourse and that orgasm can be reached
	1.
	  a. Alternative methods of sexual expression and gratification promote positive sexual function.

(continues on page 746)

Interventions continued	Rationales continued
through noncoital manual or oral stimulation. Remind client that sexual expression is not limited to intercourse but includes closeness, communication, touching, and giving pleasure to another. b. Explain the function of a penile prosthesis. Both semirigid and inflatable penile prostheses have a high rate of success. c. Suggest counseling with a certified sex therapist.	 b. Penile implants provide the erection needed for intercourse and do not alter sensations or the ability to ejaculate. c. Certain sexual problems require continuing therapy and the advanced knowledge of therapists.
2. In women: a. Suggest using a water-based vaginal lubricant for intercourse. b. Teach client to perform Kegel exercises, and instruct her to do them regularly. c. Suggest that she sit astride her partner during intercourse.	2. a. Water-based lubricant can help to prevent dyspareunia related to inadequate vaginal lubrication. b. Kegel exercises promote control of the pubococcygeal muscles around the vaginal entrance; this can ease dyspareunia. c. A woman on top can control the depth and rate of penetration; this can enhance vaginal lubrication and relaxation.

 Documentation

Progress notes
  Interventions
  Response to interventions

High Risk for Loneliness Related to Anxiety about Possible Odor and Leakage from Appliance

Focus Assessment Criteria	Clinical Significance
1. Preoperative socialization pattern 2. Anticipated changes	1,2. A client at risk for social isolation must be assessed carefully; the suffering associated with isolation is not always visible. Feelings of rejection and repulsion are common.

Goal

The client will state the intent to reestablish preoperative socialization pattern.

Indicators

- Discuss methods to control odor and appliance leakage.
- Participate in self-help groups with similar experiences.

Interventions	Rationales
1. Select an appropriate odor-proof pouching system and explain to the client how it works.	1. Fear of accidents and odor can be reduced through effective management. Some pouches have charcoal filters to reduce odor from flatus.
2. Stress the need for good personal hygiene. 3. Teach the client care of a stoma appliance.	2,3. Proper hygiene and appliance care removes odoriferous retained fecal material.

4. Discuss methods for reducing odor.
  a. Avoid odor-producing foods such as onions, fish, eggs, cheese, and asparagus.
  b. Use internal chlorophyll tablets or a liquid appliance deodorant.
  c. Empty or change the ostomy pouch regularly when pouch is one-third to one-half full.
	4. Minimizing odor improves self-confidence and can permit more effective socialization. Bacterial proliferation in retained effluent increases odor with time. A full pouch also puts excessive pressure on seals, which increases risk of leakage.

5. Encourage client to reestablish his or her preoperative socialization pattern. Help through measures such as progressively increasing client's socializing time in the hospital, role-playing possible situations that the client feels may cause anxiety, and encouraging client to visualize and anticipate solutions to "worst-case scenarios" for social situations.	5. Encouraging and facilitating socialization help to prevent isolation. Role playing can help client to identify and learn to cope with potential anxiety-causing situations in a nonthreatening environment.
6. Suggest that client meet with a person from the UOA who can share similar experiences.	6. Others in a similar situation can provide a realistic appraisal and may provide information to answer client's unasked questions.

 Documentation

Progress notes
  Dialogues
Discharge summary record
  Client teaching
Outcome achievement or status

High Risk for Ineffective Therapeutic Regimen Management Related to Insufficient Knowledge of Stoma Poaching Procedure, Colostomy Irrigation, Peristomal Skin Care, Perineal Wound Care, and Incorporation of Ostomy Care into Activities of Daily Living (ADLs)

Focus Assessment Criteria	Clinical Significance
1. Type of colostomy	1. Colostomy care differs according to type and concurrent therapies. Sigmoid and descending colostomies may be cleansed with irrigation enemas to predict the time of a

(continues on page 748)

Focus Assessment Criteria continued	Clinical Significance continued
	bowel movement. Colostomies higher in the GI tract produce mushy effluent rather than formed stool; discharge of unformed stool is never predictable. A client receiving radiation or chemotherapy is not able to predict a regular bowel pattern.
2. Desire for control of elimination by irrigation	2. Not every client is a candidate for irrigation. In addition to the type of colostomy, the client's age, physical disabilities, concurrent disease, and personal preference determine the appropriateness of colostomy irrigation. The bowel does empty without irrigation but not in a predictable pattern.
3. Usual elimination pattern	3. Irrigation should be done within the same 2- or 3-hour period each day so that the bowel becomes regulated. Regular irrigation assists in establishing a normal bowel evacuation pattern. If possible, irrigation should be timed to produce evacuation on a schedule coinciding with the client's preoperative bowel pattern.
4. Home facilities needed for irrigation	4. Adequate and accessible toileting facilities are essential to an effective elimination schedule.
5. Knowledge of colostomy care: diet, activity, hygiene, clothing, sexual expression, community resources, employment, travel, odor, skin care, appliances, and irrigation if applicable	5. Assessment identifies learning needs and guides nurse in planning effective teaching strategies.
6. Client's and support person's readiness and ability to learn and retain information	6. A family or client who fails to achieve learning goals requires a referral for assistance postdischarge.

Goals

The goals for this diagnosis represent those associated with discharge planning. Refer to the discharge criteria.

Interventions	Rationales
1. Consistently use the same sequence in client teaching.	1. Consistency reinforces learning and may enhance the client's sense of control over the situation.

(continues on page 749)

Interventions continued	**Rationales** continued
2. Teach the client basic stoma pouching principles including the following: a. Keeping peristomal skin clean and dry b. Using a well-fitting appliance c. Changing pouch when the least amount of drainage is anticipated (usually on arising) d. Emptying pouch when it is one-third to one-half full and changing routinely before a leak occurs e. Changing pouch if burning or itching occurs under the appliance f. Observing the condition of the stoma and peristomal skin during pouch changes	2. Proper pouching techniques can prevent leakage and skin problems. a. This ensures that the appliance adheres to skin. b. Proper fit protects the surrounding skin surface from contact with drainage. c. This prevents copious drainage from interfering with pouch changes. d. A pouch filled more than halfway exerts increased pressure on the seal; this increases risk of leakage. e. Burning or itching may indicate that ostomy effluent has undermined the skin barrier; prompt intervention is necessary to prevent skin breakdown. f. Regular observation enables early detection of skin problems.
3. Teach the procedure for preparing a stoma pouch (Ellis & Sadder, 2000). a. Select appropriate stoma pouching system. b. Measure stoma carefully. c. Use appliance manufacturer's stoma measuring card if possible. If the card does not accommodate stoma size or shape, teach client to make a customized stoma pattern. Place clear plastic wrap from the skin barrier wafer over the stoma, trace the stoma with a marking pen, and cut a hole in the plastic to accommodate the stoma. d. Cut an opening in the center of the skin barrier slightly larger than the stoma (approximately 1/8 inch). e. Secure an appropriate odor-proof pouch onto the skin barrier wafer (if using a two-piece appliance system).	3. Preparing a new pouch beforehand ensures that it is ready to apply as soon as the used pouch is removed; this helps to minimize drainage on the skin surface.
4. Teach the procedure for changing a disposable stoma pouch. a. Remove the old pouch by gently pushing the skin away from the paper tape and skin barrier wafer. b. Fold the old pouch over on itself and discard in a plastic bag. c. Cleanse the peristomal skin with a wash cloth and warm tap water.	4. Correct pouch removal and attachment techniques minimize irritation and injury of peristomal skin and ensure a tight, reliable seal between pouch and skin.

(continues on page 750)

Interventions continued	**Rationales** continued
d. Blot or pat the skin dry. e. Apply the new pouch to the abdomen, carefully centering the hole in the skin barrier wafer over the stoma. Press on the wafer for a few minutes. f. Secure the pouch by "picture framing" the wafer with four strips of hypo-allergenic paper tape (if the wafer does not already have tape attached).	

5. Teach the procedure for emptying a stoma pouch.
  a. Put some toilet paper in the toilet bowl and sit on the toilet seat.
  b. Remove clamp from the tail of the pouch and carefully empty pouch contents into the toilet.
  c. Clean the inside and outside of the pouch tail with toilet paper and squeeze ostomy appliance deodorant into the end of the pouch.
	5. Correct techniques can reduce spillage, soiling, and odor. Placing toilet paper in the bowl prevents water from splashing as the pouch contents are emptied.

6. Teach the ostomy irrigation procedure.
 	
  a. Assemble all equipment:
    • Water container and water
    • Irrigating sleeves and stoma
    • Items to clean skin and stoma
    • Way to dispose of old pouch
    • Clean pouch and closure
    • Skin care items
  b. Cleanse stoma and surrounding skin with water and let dry. Observe their condition and color.
  c. Apply irrigating sleeve and belt securely. If using karaya washer, dampen and apply this first. You may lubricate the inside of the irrigation sleeve with oil to help the stool slide through the sleeve.
  d. Fill the irrigating container with about 1 quart of tepid water.
  e. Suspend the irrigating container so that the bottom of the container is even with the top of the shoulder.
 	
  f. Remove all air from tubing.
	6. The purpose of colostomy irrigation is to establish a regular bowel evacuation pattern; this makes a colostomy pouch unnecessary.
	  a. Assembling all equipment beforehand prevents delays during the procedure.
	
	  b. Thorough cleansing removes drainage from skin.
	
	  c. Preapplication makes cleaning easier.
	
	  d. Hot water traumatizes the bowel; cold water causes cramping.
	  e. At a lower height, the water may not flow easily. Higher height would give too much force to the water, causing cramping or incomplete emptying.
	  f. Removing air from the tubing helps to prevent gas pains during irrigation.

(continues on page 751)

Interventions continued	**Rationales** continued
g. Gently insert the irrigating cone into the stoma, holding it parallel to the floor. Start the water slowly. If water does not flow easily, try or check the following: • Slightly adjust body position or the angle of the cone. • Check for kinks in the tubing from the irrigating container. • Check the height of the irrigating container. • Relax and take some deep breaths.	g. Gentle and slow movements help reduce tissue trauma. Relaxation decreases muscle tension and resistance.
h. Instill water into the bowel; the amount of fluid instillation varies. Do not force water into the bowel. If cramping occurs, if the flow of water stops, or if water is forcefully returning around the irrigating cone or catheter, stop the flow.	h. Forcing water can cause tissue damage.
i. If bloating or constipation develops, irrigate with about ½ quart more water in the same day or use a mild laxative.	i. Increasing the amount of water may promote evacuation.
j. Look for most of the stool to return in about 15 minutes. When most of the stool is expelled, rinse the sleeve with water, dry the bottom edge, roll it up, and close the end.	j. The clamped irrigation sleeve acts as a temporary pouch until all stool is expelled.
k. Allow 30 to 45 minutes more for the bowels to finish emptying.	k. Complete emptying helps to prevent later leakage.
l. Remove irrigation sleeve and apply a clean closed-end pouch or a stoma cover.	l. Just a stoma cover is appropriate if client can achieve total control by irrigation. Manufacturers are currently testing stoma occluding devices that can be inserted and removed intermittently to allow fecal elimination; this would serve as an alternative to an external colostomy pouch.
m. Rinse irrigation sleeve and hang it up to dry.	m. Thorough rinsing and drying decreases odor.
7. Teach strategies for prevention and management of potential peristomal skin problems. a. Shave peristomal skin with an electric razor rather than a blade; avoid using shaving cream, soap, and detergents except when showering. b. Evaluate all skin products for possible allergic reaction; patch-test all suspect products elsewhere on the abdomen. c. Do not change brands of skin barriers and adhesives casually; assess for allergic reaction before using a new brand.	7. A client with a stoma is at increased risk for peristomal skin breakdown. Factors that influence skin integrity include: composition, quantity, and consistency of the ostomy effluent; allergies; mechanical trauma; the underlying disease and its treatment (including medications); surgical construction and location of the stoma; the quality of ostomy and peristomal skin care; availability of proper supplies; nutritional status; overall health status; hygiene; and activity level.

(continues on page 752)

Interventions continued	**Rationales** continued
d. Avoid irritation from contact with ostomy effluent. e. Avoid prolonged skin pressure, especially if fair-skinned or with thin, atrophic skin due to long-term corticosteroid therapy. f. Use corticosteroid creams sparingly and briefly; they can cause dryness and irritation. g. If bacterial or fungal infection is suspected, use a specific antibacterial or antifungal cream or powder. h. Use a liquid film barrier; avoid tincture of benzoin compound that can dry skin. i. Avoid aluminum paste and greasy ointments that can mask skin problems and also interfere with pouch adherence. j. Protect the skin with barriers. k. Expect the stoma to shrink slightly over time. This necessitates re-measuring the stoma to ensure proper appliance fit.	
8. Teach the procedure for perineal wound care. a. Take sitz baths or irrigate the area with warm water to cleanse the wound thoroughly. b. Wear a peripad to protect the wound and contain drainage until healing occurs. c. Watch for and report signs and symptoms of infection or abscess (e.g., pain or purulent drainage). d. If the rectum is missing, thermometers, suppositories, and other devices cannot be inserted.	8. Removal of the rectum results in a large perineal wound that may be left open to heal by secondary intention. Some clients with a colostomy do not have the rectum and anus removed but have a rectal stump sutured across the top. This becomes a nonfunctioning internal pouch (Hartmann's pouch). In this situation, the client continues to expel mucus through the anus produced by the remaining rectal mucosa.
9. Address nutrition and diet management. a. Teach how the ostomy affects absorption and use of nutrients, and discuss dietary implications. b. Assess food tolerances by adding new foods one at a time and in small amounts. c. Teach client to eat regularly and slowly, to chew food well, and to avoid high-fiber foods that can promote stomal blockage. d. Discuss dietary modifications that can help to decrease odor and flatus.	9. Proper nutritional intake and dietary management are important factors in ostomy management.

(continues on page 753)

Interventions continued	**Rationales** continued
e. List dietary modifications to prevent or manage diarrhea and constipation as indicated. f. Instruct client to monitor weight and report any loss or gain of more than 10 pounds. g. Explain the importance of adequate fluid intake (water and juices) to prevent or manage fluid and electrolyte problems related to altered elimination	
10. Explain the effects of certain medications on ostomy function. a. Antibiotics may induce diarrhea. b. Narcotics and aluminum- or calcium-containing antacids can promote constipation. c. Internal or external deodorizers can control fecal odor. Internal deodorizers may have a mild laxative effect. d. Suppositories cannot be used after the rectum and anus are removed. Instruct client to notify a physician or pharmacist if a drug problem is suspected.	10. Counseling client about the possible harmful effects of home remedies and indiscriminate self-medication may help to prevent minor or serious problems.
11. Promote measures to help client incorporate ostomy care into ADLs (Maklebust, 1990). a. Working/traveling: Keep extra supplies at work. When traveling, carry supplies rather than pack them in a suitcase and risk losing them; keep in mind that pectin-based wafers melt in high environmental temperatures. Take a list of ostomy supplies when traveling. b. Exercise: The only limits involve contact sports during which trauma to the stoma may occur. Normal exercise is beneficial and may help to stimulate bowel evacuation and in some cases can eliminate the need for irrigation. Successful use of exercise to regulate the bowel depends on the presurgical bowel pattern and regularity of elimination. Other contributing factors include the consistency of the fecal contents, motivation, diet, ability to exercise, and practice. c. Wardrobe: Ostomy appliances are invisible under clothing. Any clothing worn preoperatively may be worn postoperatively. Dress comfortably.	11. Successful incorporation of ostomy management into ADLs allows client to resume his or her precolostomy lifestyle and pursue goals and interests before surgery. If the ostomate had a strong supportive relationship before surgery, there usually are no problems after surgery (Galis, 1996; Maklebust, 1990).

(continues on page 754)

Interventions continued	**Rationales** continued

d. Bathing/showering/swimming: These activities may be done while wearing an ostomy appliance. "Picture-frame" the skin barrier with paper tape to seal the edges and keep the barrier edge from getting wet. Showering may be done without an appliance and, in fact, is recommended on days of appliance changes.

e. Wardrobe:
- Wear two pairs of underpants. The inside pair should be low-rise or bikini-height cotton knit worn *under* the ostomy appliance to absorb perspiration and keep the pouch away from the skin. The outside pair can be cotton or nylon, should be waist high, and is worn *over* the ostomy appliance.
- The ostomy pouch can be tucked between the two pairs of underwear like a kangaroo pouch. Special pouch covers are expensive, soil rapidly, and are not necessary.
- Avoid too-tight clothing that can restrict the appliance and cause leakage. A boxer-type bathing suit is preferable for men. For women, a patterned bathing suit with shirring can camouflage the appliance well.

f. Diet:
- Chew all food well.
- Noise from passing flatus will decrease postoperatively with progression to a regular diet.
- Eat on a regular schedule to help decrease the noise from an empty gut.
- Avoid mushrooms, Chinese vegetables, popcorn, and other foods that may cause blockage. (*Note:* Pillsbury microwave popcorn is specially made to be tolerated because adequate chewing can finely ground the kernels.)
- Keep in mind that fish, eggs, and onions cause odor in the stool.
- Drink at least several 8-oz glasses of water a day to prevent dehydration in an ileostomate and constipation in a colostomate. Concentrated urine or decreased urinary output is a good indicator of dehydration.

g. Odor control:
- Explain that odor is caused from bacteria in the stool.

(continues on page 755)

Interventions continued	**Rationales** continued

- Because most ostomy appliances are made to be odor-proof, do not poke a hole in the ostomy appliance to allow flatus to escape; constant odor will result.
- Control offensive odors with good hygiene and ostomy pouch deodorants. (Super Banish appliance deodorant works best because it contains silver nitrate, which kills the bacteria.) Hydrogen peroxide and mouthwashes such as Binaca can be placed in the ostomy pouch as inexpensive appliance deodorants.
- Do not use aspirin tablets as a deodorant in the ostomy pouch; aspirin tablets coming in contact with the stoma may cause stomal irritation and bleeding.
- Avoid foods that increase flatus (beer, beans, cabbage, onions, fish).
- Avoid foods that increase odor (onions, cabbage, eggs, fish, beans).
- Eating yogurt and cranberry juice may help to reduce fecal odor. Certain oral medications reduce fecal odor, but these should be used only with the advice of a physician.

h. Hygiene:
- Use a hand-held shower spray to wash the skin around the stoma and irrigate perineal wounds.
- Showers can be taken with the ostomy appliance on or off. On days when the appliance is changed, a shower can be taken when the old pouch is removed but before the new pouch is applied.
- The new pouch should be readied before getting in the shower. On days between appliance changes, showering with the appliance on requires only that the paper tape around the wafer be covered with a liquid sealant to waterproof the tape.

i. Exercise:
- Normal activities (even strenuous sports, in most cases) can be resumed after recovery from surgery.
- Be aware that increased incidence of peristomal herniation is associated with heavy lifting.
- Also keep in mind that increased perspiration from strenuous exercise may require more frequent ostomy

(continues on page 756)

Interventions continued	**Rationales** continued

appliance changes due to increased melting of the appliance skin barrier.
j. Travel:
  • Take all ostomy supplies along when traveling.
  • Do not leave ostomy appliances in automobiles parked in the sun because the heat will melt the skin barrier.
  • When flying, always keep appliances in carry-on luggage to avoid loss.
k. Sexual activity:
  • Remember that an ostomy does not automatically make a person undesirable;
    As in any sexual encounter, the client may have to indicate sexual interest to his or her partner who may be afraid of hurting the ostomy.
  • Wearing a stretch tube top around the midriff will cover the ostomy appliance while leaving the genitals and breasts exposed.
  • If male impotence is a problem, the man can be referred to a urologist for discussion or investigation of a penile prosthesis.	

12. Discuss community resources/self-help groups.
  a. Visiting nurse
  b. United Ostomy Association
  c. Foundation for Ileitis and Colitis
  d. Recovery of male potency—help for the impotent male
  e. American Cancer Foundation
  f. Community suppliers of ostomy equipment
  g. Financial reimbursement for ostomy equipment
	12. Personal sources of information have been found to be more important than written materials (Bilodeau & Degner, 1996).

 Documentation

Discharge summary record
  Client and family teaching
  Response to teaching.

CORONARY ARTERY BYPASS GRAFTING

Indicated for clients with coronary artery disease, coronary artery bypass grafting (CABG) increases blood flow to the heart by either anastomosis of an autograft vessel (i.e., saphenous vein or inferior epigastric artery) to an area proximal and distal to the coronary artery occlusion or by use of an autograft vessel (i.e., internal mammary or gastroepiploic artery) grafted distal to the coronary artery occlusion. Surgery often involves cardiopulmonary bypass, or extracorporeal circulation, to circulate and oxygenate the blood while diverting it from the heart and lungs to provide a bloodless operative field for the surgeon. A more recent trend in cardiac surgery is a minimally invasive procedure. The heart is not stopped for suturing of bypass graft(s). Cardiopulmonary bypass is not used and the incision is smaller.

 Time Frame
Preoperative and postoperative periods (not intensive care period)

⊗ DIAGNOSTIC CLUSTER

Preoperative Period

Nursing Diagnosis

▲ Fear (individual/family) related to the client's health status, need for coronary artery bypass graft surgery, and unpredictable outcome

Postoperative Period

Collaborative Problems

• Potential Complications:

▲ Cardiovascular Insufficiency
▲ Respiratory Insufficiency
▲ Renal Insufficiency
* Hyperthermia
* Postcardiotomy Delirium

Nursing Diagnoses

△ Fear related to transfer from intensive environment of the critical care unit and potential for complications
△ Interrupted Family Processes related to disruption of family life, fear of outcome (death, disability), and stressful environment (ICU)
△ High Risk for Disturbed Self-Concept related to the symbolic meaning of the heart and changes in life style
△ High Risk for Ineffective Therapeutic Regimen Management related to insufficient knowledge of incisional care, pain management (angina, incisions), signs and symptoms of complications, condition, pharmacologic care, risk factors, restrictions, stress management techniques, and follow-up care
▲ Impaired Comfort related to surgical incisions, chest tubes, and immobility secondary to lengthy surgery (refer to General Surgery)

(continues on page 758)

Nursing Diagnoses continued
Related Care Plan General Surgery Generic Care Plan Thoracic Surgery

▲ This diagnosis was reported to be monitored for or managed frequently (75%–100%).
△ This diagnosis was reported to be monitored for or managed often (50%–74%).
* This diagnosis was not included in the validation study.

Discharge Criteria

Before discharge, the client and family will

1. Demonstrate insertion site care.
2. Relate at-home restrictions and follow-up care.
3. State signs and symptoms that must be reported to a health care professional.
4. Relate a plan to reduce risk factors as necessary.

Preoperative: Nursing Diagnosis

Fear (Individual Family) Related to the Client's Health Status, Need for Coronary Artery Bypass Graft Surgery, and Unpredictable Outcome

Focus Assessment Criteria	**Clinical Significance**

1. Understanding of coronary artery disease
2. Understanding of coronary artery bypass graft (CABG) surgery including:
  a. Reason for surgery
  b. Anticipated outcome
  c. Risks involved
  d. Type of anesthesia to be used
  e. Expected length of recovery period
3. Past experiences with CABG surgery
	1–3. Client's and family's knowledge levels guide nurse in planning appropriate teaching.

4. Concerns or fears regarding CABG surgery	4. Unknown situations produce anxiety and fear. Assessment of the degree of client's and family's responses helps nurse to plan appropriate interventions to decrease concerns.
5. Readiness and ability to learn and retain information	5. Client or family failing to meet learning goals requires a referral for assistance post discharge.

Goals

The client or family will verbalize concerns regarding surgery.

Indicators
- Verbalize, if asked, what to expect before surgery (e.g., routines and tests).
- Verbalize, if asked, an understanding of the CABG procedure.
- Verbalize, if asked, what to expect post-CABG (e.g., monitoring and care).
- Demonstrate postoperative exercises, turning, splinting, and respiratory regimen.

Interventions	Rationales
1. Reinforce previous teaching about coronary artery disease as necessary.	1–6. Preoperative teaching provides information to help reduce client's and family's fears of the unknown and enhance their sense of control over the situation.
2. Reinforce physician's explanation of CABG surgery and why it is needed as necessary. Notify physician if additional explanation is indicated.	
3. Explain necessary preoperative tests and procedures such as the following:	
a. 12-Lead electrocardiogram (ECG)	
b. Chest x-ray film	
c. Cardiac catheterization	
d. Urinalysis	
e. Blood work: electrolytes, coagulation studies, complete blood count, type and crossmatch	
f. Nuclear studies if indicated	
4. Provide instruction about preoperative routines beyond general surgery routines such as the following:	
a. Chlorhexidine gluconate (Hibiclens or Betadine) shower the night before and the morning of surgery	
b. Sending belongings home with family members	
c. Measures in operating room holding area: skin preparation, IV and other invasive line insertion, and indwelling (Foley) catheter insertion	
5. Discuss postoperative measures, routines, and expectations, including the following:	
a. Endotracheal intubation and mechanical ventilation	
b. Chest tubes	
c. Multiple IV lines	
d. Sedative the evening before	
e. Pulmonary artery catheter	
f. Arterial line	
g. Epidural cardiac pacing	
h. Cardiac monitoring	
i. Indwelling urinary catheter	
j. Autotransfusion/blood replacement	
k. Weight increase	
l. Nasogastric tube	
m. Pain	
n. Frequent assessment of vital signs, dressing, heart and lung sounds, peripheral pulses, skin, and capillary refill time	
o. TEDS stockings	
6. Discuss expectations for intensive care:	
a. Environment, noises	
b. Length of stay	
c. Care measures	
d. Visiting policies	

(continues on page 760)

Interventions continued	Rationales continued
7. Explain specific pain-relief measures that will be used and the comfort level goals.	7. Knowledge of the pain expected and the ability to control pain can reduce fear and increase pain tolerance.
8. Discuss possible emotional and mental reactions post-CABG surgery.	8. The heart is a symbol of life; cardiac dysfunction and surgery typically invoke a profound emotional reaction. Anesthesia, fluid loss from surgery, and pain medications can temporarily cloud thinking.
9. Present information or reinforce learning using written materials (e.g., booklets, posters, or instruction sheets) and audio-visual aids (e.g., slides, videotapes, models, or diagrams).	9. Using various teaching materials and approaches provides multisensory stimulation that can enhance effectiveness of teaching and learning and improve retention.
10. Offer tour of intensive care unit.	10. Individuals who have a preoperative tour of ICU report a benefit from the experience (Lynn-McHale et al., 1997).

 Documentation

Progress notes
   Present emotional status
   Interventions
   Response to interventions
Patient teaching record or discharge summary record
   Client and family teaching
   Response to teaching
   Outcome achievement or status

Postoperative: Collaborative Problems

Potential Complication: Cardiovascular Insufficiency

Potential Complication: Respiratory Insufficiency

Potential Complication: Renal Insufficiency

Potential Complication: Hyperthermia

Potential Complication: Postcardiotomy Delirium

Nursing Goal

The nurse will detect early signs and symptoms of (a) cardiovascular insufficiency, (b) respiratory insufficiency, (c) renal insufficiency, (d) hyperthermia, and (e) postcardiotomy delirium.

Indicators
• Oriented, calm (a, b, c, d, e)
• No change in vision (a)

- Normal sinus rhythm (EKG) (a, b)
- Heart rate 60–100 beats/min (a, b)
- B/P >90/60, <140/90 mm Hg (a, b)
- No c/o syncope, palpitations (a, b)
- Mean arterial pressure 70/90 mm Hg (a, b)
- Pulmonary artery wedge pressure 4–12 mm Hg (a, b)
- Cardiac output/index >2.4 (a, b)
- Pulmonary artery systolic pressure 20–30 mm Hg (a, b)
- Pulmonary artery diastolic pressure 10–15 mm Hg (a, b)
- Temperature 98–99.5°F (d)
- Minimal change in pulse pressure (a, b)
- Respirations 16–20 breaths/min (a, b)
- Urine output >30 mL/hour (a, b, c)
- Capillary refill <3 seconds (a, b)
- Skin warm, no pallor, cyanosis, or grayness (a, b)
- No c/o palpitations, syncope, chest pain (a, b)
- No neck vein distension (a, b)
- Cardiac enzymes (a)
  - Myoglobin up to 85 ng/mL
  - Creatine phosphokinase (CK)
    - Male 50–325 mU/mL
    - Female 50–250 mU/mL
  - Troponin complex (C, I, T)
- Hemoglobin (a)
  - Males 13–18 gm/dL
  - Females 12–16 gm/dL
- Hematocrit (a)
  - Males 42–50%
  - Females 40–48%
- Partial thromboplastin time (PTT) 20–45 seconds (a)
- International Normalized Ratio IRN 1.0 (a)
- Platelets 100,000–400,000/cu mm (a)
- Prothrombin time (PT) >20 seconds (a)
- Urine specific gravity 1.005–1.025 (a, b, c)
- Blood urea nitrogen 8–20 mg/dL (a, b, c)
- Creatinine 0.6–1.2 mg/dL (c)
- Potassium 3.5–5.0 mEq/L (c)
- Magnesium 1.84–3.0 mEq/L (c)
- Sodium 135–145 mEq/L (c)
- Calcium 8.5–10.5 mg/dL (c)
- Oxygen saturation (SaO_2) 4–100 mm Hg (a, b)
- Carbon dioxide ($PaCO_2$) 35–45 mm Hg (a, b)
- pH 7.35–7.45 (a, b)
- Relaxed, regular, deep, rhythmic respirations (a, b)
- Rates, crackles, wheezing (b)
- Wound approximated, minimal drainage (d)
- Chest tube drainage <200 mL/hr (d)
- Full, easy to palpate pulses (a, b)
- No evidence of petechiae (pinpoint round, reddish lesions)/ecchymoses (bruises) (a)
- No seizure activity (a, d, e)

Interventions	Rationales
1. Monitor for the following every 4 hours or more frequently if not stable: a. Dysrhythmias, abnormal rate	1. Myocardial ischemia results from reduction of oxygen to myocardial tissue. Ischemic muscle is electrically unstable,

(continues on page 762)

Interventions continued	**Rationales** continued
b. ECG changes: ST segment depression or elevation; T-wave changes; PR, QRS, or QT interval changes c. Peripheral pulses (pedal, tibial, popliteal, femoral, radial, brachial) d. Blood pressure (arterial, left atrial, pulmonary artery) e. Pulmonary artery diastolic pressure (PAD) f. Pulmonary artery wedge pressure (PAWP) g. Cardiac output/index h. Cardiac enzymes daily (e.g. creatine phosphokinase, troponin complex) i. Urine output j. Skin color, temperature k. Capillary refill l. Palpitations m. Syncope n. Cardiac emergencies (e.g., arrest or ventricular fibrillation)	leading to dysrhythmias. Dysrhythmias also may result from surgical manipulation, hypothermia, and acidosis. Atrial dysrhythmias may also be due to mechanical remodeling or injury or conductive delays (Porth, 2002).
2. Monitor select electrolytes (Porth, 2002): a. Potassium b. Magnesium c. Sodium d. Calcium	2. Specific levels of electrolytes are necessary for both extracellular and intracellular body fluids a. Inadequate intake, diuretics, vomiting, nasogastric drainage, and stress can decrease potassium. Renal insufficiency, increased intake, tissue necrosis, and adrenal cortical insufficiency can increase potassium levels. b. Decreased intake, alcoholism, excess intake of calcium, and increased excretion after surgery; diabetic ketoacidosis; primary aldosteronism; and primary hyperparathyroidism cause decreased magnesium levels. Renal failure and excess intake of medications with magnesium (antacids, cathartics) increase magnesium levels. c. Increased water intake causes decreased sodium levels. d. Alkalosis and multiple transfusions of citrated blood products cause low calcium levels. Prolonged immobility causes increased calcium levels.
3. Monitor for signs and symptoms of hypotension and low cardiac output syndrome: a. Cardiac index <2.4 b. Increased pulmonary arteriole wedge pressure (PAWP)	3. These effects can result from severe pain or greatly reduced cardiac output secondary to severe tissue hypoxia; inadequate preload and inadequate myocardial contractility; dysrhythmias; and

(continues on page 763)

Interventions continued	**Rationales** continued
c. Increased central venous pressure (CVP) d. SvO_2 <60% e. Development of S_3 or S_4 f. Neck vein distention g. Decreased systolic BP (90 mm Hg or 30 mm Hg below baseline) h. Irregular pulse i. Cool moist skin j. Decreased urine output (<5 mL/kg/hr) k. Increased pulse and respirations l. Increased restlessness m. Lethargy or confusion n. Increased rales/crackles o. Weak peripheral pulses	ventricular failure (Norris, 1993). Decreased circulating volume and cardiac output can lead to kidney hypoperfusion and overall decreased tissue perfusion, triggering a compensatory response of decreased circulation to the extremities and increased heart and respiratory rates. Cerebral hypoperfusion also may result.
4. Monitor for signs and symptoms of cardiac tamponade: a. Decreased systolic BP (90 mm Hg or 30 mm Hg below baseline) b. Muffled heart sounds c. Pericardial friction rub d. Pulsus paradoxus e. Kussmaul's respirations f. Neck vein distention g. Narrowing pulse pressure h. Anginal pain i. Restlessness or stupor j. Equalizing CVP and pulmonary arterial wedge pressure (PAWP) k. Significant increase in or cessation of chest tube drainage l. Decreased electrocardiograph (ECG) voltage	4. Cardiac tamponade is a condition in which excess fluid collects within the pericardial space and impairs cardiac filling. It occurs because of graft leakage, inadequate hemostasis, or inadequate chest tube drainage (Porth, 2002).
5. Monitor for signs and symptoms of respiratory failure: a. Increased respiratory rate b. Dyspnea c. Use of accessory muscles of respiration d. Cyanosis e. Increasing rales, crackles, or wheezing f. Increased PCO_2, decreased O_2 saturation, decreased pH g. Decreased SvO_2 h. Restlessness i. Decreased capillary refill time >3 seconds	5. In the immediate postoperative period, hypoventilation may result from central nervous system depression caused by narcotics and anesthesia, impaired respiratory effort resulting from pain, fatigue, and immobility, or incomplete reinflation of lungs collapsed during surgery (Woods & Froelicher, 1995).
6. Monitor for signs and symptoms of hypertension or hypervolemia:	6. Hypervolemia and hypertension can result from a response to circulating

(continues on page 764)

Interventions continued	**Rationales** continued

a. Systolic blood pressure >140 mm Hg
   b. Diastolic blood pressure >90 mm Hg
   c. Mean arterial pressure >90 mm Hg
   d. Increased systemic vascular resistance
	catecholamines and renin secretion following cardiopulmonary bypass, which causes sodium and water retention.

7. Monitor for signs and symptoms of hemorrhage or hypovolemia:
   a. Incisional bleeding
   b. Chest tube drainage >200 mL/hr
   c. Increased heart rate, decreased blood pressure, increased respirations
   d. Weak or absent peripheral pulses
   e. Cool, moist skin
   f. Dizziness
   g. Petechiae
   h. Ecchymoses
   i. Bleeding gums
   j. Decreased hemoglobin and hematocrit
   k. Increased prothrombin time (PT), partial thromboplastin time (PTT), international normalized ratio (INR), and decreased platelet count
	7. Hemorrhage can be caused by inadequate surgical hemostasis, inadequate heparin reversal, or hypertension.

8. Monitor for signs and symptoms of myocardial infarction:
   a. Chest pain or pressure
   b. Increased heart rate
   c. Hypotension
   d. Tachypnea
   e. Abnormal heart sounds
   f. Restlessness, lethargy, or confusion
   g. Elevated CVP and PAWP
   h. Nausea and vomiting
   i. ECG changes: ST segment elevation, abnormal Q waves
   j. Increased cardiac enzymes
   k. Decreased SvO_2
   l. Neck vein distention
   m. Weak peripheral pulses
   n. Moist, cool skin
   o. Decreased urine output (<0.5 mL/kg/hr)
	8. Cardiac pain results from cardiac tissue hypoxia secondary to narrowing or blockage of the coronary arteries, increased myocardial oxygen consumption, or collapse of the newly grafted bypass.

9. Monitor for signs and symptoms of renal failure:
   a. Elevated BUN, creatinine, and potassium
   b. Decreased urine output (<0.5 mL/kg/hr)
   c. Elevated urine specific gravity (>1.030)
   d. Weight gain
   e. Elevated CVP and PAP
	9. Cardiopulmonary bypass causes destruction of some red blood cells (RBCs), producing free hemoglobin that may occlude renal arteries. Hypovolemia or poor myocardial contractility may decrease circulation to the kidneys, resulting in hypoperfusion and eventual renal failure.

(continues on page 765)

Interventions continued	Rationales continued

10. Monitor for signs and symptoms of cerebrovascular accident (stroke):
  a. Unequal pupil size and reaction
  b. Paralysis or paresthesias in extremities
  c. Decreased level of consciousness
  d. Dizziness
  e. Blurred vision
  f. Seizure activity
	10. CVA may result from embolization or hypoperfusion that obstructs or interrupts blood flow to the central nervous system (Leahy, 1993).

11. Monitor for signs and symptoms of post-cardiotomy delirium:
  a. Disorientation
  b. Confusion
  c. Hallucinations or delusions
	11. This disorder may result from surgery-related microemboli, sensory overload or deprivation, altered sleep pattern, hypoxia, medications, metabolic disorders, or hypotension (Segatore, Putkiewicz, & Adams, 1998).

12. Monitor for hyperthermia:
  a. Increased temperature
  b. Increased heart rate
  c. Hypotension
	12. Hyperthermia can indicate infection or postpericardiotomy syndrome (pericarditis) (Porth, 2002).

◣ Related Physician-Prescribed Interventions

Medications. Antibiotics, anticoagulants, analgesics, stool softeners, diuretics, beta-blockers, aspirin (postoperatively), antidysrhythmics, calcium-channel blockers

Intravenous Therapy. Fluid/electrolyte replacement

Laboratory Studies. Complete blood count, arterial blood gas analysis, glucose, creatinine, cardiac enzymes, amylase, electrolytes, BUN, blood chemistry profile, coagulation levels

Diagnostic Studies. Ear/pulse oximetry, chest x-ray film, ECG, cardiac echocardiogram, cardiac catheterization

Nuclear Studies. Egthallium-221

Therapies. Supplemental oxygen, pulse oximetry, others dependent on symptomatology

◉ Documentation

Flow records
  Vital signs
  Cardiac rhythm
  Peripheral pulses
  Skin color, temperature, moisture
  Neck vein distention
  Respiratory assessment
  Neurological assessment
  Intake (oral, IVs, blood products)
  Incisions (color, drainage, swelling)
  Output (chest tubes, nasogastric tube)
  Bowel function (bowel sounds, distention)
  Sputum (amount, tenaciousness, color)
Progress notes
  Change in physiological status
  Interventions
  Response to interventions

Postoperative: Nursing Diagnoses

Fear Related to Transfer from Intensive Environment of the Critical Care Unit and Potential for Complications

Focus Assessment Criteria	Clinical Significance
1. Nature of concern and fears 2. Perception of progress 3. Understanding of need for transfer from critical care unit 4. Level of anxiety: a. Mild b. Moderate c. Severe d. Panic	1–4. Assessing client's fears and anxiety level enables the nurse to plan effective interventions to reduce them. This is especially important to the post-CABG client because stress, anxiety, and fear can precipitate a sympathetic nervous system response that increases heart rate, blood pressure, and myocardial oxygen demand.

Goal

The client will report a decreased level of anxiety or fear.

Indicators

- Verbalize any concerns regarding the completed surgery, possible complications, and the critical care environment.
- Verbalize the intent to share fears with one person after discharge.

Interventions	Rationales
1. Take steps to reduce client's levels of anxiety and fear. a. Reassure client that you or other nurses are always close by and will respond promptly to requests. b. Convey a sense of empathy and understanding. c. Minimize external stimuli (e.g., close the room door, dim the lights, speak in a quiet voice, decrease the volume level of equipment alarms, and position equipment so that alarms are diverted away from the client). d. Plan care measures to provide adequate periods of uninterrupted rest and sleep. e. Promote relaxation; encourage regular rest periods throughout the day. f. Explain each procedure before performing it.	1. Reducing anxiety, fear, and stress can decrease demands made on an already compromised heart.
2. Encourage client to verbalize concerns and fears. Clarify any misconceptions and provide positive feedback regarding progress.	2. This sharing allows nurse to correct any erroneous information the client may believe and validates that concerns and fears are normal; this may help to reduce anxiety.

(continues on page 767)

Interventions continued	Rationales continued
3. Encourage client to identify and call on reliable support persons and previously successful coping mechanisms.	3. Support persons and coping mechanisms are important tools in anxiety reduction.
4. Consult with physician for medications as necessary.	4. Pharmacological assistance may be necessary if anxiety is at an unmanageable level; severe pain may also be interfering with client's ability to cope.
5. Prepare client for progression through intensive care unit (ICU) and stepdown to general care unit.	5. Explanations can prevent serious complications related to unexpected relocations or transfers.

 Documentation

Progress notes
   Present emotional status
   Interventions
   Response to interventions

Interrupted Family Processes Related to Disruption of Family Life, Fear of Outcome (Death, Disability), and Stressful Environment (ICU)

Focus Assessment Criteria	Clinical Significance
1. Specific stressors 2. Nature of concerns 3. Understanding of disease, surgery, and expected outcome 4. Familiarity with the ICU 5. Family coping mechanisms and use of support systems	1–5. A CABG client's family is experiencing a life crisis and may be under extreme stress related to separation from the client and the uncertain prognosis. Assessing these factors gives the nurse information on which to base effective interventions.
6. Need for additional resources	6. Family may need referrals to assist with coping.

Goal

The family members or significant others will report continued adequate family functioning during the client's hospitalization.

Indicators

- Verbalize concerns regarding CABG outcome and client prognosis.
- Verbalize concerns regarding the discharge.

Interventions	Rationales
1. Spend time with family members or significant others and convey a sense of empathetic understanding.	1. Frequent contact and communicating a sense of caring and concern can help to reduce stress and promote learning.
2. Allow family members or significant others to express their feelings, fears, and concerns.	2. Sharing allows nurse to identify fears and concerns, then plan interventions to address them.
3. Explain the ICU environment and equipment. 4. Explain expected postoperative care measures and progress, and provide specific information on client's progress as appropriate.	3–4. This information can help to reduce anxiety associated with the unknown.
5. Teach family members or significant others ways in which they can be more supportive (e.g., show them how they can touch the client; encourage them to talk with and touch client and to maintain a sense of humor as appropriate).	5. This information can ease fears associated with doing or saying the wrong thing and can promote normal interaction with client.
6. Encourage frequent visitation and participation in care measures.	6. Frequent visitation and participation in care can promote continued family interaction and support.
7. Consult with or provide referrals to community and other resources (e.g., social service agency) as necessary.	7. Families with problems such as financial needs, unsuccessful coping, or unresolved conflicts may need additional resources to help maintain family functioning.

Documentation

Progress notes
    Present family functioning
    Interventions
    Response to interventions
Discharge summary record
    Referrals if indicated

High Risk for Disturbed Self-Concept Related to the Symbolic Meaning of the Heart and Changes in Life Style

Focus Assessment Criteria	Clinical Significance
1. Expressed self-concept	1. Heart disease and surgery pose a threat to self-concept beyond the obvious threat to life. The heart is a symbol of life and vitality; any disruption in its function may trigger negative changes in self-concept.

(continues on page 769)

Focus Assessment Criteria continued	Clinical Significance continued
2. Perceptions of and feelings about necessary post-CABG life-style changes.	2. The client's perception of post-CABG life-style changes (e.g., physical, psychological, social, spiritual, financial) influences the extent of his or her self-concept disturbance.

Goal

The client will demonstrate healthy coping skills.

Indicators

• Report realistic changes in life style.
• Appraise situation realistically.

Interventions	Rationales
1. Encourage client to express feelings and concerns about necessary life style changes and changes in level of functioning.	1. Sharing gives nurse the opportunity to correct misconceptions, provide realistic feedback, and reassure client that his or her concerns are normal.
2. Stress client's role in preventing recurrence of atherosclerosis. Emphasize steps the client can take and encourage progress.	2. Client's knowledge of control over the situation can enhance ego strength. Stressing the positive promotes hope and reduces frustration.
3. Allow client to make choices regarding daily activities.	3. A decrease in power in one area can be counter balanced by providing opportunities for choices and control in other areas.
4. Encourage client to participate actively in the care regimen.	4. Participation in self-care mobilizes client and promotes decision making, which enhances self-concept.
5. Identify a client at risk for poor ego adjustment (Shipes, 1987): a. Poor ego strength b. Ineffective problem-solving ability c. Difficulty learning new information or skills d. Lack of motivation e. External locus of control f. Poor health g. Unsatisfactory preoperative sex life h. Lack of positive support systems i. Unstable economic status j. Rejection of counseling	5. Successful adjustment to CABG surgery is influenced by factors such as the following: a. Previous coping success b. Achievement of development tasks before surgery c. The extent to which resulting life style changes interfere with goal-directed activity d. Sense of control over the situation e. Realistic perceptions by client and support persons
6. Refer an at-risk client for counseling.	6. Follow-up therapy is indicated to assist with effective adjustment.

High Risk for Ineffective Therapeutic Regimen Management Related to Insufficient Knowledge of Incisional Care, Pain Management (Angina, Incisions), Signs and Symptoms of Complications, Condition, Pharmacologic Care, Risk Factors, Restrictions, Stress Management Techniques, and Follow-up Care

Focus Assessment Criteria	Clinical Significance
1. Understanding of home care needs	1. This information guides nurse in planning teaching strategies.
2. Readiness and ability to learn and retain information	2. A client or family failing to meet learning goals requires a referral for assistance post-discharge.

Goal

The goals for this diagnosis represent those associated with discharge planning. Refer to the discharge criteria.

Interventions	Rationales
1. Explain and demonstrate care of uncomplicated surgical incisions. a. Wash with soap and water (bath and shower permitted; use lukewarm water). b. Wear loose clothing until incision areas are no longer tender.	1. Correct technique is needed to reduce the risk of infection.
2. Provide instruction for pain management. a. For incision pain (sore, sharp, stabbing): • Take pain medication as prescribed and before activities that cause discomfort. • Continue to use the splinting technique as needed. b. For angina (tightness, squeezing, pressure, pain, or mild ache in chest; indigestion; choking sensation; pain in jaw, neck, and between shoulder blades; numbness, tingling, and aching in either arm or hand): • Stop whatever you are doing and sit down. • Take nitroglycerin as prescribed (e.g., one tablet every 5 minutes sublingually until pain subsides or a maximum of three tablets have been taken). • If pain is unrelieved by three nitroglycerin tablets, call for immediate transportation to the emergency room.	2. a. Adequate instruction in pain management can reduce the fear of pain by providing a sense of control. Combining analgesics and nonsteroidal anti-inflammatory agents may increase the effectiveness of pain management (Watt-Watson & Stevens, 1998). b. Angina is a symptom of cardiac tissue hypoxia. Immediate rest reduces the tissues' oxygen requirements. Nitroglycerin causes coronary vasodilatation, which increases coronary blood flow in an attempt to increase myocardial oxygen supply.

(continues on page 771)

Interventions continued	Rationales continued

3. Provide instruction regarding condition and reduction of risk factors.
   a. Reinforce purpose and outcome of CABG surgery.
 	
   b. Explain the risk factors that need to be eliminated or reduced (e.g., obesity, smoking, high-cholesterol, sedentary life style, regular heavy alcohol intake, excessive stress, hypertension, or uncontrolled diabetes mellitus).
	3. Surgery does not replace the need to reduce risk factors.
	   a. Preoperative anxiety may have interfered with retention of preoperative teaching.
	   b. Emphasizing those risk factors that can be reduced may decrease client's sense of powerlessness regarding those factors that cannot be reduced such as heredity.

4. Teach client about safe and effective weight loss methods if indicated. Consult a dietitian, and refer client to appropriate community resources.	4. Weight reduction reduces peripheral resistance and cardiac output.
5. Provide instruction about smoking cessation if indicated; refer to a community program.	5. Smoking's immediate effects include vasoconstriction and decreased blood oxygenation, elevated blood pressure, increased heart rate, and possible dysrhythmias, and increased cardiac workload. Long-term effects include an increased risk of coronary artery disease and myocardial infarction. Smoking also contributes to hypertension, peripheral vascular disease (e.g., leg ulcers), and chronically abnormal arterial blood gases (low oxygen, or PO_2, and high carbon dioxide, or PCO_2).
6. Teach about a low-fat, high-fiber, low-cholesterol diet; consult with a dietitian.	6. A low-fat, high-fiber, and low-cholesterol diet can reduce or prevent arteriosclerosis in some clients.

7. Provide instruction in a progressive activity program.
   a. Increase activity gradually.
 	
   b. Consult with physical therapist and cardiac rehabilitation specialist.
   c. Schedule frequent rest periods throughout the day for the first 6 to 8 weeks. Balance periods of activity with periods of rest.
   d. Consult with physician before resuming work, driving, strenuous recreational activities (e.g., jogging, golfing, and other sports), and travel (airplane or automobile).
	7.
	
	   a. Progressive regular exercise increases cardiac stroke volume, thus increasing the heart's efficiency without greatly altering rate.
	   b. These professionals can provide specific guidelines.
	   c. Rest periods reduce myocardial oxygen demands.
	
	   d. Caution is needed to reduce risk of myocardial hypoxia from overexertion.

(continues on page 772)

Interventions continued	**Rationales** continued
e. Try to get 8 to 10 hours of sleep each night.	e. Sleep allows the body restorative time.
f. Avoid isometric exercises (e.g., lifting anything over 10 lb). Avoid pushing anything weighing more than 10 lb (e.g., vacuum cleaner, grocery cart) for 6 to 8 weeks.	f. Isometric exercises and straining increase cardiac workload and peripheral resistance. They also place stress on the healing sternum.
g. Limit stair climbing to once or twice a day.	g. Stair climbing increases cardiac workload.
8. Provide instructions for stress management strategies. a. Identify stressors. b. Avoid stressors if possible. c. Use techniques to reduce stress response (e.g., deep breathing, progressive relaxation, guided imagery, or exercise within postoperative constraints).	8. Although the relationship of stress and atherosclerotic changes is not clear, stress may increase cardiac workload.
9. Provide instructions for sexual activity. a. Consult with physician about when sexual activity can be resumed. b. Rest before and after engaging in sexual activity. c. Stop sexual activity if angina occurs. d. Try different positions to decrease exertion (e.g., both partners side-lying or client on bottom). e. If prescribed, take nitroglycerin before sexual activity. f. Avoid sexual activity in very hot or cold temperatures, within 2 hours of eating or drinking, when tired, after alcohol intake, with an unfamiliar partner, and in an unfamiliar environment.	9. Although resumption of sexual activity is encouraged, client needs specific instructions focusing on reducing cardiac workload and avoiding certain situations that increase anxiety or vasoconstriction.
10. Provide instructions regarding prescribed medications (i.e., purpose, dosage and administration techniques, and possible side effects).	10. Understanding can help to improve compliance and reduce the risk of overdose and morbidity.
11. Teach client and family to report these signs and symptoms of complications to the physician: a. Redness, drainage, warmth, or increasing pain at incision site b. Increasing weakness, fatigue c. Elevated temperature	11. Early reporting of complications enables prompt interventions to minimize their severity. a–c. These signs and symptoms may indicate infection.

(continues on page 773)

Interventions continued	Rationales continued
d. Anginal pain	d. Anginal pain indicates myocardial hypoxia.
e. Difficulty breathing f. Weight gain exceeding 3 lb in 1 day or 5 lb in 1 week	e,f. Difficulty breathing and abnormal weight gain may point to fluid retention.
g. Calf swelling, tenderness, warmth, or pain	g. These signs and symptoms may indicate thrombophlebitis.
12. Provide information regarding community services (e.g., American Heart Association, "Mended Heart Club").	12. Community resources after discharge can assist with adaptation and self-help strategies.

 Documentation

Discharge summary record
   Client and family teaching
   Response to teaching
   Referrals if indicated

For a Care Path on Cardiac Surgery, visit http://connection.lww.com.

CRANIAL SURGERY

Involving surgical access through the skull to the intracranial structures, cranial surgery is indicated to remove a tumor, control hemorrhage, remove hematomas or clippings, excise vascular abnormalities, or reduce increased intracranial pressure. The surgical approach depends on the location of the lesion.

 Time Frame

Preoperative and postoperative periods
Postintensive care unit

 DIAGNOSTIC CLUSTER

Preoperative Period

Nursing Diagnosis

△ Anxiety related to impending surgery and perceive negative effects on life style

Postoperative Period

Collaborative Problems

▲ PC: Increased Intracranial Pressure
▲ PC: Brain Hemorrhage, Hematoma, Hygroma
▲ PC: Cranial Nerve Dysfunctions
▲ PC: Fluid/Electrolyte Imbalances
△ PC: Meningitis/Encephalitis
▲ PC: Sensory/Motor Losses
▲ PC: Cerebral/Cerebellar Dysfunction
▲ PC: Hypo or Hyperthermia
△ PC: Diabetes Insipidus
　　SIADH
▲ PC: Cerebrospinal Fluid (CSF) Leaks
▲ PC: Seizures

Nursing Diagnoses

▲ Acute Pain related to compression/displacement of brain tissue and increased intracranial pressure
△ High Risk for Impaired Corneal Tissue Integrity related to inadequate lubrication secondary to tissue edema
△ High Risk for Ineffective Therapeutic Regimen Management related to insufficient knowledge of wound care, signs and symptoms of complications, restrictions, and follow-up care

Related Care Plan

General Surgery Generic Care Plan

▲ This diagnosis was reported to be monitored for or managed frequently (75%–100%).
△ This diagnosis was reported to be monitored for or managed often (50%–74%).

Discharge Criteria

Before discharge, the client or family will

1. Explain surgical site care.
2. Discuss management of activities of daily living (ADLs).

3. Verbalize precautions to take for medication use.
4. State the signs and symptoms that must be reported to a health care professional.

Preoperative: Nursing Diagnosis

Anxiety Related to Impending Surgery and Perceived Negative Effects on Life Style

Focus Assessment Criteria	Clinical Significance
1. Understanding condition 2. Knowledge of structure and function of affected area. 3. Understanding anticipated surgical procedure	1–3. Assessing client's knowledge level guides the nurse in planning effective teaching strategies.
4. Previous exposure to person(s) experiencing cranial surgery	4. Often a client is positively or negatively influenced by information from others who have undergone cranial surgery.
5. Client and family concerns	5. To prepare client and family for surgery, these concerns must be assessed (Hickey, 2002).

Goal

The client will verbalize decreased anxiety related to impending surgery.

Indicators
- State the reason for surgery.
- Describe postoperative restrictions.

Interventions	Rationales

1. Elicit from client and family their concerns regarding
  a. Surgical procedure
  b. Prognosis
  c. Postoperative period
  d. Function (loss or return)
  e. Current disability
	1. These concerns were most frequently cited (Hickey, 2002).

2. Reinforce the effects of disease on the affected brain area and the need for surgery.	2. This information can help client accept the need for surgery and ready himself or herself psychologically, which may reduce anxiety.

3. Explain the specific postoperative experience that may include the following:
  a. A large head dressing
  b. Swollen eyes
  c. Tracheostomy or endotracheal intubation
	3. Information about what to expect can reduce anxiety associated with the unknown.

(continues on page 776)

Interventions continued	**Rationales** continued

4. Discuss the possibility of cognitive and behavioral changes related to site of surgery.
  a. Frontal—lack of spontaneity, initiative, child-like, impulsivity, decreased concentration and attention loss of recent memory, inability to plan/organize
  b. Temporal:
    • Dysnomia
    • Aphasia
    • Test taking
    • Impairments
    • Apathy
    • Placidity
  c. Parietal:
    • Cognitive deficits
    • Inattention
    • Language disorders
    • Astereognosis
    • Apraxia
    • Apathy
  d. Occipital:
    • Visual agnosia
    • Alexia
	4. Cognitive and behavioral changes have been reported in 50% to 70% of clients postcraniotomy (Hickey, 2002).

5. Discuss the uncertainty of resolution of previous cognitive or behavior patterns.	5. Cognitive and behavior changes frequently diminish or disappear 6 weeks to 6 months after surgery (Hickey, 2002).

6. Assess and document cognitive function preoperatively.
  a. Orientation (place, person, and time)
  b. Short-term memory (ask to repeat a set of words)
  c. Long-term memory (ask to identify name of high school)
  d. Affect (apathetic, hostile, or labile)
  e. General behavior (appropriate/inappropriate)
  f. Abstract reasoning (ask to relate the meaning of a proverb)
  g. Ability to calculate
  h. Attention (easily distracted or attentive)
	6. Baseline data will permit clear and accurate communication of the client's condition changes postoperatively.

7. Inform client if an alternate form of communication to speech (e.g., note pad and pencil or hand signals) will be necessary postoperatively.	7. Client may require another means of communication if large head dressings inhibit hearing, periorbital edema impairs sight, or speech is prevented by tracheostomy or endotracheal intubation. Preoperative teaching prepares client for this possibility and may decrease anxiety.
8. Refer to the General Surgery Care Plan for more interventions and rationales.	

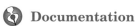 **Documentation**

Progress notes
  Present emotional status
  Interventions
  Response to interventions

Postoperative: Collaborative Problems

Potential Complication: Increased Intracranial Pressure

Potential Complication: Brain Hemorrhage, Hematoma, Hygroma

Potential Complication: Cranial Nerve Dysfunction

Potential Complication: Fluid and Electrolyte Imbalances

Potential Complication: Meningitis or Encephalitis

Potential Complication: Sensory and Motor Losses

Potential Complication: Cerebral or Cerebellar Dysfunction

Potential Complication: Hypothermia or Hyperthermia

Potential Complication: Diabetes Insipidus

Potential Complication: SIADH

Potential Complication: Cerebrospinal Fluid Leakage

Potential Complication: Seizure Activity

Nursing Goal

The nurse will detect early signs and symptoms of (a) increased ICP; (b) brain hemorrhage, hematoma, hygroma; (c) cranial nerve dysfunction; (d) fluid and electrolyte imbalances; (e) meningitis, encephalitis; (f) sensory and motor losses; (g) cerebellar dysfunction; (h) hypothermia or hyperthermia; (i) diabetes insipidus; (j) SIADH; (k) cerebrospinal fluid leakage; and (l) seizure activity and collaboratively intervene to stabilize client.

Indicators
- Alert, calm, oriented (a, b)
- No seizures (l)
- Appropriate speech (a, b)
- Pupils equal; reactive to light and accommodation (a, b)
- Intact extraocular movements (a, b)
- Pulse 60–100 beats/min (a, b)
- Respirations 16–20 breaths/min (a, b)
- Respirations regular, easy (a, b)
- BP >90/60, <140/90 mm Hg (a, b)
- Stable pulse pressure (difference between diastolic and systolic readings) (a, b)
- Temperature 98–99.5°F (e, h)
- No shivering (e, h)
- No c/o nausea/vomiting (a, b)
- Mild or no headache (a, b)
- Intact gag reflex (c)
- Intact swallowing (c)
- Symmetrical face (c)
- Symmetrical tongue movements (c)
- Intact sensory function (c, f)

- Full range of motion (c, f)
- Intact strength (c, f)
- Stable gait (c, g, f)
- Wound approximated (b, k)
- No or minimal bleeding/drainage (b, k)
- Urine output > 30mL/hr (d, i, j)
- Urine specific gravity 1.005–1.025 (d, i, j)
- Urine osmolality
  - Male 390–1090 mM/kg
  - Female 300–1090 mM/kg
- Electrolytes
  - Sodium 135–145 mEq/L (d, i, j)
  - Potassium 3.5–5.0 mEq/L (d)
  - White blood count 4,000–10,800 cu mm (e)
- Hemoglobin (b)
  - Males 13–15 gm/dL
  - Females 12–16 gm/dL
- Hematocrit (b)
  - Males 42–50%
  - Females 40–48%
- ICP monitoring (a)
- Mean arterial pressure 60–160 mm/Hg (a)
- Oxygen saturation (SaO_2) 94–100 mm/Hg (a)
- Carbon dioxide ($PaCo_2$) 35–45 mm/Hg (a)
- pH 7.35–7.45 (a)

Interventions	Rationales
1. Maintain and monitor increased intracranial pressure (ICP) (McCabe, 2000): a. A waves b. B waves c. C waves	
2. Follow institutions procedures regarding ICP monitoring (e.g., calibration, draining, maintenance).	2. ICP can be monitored by an intraventricular catheter or a fiberoptic transducer-tipped catheter inserted in the brain tissue or the ventricle a. A waves are transient, paroxysmal wanes that may last 5 to 20 minutes with amplitudes from 50 to 100 mmHg. They indicate cerebral ischemia. b. B waves have a shorter duration (30 seconds to 2 minutes) with amplitude of up to 50 mm Hg. They may precede A waves and indicate intracranial hypertension. c. C waves are small oscillations (about 6 per minute) that are rhythmic to respirations and systemic arterial blood pressure.

(continues on page 779)

Interventions continued	**Rationales** continued
3. Monitor for signs and symptoms of increased intracranial pressure (ICP).	3. Cerebral tissue is compromised by deficiencies of cerebral blood supply caused by hemorrhage, hematoma, cerebral edema, thrombus, or emboli. Monitoring intracranial pressure (ICP) serves as an indicator of cerebral perfusion (Ropper, 1998).
a. Assess the following: • Best eye opening response: spontaneously to auditory stimuli, to painful stimuli, or no response • Best motor response: obeys verbal commands, localizes pain, flexion-withdrawal, flexion-decorticate, extension-decerebrate, or no response • Best verbal response: oriented to person, place, and time; confused conversation; inappropriate speech; incomprehensible sounds; or no response	a. These responses evaluate client's ability to integrate commands with conscious and involuntary movement. Cortical function can be assessed by evaluating eye opening and motor response. No response may indicate damage to the midbrain (Hickey, 2002).
b. Assess for changes in vital signs: • Pulse changes: slowing rate to 60 or below or increasing rate to 100 or above • Respiratory irregularities: slowing of rate with lengthening periods of apnea	b. These vital sign changes may reflect increasing ICP (Hickey, 2002). • Changes in pulse may indicate brain-stem pressure—slowed at first then increasing to compensate for hypoxia. • Respiratory patterns vary with impairments at various sites. Cheyne-Stokes breathing (a gradual increase followed by a gradual decrease, then a period of apnea) points to damage in both cerebral hemispheres, midbrain, and upper pons. Ataxic breathing (irregular with random sequence of deep and shallow breaths) indicates medullar dysfunction.
• Rising blood pressure or widening pulse pressure • Decreased oxygen saturation (pulse oximetry)	• Blood pressure and pulse pressure changes are late signs indicating severe hypoxia. • Pulse oximetry provides ongoing assessment of cardiovascular and respiratory status.
c. Assess pupillary response: • Inspect pupils with a bright pinpoint light to evaluate size, configuration, and reaction to light. Compare both eyes for similarities and differences.	c. Pupillary changes indicate pressure on oculomotor or optic nerves (Hickey, 2002). • Pupil reactions are regulated by the oculomotor nerve (cranial nerve III) in the brain stem.

(continues on page 780)

Interventions continued	**Rationales** continued
• Evaluate gaze to determine whether it is conjugate (paired, working together) or if eye movements are abnormal. • Evaluate ability of eyes to adduct and abduct. d. Note the presence of the following: • Vomiting • Headache (constant, increasing in intensity, or aggravated by movement or straining) • Subtle changes (e.g., lethargy, restlessness, forced breathing, purposeless movements, and changes in mentation)	• Conjugate eye movements are regulated from parts of the cortex and brain stem. • Cranial nerve VI, or the abducens nerve, regulates abduction and adduction of the eyes. Cranial nerve IV, or the trochlear nerve, also regulates eye movement. d. • Vomiting results from pressure on the medulla that stimulates the brain's vomiting center. • Compression of neural tissue movement increases ICP and increases pain. • These changes may be early indicators of ICP changes.
4. Assist with cerebrospinal fluid (CSF) drainage through ventriculostomy drain.	4. Decreasing CSF will rapidly decrease ICP.
5. Elevate the head of the bed 15 to 30 degrees unless contraindicated. Avoid changing position rapidly.	5. Slight head elevation can aid venous drainage to reduce cerebrovascular congestion (Simmons, 1997).
6. Avoid the following: a. Carotid massage b. Neck flexion or extreme rotation c. Digital anal stimulation d. Breath holding e. Straining f. Extreme flexion of hips and knees	6. These situations or maneuvers can increase ICP (Sullivan, 1989). a. Carotid massage slows heart rate and reduces systemic circulation, which is followed by a sudden increase in circulation. b. Neck flexion or extreme rotation disrupts circulation to the brain. c–e. These activities initiate Valsalva's maneuver, which impairs venous return by constricting the jugular veins and increases ICP.
7. Consult with physician for stool softeners if needed.	7. Stool softeners prevent constipation and straining, which initiates Valsalva's maneuver.
8. Maintain a quiet, calm, softly lit environment. Plan activities to minimize interruptions.	8. These measures promote rest and decrease stimulation, helping decrease ICP.

(continues on page 781)

Interventions continued	**Rationales** continued
9. Assess cranial nerve function by evaluating the following: a. Pupillary responses b. Corneal reflex c. Gag reflex d. Cough e. Swallow f. Facial movements g. Tongue movements	9. Cranial nerve pathways may be damaged directly by ischemia, trauma, or increased pressure.
10. Assess motor and sensory functions by observing each extremity separately for strength and normalcy of movement, response to stimuli.	10. The frontal and parietal lobes contain the neurons responsible for motor and sensory functions and may be affected by ischemia, trauma, or increased pressure.
11. Assess cerebellar function by observing for the following: a. Ataxic movements b. Loss of equilibrium	11. Cerebellar function may be affected by ischemia, trauma, or increased pressure.
12. Carefully monitor hydration status; evaluate fluid intake and output, electrolytes, serum osmolality, and urine specific gravity and osmolality.	12. Fluid and electrolyte imbalances are not uncommon after cranial surgery. They result when water load exceeds renal excretion (hyposmolar) from excess fluid loss or inadequate intake (hyperosmolar) (Parobek & Alaimo, 1996).
13. Identify possible causes of hyposmolar state. a. Excess IV fluids b. Inappropriate antidiuretic hormone secretion	13. A lowered serum osmolarity releases the antidiuretic hormone.
14. Identify possible causes of hyperosmolar state. a. Fever b. Diarrhea c. Osmotic diuretic d. High-protein tube feeding e. Surgically induced diabetes insipidus f. Hyperglycemia	14. Fever and diarrhea increase fluid losses. High solute tube feeding draws water from tissues by osmosis (Parobek & Alaimo, 1996).
15. Monitor intake and administer necessary IV fluids via infusion pump.	15. Strict control of infusion is imperative to prevent fluid overload or dehydration.

(continues on page 782)

Interventions continued	**Rationales** continued
16. Monitor for diabetes insipidus. 　a. Excessive urinary output 　b. Excessive thirst 　c. Increased serum sodium 　d. Prolonged capillary filling	16. Surgery around the pituitary gland and hypothalamus can cause a deficiency of ADH, resulting in diabetes insipidus. Increased ICP causes cessation of blood flow to the brain. One result is decreased secretion of ADH, causing excessive urine output (Porth, 2002).
17. Monitor for Syndrome of Inappropriate Antidiuretic Hormone (SIADH). 　• Decreased urine output 　• Decreased serum sodium 　• Decreased BUN	17. Surgery can cause direct pressure on the hypothalamic-posterior pituitary structures, stimulating secretion of ADH (Porth, 2002).
18. Monitor urinary output and urine specific gravity every hour.	18. Trauma to the brain results in increased aldosterone production and sodium retention, which intensifies hypertonicity and decreases urine output.
19. Monitor temperature for elevations and use cooling blanket as needed.	19. Hyperthermia increases cerebral metabolic demands and leads to depletion of energy stores in the brain. Fever can result from impaired hypothalamic function, urinary tract infections, atelectasis, or wound infection (Hickey, 2002).
20. If shivering occurs, notify physician for a pharmacological treatment.	20. Shivering will increase cranial pressure. Thorazine may be prescribed (McCabe, 2000).
21. Monitor wound site for the following: 　a. Bleeding 　b. Bulging 　c. CSF leakage 　d. Infection	21. A visible bulge under the wound may indicate localized bleeding or hygroma (collection of CSF). CSF leakage through the incision must be dealt with using strict asepsis to avoid ascending infection.
22. Consult with physician if client experiences seizure activity.	22. Seizures must be controlled to avoid hypoxia and resultant increased PCO_2 and increased ICP.
23. Teach client to avoid the following: 　a. Coughing 　b. Neck hyperextension 　c. Neck hyperflexion 　d. Neck turning	23. Head and neck alignment must be maintained to prevent jugular vein compression that can inhibit venous return and result in increased ICP. Coughing increases intrathoracic pressure, which also has these effects (Ropper, 1998).

(continues on page 783)

Interventions continued	Rationales continued
24. Avoid sequential performance of activities that increase ICP (e.g., coughing, suctioning, repositioning, and bathing).	24. Research has validated that such sequential activities can cause a cumulative increase in ICP (Hickey, 2002).
25. Limit suctioning time to 10 seconds at a time; hyperoxygenate and hyperventilate client both before and after suctioning.	25. These measures help to prevent hypercapnia, which can increase cerebral vasodilation and raise ICP and prevent hypoxia that may increase cerebral ischemia (Ropper, 1998)
26. Prevent hypoxia and atelectasis.	26. Hypoxia is the most common cause of decreased level of consciousness.

Related Physician-Prescribed Interventions

Medications. Antihypertensives, stool softeners, peripheral vasodilators, osmotic diuretics, anticoagulants, corticosteroids, anticonvulsants

Intravenous Therapy. Fluid and electrolyte replacement

Laboratory Studies. Complete blood count, urinalysis, blood chemistry profile, drug levels, prothrombin time, urine chemistries

Diagnostic Studies. Computed tomography (CT) scan of head, lumbar puncture, cerebral angiography, magnetic resonance imaging (MRI), positron emission tomography (PET) scan, brain scan, Doppler ultrasonography, electroencephalography, skull x-ray film

Therapies. Antiembolism stockings, speech therapy, physical therapy, enteral feedings, occupational therapy, ventriculostomy drain, pulse oximetry, CP monitor

Documentation

Flow records
  Vital signs
  Intake and output
  Body systems assessment findings
  Neurologic assessment findings
Progress notes
  Assessment findings deviating from normal
  Seizures
  Complaints of vomiting, headache

Postoperative: Nursing Diagnoses

Acute Pain Related to Compression/Displacement of Brain Tissue and Increased Intracranial Pressure

Focus Assessment Criteria	Clinical Significance
1. Complaints of pain location description intensity duration	1,2. Client is the best source of information about this pain and the degree of relief obtained from interventions.
2. Effects of pain relief interventions	

Goal

The client will report progressive pain reduction after pain relief measures.

Indicators

- Report strategies that reduce pain.
- Report position restrictions.

Interventions	Rationales
1. Ascertain the location, nature, and intensity of the pain.	1. Pressure exerted on the baroreceptors in blood vessel walls causes generalized headache. Other sources of discomfort may include dressings, IV lines, edema, and poor positioning.
2. If the pain is a headache, slightly raise the head of the bed, reduce bright lights and room noise, and loosen head dressings if constrictive.	2. These measures may help to reduce increased ICP and relieve headache.

3. Provide nonpharmacologic relief measures as appropriate:
  a. For eye edema: eye patches
  b. For immobility: frequent position changes and back rubs
	3. Nurse should make every attempt to minimize the use of narcotic analgesics.

4. Observe for a decrease in level of consciousness (LOC) and respiratory rate after narcotic administration. (*Note:* Nurse must be able to arouse the client fully to ascertain actual LOC.)	4. Narcotics constrict pupils, may mask eye sign changes, and depress respiration.
5. Refer to General Surgery care plan under Pain.	

 Documentation

Medication administration record
   Type, dosage, and route of all medications
Progress notes
   Unsatisfactory pain relief

High Risk for Impaired Corneal Tissue Integrity Related to Inadequate Lubrication Secondary to Tissue Edema

Focus Assessment Criteria	Clinical Significance
1. Eyes moisture lid closure drainage abrasions	1. Assessment is indicated to establish a baseline and detect early changes.

Goal

The client will demonstrate continued corneal integrity.

Indicators

- Relate rationale for eye drops.
- Relate why eyes are at risk.

Interventions	Rationales
1. If eyelids do not close completely, use an eye shield or tape lids closed per protocol.	1. Corneal abrasion or erosion can occur within 4 to 6 hours if eyelids do not close completely (Hickey, 2002).
2. Loosen any tight dressings over eyes.	2. Direct pressure on eyes should be reduced.
3. Instill normal saline or hydroxyethylcellulose (Artificial Tears) as necessary.	3. Moisture provides lubrication and prevents dryness (Hickey, 2002).
4. Assess for irritation and drainage.	4. Early recognition of inflammation enables prompt intervention to prevent serious damage.
5. Apply cool compresses to the eye area if necessary.	5. This can help to reduce periocular edema by decreasing lymphatic response to injured tissue.

 Documentation

Flow records
   Eye assessment findings (vision, edema)

High Risk for Ineffective Therapeutic Regimen Management Related to Insufficient Knowledge of Wound Care, Signs and Symptoms of Complications, Restrictions, and Follow-up Care

Focus Assessment Criteria	Clinical Significance
1. Readiness and ability to learn and retain information	1. A client or family failing to meet learning goals requires a referral for assistance post-discharge.

Goals

The goals for this diagnosis represent those associated with discharge planning. Refer to the discharge criteria.

Interventions	Rationales
1. Explain that mild headaches will persist but gradually decrease.	1. Knowing what to expect can reduce client's anxiety associated with headaches.

2. Explain surgical site care
 	
   a. Wear a cap after bandages are removed.
   b. Hair can be shampooed after suture removal, but avoid scrubbing near the incision.
   c. Pat the incision area dry.
	2. This knowledge enables client and family to participate in care.
	   a. This helps to protect incision site.
	
	   b. Hair regrowth indicates adequate wound closure.
	
	   c. Vigorous rubbing can separate the wound edges.

3. Explain the need to avoid hair dryers or hot curlers until hair has regrown.	3. Direct heat can burn the unprotected surgical site.

4. Teach client not to do the following:
   a. Hold breath
   b. Strain during defecation
   c. Lift heavy objects
   d. Blow nose
   e. Cough, sneeze
	4. These activities activate Valsalva's maneuver, which impairs venous return by compressing the jugular veins and can increase ICP.

5. Teach client to exhale during certain activities (e.g., defecating, turning, or bending).	5. Exhaling causes the glottis to open, which prevents Valsalva's maneuver (Hickey, 2002).

6. Teach client and family to watch for and report the following:
 	
   a. Drainage from surgical site, nose, or ear
   b. Increasing headaches
 	
   c. Elevated temperature, stiff neck, photophobia, hyperirritability
	6. Early detection enables prompt intervention to prevent serious complications (Ropper, 1998).
	   a. Leakage may be CSF, which represents an entry route for microorganisms.
	   b. Increasing headaches may point to increasing ICP.
	   c. These signs may indicate infection or meningitis.

7. If motor-sensory deficits remain, refer to the index for specific nursing diagnoses (e.g., Impaired Communication, Self-Care Deficits, Caregiver Role Strain, and Disturbed Thought Processes).	
8. Discuss with client and family their perceptions of cognitive and behavior changes.	8. Evaluation of client's personal system is essential to plan interventions (Hickey, 2002).

(continues on page 787)

Interventions continued	**Rationales** continued

9. Depending on client's and family's readiness for more information, explain the following:
  a. Specific problems that may arise:
    • Decreased concentration
    • Difficulty with multiple stimuli
    • Emotional lability
    • Easy fatigability
    • Decreased libido
    • Allusiveness
  b. Different problems can occur throughout the recovery period.
	9. Family caregivers who are more informed are better prepared to help client to compensate (Hickey, 2002).

10. Discuss need to evaluate the effects of changes on the following:
  a. Safety
  b. Self-care ability
  c. Communication
  d. Family system
	10. The negative impact of deficits can be decreased by identifying strategies to be used at home (Hickey, 1996).

11. Expand community services that may be indicated:
  • Home health care
  • Respite care
  • Counseling
  • National Head Injury Foundation
	11. More intensive therapy may be necessary for adaptation.

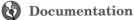 **Documentation**

Discharge summary record
  Client and family teaching
  Outcome achievement or status

ENUCLEATION

Surgical removal of the eyeball, enucleation, is indicated for post-trauma, severe infections, malignant tumors, blind painful eye, or cosmetic improvement (blind eye). After the eyeball is excised, the ocular muscles are sutured on to a hydroxyapatite sphere that has been covered with donor sclera of fascia, or a synthetic porous sphere is inserted in the ocular cavity. A temporary conformer is inserted to maintain the natural shape of the eyelids. Between 4 and 6 weeks after surgery, an ocular prosthesis can be created for the client to insert; this restores natural appearance and some movement.

 Time Frame

Preoperative and postoperative periods

 DIAGNOSTIC CLUSTER

Preoperative Period

Nursing Diagnosis

▲ Fear related to upcoming surgery, uncertain cosmetic outcome of surgery

Preoperative Period

Collaborative Problem

PC: Bleeding (refer to General Surgery)

Nursing Diagnoses

△ Risk for Infection related to increased susceptibility secondary to surgical interruption of body surface and use of prosthesis (ocular)
▲ Acute Pain related to surgical interruption of body surfaces
△ Grieving related to loss of eye and its effects on life style
△ High Risk for Disturbed Self-Concept related to effects of change in appearance on life style (acute)
△ High Risk for Impaired Home Maintenance Management related to inability to perform activities of daily living (ADLs) secondary to change in visual abilities and loss of depth perception
△ High Risk for Ineffective Therapeutic Regimen Management related to insufficient knowledge of activities permitted, self-care activities, medications, complications, and plans for follow-up care

---

▲ This diagnosis was reported to be monitored for or managed frequently (75%–100%).
△ This diagnosis was reported to be monitored for or managed often (50%–74%).

Discharge Criteria

Before discharge, the client and family will

1. Demonstrate site care.
2. Verbalize precautions to take to protect the remaining eye (e.g., wearing protective glasses at all times).
3. State the signs and symptoms that must be reported to a health care professional.
4. Verbalize an intent to share feelings and concerns related to surgery with significant others.
5. Identify available community resources and self-help groups.

Preoperative: Nursing Diagnosis

Fear Related to Upcoming Surgery, Uncertain Cosmetic Outcome of Surgery

Focus Assessment Criteria	Clinical Significance
1. Verbal and nonverbal indicators of anxiety	1. Most surgical clients express anxiety and fear. A client awaiting enucleation also may have additional fears related to the impact of surgery on his or her appearance and life style (e.g., occupation and financial status), the underlying reason for the procedure (e.g., cancer), and other concerns. The nurse needs to delve into the source of the fears to plan effective interventions to reduce them.
2. Knowledge of surgical procedure and its risks and benefits	2. This assessment guides the nurse in planning teaching strategies.
3. Amount of information the client seeks	3. Providing just the amount of information sought by the client affords him or her a measure of control over the situation. Some clients may find detailed information overwhelming and confusing; others may experience reduced anxiety from receiving detailed information.

Goal

The client will express concerns regarding upcoming surgery during dialogues.

Indicators

- Describe postoperative restrictions.
- Describe expected postoperative cause.

Interventions	Rationales
1. Promote an environment in which client will express feelings and concerns. Listen actively, validate client's fears, and reassure client that anxiety and fear are normal and expected responses to the upcoming surgery.	1. Verbalizing feelings and concerns increases the client's self-awareness and helps the nurse to identify sources of anxiety. Validation and reassurance promote self-esteem and may help to reduce anxiety.
2. Present information using a variety of instructional methods and media such as the following: a. Audiovisual programs b. Ball implant and conformer models c. Sample prosthesis	2. Simultaneous stimulation of multiple senses enhances the teaching-learning process. Written materials also provide a source to refer to after discharge.

(continues on page 790)

Interventions continued	Rationales continued

3. Explain required preadmission activities:
  a. Adherence to dietary instructions provided by anesthesia services
  b. Adjustments in medication regimen as ordered by surgeon, anesthesiologist, or client's physician
	3. Depending on the client's general health status, presence of concurrent medical problems, time of surgery, and physician's preferences, adjustments may be needed in diet (nothing by mouth for a specified period) and medications (e.g., withholding diuretics, decreasing insulin dose).

4. Discuss expected preoperative care measures including the following:
  a. Preoperative sedation
  b. IV fluid infusion for medications
  c. Bladder emptying
	4. Information about what to expect can help to reduce anxiety associated with fear of the unknown. Knowledge also enables the client to participate better in care measures and enhances his or her sense of control.

5. Explain when the pressure dressing will be removed.
 	
6. Explain general postoperative care measures such as
  a. Ice compresses
  b. Antibiotic/steroid eye drops/ointment
	5,6. Information about what to expect can reduce fear of the unknown. Explaining postoperative care before surgery allows the client to absorb the information while not under the effects of sedation. It also can help to improve compliance and facilitates the discharge planning process.

 Documentation

Progress notes
  Client teaching
  Client's understanding of teaching and response
Progress notes
  Dialogues

Postoperative: Collaborative Problem

Potential Complication: Bleeding

Nursing Goal

The nurse will detect early signs and symptoms of bleeding and collaboratively intervene to stabilize client.

Indicators
- No bleeding on dressing
- Urine output > 30 mL/hr

Interventions	Rationale
1. Monitor for bleeding through pressure patch.	1. Surgical disruption can cause trauma and bleeding. The pressure patch usually is removed in 1 week.

Related Physician-Prescribed Interventions

Medications. Antibiotics/steroid drops/ointment

Laboratory Studies. Liver function studies, refer to the General Surgery Care Plan (Appendix II)

Diagnostic Studies (preoperative). Dependent on underlying etiology, CT scan, MRI, A scan, B scan

Therapies. Ophthalmic site care

Documentation

Flow records
  Vital signs
Progress notes
  Unusual complaints

Postoperative: Nursing Diagnoses

Risk for Infection Related to Increased Susceptibility Secondary to Surgical Interruption of Body Surface and Use of Prosthesis (Ocular)

Focus Assessment Criteria	Clinical Significance

1. Signs of infection:
  a. Periorbital redness
  b. Drainage on eyelids or eyelashes
  c. Drainage from eye socket
  d. Elevated temperature
  e. Laboratory values: increased WBC count, change in WBC differential abnormal culture and sensitivity results
	1. A client receiving a prosthetic device, such as a ball implant inserted immediately after enucleation and a conformer placed between the eyelids and conjunctiva, is at risk for infection. Postoperative care must focus on prevention, early detection, and prompt treatment of conjunctival infection.

Goal

The client will demonstrate evidence of wound healing without infection.

Indicators
• Demonstrate aseptic technique with eye care.
• Explain precautions.

Interventions	Rationales

1. Promote wound healing.
  a. Encourage a well-balanced diet and adequate fluid intake.
  b. Instruct client to keep the pressure dressing over the eye for either 12 to 15 hours for hydroxyapatite implants or 4 to 5 days for synthetic Porex implants.
	1. Optimal nutrition and hydration improve overall good health that promotes healing of any surgical wound. Wearing pressure patch decreases swelling.

2. Instruct client to use aseptic technique to care for the socket and prosthesis. a. Wash hands first.	2. Aseptic technique minimizes introduction of microorganisms and reduces risk of infection.

(continues on page 792)

Interventions continued	Rationales continued
b. Gently clean the eyelids if there is a discharge by wiping the lashes from nose to cheek. c. Once the prosthesis is in place, remove it weekly and clean as ordered. d. With the prosthesis removed, inspect the cavity for signs of conjunctival infection or other problems.	

Documentation

Progress notes
   Client teaching
   Signs of infection

Acute Pain Related to Surgical Interruption of Body Surfaces

Focus Assessment Criteria	Clinical Significance
1. Location of pain	1. Incising ocular tissues during enucleation injures surrounding tissues as well. Generally, the greater the tissue manipulation, the greater the post-operative pain.
2. Severity of pain based on a scale of 0 to 10 (0 = no pain, 10 = greatest pain) rated as follows: a. Before pain relief interventions b. One half hour after intervention	2. This rating scale provides an objective method of evaluating the subjective experience of pain.
3. Previous experiences with and usual response to pain 4. Verbal and nonverbal indicators of pain, such as the following: a. Grimacing b. Rubbing the eye c. Withdrawal d. Vital sign changes e. Altered disposition	3,4. Each client responds to pain in a personal manner. Assessing the client's usual response to pain helps the nurse to plan effective pain relief interventions.

Goal

The client will voice progressive pain reduction and pain relief after interventions.

Indicators

• State pain-relief measures.
• Report what increases pain.

Interventions	Rationales
1. Assist client in identifying effective pain relief measures.	1. The client has the most intimate knowledge of his or her pain and the effectiveness of relief measures.

2. Provide information to allay anxiety and fear such as the following:
  a. Give reassurance that pain is not always directly related to the development of complications.
  b. Explain how and when pain reduction interventions will begin working.
	2. This information can help to reduce anxiety associated with the unexpected; anxiety and fear actually can increase pain.

3. Use ice compresses over enucleation site 3 to 4 times a day.	3. Ice compresses will decrease swelling.
4. Support pain relief measures with prescribed analgesics as necessary.	4. For some clients, pharmacologic therapy may be needed to provide adequate pain relief.
5. Notify physician if pain is unrelieved within ½ hour of drug administration, if pain is accompanied by nausea, or if there is drainage on the eye patch or shield.	5. These signs may indicate increased intra-ocular pressure or other complications.

 Documentation

Progress notes
  Complaints of pain
  Interventions
  Response to interventions

*Grieving Related to Loss of Eye and Its Effects on Life Style

Focus Assessment Criteria	Clinical Significance
1. Response to loss of eye	1. Grieving over the loss of vision secondary to removal of an eye is a difficult situation through which to assist a client.
2. Independence in activities	2. Increased dependency can indicate depression.

Goal

The client will express grief.

Indicators
• Report an intent to discuss feelings with significant others.
• Describe meaning of loss.

*This diagnosis is not currently on the NANDA list but has been included for clarity and usefulness.

Interventions	Rationales
1. Provide opportunities for client and family members to vent feelings, discuss the loss openly, and explore the personal meaning of the loss. Explain that grief is a common and healthy reaction.	1. Loss of an eye and vision may give rise to feelings of powerlessness, anger, profound sadness, and other grief responses. Open, honest discussions can help the client and family members to accept and cope with the situation and their responses to it.
2. Encourage use of positive coping strategies that have proved successful in the past.	2. Positive coping strategies can help to decrease feelings of hopelessness and aid with problem solving.
3. Encourage client to express positive self-attributes.	3. Focusing on positive attributes increases self-acceptance.
4. Implement measures to support the family and promote cohesiveness. a. Support the family at its level of functioning. b. Encourage members to reevaluate their feelings and to support one another.	4. Family cohesiveness is important to client support.

 Documentation

Progress notes
    Present emotional status
    Interventions
    Response to interventions

High Risk for Disturbed Self-Concept Related to Effects of Change in Appearance on Life Style (Acute)

Focus Assessment Criteria	Clinical Significance
1. Client's expressed self-concept before and after enucleation	1–3. Appearance is a critical component of self-concept; any change in appearance affects self-concept to some degree. Enucleation can have a dramatic negative impact on self-concept. Assessing the client's self-concept before surgery allows the nurse to evaluate adaptation to the change. Others' perceptions of the client's self-concept and any change after surgery may provide even more useful information than that obtained from the client. Others may provide insight into factors that may have affected the client's self-concept development and, from their more objective viewpoint, be sensitive to subtle changes.
2. Support persons' perceptions of client's self-concept	
3. Reaction to changes in self-concept	

Goal
The client will demonstrate self-care.

Indicators
- Acknowledge the change in appearance.
- Communicate feelings regarding the effects of loss of an eye and changes in appearance on his or her life style.
- Participate in self-care.

Interventions	Rationales
1. Encourage client to verbalize feelings about surgery and altered appearance and self-concept.	1. Interactions seeking to improve a client's self-concept must begin with assessing how the client feels about the illness, surgery, and self at this stress-producing time.
2. Help client to identify personal attributes and strengths.	2. This may help client to shift focus from the change in appearance to all the positive aspects that contribute to self-concept.
3. Facilitate adjustment through active listening.	3. By doing so, nurse can reinforce positive attributes and help the client to reincorporate them into his or her new self-concept.
4. Encourage regular hygiene, grooming, and other self-care activities; assist as necessary. Allow client to make decisions about care and participate in planning as appropriate.	4. Participation in self-care and planning helps to facilitate positive coping with the change.
5. Encourage visitors and telephone conversations.	5. Maintaining social contacts can promote positive coping.
6. Reinforce that an ocular prosthesis (usually fitted 2 to 6 weeks after surgery) restores cosmetic appearance.	6. This information can minimize anxiety related to fear of a radical change in appearance.
7. Discuss strategies for socialization as necessary (e.g., continued involvement in presurgical activities on exploration of new activities and interests).	7. Minimizing life style changes promotes adjustment and coping. Isolation can contribute to negative self-concept.
8. Assess for signs of negative adjustment to change in appearance. a. Refusal to discuss the loss b. Refusal to discuss future care including prosthesis fitting	8. These signs may indicate that the client is at high risk for unsuccessful adjustment.
9. Refer an at-risk client for professional counseling.	9. Client may need follow-up counseling to assist with successful adjustment.

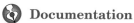 **Documentation**

Progress notes
  Present emotional status
  Interventions
    Response to interventions

High Risk for Impaired Home Maintenance Management Related to Inability to Perform Activities of Daily Living (ADLs) Secondary to Change in Visual Ability and Loss of Depth Perception

Focus Assessment Criteria	Clinical Significance

1. Home environment
  a. Layout
  b. Stairs
  c. Obstacles or hazards to ambulation (e.g., throw rugs, low furniture, pets, clutter)
 	
2. Available support systems (e.g., family, friends visiting nurse, Meals-on-Wheels, Lions Club, or Center for the Visually Impaired)
 	
3. Services currently used
	1–3. This assessment identifies whether home adaptations or referral to community resources is indicated.

Goal

Before discharge, the client and family will verbalize ways to adjust the home environment to accommodate the client's current abilities.

Indicators

- Review safety risks.
- Identify community resources available.

Interventions	Rationales
1. Help client identify problem areas such as stairs, curbs.	1. A client experiencing a vision loss needs to adapt the home environment to his or her current ability. As the client adjusts to altered depth perception and other changes, home maintenance abilities will improve.

2. Assist with adaptations to address problems.
  a. Transportation needs: Call on family, friends, or public transportation.
  b. Shopping: Arrange for delivery from the market; call on community resources.
  c. Food preparation: Obtain assistance from friends and family; arrange for Meals-on-Wheels.
	2. The nurse should make every feasible attempt to promote self-care and independence.

3. Refer client to community agencies as necessary (e.g., Lion's Club for financial aid).	3. Specialized assistance may be required.

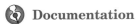 **Documentation**

Progress notes
  Needs identified
  Interventions
  Response to interventions

High Risk for Ineffective Therapeutic Regimen Management to Insufficient Knowledge of Activities Permitted, Self-care Activities, Medications, Complications, and Plans for Follow-up Care

Focus Assessment Criteria	Clinical Significance
1. Knowledge of and ability to comply with the therapeutic regimen	1. The client's understanding of the regimen and physical ability to perform necessary activities is essential to optimal compliance.
2. Readiness and ability to learn and retain information	2. A client or family failing to achieve learning goals requires a referral for assistance post-discharge.

Goals

The goals for this diagnosis represent those associated with discharge planning. Refer to the discharge criteria.

Interventions	Rationales
1. Reinforce postoperative activity restrictions such as avoiding the following: a. No swimming for 2 weeks b. Driving too close to other cars	1. Activity restrictions are aimed at reducing strain on the suture line and, in the case of driving, at eliminating situations that could be hazardous owing to impaired depth perception and visual field loss.
2. Reinforce required self-care activities. a. Wear eye protection at all times during waking hours. Suggest wearing glasses even when no vision correction is required. b. Cleanse eyelids and eyelashes of mucous threads as necessary.	2. a. Because only one operative eye remains, that eye must be protected to preserve vision. b. Daily face washing reduces risk of infection.
3. Instruct client to notify physician of the following: a. Periorbital redness and edema b. Purulent drainage c. Pain	3. These signs and symptoms can indicate infection; early detection enables prompt intervention to prevent serious infection.
4. Provide information about scheduled follow-up care. Stress the importance of	4. Follow-up care enables early detection of problems.

(continues on page 798)

Interventions continued	Rationales continued
keeping appointments with surgeon and ocularist. Make sure client has the date and time of the first scheduled appointment after discharge.	
5. Review instructions on how to reinsert conformers if dislodged.	5. The conformer maintains the integrity of the eyelids.
6. Explain to client that the ocularist will give specific instructions on prosthetic care.	6. Specific instructions and return demonstrations will provide practical instructions.

 Documentation

Discharge summary record
   Client teaching
   Outcome achievement or status

FRACTURED HIP AND FEMUR

A fractured hip may be intracapsular, which involves the neck of the femur, or extra-capsular, which involves the trochanteric region. Intracapsular fractures tend to heal poorly because the fracture damages circulation to the area. Surgical treatment will be open reduction of the fracture and internal fixation or replacement of the femoral head with a prosthesis (hemiarthroplasty). Elderly persons are more vulnerable to hip fractures because of osteoporosis and mobility problems. Between 38% and 60% of hip fractures result in permanent institutional care.

 Time Frame
Preoperative and postoperative periods

⊗ **DIAGNOSTIC CLUSTER**

Preoperative Period

Nursing Diagnosis	Refer to
▲ Anxiety related to recent trauma, upcoming surgery and insufficient knowledge of preoperative routines, postoperative routines, and postoperative sensations	General Surgery

Postoperative Period

Collaborative Problems

	Refer to
PC: Fat Emboli	
PC: Compartment Syndrome	
PC: Peroneal Nerve Palsy	
PC: Displacement of Hip Joint	
PC: Venous Stasis/Thrombosis	
PC: Avascular Necrosis of Femoral Head	
PC: Sepsis	
PC: Hemorrhage/Shock	General Surgery
PC: Pulmonary Embolism	General Surgery

Nursing Diagnoses	Refer to
▲ Acute Pain related to trauma and muscle spasms	
▲ Impaired Physical Mobility related to pain, impaired gait, and postoperative position restrictions	
▲ (Specify) Self-Care Deficit related to prescribed activity restrictions	

(continues on page 800)

Nursing Diagnoses continued	Refer to continued
▲ Fear related to anticipated dependence postoperatively	
△ Acute Confusion related to the multiple stressors associated with fractured hip and surgery	
▲ High Risk for Ineffective Therapeutic Regimen Management related to insufficient knowledge of activity restrictions, assistive devices, home care, follow-up care, and supportive services	
▲ High Risk for Constipation related to immobility	Immobility or Unconsciousness
▲ High Risk for Impaired Skin Integrity related to immobility and urinary incontinence secondary to inability to reach toilet quickly enough between urge to void and need to void	Immobility or Unconsciousness

Related Care Plan
- General Surgery Generic Care Plan

▲ This diagnosis was reported to be monitored for or managed frequently (75%–100%).
△ This diagnosis was reported to be monitored for or managed often (50%–74%).

Discharge Criteria

Before discharge, the client and family will

1. Demonstrate care of the surgical site and use of assistive devices.
2. Relate at-home restrictions and follow-up care.
3. State the signs and symptoms that must be reported to a health care professional.

Postoperative: Collaborative Problems

Potential Complication: Fat Emboli

Potential Complication: Compartment Syndrome

Potential Complication: Peroneal Nerve Palsy

Potential Complication: Hip Joint Displacement

Potential Complication: Venous Stasis/Thrombosis

Potential Complication: Avascular Necrosis of the Femoral Head

Potential Complication: Sepsis

Nursing Goal

The nurse will detect early signs and symptoms of (a) fat emboli, (b) compartmental syndrome, (c) peroneal nerve palsy, (d) hip joint displacement, (e) venous stasis/thrombosis, (f) avascular necrosis of femoral head, and (g) sepsis and will collaboratively intervene to stabilize client.

Indicators

- Alert, calm, oriented (g)
- Temperature 98.5–99°F (a, f, g)
- Heart rate 60–100 beats/min (a, g)
- Respirations 16–20 breaths/min (a, g)
- Deep relaxed respirations (a, g)
- BP > 90/60, <140/90 mm Hg (a, g)
- Peripheral pulses: full, equal, strong (h)
- Sensation intact (b)
- No pain with passive dorsiflexion (calf, toes) (b)
- Mild edema (b)
- Pain relieved by analgesics (b)
- No tingling in legs (b, c)
- Can move legs (b, c, d)
- No calf or thigh redness, warmth (e)
- Negative Homans' sign (e)
- Affected extremity aligned (d)
- No petechiae (upper trunk, axilla) (a)
- Urine output > 30 ml/hour (a, g)
- White blood cells 4,000–10,800 (g)
- Oxygen saturation 94–100% (a, g)
- Capillary refill < 3 seconds (b)
- Blood urea nitrogen 10–20 mg/dL (g)
- Creatinine 0.7–1.4 mg/dL (g)

Interventions	Rationales
1. Assess high-risk individuals for post-operative complications. a. Low serum albumin b. Co-mobilities of cardiac disease, COPD, serum creatinine > 1.7, pneumonia, digestive system disorder	1. a. Low serum albumin is a stronger predictor of death, length of stay, and readmission than age. b. These factors increase (in decreasing order) mortality after hip fracture.
2. Monitor for signs and symptoms of fat emboli: a. Fever b. Tachycardia c. Dyspnea d. Cough e. Petechiae (pinpoint reddish lesions) on upper trunk and axillae	2. Fat emboli can occur after long bone fractures especially in older clients. Signs and symptoms indicate an inflammatory response or obstruction (Pellino, Polacek, Preston, Bell, Evans, 1998).
3. Monitor for signs and symptoms of compartment syndrome. a. Deep, throbbing pain at the fracture site	3. Edema at the fracture site can compromise muscular vascular perfusion. Stretching damaged muscle causes pain. Sensory deficit is an early sign of nerve

(continues on page 802)

Interventions continued	**Rationales** continued
b. Increasing pain with passive movement c. Decreased sensation to light touch d. Inability to distinguish between sharp and dull sensation in first web space of toes, sole, and dorsum and lateral aspect of foot e. Diminished or absent pedal pulses f. Increased edema and induration in extremity g. Increased capillary refill >3 seconds	ischemia; the specific area of change indicates the affected compartment (Tumbarrello, 2000).
4. a. Before surgical treatment, turn toward fracture with pillows between legs. b. Post-surgery, turn away from fracture until able to tolerate operative side with pillow between legs.	4. This will avoid dislocation or further displacement.
5. Monitor for signs and symptoms of peroneal nerve palsy. a. Decreased sensation to light touch b. Inability to distinguish between sharp and dull sensations c. Tingling in extremity d. Paralysis	5. Pressure of the strap from skeletal traction (Buck's traction) over the fibular head can compress the peroneal nerve, resulting in paresthesias and ultimately paralysis due to nerve ischemia. (Buck's traction is not commonly used in acute care settings.)
6. Reduce dislocation during turning by placing a pillow between legs.	6. The pillow will maintain abduction and alignment.
7. Monitor for signs and symptoms of hip joint displacement. a. External rotation of affected extremity b. Affected extremity shorter than unaffected extremity c. Increased pain	7. Damaged tissue and muscles may not provide adequate support of the hip joint, resulting in displacement.
8. Monitor for signs and symptoms of venous stasis thrombosis. a. Calf pain b. Inflammation with redness and warm to touch c. Positive Homans' sign	8. The incidence of DVT in individuals with hip fractures ranges from 40% to 74% (Pellino et al., 1998). The rate of pulmonary embolus in patients after hip surgery is as much as 15% with the incidence of fatality being as high as 10%. Aspirin, subcutaneous or IV heparin, and low-dose coumarin are the most commonly used therapies; aspirin is used most often.

(continues on page 803)

Interventions continued	**Rationales** continued
9. Maintain external compression devices (graded compression elastic stockings, intermittent external pneumatic compression [IPC], impulse boots).	9. Venous return is increased; pooling is decreased. Some devices (IPC and impulse) increase rate and velocity of venous flow that promote clearance and decrease hypercoagulability (Pellino et al., 1998).
10. Institute measures to decrease risks of DVT (Pellino et al., 1998). a. Discourage smoking pre- and postoperation. b. Elevate foot of the bed without bending knee. c. Encourage rhythmic and plantar flexion of foot each hour. d. Ambulate as soon as possible.	10. a. Nicotine causes vasoconstriction. b. Elevation promotes venous return. c. This increases blood flow in lower extremities and through femoral vein.
11. Monitor for signs and symptoms of avascular necrosis of the femoral head: a. Redness b. Warmth	11. Hematoma formation results from tearing and rupture of blood vessels within the bone. Extensive blood loss with disruption of blood supply can result in bone death.
12. Monitor for signs and symptoms of sepsis: a. Temperature >101°F or <98.6°F b. Abnormal laboratory values: increased creatinine, decreased pH, increased WBC count c. Decreased urine output d. Heart rate >90 per minute e. Respiratory rate >20 minute f. Change in mentation (elderly)	12. Sepsis results in massive vasodilatation and hypovolemia, leading to tissue hypoxia with decreased renal function and cardiac output. This triggers a compensatory response of increased heart and respiratory rates in an attempt to correct hypoxia and acidosis.

Related Physician-Prescribed Interventions

Medications. Anticoagulant use (low-weight heparin, warfarin); antibiotic prophylaxis (cephalosporin IM 2 hours prior to surgery); also refer to the General Surgery Care Plan

Intravenous Therapy. Refer to the General Surgery Care Plan

Laboratory Studies. Coagulation studies; also refer to the General Surgery Care Plan

Diagnostic Studies. Femur X-ray film, bone scans, MRI, computed tomography (CT) scan

Therapies. Wound care, compression stocking, external pneumatic compression, assistive devices, anticoagulant therapy, physical therapy, impulse devices, pulse oximetry, Buck's traction

Documentation

Flow records
  Vital signs
  Distal limb sensation, paresthesias, circulation
  Intake (oral, parenteral)
  Output (urine, urine specific gravity)
  Wound (color, drainage, swelling, rate of health)

Postoperative: Nursing Diagnoses

Acute Pain Related to Trauma and Muscle Spasms

Focus Assessment Criteria	Clinical Significance

1. Source of pain:
  a. Fracture site with hematoma
  b. Groin
  c. Medial aspect of knee
	1. External rotation resulting from a shortened leg after fracture may cause muscle spasms. These spasms are more pronounced in intracapsular fracture because of the greater extent of external rotation involved.

Goal

The client will participate in self-care to the greatest extent possible considering his or her condition and status.

Interventions	Rationales
1. Position client in proper alignment. Handle gently, supporting client's leg with your hands or a pillow.	1. Optimal alignment reduces pressure on nerves and tissue; this reduces pain. Muscle spasms accompany movement.
2. Use a trochanter roll to support the involved extremity in the neutral position (Sanford, 1989).	2. The trochanter roll prevents or minimizes external rotation.
3. Preoperatively, roll only on affected side with pillow between legs.	3. This will avoid dislocation or further displacement.

4. Take steps to maintain the effectiveness of Buck's traction:
  a. Evaluate for appropriate use of weights.
  b. Ensure that weights hang freely.
  c. Ensure proper pulley functioning.
  d. Ensure that the heel does not rest on the mattress.
  e. Assess for paresthesias in the involved extremity.
	4. Proper use of Buck's traction immobilizes the involved extremity, reducing muscle spasms and minimizing further tissue destruction from bone fragments. Recent research found that skeletal and skin traction showed no benefits compared with no treatment (Pellino et al., 1998).

5. Provide an orthopedic (fracture) bedpan rather than a standard bedpan.	5. Use of an orthopedic bedpan helps to maintain proper body alignment during elimination.
6. Explain and demonstrate patient-controlled analgesia (PCA).	6. PCA provides control and decreases fear and anxiety (Seeman, 2000).

(continues on page 805)

Interventions continued	Rationales continued
7. Encourage client to use PCA before pain is unbearable.	7. A steady blood level of analgesia can prevent severe pain.
8. Consult with physician/advanced practice nurse if relief from pain is not achieved.	8. A change in the pain management plan is indicated.
9. Refer to the General Surgery Care Plan for general pain relief interventions.	

 Documentation

Flow records
  Participation in self-care

Impaired Physical Mobility Related to Pain, Impaired Gait, and Postoperative Position Restrictions

Goal

The client will report progressive increase in range of motion and ambulation.

Indicators
- Demonstrate use of assistive devices.
- Demonstrate measures to increase mobility.
- Report pain is tolerable during physical therapy.

Interventions	Rationales
1. Explain the rationale for bed exercises and early ambulation.	1. Aggressive pursuit of range-of-motion exercises and early ambulation can decrease deep-vein thrombosis and muscle wasting and increase strength.
2. Implement physical therapy (PT) plan on unit. Progress client per PT treatment program (e.g., gait training, transfers).	2. PT is an important intervention to help with early mobilization.
3. Stress the importance of pain management.	3. Pain must be controlled for client to actively participate in exercise.
4. Explain the importance of aggressive post-discharge PT and at-home exercises.	4. The literature reports that less than 50% of people with hip fractures achieve this pre-injury status (Ward, Renni, & Hager, 1998).
5. Encourage use of trapeze.	5. Shoulder and arm muscles need strengthening to use assistive device.

(continues on page 806)

Interventions continued	Rationales continued
6. Refer to discharge instructions under Ineffective Therapeutic Regimen Management.	
7. Arrange for home visit (nursing, PT) to evaluate adaptations needed (e.g. raised toilet seat, throw rugs).	7. Adaptations will be needed to reduce injury and prevent dislocation.

(Specify) Self-Care Deficit Related to Prescribed Activity Restrictions

Focus Assessment Criteria	Clinical Significance
1. Preoperative self-care ability 2. Preoperative endurance level 3. Preoperative mobility 4. Home environment: barriers to access	1–4. Pain and limited mobility affect a client's self-care ability. An elderly client may have had mobility problems before surgery (e.g., arthritis), further compromising self-care ability.

Goal

The client will report pain relief after pain relief measures.

Interventions	Rationales
1. Collaborate with client to prioritize self-care tasks.	1. Client is more likely to participate in the self-care activities that he or she values. Prioritizing activities also gives client a sense of control over the situation.
2. Encourage client to participate in doable high-priority self-care tasks to the fullest extent possible.	2. Achieving success at some tasks encourages client to attempt other activities that can promote progression in self-care ability.
3. Provide physical therapy (e.g., ROM exercises, instruction in proper transfer techniques, and use of assistive devices). *Note:* The client, particularly if elderly, may have other problems that require modifications to standard assistive devices.	3. This can help to increase muscle strength, endurance, and mobility.
4. Pace activities to ensure adequate rest periods.	4. Pacing activities helps to avoid fatigue and ensure sufficient energy to perform tasks.

(continues on page 807)

Interventions continued	Rationales continued
5. Evaluate progression of ability and refer to a rehabilitation center if necessary.	5. Client needs referral if he or she is unable to return to his or her former setting safely.
6. As necessary, consult with occupational therapy for assistance in adapting self-care activities such as dressing and cooking. 7. Instruct client or family in ways to modify the home environment to ease access to the bathroom, kitchen, and other areas.	6,7. Assistance with tasks can help client to perform them; this promotes independence. In turn, independence increases motivation and decreases feelings of helplessness.

Documentation

Medication administration record
  Type, dosage, route of all medications
Progress notes
  Unsatisfactory response
    Positioning

Fear Related to Anticipated Dependence Postoperatively

Focus Assessment Criteria	Clinical Significance
1. Emotional status	1. Assessment is needed to establish a baseline and to determine interventions needed.

Goal

The client will express a progressive reduction in fear.

Interventions	Rationales
1. Encourage client to express his or her feelings regarding the impact of the fracture and surgery on self-care ability and life style.	1. Fear of adverse health impacts and loss of independence has a significant impact on a client's psychosocial functioning. Encouraging client to share these fears gives nurse the opportunity to validate them and possibly to correct any misconceptions.
2. If appropriate, tell client that persons with active life styles before surgery have high recovery rates.	2. Several studies have supported this (Poor, Alkinson, & O'Fallon, 1995; Williams, Oberst, & Bjorklund, 1994).
3. Stress the importance of complying with the treatment regimen.	3. Compliance can decrease the length of rehabilitation and promote a return to preoperative functioning.

(continues on page 808)

Interventions continued	Rationales continued
4. Encourage the highest possible level of independent functioning.	4. Self-care promotes self-esteem and reduces feeling of dependency.
5. Involve family members or significant others in the care regimen to the fullest extent possible.	5. Support systems involvement has been shown to promote a greater recovery (Magaziner, 1990).
6. Plan diversional activities for stress management.	6. Diversional activities can help client to refocus on matters other than his or her condition and associated fears.

Documentation

Progress notes
  Interventions
  Response to interventions

Acute Confusion Related to the Multiple Stressors Associated With Fractured Hip and Surgery

Focus Assessment Criteria	Clinical Significance
1. Preoperative level of orientation 2. Age 3. Preoperative level of activity	1–3. Elderly clients, who tend to have a lowered preinjury activity pattern and some errors in mental tests on admission, are at high risk for confusion postsurgery and increased mobility and mortality (O'Brien, Grisso, & Maislin, 1993).

Goal

The client will resume presurgical orientation postoperatively.

Interventions	Rationales
1. Provide education to family, significant others, and caregivers regarding the situation and methods of response.	1. Explanations regarding causes of acute confusion can help to alleviate fears.

2. Maintain standards of empathetic, respectful care.
  a. Be an advocate when other caregivers are insensitive to the individual's needs.
  b. Function as a role model with coworkers.
	2. "Confusion" is a term frequently used by nurses to describe an array of cognitive impairments. Identifying a person as confused is just an initial step.

(continues on page 809)

Interventions continued	**Rationales** continued
c. Provide other caregivers with up-to-date information on confusion. d. Expect empathetic, respectful care and monitor its administration.	
3. Attempt to obtain information that will provide useful and meaningful topics for conversations (likes, dislikes; interests, hobbies; work history).	3. Assessing the individual's personal history can provide insight into current behavior patterns and communicates interest in the individual (Hall, 1994).
4. Encourage significant others and caregivers to speak slowly with a low voice pitch and at an average volume (unless hearing deficits are present) as one adult to another, with eye contact, and as if expecting person to understand.	4. Sensory input is carefully planned to reduce excess stimuli that increase confusion.
5. Provide respect and promote sharing. a. Pay attention to what person is saying. b. Pick out meaningful comments and continue talking. c. Call person by name and introduce yourself each time contact is made; use touch if welcomed. d. Use name the person prefers; avoid "Pops" or "Mom," which can increase confusion and is unacceptable. e. Convey to person that you are concerned and friendly (through smiles, an unhurried pace, humor, and praise; do not argue). f. Focus on feeling behind the spoken word or action.	5. This demonstrates unconditional positive regard and communicates acceptance and affection to a person who has difficulty interpreting the environment (Hall, 1994).
6. Keep person oriented to time and place. a. Refer to time of day and place each morning. b. Provide person with a clock and calendar large enough to see. c. If dementia is severe, remove all visual mirrors. d. Use night lights or dim lights at night. e. Use indirect lighting. f. Turn lights on before dark. g. Provide person with opportunity to see daylight and dark through a window or take person outdoors. h. Single out holidays with cards or pins (e.g., lighting, glasses, hearing aids).	6. Overstimulation, understimulation, or misleading stimuli can cause dysfunctional episodes because of impaired sensory interpretation (Hall, 1994).

(continues on page 810)

Interventions continued	Rationales continued
7. Encourage family to bring in familiar objects from home (e.g., photographs with non-glare glass, afghan).	7,8. Topics and objects that the person has experiences with can increase orientation.
8. Discuss current events, seasonal events (snow, water activities); share your interests (travel, crafts).	

9. Explain all activities.
  a. Offer simple explanations of tasks.
  b. Allow individuals to handle equipment related to each task.
  c. Allow individual to participate in task such as washing his or her face.
  d. Acknowledge that you are leaving and say when you will return.
	9. Assessing the individual's personal history can provide insight into current behavior patterns and communicates interest in the individual (Hall, 1994).

10. Do not endorse confusion.
  a. Do not argue with person.
  b. Never agree with confused statements.
  c. Direct person back to reality; do not allow him or her to ramble.
  d. Adhere to the schedule; if changes are necessary, advise the person of them.
  e. Avoid talking to coworkers about other topics in person's presence.
  f. Provide simple explanations that cannot be misinterpreted.
  g. Remember to acknowledge your entrance with a greeting and your exit with a closure ("I'll be back in 10 minutes.")
  h. Avoid open-ended questions.
  i. Replace five- to six-step tasks with two- or three-step tasks.
	10. Overstimulation, understimulation, or misleading stimuli can cause dysfunctional episodes because of impaired sensory interpretation (Hall, 1994).

11. Avoid use of restraints; explore other alternatives.
  a. Put person in a room with others who can help watch him or her.
  b. Enlist aid of family or friends to wash person during confused periods.
  c. If person is pulling out tubes, use mitts instead of wrist restraints.
	11. Research has validated that restraints increase fear, which increases confusion (Hall, 1994).

Documentation

Progress notes
  Level of orientation

High Risk for Ineffective Therapeutic Regimen Management Related to Insufficient Knowledge of Activity Restrictions, Assistive Devices, Home Care, Follow-up Care, and Supportive Services

Focus Assessment Criteria	Clinical Significance
1. Readiness and ability to learn and retain information.	1. A client or family failing to meet learning goals requires a referral for assistance postdischarge.

Goals

The goals for this diagnosis represent those associated with discharge planning. Refer to the discharge criteria.

Interventions	Rationales
1. Evaluate client's ability to ambulate and perform ADLs.	1. Nurse must evaluate client's self-care abilities before discharge to determine the need for referrals.
2. Evaluate mental status and presence of depression.	2. Individuals with confusion and depressive symptomatology have very high risk for prolonged disability and death (Magaziner, 1990; O'Brien et al., 1993).
3. Consult with specialist for management of depression.	3. Early detection and treatment of depression can reduce hospital stay and long-term disabilities.

4. Provide instruction on postoperative exercises per PT plan; these may include the following:
  a. Quadriceps setting
  b. Gluteal strengthening
  c. Dorsiplantar flexion
  d. Range-of-motion for upper and non-affected lower extremities
	4. Exercises facilitate use of assistive devices by maintaining or enhancing present level of muscle function in unaffected limbs.

5. Teach client how to ambulate without weightbearing using crutches or a walker; request a return demonstration to evaluate ability. Consult with physician regarding amount of weightbearing allowed.	5. The client—particularly if elderly—may have impaired balance or decreased upper body strength that necessitates the use of a walker to maintain mobility. Depending on the internal fixation device used, this need may persist for 3 to 7 days after surgery.
6. Teach client and family to do the following:	6. These measures may help to reduce risk of injury.

(continues on page 812)

Interventions continued	**Rationales** continued
a. Use proper transfer techniques to a chair: Place chair on the affected side, abduct and support the affected leg, and pivot on the unaffected leg.	a. Proper transfer technique prevents weightbearing on the affected side.
b. Use pillows to maintain abduction while seated.	b. Leg abduction relieves stress on the internal fixation device and fracture site.
c. For 5 to 10 days after surgery, sit without flexing the hip more than 60 degrees.	c. Hip flexion puts stress on the internal fixation device and fracture site.
d. Avoid adducting the affected extremity beyond the midline for at least 2 months after surgery.	d. Leg adduction puts stress on the internal fixation device and fracture site.
e. Use proper body mechanics within limitations.	e. Proper body mechanics prevent injury to muscles and ligaments.
f. Use an elevated toilet seat.	f. Using an elevated toilet seat decreases flexion and minimizes stress on fracture site. It also facilitates independent toileting.
7. Present information or reinforce learning using written materials (e.g., booklets on instruction sheets) and audiovisual aids (e.g., slides, videotapes, models, or diagrams).	7. Using a variety of teaching materials stimulates learning and enhances retention, particularly for an elderly client who may have visual or hearing impairment.
8. Explain the importance of progressive care, i.e., early nonweightbearing ambulation, self-care within abilities.	8. The risk for complications increases with each day of immobility, particularly in an elderly client.
9. Teach client and family to watch for and report subtle signs of infection: a. Increased temperature, chills b. Malaise	9. Hip fracture typically affects elderly clients who have a decreased ability to compensate for physiological changes and immunologic system changes that may mask pronounced signs and symptoms of infection.
10. Explain anticoagulation therapy. Refer to Anticoagulation Care Plan.	

🕮 Documentation

Discharge summary record
  Client and family teaching
  Outcome achievement or status
  Referrals if indicated

For a Clinical Pathway on an Operable Fractured Femur, visit http://connection.lww.com

HYSTERECTOMY

*S*ubtotal hysterectomy involves removal of the uterus only; *total hysterectomy,* removal of the uterus and cervical stump; *salpingectomy,* removal of these structures plus the fallopian tubes; and *oophorectomy,* removal of the uterus, cervix, fallopian tubes, and ovaries. Surgery is performed either through a lower abdominal incision, through the vagina, or via various sites with laparoscopic techniques (Reich, 2001).

 Time Frame

Preoperative and postoperative periods

 DIAGNOSTIC CLUSTER

Preoperative Period

Refer to General Surgery Generic Care Plan

Postoperative Period

Collaborative Problems

▲ PC: Ureter, Bladder, Bowel Trauma
▲ PC: Vaginal Bleeding
▲ PC: Deep Vein Thrombosis

Nursing Diagnoses

△ High Risk for Disturbed Self-Concept related to perceived effects on sexuality and feminine role
△ High Risk for Ineffective Therapeutic Regimen Management related to insufficient knowledge of perineal/incisional care, signs of complications, activity restrictions, loss of menses, hormone therapy, and follow-up care

---

▲ This diagnosis was reported to be monitored for or managed frequently (75%–100%).
△ This diagnosis was reported to be monitored for or managed often (50%–74%).

Discharge Criteria

Before discharge, the client and family will

1. State wound care procedures to follow at home.
2. Verbalize precautions to take regarding activities.
3. State the signs and symptoms that must be reported to a health care professional.
4. Verbalize an intent to share feelings and concerns with significant others.

Postoperative: Collaborative Problems

Potential Complication: Ureter, Bladder, Bowel Trauma

Potential Complication: Vaginal Bleeding

Potential Complication: Deep Vein Thrombosis

Nursing Goal

The nurse will detect early signs and symptoms of (a) ureter, bladder, and bowel trauma; (b) vaginal bleeding; and (c) deep vein thrombosis and collaboratively intervene to stabilize client.

Indicators

- Urine output > 30 mL/hr (a)
- Clear urine (a)
- Intact bowel sounds all quadrants (a)
- Flatus present (a)
- No leg pain (c)
- No leg edema (c)
- No pain with dorsiflexion of feet (Homans' sign) (c)
- Light-colored vaginal drainage (b)
- Patent suprapubic catheter (a)
- Intact, minimal erythema at catheter site (a)

Interventions	Rationales

1. Monitor for signs and symptoms of ureter, bladder, or rectal trauma.
  a. Urinary retention
  b. Prolonged diminished bowel sounds
  c. Bloody, cloudy urine
  d. Absence of flatus
	1. Proximity of these structures to the surgical site may predispose them to atony because of edema or nerve trauma.

2. Monitor for signs and symptoms of deep venous thrombosis (DVT).
  a. Leg pain or calf pain
  b. Leg swelling
  c. Referred pain in abdomen or buttocks
  d. Positive Homans' sign
	2. Gynecological surgery increases the risk of DVT because of operative time and surgical positioning.

3. Apply elastic stockings as ordered.	3. Stockings provide even compression to increase venous return.
4. Perform leg exercises every hour while client is in bed. Ambulate client early.	4. Leg exercises and ambulation contract leg muscles, stimulate the venous pump, and reduce stasis.
5. Provide frequent position changes; avoid putting pressure under the knees.	5. Movement reduces stasis and vascular pooling in legs; pressure under knees can interfere with peripheral circulation (Porth, 2002).

6. If vaginal route, monitor vaginal bleeding every 2 to 4 hours.
  a. Monitor vaginal drainage. Record amount and color.
	6.
	
	  a. Drainage is expected. Frank vaginal bleeding, if it occurs, should be light (Porth, 2002).

(continues on page 815)

Interventions continued	Rationales continued
b. If packing is used, notify physician if packing is saturated or clots are passed. c. Notify physician if perineal pad is saturated.	b,c. Packing is used if hemostasis is a problem during surgery. Excess bleeding or clots can indicate abnormal bleeding (Porth, 2002).
7. If the route is abdominal, monitor for incisional and vaginal bleeding every 2 hours.	7. The female pelvis has an abundant supply of blood vessels, creating a high risk for bleeding.

8. If suprapubic catheter is used, do the following:
  a. Evaluate in what position the catheter drains best.
  b. Monitor intake and output.
  c. Clean insertion site at least once a day.
  d. Check catheter potency (e.g., kinks or blockage) every 2 hours.
	8. Suprapubic catheters are used to decrease urethra swelling; this will promote healing.

 Related Physician-Prescribed Interventions

Medications. Estrogen therapy (selected cases)

Intravenous Therapy. Refer to the General Surgery Care Plan

Laboratory Studies. STD screening; also refer to the General Surgery Care Plan

Diagnostic Studies. Ultrasound or computed tomography (CT) scan

Therapies. Urinary or suprapubic catheter; pelvic ultrasound; hysterosalpingography; also refer to the General Surgery Care Plan

 Documentation

Flow records
  Vital signs
  Perineal drainage
  Intake and output
  Turning, ambulation

Postoperative: Nursing Diagnoses

High Risk for Disturbed Self-Concept Related to Significance of Loss

Focus Assessment Criteria	Clinical Significance
1. Exposure to others who have undergone hysterectomy 2. Ability to express feelings about the hysterectomy	1,2. This information can be used to measure present response and progress. Discussions can detect misinformation and fears.

(continues on page 816)

Focus Assessment Criteria continued	Clinical Significance continued
3. Evidence of negative self-concept	3. A client with a previous negative self-concept is at higher risk for impaired adjustment.
4. Participation in self-care	4. Participation in self-care indicates an attempt to cope positively with the changes.

Goal

The client will acknowledge change in body structure and function.

Indicators

• Communicate feelings about the hysterectomy.
• Participate in self-care.

Interventions	Rationales
1. Contact the client frequently and treat her with warm, positive regard.	1. Frequent contact by caregiver indicates acceptance and may facilitate trust. Client may be hesitant to approach staff because of a negative self-concept.
2. Incorporate emotional support into technical care teaching sessions (e.g., wound care and bathing).	2. This encourages resolution of emotional issues while teaching technical skills.
3. Encourage client to verbalize her feelings about surgery and perceptions of life style impact. Validate her perceptions and reassure her that the responses are normal and appropriate.	3. Sharing concerns and ventilating feelings provides an opportunity for nurse to correct any misinformation. Validating the client's perceptions increases self-awareness (Webb & Wilson-Barnet, 1983).
4. Replace myths with facts (e.g., hysterectomy usually does not affect physiologic sexual response).	4. Misinformation may contribute to unfounded anxiety and fear. Providing accurate information can help to reduce these emotional stressors.
5. Discuss the surgery and its effects on functioning with family members or significant others; correct any misconceptions. Encourage client to share her feelings and perceptions with family and significant others.	5. The support of family members or significant others often is critical to client's acceptance of changes and positive self-concept (Webb & Wilson-Barnet, 1983).
6. Refer the client at high risk for unsuccessful adjustment for professional counseling.	6. Follow-up therapy to assist with effective adjustment may be indicated.

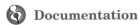 **Documentation**

Progress notes
  Present emotional status
  Interventions
    Response to interventions

High Risk for Ineffective Therapeutic Regimen Management Related to Insufficient Knowledge of Perineal/Incisional Care, Signs of Complications, Activity Restrictions, Loss of Menses, Hormone Therapy, and Follow-up Care

Focus Assessment Criteria	Clinical Significance
1. Readiness and ability to learn and retain information	1. A client or family failing to meet learning goals requires a referral for assistance postdischarge.

Goals

The goals for this diagnosis represent those associated with discharge planning. Refer to the discharge criteria.

Interventions	Rationales
1. Discuss expectations for recovery based on type and extent of surgery. Explain that vaginal hysterectomy generally affords more rapid recovery and causes less postoperative discomfort but has several disadvantages, including the following: a. Greater risk of postoperative infection. b. Reduced ability (as compared with abdominal hysterectomy) to deal with unexpected difficulties of surgery or complications. Explain that abdominal hysterectomy allows better visualization during surgery and has fewer contraindications, but it involves longer recovery periods, increased use of anesthesia, and increased postoperative pain.	1. Understanding expectations for recovery can help client and family to plan strategies for complying with the postoperative care regimen.
2. Explain care of an uncomplicated wound (abdominal hysterectomy); teach client to do the following: a. Wash with soap and water (bath or shower when able). b. Towel-dry thoroughly; separate skin folds to ensure complete drying. Consult with physician for care of a complicated wound.	2. Proper wound care helps to reduce microorganisms at incision site and prevent infection.

(continues on page 818)

Interventions continued	Rationales continued
3. Explain perineal care (vaginal hysterectomy); teach client to do the following: a. Maintain good hygiene. b. Wash thoroughly with soap and water. c. Change the peripad frequently. d. After elimination, wipe from the front to back using a clean tissue for each front-to-back pass.	3. Proper perineal care reduces microorganisms around the perineum and minimizes their entry into the vagina.
4. Explain the need to increase activity as tolerated.	4. Physical activity, especially early and frequent ambulation, can help to prevent or minimize abdominal cramps, a common complaint during recovery from abdominal hysterectomy.
5. Teach client and family to watch for and report the following: a. Changes in perineal drainage (e.g., unusual drainage, bright red bleeding, foul odor) b. Urinary retention, burning, frequency c. Cloudy, foul-smelling urine d. Blood in urine e. Change in bowel function (constipation, diarrhea)	5. Because of the abundance of blood vessels in the female pelvis, hysterectomy carries a higher risk of postoperative bleeding than most other surgeries. Bleeding most often occurs within 24 hours after surgery, but high risk also occurs on the fourth, ninth, and 21st postoperative days when sutures dissolve. A small amount of pink, yellow, or brown serous drainage or even minor frank vaginal bleeding (no heavier than normal menstrual flow) is normal and expected (Kramer & Reiter, 1992).
6. Explain the effects of surgery on menstruation and ovulation. Instruct client to report symptoms of the climacteric (cessation of menses). a. Hot flashes b. Headache c. Nervousness d. Palpitations e. Fatigue f. Depression, feelings of uselessness, and other emotional reactions	6. Removal of the uterus (leaving the ovaries) theoretically should not produce menopausal symptoms; however, the client may experience them temporarily apparently because of increased estrogen levels resulting from surgical manipulation of the ovaries. Removal of both ovaries artificially induces menopause; this causes more severe symptoms than typically experienced in a normal climacteric. To help reduce these symptoms, a portion of the ovary often is left in place unless contraindicated. Estrogen therapy relieves symptoms and may be indicated except in cases of malignancy.
7. Explain activity restrictions; teach client to do the following: a. Expect fatigue and weakness during the recovery period. b. Delegate tasks to others (e.g., vacuuming or lifting) for at least 1 month.	7. Adequate rest allows the body to repair surgical tissue trauma. Walking improves muscle strength and endurance that speed recovery. Prolonged sitting or standing may cause pelvic congestion and thrombosis formation. Repetitive activities also cause pelvic congestion.

(continues on page 819)

Interventions continued	**Rationales** continued
c. Walk in moderation; gradually increase distance and pace. d. Resume driving 2 weeks after surgery if the car is equipped with an automatic transmission. e. Avoid sitting and standing for prolonged periods. f. Avoid aerobic activity. g. Avoid horseback riding.	
8. Explore client's concerns regarding the impact of surgery on sexual feelings and function. Explain that she should be able to resume intercourse anywhere from 3 weeks (with a vaginal hysterectomy) to 16 weeks after surgery; confirm a specific time frame with physician.	8. In most cases, hysterectomy should not affect sexual response or functioning. For 3 to 4 months after surgery, intercourse may be painful owing to abdominal soreness and temporary shrinking of the vagina. Intercourse helps to stretch the vaginal walls and eventually relieves the discomfort.
9. If a subtotal hysterectomy was performed, explain that menses will continue because a portion of the uterus and its endometrial lining remain. 10. Explain that total removal of the uterus prevents pregnancy and results in loss of menses, but as long as even a portion of an ovary remains, client may experience monthly premenstrual symptoms such as bloating and abdominal cramps.	9,10. Explanations of what to expect from surgery can help reduce anxiety associated with the unknown and allow effective coping (Redman & Thomas, 1996).
11. If estrogen replacement therapy is indicated, provide client teaching. a. Explain that estrogen typically is administered in low doses on a cyclical basis—5 days on, 2 days off—until she reaches the average age of menopause. b. Discuss the rationale for therapy: to provide a feeling of well-being, to decrease risk of cardiovascular disease, to decrease risk of osteoporosis. c. Explain risks associated with therapy.	11. Client's understanding of estrogen therapy may encourage compliance with the prescribed regimen. c. Nulliparous women were found to be at high risk for breast cancer during the first 10 years of therapy. Women older than 55 years and women experiencing late menopause also were found to be at increased risk for breast cancer. The study recommended that physicians give these clients special consideration before prescribing estrogen therapy.

(continues on page 820)

Interventions continued	Rationales continued
d. Teach client to report the following: • Mood changes especially depression • Signs and symptoms of throm-bophlebitis (warmth and pain in the calf, abdominal pain, and pain, numbness, or stiffness in the legs and buttocks) • Excessive fluid retention • Jaundice • Excessive nausea and vomiting • Dizziness, frequent headaches • Hair loss • Visual disturbances • Breast lumps e. Explain the need for regular follow-up visits (at least yearly) and monthly breast self-examination.	d. Estrogen replacement therapy can cause adverse effects such as hyperten-sion, embolic disorders, or hepatic and gallbladder disease.
12. Discuss follow-up care; explain that dis-charge usually occurs in 5 to 7 days and that a postoperative check is scheduled for 4 to 6 weeks after discharge. Reinforce the importance of keeping scheduled appointments.	12. Regular follow-up care is necessary to evaluate the results of surgery and estro-gen therapy, if indicated, and to detect any complications.

 Documentation

Discharge summary record
   Client and family teaching
   Outcome achievement or status

ILEOSTOMY

Ileostomy is the surgical creation of an opening between the ileum and the abdominal wall for the purpose of fecal diversion. An ileostomy may be temporary or permanent and may be constructed as an end stoma, a loop stoma, or a double-barrel stoma. Ileostomy differs from colostomy in that the feces have a more liquid consistency, digestive enzymes are present, and the flow of contents is uncontrolled, so that a collection appliance must be used continuously.

Two internal pouching procedures can replace the external ostomy pouch that must be worn following a standard ileostomy. A *Kock continent ileostomy* pouch is an internal fecal reservoir constructed of ileum and containing a nipple valve that maintains continence of stool and flatus. An *ileoanal reservoir* is an ileal pouch located in the pelvis. Various pouch configurations are possible, the most common being an S- or J-shaped pouch. Ileostomy surgery is done in two stages. The first operation involves an abdominal colectomy, construction of an ileal pouch, mucosectomy of the rectum, ileoanal anastomosis, and creation of a diverting ileostomy. The second operation is performed to take down the temporary ileostomy to restore the continuity of the fecal stream. Ileostomy is typically indicated for clients with pathologic small bowel conditions (e.g., ulcerative colitis and regional enteritis) (Hoebler, 1997).

 Time Frame

Preoperative and postoperative periods

 DIAGNOSTIC CLUSTER

Preoperative Period

Nursing Diagnoses

▲ Anxiety related to lack of knowledge of ileostomy care and perceived negative effects on life style

Postoperation Period

Collaborative Problems

▲ PC: Peristomal Ulceration/Herniation
▲ PC: Stomal Necrosis, Retraction Prolapse, Stenosis, Obstruction
▲ PC: Fluid and Electrolyte Imbalances
   PC: Ileal Reservoir Pouchitis (Kock Pouch)
   PC: Failed Nipple Valve (Kock Pouch)
   PC: Ileoanal Kock Pouchitis
   PC: Cholelithiasis
   PC: Urinary Calculi

Nursing Diagnoses

▲ High Risk for Disturbed Self-Concept related to effects of ostomy on body image and lifestyle
△ High Risk for Ineffective Sexuality Patterns related to perceived negative impact of ostomy on sexual functioning and attractiveness
△ High Risk for Sexual Dysfunction related to physiologic impotence secondary to damaged sympathetic nerve damage (male) or inadequate vaginal lubrication (female)
△ High Risk for Loneliness related to anxiety over possible odor and leakage from appliance
△ High Risk for Ineffective Therapeutic Regimen Management related to insufficient knowledge of stoma pouching procedure, peristomal skin care, perineal wound care, and incorporation of ostomy care into activities of daily living (ADLs)

(continues on page 822)

Nursing Diagnoses continued

△ High Risk for Ineffective Therapeutic Regimen Management related to insufficient knowledge of care of ileoanal reservoir

High Risk for Ineffective Therapeutic Regimen Management related to insufficient knowledge of intermittent intubation of Kock continent ileostomy

Related Care Plan

General Surgery Generic Care Plan

▲ This diagnosis was reported to be monitored for or managed frequently (75%–100%).
△ This diagnosis was reported to be monitored for or managed often (50%–74%).

Discharge Criteria

Before discharge, the client and family will

1. State conditions of ostomy care at home: stoma, pouching, irrigation, skin care.
2. Discuss strategies for incorporating ostomy management into ADLs.
3. Verbalize precautions for medication use and food intake.
4. State signs and symptoms that must be reported to a health care professional.
5. Verbalize an intent to share feelings and concerns related to ostomy with significant others.
6. Identify available community resources and self-help groups:
   a. Visiting nurse
   b. UOA
   c. Recovery of Male Potency: Help for Impotent Male
   d. American Cancer Foundation
   e. Community supplier of ostomy equipment
   f. Financial reimbursement for ostomy equipment
7. If the client has a Kock continent ileostomy, he or she should demonstrate ability to perform intermittent self-intubation.

Preoperative: Nursing Diagnosis

Anxiety Related to Lack of Knowledge of Ileostomy Care and Perceived Negative Effects on Life Style

Focus Assessment Criteria	Clinical Significance
1. Understanding underlying disorder necessitating ileostomy 2. Knowledge of structure and function of affected organs 3. Anticipated surgical procedure and stoma location 4. Previous exposure to a client with an ostomy 5. Familiarity with stoma pouching equipment 6. Emotional status, cognitive ability, memory, vision, manual dexterity 7. Life style, strengths, coping mechanisms, available support systems 8. Fears	1–8. Assessing client's knowledge of ileostomy identifies learning needs and guides nurse in planning effective teaching strategies. Assessing client's emotional status, mental and physical ability, and other relevant factors helps nurse to evaluate client's ability to accept, adjust to, and manage ostomy and stoma (Pieper & Mikols, 1996).

Goal

The client will verbalize decreased anxiety related to fear of the unknown.

Indicators
- State reason for ileostomy.
- Describe anatomic changes following ileostomy surgery.
- Identify his or her own type of ileostomy.

Interventions	Rationales
1. Identify and dispel any misinformation or misconceptions the client has regarding ostomy.	1. Replacing misinformation with facts can reduce anxiety.
2. Explain the normal anatomical structure and function of the gastrointestinal (GI) tract.	2. Knowledge increases confidence; confidence produces control and reduces anxiety.
3. Explain the effects of the client's particular disorder on affected organs.	3. Understanding the disorder can help the client accept the need for ileostomy.
4. Use an anatomic diagram or model to show the resultant altered route of elimination.	4. Understanding how body waste elimination occurs after the rectum and the anus are removed can help to allay anxiety related to altered body function.
5. Describe the stoma's appearance and anticipated location. Explain the following about the stoma: a. It will be the same color and moistness as oral mucous membrane. b. It will not hurt when touched because it has no sensory endings. c. It may bleed slightly when wiped; this is normal and not of concern. d. It will become smaller as the surgical area heals; color will remain the same. e. It may change in size depending on illness, hormone levels, and weight gain or loss.	5. Explaining expected events and sensations can help to reduce anxiety associated with the unknown and unexpected. Accurate descriptions of the stoma appearance help to ease shock at the first sight of it after ostomy surgery.
6. Discuss function of the stoma pouch. Explain that it serves as an external receptacle for storage of feces much as the colon acts as an internal storage receptacle.	6. Understanding the purpose and need for a pouch encourages client to accept it and participate in ostomy management.
7. Encourage client to handle the stoma pouching equipment.	7. Many clients are relieved to see the actual size and material of a stoma pouch. Often, the uninformed client's visions of large bags and complicated, difficult-to-manage equipment can produce anxiety.

Documentation

Progress notes
Present emotional status
Teaching records
   Client teaching

Postoperative: Collaborative Problems

Potential Complication: Peristomal Ulceration/Herniation

Potential Complication: Stomal Necrosis, Retraction, Prolapse, Stenosis, Obstruction

Potential Complication: Fluid and Electrolyte Imbalances

Potential Complication: Ileal Reservoir Pouchitis (Kock Pouch)

Potential Complication: Failed Nipple Valve (Kock Pouch)

Potential Complication: Ileoanal Kock Pouchitis

Potential Complication: Cholelithiasis

Potential Complication: Urinary Calculi

Nursing Goal

The nurse will detect early signs and symptoms of (a) peristomal ulceration/herniation; (b) stomal necrosis, retraction; (c) prolapse, stenosis, obstruction; (d) fluid and electrolyte imbalances; (e) ileal reservoir pouchitis (Koch pouch); (f) failed nipple valve (Koch pouch); (g) ileoanal Koch pouchitis; (h) cholelithiasis; and (i) urinary calculi and collaboratively intervene to stabilize client.

Indicators
- Intact peristomal muscle tone (a)
- No stomal ulceration (a)
- No c/o abdominal cramping or pain (b, e, g)
- No abdominal or flank pain (h, i)
- No nausea or vomiting (b, d, e, g)
- No abdominal distention (b, d, h)
- Urine output > 30 mL/hr (d, e, g)
- Minimal or no weight loss (d, e, g)
- Clear, pale urine (d, e, g)
- Urine specific gravity 1.005–1.030 (d, e, g)
- No change in stool color (d, e, g)
- Serum sodium (d, e, g)
- Serum potassium (d, e, g)
- Serum magnesium (d, e, g)
- Serum cholesterol (d, e, g)
- No epigastric fullness (h)
- No jaundice (h)
- Temperature 98.5–99°F (e, g)

Interventions	Rationales

1. Monitor for signs of peristomal ulceration or herniation.
  a. Decreased peristomal muscle tone
  b. Bulging beyond normal skin surface and musculature
  c. Persistent ulceration
	1. Early detection of ulcerations and herniation can prevent serious tissue damage.

(continues on page 825)

Interventions continued	**Rationales** continued
2. Monitor for stomal necrosis, prolapse, retraction, stenosis, and obstruction. Assess the following: a. Color, size, and shape of stoma b. Color, amount, and consistency of ostomy effluent c. Complaints of cramping, abdominal pain, nausea and vomiting, abdominal distension d. Ostomy appliance and appliance belt fit	2. Daily assessment is necessary to detect early changes in stoma condition. a. Changes can indicate inflammation, retraction, prolapse, or edema. b. Changes can indicate bleeding or infection. Decreased output can indicate obstruction. c. These complaints may indicate obstruction. d. Improperly fitting appliance or belt can cause mechanical trauma to the stoma.
3. Monitor for signs of fluid and electrolyte imbalance. a. High volume of watery ostomy output (more than five one-third to one-half filled pouches or >1,000 mL daily) b. Decreased serum sodium, potassium, and magnesium levels c. Weight loss d. Nausea and vomiting, anorexia, abdominal distention	3. Fluid and electrolyte imbalances most commonly result from diarrhea. Major causes of acute diarrhea include infection, diuretic therapy, obstruction, and hot weather. Chronic diarrhea can result from ileal resection or "short gut syndrome," radiation therapy, or chemotherapy (Ellis & Saddler, 2000).
4. Administer fluid and electrolyte replacement therapy as ordered.	4. Replacement therapy may be needed to prevent serious electrolyte imbalance or fluid deficiency.
5. Monitor for signs and symptoms of ileal reservoir or ileoanal pouchitis: a. Acute increase in effluent flow b. Evidence of dehydration c. Abdominal pain and bloating, nausea and vomiting d. Fever	5. Pouchitis or ileitis involves inflammation of the ileal pouch. The cause is unknown, but bacterial growth in the pouch is a suspected causative factor. Insufficiently frequent pouch emptying increases the risk; it occurs in about 10% of clients with a Kock ileostomy.
6. Connect an indwelling catheter to continuous straight drainage.	6. This measure promotes continuous urine drainage of the Kock Pouch.
7. Monitor for stool leakage from a stoma with a nipple valve.	7. Nipple valve failure—pulling apart of the bowel segment forming the valve—most commonly occurs within the first 3 months after surgery.
8. Irrigate the ileoanal reservoir daily to flush out mucus.	8. Daily irrigation helps to prevent stomal obstruction.

(continues on page 826)

Interventions continued	Rationales continued

9. Monitor for cholelithiasis (gallstones):
  a. Epigastric fullness
  b. Abdominal distention
  c. Vague pain
  d. Very dark urine
  e. Grayish or clay colored stools
  f. Jaundice
  g. Elevated cholesterol
	9. Changes in absorption of bile acids post-operatively increase cholesterol levels and can cause gallstones.

10. If symptoms occur, collaborate with physician or advanced practice nurse for preparation for a diagnostic evaluation (e.g., ultrasound, cholecystography).	10. Diagnostic studies will be indicated to confirm gallstones and to determine severity.

11. Monitor for urinary calculi (stones):
  a. Lower abdominal pain
  b. Flank pain
  c. Hematuria
  d. Decreased urine output
  e. Increased urine specific gravity
	11. Large volumes of fluid lost through the ileostomy can cause urinary stones as a result of dehydration.

 Related Physician-Prescribed Interventions

Dependent on the underlying problem. Refer also to the General Surgery Care Plan in Appendix II.

Documentation

Flow records
  Intake and output
  Bowel sounds
  Wound status
Progress notes
Stoma condition
Changes in physiological status

Postoperative: Nursing Diagnoses

High Risk for Disturbed Self-Concept Related to Effects of Ostomy on Body Image

Focus Assessment Criteria	Clinical Significance
1. Previous exposure to person(s) with an ostomy	1–7. This assessment information helps the nurse evaluate present responses and progress. Participation in self-care and planning indicates positive attempts to cope with the changes.
2. Ability to visualize the stoma	
3. Ability to express feelings about the stoma	
4. Ability to share feelings about the ostomy with significant others	

(continues on page 827)

Focus Assessment Criteria continued	**Clinical Significance** continued
5. Ability to participate in the stoma pouching procedure	
6. Ability to discuss plans to incorporate ostomy management into body image and life style	
7. Evidence of negative self-concept	

Goal

The client will acknowledge change in body structure and function.

Indicators

- Communicate feelings about the ostomy.
- Participate in stoma care.

Interventions	**Rationales**
1. Contact client frequently and treat him or her with warm, positive regard.	1. Frequent contact by the caregiver indicates acceptance and may facilitate trust. The client may be hesitant to approach the staff because of negative self-concept (Dudas, 1993).
2. Incorporate emotional support into technical ostomy self-care sessions.	2. This allows resolution of emotional issues during acquisition of technical skills. Shipes (1987) identified four stages of psychological adjustment that ostomy clients experience. a. *Narration.* Each client recounts his or her illness experience and reveals understanding of how and why he or she finds self in this situation. b. *Visualization and verbalization.* Client looks at and expresses feelings about his or her stoma. c. *Participation.* Client progresses from observer to assistant, then to independent performer of the mechanical aspects of ostomy care. d. *Exploration.* Client begins to explore methods of incorporating the ostomy into life style. Use of this adjustment framework helps to establish guidelines for planning the client's experiences in an organized manner.

(continues on page 828)

Interventions continued	**Rationales** continued
3. Have client look at and touch the stoma.	3. Nurse should not make assumptions about a client's reaction to ostomy surgery. Client may need help accepting the reality of the altered body appearance and function or dealing with an overwhelming situation.
4. Encourage client to verbalize feelings about the stoma and perceptions of its anticipated effects on his or her life style.	4. Sharing gives the nurse an opportunity to identify and dispel misconceptions and allay anxiety and self-doubt.
5. Validate client's perceptions and reassure client that such responses are normal and appropriate.	5. Validating the client's perceptions promotes self-awareness and provides reassurance.
6. Have client practice using a pouch clamp on an empty pouch.	6. Beginning client teaching with a necessary skill that is separate from the body may be less threatening and may ease the fear of failure when performing on his or her own body.
7. Assist the client with pouch emptying as necessary.	7. During ostomy care procedures, the client watches health care professionals for signs of revulsion. The nurse's attitude and support are of primary importance (Dudas, 1993).
8. Have client participate in pouch removal and pouch application. Provide feedback on progress; reinforce positive behavior and proper techniques.	8. Effective, thorough teaching helps client learn to master procedures.
9. Have client demonstrate the stoma pouching procedure independently in the presence of support persons.	9. Return demonstration lets nurse evaluate the need for any further teaching.
10. Involve support persons in learning ostomy care principles. Assess client's interactions with support persons.	10. Others' response to the ostomy is one of the most important factors influencing the client's acceptance of it.
11. Encourage client to discuss plans for incorporating ostomy care into his or her life style.	11. Evidence that client will pursue his or her goals and life style reflects positive adjustment.
12. Encourage client to verbalize positive self-attributes.	12. Identifying personal strengths promotes self-acceptance and positive self-concept.

(continues on page 829)

Interventions continued	Rationales continued
13. Suggest that client meet with a person from the UOA who can share similar experiences.	13. In addition to the professional nurse's clinical expertise, the ostomy client may choose to take advantage of a UOA visitor's actual experience with an ostomy (Maklebust, 1985).
14. Identify a client at risk for unsuccessful adjustment (Shipes, 1987): a. Poor ego strength b. Ineffective problem-solving ability c. Difficulty learning new skills d. Lack of motivation e. External focus of control f. Poor health g. Unsatisfactory preoperative sex life h. Lack of positive support systems i. Unstable economic status j. Rejection of counseling	14. Successful adjustment to ostomies is influenced by factors such as the following: a. Previous coping success b. Achievement of developmental tasks presurgery c. Extent to which the disability interferes with goal-directed activity d. Sense of control e. Realistic perception of the event by the client and support persons
15. Refer an at-risk client for professional counseling.	15. In such a client, follow-up therapy is indicated to assist with effective adjustment.

 Documentation

Progress notes
　Present emotional status
　Interventions
　Response to interventions

High Risk for Ineffective Sexuality Patterns Related to Perceived Negative Impact of Ostomy on Sexual Functioning and Attractiveness

Focus Assessment Criteria	Clinical Significance
1. Importance of sex to the client 2. Availability of a partner 3. Concerns about resuming intercourse 4. Preferred methods of sexual expression 5. Acceptability of alternative pleasuring activities to the client and partner	1–5. Assessing current concerns and past sexual patterns provides direction for planning effective nursing interventions.

Goal

The client will discuss own feelings and partner's concerns regarding the effect of ostomy surgery on sexual functioning.

Indicators
- Verbalize the intent to discuss concerns with partner before discharge.
- Discuss own feelings and partner's concerns regarding the effect of ostomy surgery on sexual functioning.

Interventions	Rationales
1. Reaffirm the need for frank discussion between sexual partners and the need for time for the partner to become accustomed to changes in the client's body.	1. Individuals report that their lives have suffered as the result of their surgeries (Sprangers, Taal, Aaronson et al., 1995).
2. Role-play ways for client and partner to discuss concerns about sex.	2. Role-playing helps a person to gain insight by placing him or her in the position of another. It also may promote more spontaneous sharing of fears and concerns.
3. Discuss the possibility that client may project his or her own feelings onto the partner. Encourage frequent validation of feelings between partners.	3. Client may have erroneous assumptions about the partner (e.g., he or she may erroneously assume that the partner is "turned off" by the ostomy).
4. Reaffirm the need for closeness and expressions of caring; involve client and partner in touching, stroking, massage, and so on.	4. Sexual pleasure and gratification are not limited to intercourse. Other expressions of caring may prove more meaningful.
5. Explore any fears the client may express regarding mutilation, unacceptability, and other concerns that might limit his or her involvement in relationships.	5. These fears might limit involvement in relationships.
6. Discuss the possible availability of a penile prosthesis if the client is physiologically unable to maintain or sustain an erection sufficient for intercourse. Explain that a penile implant provides the erection needed for intercourse and does not alter sensations or the ability to ejaculate.	6. Realizing that a prosthesis may be available may reassure the client and reduce anxiety about performance; this actually could help to improve function.
7. Refer client to a certified sex or mental health counselor if desired.	7. Certain sexual problems require continuing therapy and the advanced knowledge of therapists.

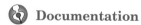 **Documentation**

Progress notes
    Assessment data
    Interventions
    Response to interventions
    Referrals if indicated

High Risk for Sexual Dysfunction Related to Physiologic Impotence Secondary to Damaged Sympathetic Nerve Damage (Male) or Inadequate Vaginal Lubrication (Female)

Focus Assessment Criteria	Clinical Significance
1. Knowledge of the effects of surgery on sexual function. 　a. In men, a wide resection for Crohn's disease occasionally damages sympathetic nerves in the presacral area that control emission. This may result in retrograde ejaculation into the bladder and a "dry" orgasm. During abdominoperineal surgery, the parasympathetic nerves that control blood flow to the penis can be damaged, possibly resulting in erectile dysfunction (Maklebust, 1990; Krebs, 2000). 　b. In women, body image fears are focused on aesthetics (e.g., appearance, odor).	1. Assessment of client's knowledge of possible effects on sexual function guides nurse in planning effective interventions. 　b. One study reported that women pre/post ostomy surgery related fear of stool leakage, odor, and change in body appearance, sexual love play, and intercourse (Pieper & Mikols, 1996).

Goal

The client will state alternatives to deal with physiologic impotence.

Indicators

- Explain surgical effects on erections.
- Report community resources available.

Interventions	Rationales
1. Allow individual opportunities to share their fears and concerns.	1. Refer to clinical significance, 1b.
2. In men 　a. Suggest that sexual activity need not always culminate in vaginal intercourse and that orgasm can be reached through noncoital manual or oral stimulation. Remind client that sexual expression is not limited to intercourse but includes closeness, communication, touching, and giving pleasure to another (Krebs, 2000). 　b. Suggest counseling with a certified sex therapist.	2. 　a. Alternative methods of sexual expression and gratification promote positive sexual function. 　b. Certain sexual problems require continuing therapy and the advanced knowledge of therapists.

(continues on page 832)

Interventions continued	Rationales continued

3. In women
   a. Suggest using a water-based vaginal lubricant for intercourse.
 	
   b. Teach client to perform Kegel exercises and instruct her to do them regularly.
 	
   c. Suggest that she sit astride her partner during intercourse.
	3.
	   a. Water-based lubricant can help to prevent dyspareunia related to inadequate vaginal lubrication.
	   b. Kegel exercises promote control of the pubococcygeal muscles around the vaginal entrance; this can ease dyspareunia.
	   c. A woman on top can control the depth and rate of penetration; this can enhance vaginal lubrication and relaxation.

✽ Documentation

Progress notes
  Interventions
  Response to interventions

High Risk for Loneliness Related to Anxiety Over Possible Odor and Leakage from Appliance

Focus Assessment Criteria	Clinical Significance
1. Preoperative socialization pattern 2. Anticipated changes	1,2. A client at risk for loneliness must be assessed carefully; the suffering associated with isolation is not always visible. Feelings of rejection and repulsion are common.

Goal

The client will state the intent to re-establish preoperative socialization pattern.

Indicators

- Discuss methods to control odor and appliance leakage.
- State foods that increase odor and gas.

Interventions	Rationales
1. Select an appropriate odor-proof pouching system, and explain to client how it works.	1. Fear of accidents and odor can be reduced through effective management. Some pouches have charcoal filters to reduce odor from flatus.
2. Stress the need for good personal hygiene. 3. Teach the client care of a stoma appliance.	2,3. Proper hygiene and appliance care remove odoriferous retained fecal material.
4. Discuss methods for reducing odor: a. Avoid odor-producing foods such as onions, fish, eggs, cheese, asparagus.	4. Minimizing odor improves self-confidence and can permit more effective socialization. Bacterial proliferation in retained effluent

(continues on page 833)

Interventions continued	Rationales continued
b. Use internal chlorophyll tablets or a liquid appliance deodorant. c. Empty or change the ostomy pouch regularly—when it is one-third to one-half full.	increases odor with time. A full pouch also puts excessive pressure on seals, which increases risk of leakage.
5. Encourage client to reestablish his or her preoperative socialization pattern. Help through measures such as progressively increasing client's socializing time in the hospital, role-playing possible situations that client feels may cause anxiety, and encouraging client to visualize and anticipate solutions to "worst-case scenarios" for social situations.	5. Encouraging and facilitating socialization help to prevent isolation. Role-playing can help the client to identify and learn to cope with potential anxiety-causing situations in a nonthreatening environment.
6. Suggest that client meet with a person from the UOA who can share similar experiences.	6. Others in a similar situation can provide a realistic appraisal of the situation and may provide information to answer client's unasked questions.

 Documentation

Progress notes
   Dialogues
Discharge summary record
   Client teaching
   Outcome achievement or status

High Risk for Ineffective Therapeutic Regimen Management Related to Insufficient Knowledge of Stoma Pouching Procedure, Peristomal Skin Care, Perineal Wound Care, and Incorporation of Ostomy Care into Activities of Daily Living (ADLs)

Focus Assessment Criteria	Clinical Significance
1. Type of ileostomy	1. Ostomy care differs according to its type. Some have continuous drainage while others can be emptied intermittently.
2. Knowledge of ileostomy care: diet, activity, hygiene, clothing, sexual expression, community resources, employment, travel, odor, skin care, appliances	2. Assessment identifies learning needs and guides the nurse in planning effective teaching strategies.
3. Client's and support persons readiness and ability to learn and retain information	3. A family or client failing to achieve learning goals requires a referral for assistance postdischarge.

Goals

The goals for this diagnosis represent those associated with discharge planning. Refer to the discharge criteria.

Interventions	Rationales
1. Consult with wound care/ostomy specialist.	1. Experts in intervening with people with ostomies are needed to increase client and family confidence and to provide specific information on what to expect.
2. Teach client the basic stoma pouching principles. a. Keeping the peristomal skin clean and dry b. Using a well-fitting appliance c. Changing the pouch when the least amount of drainage is anticipated (usually on arising) d. Emptying the pouch when it is one-third to one-half full and changing routinely before a leak occurs e. Changing the pouch if burning or itching occurs under the appliance f. Observing the condition of the stoma and peristomal skin during pouch changes	2. Proper pouching techniques can prevent leakage and skin problems. a. This ensures that the appliance adheres to the skin. b. Proper fit protects the surrounding skin surface from contact with drainage. c. This prevents copious drainage from interfering with pouch changes. d. A pouch filled more than halfway exerts increased pressure on the seal, which increases risk of leakage. e. Burning or itching may indicate that ostomy effluent has undermined the skin barrier; prompt intervention is necessary to prevent skin breakdown. f. Regular observation enables early detection of skin problems.
3. Teach the procedure for preparing a stoma pouch. a. Select the appropriate stoma pouching system. b. Measure stoma carefully. c. Use the appliance manufacturer's stoma measuring card if possible. If the card does not accommodate stoma size or shape, teach client to make a customized stoma pattern. Place clear plastic wrap from the skin barrier wafer over the stoma, trace the stoma with a marking pen, and cut a hole in the plastic to accommodate the stoma. d. Cut an opening in the center of the skin barrier slightly larger than the stoma (approximately $\frac{1}{8}$ inch). e. Secure an appropriate odorproof pouch onto the skin barrier wafer (if using a two-piece appliance system).	3. Preparing a new pouch beforehand ensures that it is ready to apply as soon as the used pouch is removed; this helps to minimize drainage on skin surface.

(continues on page 835)

Interventions continued	Rationales continued

4. Teach the procedure for changing a disposable stoma pouch.
   a. Remove the old pouch by gently pushing the skin away from the paper tape and skin barrier wafer.
   b. Fold the old pouch over on itself and discard in a plastic bag.
   c. Cleanse peristomal skin with a washcloth and warm tap water.
   d. Blot or pat skin dry.
   e. Apply the new pouch to the abdomen, carefully centering the hole in the skin barrier wafer over the stoma. Press on the wafer for a few minutes.
   f. Secure the pouch by "picture framing" the wafer with four strips of hypoallergenic paper tape (if the wafer does not already have tape attached).
	4. Correct pouch removal and attachment techniques minimize irritation and injury of peristomal skin and ensure a tight, reliable seal between pouch and skin.

5. Teach the procedure for emptying a stoma pouch.
   a. Put some toilet paper in the toilet bowl and sit on the toilet seat.
   b. Remove the clamp from the tail of the pouch, and carefully empty pouch contents into the toilet.
   c. Clean the inside and outside of the pouch tail with toilet paper and squeeze ostomy appliance deodorant into the end of the pouch.
	5. Correct techniques can reduce spillage, soiling, and odor. Placing toilet paper in the bowl prevents water from splashing as the pouch contents are emptied.

6. Teach strategies for prevention and management of potential peristomal skin problems.
   a. Shave the peristomal skin with an electric razor rather than a blade; avoid using shaving cream, soap, and detergents except when showering.
   b. Evaluate all skin products for possible allergic reaction; patch-test all suspect products elsewhere on the abdomen.
   c. Do not change brands of skin barriers and adhesives casually; assess for allergic reaction before using a new brand.
   d. Avoid irritation from contact with ostomy effluent.
   e. Avoid prolonged skin pressure, especially if skin is fair or thin and atrophic resulting from long-term corticosteroid therapy.
	6. A client with a stoma is at increased risk for peristomal skin breakdown. Factors that influence skin integrity include the following: composition, quantity, and consistency of the ostomy effluent; allergies; mechanical trauma; the underlying disease and its treatment (including medications); surgical construction and location of the stoma; the quality of ostomy and periostomal skin care; availability of proper supplies; nutritional status; overall health status; hygiene; and activity level.

(continues on page 836)

Interventions continued	**Rationales** continued
f. Use corticosteroid creams sparingly and briefly; they can cause dryness and irritation. g. If bacterial or fungal infection is suspected, use a specific antibacterial or antifungal cream or powder. h. Use a liquid film barrier; avoid tincture of benzoin compound, which can dry skin. i. Avoid aluminum paste and greasy ointments that can mask skin problems and interfere with pouch adherence. j. Protect the skin with barriers. k. Expect the stoma to shrink slightly over time. This will necessitate remeasuring the stoma to ensure proper appliance fit.	
7. Address nutrition and diet management. a. Teach how the ostomy affects absorption and use of nutrients; discuss dietary implications. b. Assess food tolerances by adding new foods one at a time and in small amounts. c. Teach client to eat regularly and slowly, to chew food well, and to avoid high-fiber foods that can promote stomal blockage. d. Discuss dietary modifications that can help decrease odor and flatus. e. List dietary modifications to prevent or manage diarrhea and constipation as indicated. f. If fecal discharge is too watery, increase fibrous foods (whole grain cereals, fresh fruit skins, beans, corn). g. If fecal discharge is too dry, increase salt intake if not contraindicated. h. Instruct client to monitor weight and report any loss or gain of more than 10 pounds. i. Explain the importance of adequate fluid intake (water, sports drinks, juices) to prevent or manage fluid and electrolyte problems related to excessive perspiration and diarrhea.	7. Proper nutritional intake and dietary management are important factors in ostomy management.
8. Explain the effects of certain medications on ostomy function. a. Antibiotics may induce diarrhea.	8. Counseling the client about the possible harmful effects of home remedies and indiscriminate self-medication may help to prevent minor or serious problems.

(continues on page 837)

Interventions continued	**Rationales** continued
b. Fecal odor may be controlled by internal or external deodorizers. Internal deodorizers may have a mild laxative effect. c. Suppositories cannot be used if the rectum and anus are removed. Instruct the client to notify a physician or pharmacist if a drug problem is suspected.	

9. Promote measures to help client incorporate ostomy care into ADLs (Maklebust, 1990).
 	
   a. Working/traveling: Keep extra supplies at work. When traveling, carry supplies rather than pack them in a suitcase and risk losing them; keep in mind that pectin-based wafers melt in high environmental temperatures. Take a list of ostomy supplies when traveling.
 	
   b. Exercise: The only limits involve contact sports during which trauma to the stoma may occur. Normal exercise is beneficial and may help to stimulate bowel evacuation; in some cases exercise can eliminate the need for irrigation. Successful use of exercise to regulate the bowel depends on the presurgical bowel pattern and regularity of elimination. Other contributing factors include the consistency of fecal contents, motivation, diet, ability to exercise, and practice.
 	
   c. Wardrobe: Ostomy appliances are invisible under clothing. Any clothing worn preoperatively may be worn postoperatively. Dress comfortably.
 	
   d. Bathing/showering/swimming: These activities may be done while wearing an ostomy appliance. "Picture-frame" the skin barrier with paper tape to seal the edges and keep the barrier edge from getting wet. Showering may be done without an appliance and, in fact, is recommended on days of appliance changes.
 	
   e. Wardrobe:
    • Wear two pairs of underpants. The inside pair should be low-rise or bikini-height cotton knit worn *under* the ostomy appliance to absorb
	9. Successful incorporation of ostomy management into ADLs allows client to resume pre-ileostomy life style and pursue goals and interests.

(continues on page 838)

Interventions continued	**Rationales** continued

perspiration and keep the pouch away from the skin. The outside pair can be cotton or nylon, should be waist-high, and is worn *over* the ostomy appliance.

- The ostomy pouch can be tucked between the two pairs of underwear like a kangaroo pouch. Special pouch covers are expensive, soil rapidly, and are not necessary.
- Avoid too-tight clothing that can restrict the appliance and cause leakage. A boxer-type bathing suit is preferable for men. For women, a patterned bathing suit with shirring can camouflage the appliance well.

f. Diet:
- Chew all food well.
- The noise from passing flatus will decrease postoperatively with progression to a regular diet.
- Eat on a regular schedule to help decrease the noise from an empty gut.
- Avoid mushrooms, Chinese vegetables, popcorn, and other foods that may cause blockage. (*Note:* Pillsbury microwave popcorn is specially made to be tolerated because adequate chewing can finely grind the kernels.)
- Keep in mind that fish, cabbage, eggs, and onions cause odor in the stool.
- Drink at least several 8-oz glasses of water a day to prevent dehydration in an ileostomate and constipation in a colostomate. Concentrated urine or decreased urinary output is a good indicator of dehydration.

g. Odor control:
- Explain that odor is caused from bacteria in the stool.
- Because most ostomy appliances are made to be odorproof, do not poke a hole in the ostomy appliance to allow flatus to escape; constant odor will result.
- Control offensive odors with good hygiene and ostomy pouch deodorants. (Super Banish appliance deodorant works best because it contains silver nitrate, which kills the

(continues on page 839)

Interventions continued	**Rationales** continued

bacteria.) Hydrogen peroxide and mouthwashes such as Binaca can be placed in the ostomy pouch as inexpensive appliance deodorants.
- Do not use aspirin tablets as a deodorant in the ostomy pouch; aspirin tablets coming in contact with the stoma may cause stomal irritation and bleeding.
- Eating yogurt and cranberry juice may help to reduce fecal odor. Certain oral medications reduce fecal odor, but these should be used only with the advice of a physician.

h. Hygiene:
- Use a hand-held shower spray to wash skin around stoma and irrigate perineal wounds.
- Showers can be taken with the ostomy appliance on or off. On days when the appliance is changed, a shower can be taken when the old pouch is removed but before the new pouch is applied.
- The new pouch should be readied before getting in the shower. On days between appliance changes, showering with the appliance on requires only that the paper tape around the wafer be covered with a liquid sealant to waterproof the tape.

i. Exercise:
- Normal activities (even strenuous sports, in most cases) can be resumed after recovery from surgery.
- Be aware that increased incidence of peristomal herniation is associated with heavy lifting.
- Also keep in mind that increased perspiration from strenuous exercise may require more frequent ostomy appliance changes because of increased melting of the appliance skin barrier.

j. Travel:
- Take all ostomy supplies along when traveling.
- Do not leave ostomy appliances in automobiles parked in the sun because the heat will melt the skin barrier.
- When flying, always keep appliances in carry-on luggage to avoid loss.

(continues on page 840)

Interventions continued	**Rationales** continued
k. Sexual activity: • Remember that an ostomy does not automatically make the person undesirable; as in any sexual encounter, the client may have to indicate sexual interest to his or her partner, who may be afraid of hurting the ostomy. • Wearing a stretch tube top around the midriff will cover the ostomy appliance while leaving the genitals and breasts exposed. • If male impotence is a problem, the man can be referred to a urologist for discussion or investigation of a penile prosthesis. • Keep in mind that in many cases, sexual problems following ostomy surgery are manifestations of problems that existed before surgery. If the ostomate had a strong supportive relationship before surgery, there usually are no problems after surgery.	
10. Teach client to monitor the stoma and adjacent skin for changes: Color, size, and shape Color, amount, and consistency of effluent Ulceration	10. Changes can indicate inflammation, retraction, prolapse, edema, or obstruction.
11. Instruct client to call physician, advanced practice nurse, or ostomy specialist if changes occur.	11. The client will be informed if the change is expected or an intervention is needed.
12. Discuss community resources/self-help groups. a. Visiting nurse b. United Ostomy Association c. Foundation for Ileitis and Colitis d. Recovery of male potency—help for the impotent male e. American Cancer Foundation f. Community suppliers of ostomy equipment g. Financial reimbursement for ostomy equipment	

 Documentation

Discharge summary record
  Client and family teaching
  Outcome achievement or status

High Risk for Ineffective Therapeutic Regimen Management Related to Insufficient Knowledge of Care of Ileoanal Reservoir

Focus Assessment Criteria	Clinical Significance
1. Perianal skin condition 2. Anal sphincter competence 3. Frequency and consistency of stools	1–3. Because stools are loose and frequent (initially 10 to 20/day, progressively decreasing to 3 to 4/day after the first post-operative year), good sphincter control is essential to bowel management.
4. Readiness and ability to learn and retain information	4. A client or family failing to achieve learning goals requires a referral for assistance postdischarge.

Goals

The goals for this diagnosis represent those associated with discharge planning. Refer to the discharge criteria.

Interventions	Rationales
1. Instruct client to practice Kegel exercises regularly.	1. Regular performance of Kegel exercises can strengthen sphincter muscle tone.
2. Teach client how to intubate the anus and irrigate the ileoanal pouch.	2. Irrigation is needed to remove mucus and prevent clogging.
3. Teach client to protect perianal skin by using liquid skin sealant prophylactically and wearing minipads at night to absorb anal drainage.	3. These measures can help to protect against perianal skin denudation resulting from frequent stools.

 Documentation

Discharge summary record
   Client teaching
      Outcome achievement or status

High Risk for Ineffective Therapeutic Regimen Management Related to Insufficient Knowledge of Intermittent Intubation of Kock Continent Ileostomy

Focus Assessment Criteria	Clinical Significance
1. Readiness and ability to learn and retain information	1. A client or family failing to achieve learning goals requires a referral for assistance post-discharge.

Goals

The goals for this diagnosis represent those associated with discharge planning. Refer to the discharge criteria.

Interventions	Rationales
1. Explain the reason for continuous drainage postoperatively.	1. Continuous drainage is needed to decrease pressure on the suture line.
2. If indicated, teach client intermittent self-intubation to drain the pouch; cover such measures as the following: a. Gradually decreasing the number of intubations to 3 to 4 times/day b. Irrigating if stool is thick c. Using lubricant on a large-bore catheter	2. Proper intubation technique helps to maximize pouch capacity, provides complete drainage, and prevents tissue trauma.
3. Encourage thorough chewing of food before swallowing; caution client against eating high-fiber foods.	3. Bulk in diet increases irritation to the bowel and risk of obstruction.
4. Notify physician immediately if unable to intubate client.	4. Inability to intubate puts client at high risk for bowel obstruction.

 Documentation

Discharge summary record
   Client teaching
   Response to teaching
   Outcome achievement or status

LAMINECTOMY

Surgical excision of a herniated disk can be done with one of the following techniques:

- Discectomy—removal of herniated or fragments of intervertebral disk
- Laminectomy—removal of lamina (part of vertebra) to expose spinal canal and to remove pathology and relieve compression
- Hemilaminectomy—removal of part of lamina and part of the posterior arch
- Discectomy with fusion—small discectomy with a bone graft (donor or from client) to fuse the spinous process to stabilize the spine
- Foraminotomy—removal of the intervertebral foramen to increase space for spinal nerve to reduce compression

Microsurgical techniques make removal of tissue more precise with less damage to normal tissue.

 Time Frame

Preoperative and postoperative periods

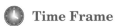 DIAGNOSTIC CLUSTER

Preoperative Period

Nursing Diagnoses

▲ High Risk for Injury related to lack of knowledge of postoperative position restrictions and log-rolling technique

Postoperative Period

Collaborative Problems

▲ PC: Neurosensory Impairments
▲ PC: Urinary Retention
▲ PC: Paralytic Ileus
△ PC: Cerebrospinal Fistula

Nursing Diagnoses

▲ Acute Pain related to muscle spasms (back, thigh) secondary to nerve irritation during surgery, edema, skeletal malalignment, or bladder distention
▲ High Risk for Ineffective Therapeutic Regimen Management related to insufficient knowledge of home care, activity restrictions, and exercise program

Related Care Plan

General Surgery Generic Care Plan

▲ This diagnosis was reported to be monitored for or managed frequently (75%–100%).
△ This diagnosis was reported to be monitored for or managed often (50%–74%).

Discharge Criteria

Before discharge, the client or family will

1. Describe proper wound care at home.
2. Verbalize necessary activity precautions.
3. State signs and symptoms that must be reported to a health care professional.

Preoperative: Nursing Diagnosis

High Risk for Injury Related to Lack of Knowledge of Postoperative Position Restrictions and Log-rolling Technique

Focus Assessment Criteria	Clinical Significance
1. Reading and ability to learn and retain information	1. A client failing to achieve learning goals requires a referral for assistance postdischarge.

Goal

The client will demonstrate correct positioning and log-rolling technique.

Indicators
- State why precautions are needed.
- State restrictions needed.

Interventions	Rationale

1. Teach client the correct body alignment to maintain while lying in bed, sitting, and standing. Teach the correct log-rolling technique to use to get in and out of bed; show client how to do the following:
  a. Roll to the edge of the bed, keeping the lower back flat and the spine straight.
  b. Raise the head and simultaneously swing both legs (bent at the knees) over the side of the bed.
  c. Use the upper hand to support the stomach muscles and the lower arm to push oneself away from the mattress.
	1. Maintaining proper positioning and good posture and using proper procedure for getting in and out of bed will minimize back strain, muscle spasms, and discomfort.

 Documentation
Discharge summary record
  Client teaching
  Outcome achievement or status

Postoperative: Collaborative Problems

Potential Complication: Neurosensory Impairment

Potential Complication: Urinary Retention

Potential Complication: Paralytic Ileus

Potential Complication: Cerebrospinal Fistula

Nursing Goal

The nurse will detect early signs and symptoms of (a) sensory/motor, (b) urinary retention, (c) paralytic ileus, (d) cerebrospinal fistula and collaboratively intervene to stabilize client.

Indicators

- Motor function equal and intact (a)
- Sensory function equal and intact (a)
- Strength equal and intact (a)
- Urinary output > 30 mL/hr (a, b)
- Can verbalize bladder fullness (a, b)
- No c/o of lower abdominal pain (a, b)
- Bowel sounds present and all quadrants (c)
- Reports flatus (c)
- Bowel movement by third day (c)
- Minimal or no drainage (d)
- Negative glucose test of drainage (d)
- No c/o of headaches (d)

Interventions	Rationales
1. Monitor symmetry of sensory and motor function in extremities. a. To touch, pin scratch b. Strength (Have client push your hand away from the soles then pull up against resistance.) Compare findings from right side to left side and preoperative baseline.	1. Cord or nerve root edema, pressure on a nerve root from herniated disc fragments, or hematoma at the operative site can cause or exacerbate deficits in motor and sensory functions postoperatively. Surgical manipulation can result in nerve damage causing paresthesias, paralysis, and possibly respiratory insufficiency.
2. Monitor bladder function. a. Ability to void sufficient quantities and empty bladder completely b. Ability to sense sensation of bladder fullness	2. Cord edema or disruption of autonomic pathways during surgery can cause a temporary loss of bladder tone (Hickey, 2002).
3. If possible, stand a male client 8 to 12 hours after surgery to void.	3. Urinary retention especially when client lies flat may be due to difficulty voiding in a horizontal position, the depressant effects of perioperative drugs, or sympathetic fiber stimulation during surgery (Hickey, 2002).
4. Monitor bowel function. a. Bowel sounds in all quadrants returning within 24 hours of surgery b. Flatus and defecation resuming by the second or third postoperative day	4. Surgery on the lumbosacral spine decreases innervation of the bowels, reducing peristalsis and possibly leading to transient paralytic ileus.
5. Monitor for signs and symptoms of cerebrospinal fistula. a. Clear or pink ring around bloody drainage b. Positive glucose test of drainage c. Severe headache	5. Incomplete closure of the dura causes CSF drainage. Glucose is present in CSF but not in normal wound drainage. Changes in CSF volume cause headache.

(continues on page 846)

Interventions continued	Rationales continued
6. Monitor incisional dressing for drainage. Report any drainage.	6. There should be little or no drainage. Suspect bleeding or cerebrospinal fluid leakage if drainage occurs.
7. If person smokes, advise him or her of increased risks. Discuss the possibility of quitting or cutting back.	7. Smokers are at high risk for postoperative cardiopulmonary complications and the risk of developing pseudoarthrosis or delayed healing.
8. Monitor output from drains. Expect 20 to 250 mL/8 hr during the first 24 hours with fusions.	8. Hypovolemia can cause decreased cardiac output.

9. Monitor for and report the following:
  a. Restlessness, confusion, apprehension, tachypnea
  b. Progressive weakness of lower extremities
	9.
	  a. Symptoms of fat embolism can occur during surgery or 72 hours postoperatively.
	  b. Surgical trauma, hematoma formation, or vascular injury can cause cauda equina syndrome.

 Related Physician-Prescribed Interventions

Medications. Corticosteroids, nonsteroidal anti-inflammatory drugs, muscle relaxants, narcotics

Intravenous Therapy. Refer to the General Surgery Care Plan

Laboratory Studies. Refer to the General Surgery Care Plan

Diagnostic Studies. CT scan, spinal X-ray film, myelography

Therapies. Brace, refer to the General Surgery Care Plan, electromyelography, MRI

 Documentation

Flow records
  Vital signs
  Intake and output
  Circulation (color, peripheral pulses)
  Neurosensory status (reflexes, sensory and motor function)
  Bowel function (bowel sounds, defecation)
  Wound condition (color, drainage, swelling)
Progress notes
  Changes in status

Postoperative: Nursing Diagnoses

Acute Pain Related to Muscle Spasms (Back or Thigh) Secondary to Nerve Irritation During Surgery, Edema, Skeletal Misalignment, or Bladder Distention

Focus Assessment Criteria	Clinical Significance
1. Pain at operative site	1–3. Nerve root irritation from surgery is the primary cause of postoperative pain. Pain

(continues on page 847)

Focus Assessment Criteria continued	Clinical Significance continued
2. Muscle spasms radiating to thigh, lower leg, foot, or arm; or to hand, in cervical spinal laminectomy	management should focus on proper positioning and activity in conjunction with narcotic or antispasmodic agents. Nurse must differentiate pain due to bladder distention from operative site pain and muscle spasms.
3. Voiding patterns (times and amounts)	

Goal

The client will report progressive pain reduction and relief after pain relief interventions.

Indicators

- Demonstrate techniques to reduce pain.
- Report movements to avoid.

Interventions	Rationales
1. Explain to client that muscle spasms and paresthesias commonly occur after surgery.	1. Surgical trauma and edema cause pain and muscle spasms. Spasms may begin on the third or fourth postoperative day. Postoperative paresthesias in the affected leg and back may result from impaired neural function due to edema. As edema subsides, normal sensation returns.
2. Teach the importance of complying with the brace regimen.	2. Wearing a brace can prevent future hardware failure and pseudoarthrosis.
3. Evaluate if casts or brace fits properly.	3. Mobilizing devices can cause sustained pressure on tissues leading to ischemia and tissue necrosis.
4. Teach client the need to evaluate if pressure areas are present.	4. Low pressure for long periods can cause damage and may not be noticed by client.
5. Teach client to use arms and legs to transfer weight properly when getting out of bed.	5. Using the stronger muscles of the arms and legs can reduce strain on the back.
6. Encourage walking, standing, and sitting for short periods from the first postoperative day or as soon as possible after surgery. Assess carefully the first few days after surgery to ensure proper use of body mechanics and to detect any gait or posture problems.	6. Activity goals depend on the client's pain level and functional ability. Gait or posture problems can contribute to pain on walking, standing, or sitting.

(continues on page 848)

Interventions continued	Rationales continued
7. Teach client the following precautions to maintain proper body alignment: a. Use the log-rolling technique with the help of two persons for the first 48 hours after surgery. (Refer to the nursing diagnosis High Risk for Injury in this care plan for details.) b. Avoid stress or strain on the operative site. c. Use the side-lying position in bed with the legs bent up evenly and the abdomen and back supported by pillows. d. Teach client to keep spine straight and when on side to place a pillow between legs. Place pillow to support upper arm and prevent shoulder from sagging. e. Sit with knees higher than hips. f. When standing, regularly shift weight-bearing from one foot to the other.	7. Proper body alignment avoids tension on the operative site and reduces spasms. Techniques are taught to keep the lower spine as flat as possible and prevent twisting, flexing, or hyperextending.
8. Ask to rate pain (from 0 to 10) before and after medication administration. Consult with physician or advanced practice nurse if relief is unsatisfactory.	8. An objective rating scale can help to evaluate the subjective experience of pain.
9. Refer to the General Surgery Care Plan for general pain-relief techniques.	

 Documentation

Medication administration record
  Type, dose, route, frequency of all medications
Progress notes
  Activity level
  Patient's response to pain medication

High Risk for Ineffective Therapeutic Regimen Management Related to Insufficient Knowledge of Home Care, Activity Restrictions, and Exercise Program

Focus Assessment Criteria	Clinical Significance
1. Readiness and ability to learn and retain information	1. A client or family failing to achieve learning goals requires a referral for assistance post-discharge.

Goals

The goals for this diagnosis represent those associated with discharge planning. Refer to the discharge criteria.

Interventions	Rationales
1. Explain the rationale for activity restrictions and for gradual activity progression as tolerance increases.	1. Activity restrictions allow the spinal supporting structures time to heal. Complete healing of ligaments and muscles takes approximately 6 weeks.
2. Teach client to avoid the following: a. Prolonged sitting b. Twisting the spine c. Bending at the waist d. Climbing stairs e. Automobile trips	2. These activities increase spinal flexion and create tension at the surgical site.
3. Teach client the proper use of a back brace if indicated.	3. A brace may be indicated to stabilize the spine and reduce pain; instruction in proper use is necessary.
4. Explain the importance of following a regular exercise program after recovery.	4. Regular, safe exercise increases spinal muscle strength and flexibility, helping protect against future injury.
5. Encourage the use of heat on the operative area as indicated.	5. Heat increases circulation to the operative site; this promotes healing and removal of wound exudate.
6. Teach client the precautions for after recovery such as the following: a. Sleeping on a firm mattress b. Maintaining proper body mechanics c. Wearing only moderately high-heeled shoes d. Avoiding lifting heavy objects over 10 lb. e. Sit in straight-backed chair with feet on stool and knees flexed slightly higher than hips f. For at least 3 weeks post-surgery; limit time in sitting position to 15 to 20 minutes.	6. Techniques that reduce stress and strain on the lumbosacral spine can decrease spasms and help to prevent other disc herniations.
7. As appropriate, explain the connection between obesity and lower back problems; encourage weight loss.	7. Excess weight, particularly in the abdomen, strains and stretches muscles that support the spine, predisposing the client to spinal injury. Explaining these effects may encourage client to lose weight.
8. Explain that normal neurologic status may not return immediately.	8. Irritation of the nerve root during surgery may increase deficits temporarily (Hickey, 2002).

(continues on page 850)

Interventions continued	Rationales continued

9. Teach client and family to report the following:
  a. Change in mobility, sensation, color, or pain in extremities
  b. Increased pain at the operative site
  c. Persistent headaches
  d. Elevated temperature
  e. Change in bowel or bladder function
  f. Drainage at incision site
	9. Early detection and reporting enable prompt intervention to prevent or minimize serious complications such as infection (marked by headache, fever, and increased pain) and cord compression (indicated by changes in bowel and bladder functions, movement, and sensation).

 Documentation

Discharge summary record
  Client and family teaching
  Outcome achievement or status

For a Clinical Pathway for Laminectomy, refer to http://connection.lww.com

LARYNGECTOMY

Laryngectomy is the surgical excision of the larynx and the removal of affected structures. Laryngectomy is indicated for advanced-stage cancer of the vocal cords and surrounding area. The removal of the larynx causes loss of voice and speech, altered respirations via tracheostomy, and diminished sense of smell and taste (Blom, 2000).

 Time Frame

Preoperative and postoperative periods

 DIAGNOSTIC CLUSTER*

Preoperative Period

Nursing Diagnoses

Anxiety related to lack of knowledge of impending surgical experience and implications of condition on life style

Postoperative Period

Collaborative Problems

Refer to Tracheostomy Care Plan.
Refer to Radical Neck Dissection Care Plan.

Related Care Plan

Enteral Nutrition
General Surgery

---

*This surgical procedure was not included in the validation study.

Discharge Criteria

Before discharge, the client and family will

1. Describe and demonstrate proper wound care techniques.
2. Discuss strategies for performing ADLs.
3. State the signs and symptoms that must be reported to a health care professional.
4. Verbalize an intent to share feelings and concerns with significant others.
5. Identify appropriate community resources and self-help groups.

Postoperative: Nursing Diagnosis

Anxiety Related to Lack of Knowledge of Impending Surgical Experience and Implications of Condition on Life Style

Focus Assessment Criteria	Clinical Significance
1. Understand condition, surgery, expected outcome, expected postoperative limitations, and care measures	1,2. Disfigurement from a permanent stoma with a tracheostomy or laryngectomy tube can pose a significant threat to a client's

(continues on page 852)

Focus Assessment Criteria continued	Clinical Significance continued
2. Readiness and ability to learn and retain information	body image and self-esteem. Assessing client's level of understanding allows nurse to identify learning needs and plan effective teaching strategies. A client who does not achieve learning goals requires a referral for assistance postdischarge (Bildstein & Blendowski, 1997).

Goal

The client will

1. State the reason for surgery and its expected outcome.
2. Describe expected limitations on speech and swallowing.
3. Describe immediate postoperative care and self-care measures.

Interventions	Rationales
1. Explain commonly used terms and procedures. Provide written information to reinforce teaching, and introduce actual equipment. Cover these topics: a. Laryngectomy tube b. Stoma c. Drains, suctioning, and suction catheter d. Mucus e. Humidity collar f. Pharynx g. Laryngectomy ties h. Trachea	1. Effective client teaching enhances positive coping mechanisms, provides an opportunity for client to express concerns and ask questions, and enables nurse to correct misconceptions—all of which can help to decrease preoperative anxiety (Padberg & Padberg, 1997).
2. Explain the postoperative changes in appearance and body function that client can expect (e.g., loss of ability to blow nose, suck, gargle, and whistle, decreased smell and taste sensations). If possible after discussion with client, arrange for a visit by a person who has already undergone laryngectomy. Inform client and significant others of any support groups and community resources available for laryngeal clients (e.g., International Association of Laryngectomees) and Web-based support groups (e.g., www.webwhispers.org).	2. This information and contact with a person who has successfully adapted to the postoperative changes in appearance and functioning may to help reduce client's anxiety associated with fear of the unknown (List, 1995).
3. Instruct client in alternative communication techniques (e.g., flip chart, picture board, electrolarynx, and esophageal speech). Request return demonstration to ensure client's mastery of the chosen technique(s).	3,4. Learning alternative communication techniques to speech lets client maintain the ability to communicate. This can help to decrease client's sense of alienation, isolation, and anxiety while enhancing

(continues on page 853)

Interventions continued	**Rationales** continued
4. Explain various methods of voice restoration (Blom, 2000):	client's sense of control over the situation. Evaluating client's performance of these techniques can also alert the nurse to possible cognitive or motor deficits (e.g., vision or hearing problems, facial nerve impairment, altered mentation) that may require further evaluation by a specialist (Logemann, 1994).
a. Artificial larynx	a. A hand-held artificial larynx (electronic or pneumatic) transforms tone articulated by the tongue, lips, and teeth into fluent, intelligible speech.
b. Esophageal speech	b. Client ingests air into the esophagus and releases it to produce a pseudovoice.
c. Tracheoesophageal puncture (TEP)	c. A valved "voice" prosthesis (a hollow French silicone tube with a one-way flags valve) produces a voice when the user inhales, occludes the tracheostomal neck opening with the thumb, and exhales. Vibrations along the pharyngoesophagus produce a husky or hoarse voice. An alternative prosthesis (tracheostoma) has a valve that closes when the person exhales to speak, eliminating the need to use a finger to occlude.
5. Explain effects of surgery on eating, taste, and smell. Refer to care plan on Neck Dissection, Risk for Imbalanced Nutrition related to swallowing difficulties and decreased sense of smell and taste.	

 Documentation

Progress notes
    Current knowledge level
    Ability to use alternative communication technique
    Response to laryngectomy visit
Discharge summary record
    Client teaching

NECK DISSECTION

Surgical removal of specific cervical lymph node groups and anatomic structures in the treatment of head and neck cancer is called a neck dissection. According to the American Academy of Otolaryngology and Head and Neck Surgeons, there are three broad categories of neck dissections: comprehensive, selective, and extended.

Comprehensive neck dissections are classified into two categories: (1) *radical neck dissection,* which involves removal of all cervical lymph node-bearing tissues, the spinal accessory nerve, the internal jugular, the omohyoid, and sternocleidomastoid muscles; and (2) *modified radical neck dissection,* which involves removal of all cervical lymph node-bearing tissues and the omohyoid muscle while preserving the spinal accessory nerve (type I); spinal accessory nerve and internal jugular (type II); spinal accessory nerve, internal jugular vein, and sternocleidomastoid muscle (Type III) or functional neck dissection.

Selective neck dissections are classified into three categories that involve the resection of only those nodal regions types (I-V) at highest risk for containing metastasis resulting from location of the primary tumor; the spinal accessory nerve, internal jugular, and sternocleidomastoid muscle are all preserved.

Extended neck dissections include any of the comprehensive or selective neck dissections "extended" to include either lymph node groups not routinely excised (e.g., paratracheal or retropharyngeal nodes) or structures not routinely removed (e.g., the carotid artery or levator scapulae) (Bildstein & Blendowski, 1997).

The spinal accessory innervates the trapezius muscle, one of the most important shoulder abductors. Neck dissections that preserve the nerve typically do not result in scapular destabilization with progressive drooping as well as anterior and lateral rotation of the scapular (Bildstein & Blendowski, 1997).

 Time Frame

Preoperative and postoperative periods
Postintensive care

 DIAGNOSTIC CLUSTER

Preoperative Period

Nursing Diagnoses (refer to Laryngectomy and Cancer: Initial Diagnosis Care Plans)

- Anxiety related to lack of knowledge of impeding surgical experience and implications of condition on life style
- Grieving related to losses associated with surgery and perceived effects on life style

Collaborative Problems

▲ PC: Flap Rejection (development of a hematoma, seroma, or infection with resulting flap necrosis)
* PC: Fistula Formation
* PC: Facial and CNS Edema (particularly after bilateral neck dissection)
▲ PC: Carotid Artery Rupture
▲ PC: Hemorrhage

Nursing Diagnoses

▲ High Risk for Impaired Physical Mobility: Shoulder, Head, related to removal of muscles, nerves, flap graft reconstruction, trauma secondary to surgery
▲ High Risk for Disturbed Self-Concept related to change in appearance

---

Nursing Diagnoses continued

Risk for Imbalanced Nutrition related to swallowing difficulties, decreased salivation, decreased sense of smell and taste, and impaired tongue movement

▲ High Risk for Ineffective Therapeutic Regimen Management related to insufficient knowledge of wound care, signs and symptoms of complications, exercises, and follow-up care

Related Care Plans

General Surgery Generic Care Plan
Tracheostomy
Laryngectomy
Chemotherapy
Radiation
Cancer: Initial Diagnosis

▲ This diagnosis was reported to be monitored for or managed frequently (75%–100%).
* This diagnosis was not included in the validation study.

Discharge Criteria

Before discharge, the client and family will

1. Demonstrate wound care.
2. Verbalize the need to continue exercises and follow-up care.
3. Discuss management of activities of daily living (ADLs).
4. State signs and symptoms that must be reported to a health care professional.
5. Verbalize an intent to share feelings and concerns related to appearance with significant others.
6. Identify available community resources and self-help groups.

Collaborative Problems

Potential Complication: Flap Rejection (development of a hematoma, seroma, or infection with resulting flap necrosis)

Potential Complication: Fistula Formation

Potential Complication: Facial and Central Nervous System Edema (particularly after bilateral neck dissection)

Potential Complication: Carotid Artery Rupture

Potential Complication: Hemorrhage

Nursing Goal

The nurse will monitor to detect early signs and symptoms of (a) flap rejection, (b) fistula formation, (c) facial/central nervous system edema, (d) carotid artery rupture, and (e) hemorrhage, and collaboratively intervene to stabilize client.

Indicators
- Pink, warm skin flap (a)
- Capillary refill < 3 seconds (a)
- Minimal or no edema (a, c)
- Temperature 98.5–99°F (a, b, e)
- Pulse 60–100 beats/min (a, d, e)
- BP >90/60, <140/90 mm Hg (a, d, e)
- Respiration 16–20 breaths/min (a, d, e)
- Oxygen saturation (pulse oximeter) > 95% (a, d, e)
- Continuous drainage of clear or pinkish fluid (200–300 ml the first 24 hours) (a, b, c)
- No bloody sputum (a, b, e)
- No epigastric distress (d, e)

Interventions	Rationales
1. Monitor the pectoralis myocutaneous flap and surrounding tissue every hour for the first 48 hours postsurgery, then every 4 hours until post-op day 5 for the following (Bildstein & Blendowski, 1997): a. Color: redness, pallor, blackness, cyanosis b. Increased capillary refill (> 3 seconds); blanching c. Temperature changes, edema	1. Abnormal findings may indicate impending flap rejection and call for immediate medical evaluation. Maximum redness should occur within the first 8 to 12 hours postsurgery and slowly decrease over the next 2 to 3 days. A healthy flap is pink and warm to the touch, has minimal edema, and recovers color slowly after exposure to blanching. Increasing edema and erythema of skin flap postoperative days 3 to 5 or later associated with odor, fever, and elevated WBC is indicative of infection; when associated with salivary drainage, it indicates fistula (Harris, 2000).
2. Report assessment changes promptly to surgeon.	2. Flaps can tolerate only 4 hours of ischemia before irreversible tissue necrosis results (Bildstein & Blendowski, 1997).
3. Monitor vital signs and pulse oximetry.	3. Vital signs are monitored to determine circulatory and respiratory status.
4. Monitor surgical drainage tubes for presence of air; foul-smelling, bloody, milky, or opaque drainage; or absence of drainage. Record amount every hour.	4. Drains prevent development of dead space (air or fluid accumulation between flap and underlying tissue) and help to prevent approximation. Air in the drains indicates dead space. Milky drainage may point to a chylous fistula. Opaque or chyle leaks particularly from the thoracic duct can lead to severe fluid and electrolyte imbalance. Continuous bloody drainage may indicate small vessel rupture requiring surgical ligation. Over the first 24 hours postsurgery, drainage should be between 200 and 300 mL and should decline daily thereafter.
5. Report increased drainage immediately.	5. Increased drainage may indicate development of a hematoma. It must be drained immediately to preserve viability of the flaps.
6. If grafts are used, monitor graft site for bleeding and infection.	6. Prompt attention to bleeding or infection can prevent systemic hypovolemia and sepsis.
7. Maintain proper body positioning. a. Elevate the head of bed 30 to 45 degrees.	7. Semi-Fowler's and high-Fowler's positions prevent hyperextension of the neck and they position the base of the flap

(continues on page 857)

Interventions continued	**Rationales** continued
b. Use pillows or sandbags to maintain proper alignment. c. Instruct client not to lay on the operative side.	inferior to the tip of the flap. This positioning limits tension of the flap and incision line and promotes venous drainage through the flap to minimize/alleviate flap, facial, cerebral, and laryngeal edemas (Bildstein & Blendowski, 1997). The position is dependent on flap location.
8. Monitor for external pressure on the reconstruction/flap from any of these: a. IV lines b. Feeding tubes c. Drainage tubes d. Tracheostomy or laryngectomy ties	8. External pressure on the flap compromises circulation, promotes venous congestion, and may lead to increased permeability and occlusion of the lymphatics. Fluid accumulation may result in dehiscence of the incision and failure of the graft to adhere to the underlying tissue; this provides a medium for bacterial growth potentiating abscess formation. Both circulatory compromise and problems resulting from accumulating fluid within the flap may potentiate wound and flap necrosis.
9. Monitor for signs of carotid artery rupture. a. Evidence of arterial erosion b. Change in color: redness, pallor, blackness c. Evidence of bleeding or bruising, pulsations, arterial exposure d. Temperature changes	9. Exposure of the adventitial layer of the artery to the atmosphere causes drying and interrupts blood supply to the flap. Once the artery is exposed to air, arterial destruction occurs in approximately 6 to 10 days. Factors contributing to arterial erosion include poor wound healing, exposure of the artery during surgery, tumor growth or invasion, radiation therapy, fistula formation, and infection.
10. Observe strict aseptic dressing technique using nonocclusive, fine-mesh, non-adherent gauze dressings with nonporous tape.	10. Dressings protect the wound from trauma and contamination, absorb drainage, and provide an aesthetic covering. Fine-mesh gauze inhibits interweaving of granulation tissue into dressing material, thus preventing mechanical debridement. Non-adherent dressings prevent growth of fungus and yeast infections that require a dark, moist environment.
11. If the carotid artery is exposed, do the following: a. Keep the wound moistened (e.g., with loosely packed saline moistened gauze or Vaseline gauze). If gauze dries while	11. Removal of a dry dressing from an exposed artery with inadvertent debridement of the arterial wall can precipitate an acute bleed.

(continues on page 858)

Interventions continued	**Rationales** continued
in the wound, it should be moistened with sterile saline before removal. b. Keep the following emergency supplies available at the bedside: • Two to three clean towels • Box of 4 × 4's • Vaginal packing or fluffs • Cuffed tracheostomy tube or a No. 8 endotracheal tube • 10-mL syringe to inflate cuff as needed c. Type and hold for 2 units of packed red blood cells. d. Suction apparatus and catheters	
12. When initial postoperative dressing is removed, change a saturated external dressing over draining wounds every 24 hours per prescribed orders. Initial dressing may remain several days.	12. Secretion saturated dressings over wounds with extensive tissue loss should be changed frequently because lack of a skin barrier increases risk of infection. Drains and initial dressings are placed in a manner to protect blood supply to flaps yet maximize drainage away from the surgical site to prevent hematoma and seroma formation (Sigler, Edwards, & Wilkerson, 1996).
13. Promote efforts to clear secretions without coughing. a. Position to maximize respiratory excursion. b. Encourage deep breathing. c. Provide gentle nasotracheal, tracheal, or oropharyngeal suctioning only when absolutely needed.	13. Coughing increases intrathoracic pressure, which stresses the wound. Because suctioning also increases intrathoracic pressure, suction only when the presence of secretions is identified on chest auscultation.
14. Monitor for nausea and vomiting.	14. Contraction of the diaphragm and abdominal muscles during vomiting raises intra-abdominal and intrathoracic pressure that stresses the wound.
15. Monitor for constipation/abdominal distention and take steps to prevent or treat constipation: a. Administer stool softener with wetting agent or glycerin suppository or gentle laxative. b. Encourage adequate dietary fiber and fluid intake.	15. a. Valsalva's maneuver, which accompanies straining on defecation related to constipation or fecal impaction, increases intrathoracic pressure that stresses the wound. b. Adequate fiber and fluid intake helps to decrease the potential for constipation.

(continues on page 859)

Interventions continued	Rationales continued
16. Monitor for bleeding at the wound site, a sudden increase in the output from external drainage apparatus, or an acute development of bloody sputum.	16. A small amount of blood or pink-tinged drainage at the wound site or on the dressing may herald major rupture. Typically a small prodromal bleed occurs 24 to 48 hours before a major rupture (Bildstein & Blendowski, 1997).
17. Monitor for complaints of sternal or high epigastric distress.	17. These complaints may indicate carotid rupture.

18. During episodes of bleeding, maintain a patent airway, prevent aspiration, and stop the hemorrhage.
  a. For external hemorrhage:
  • Apply firm pressure directly to the bleed site or secondary over the artery that is the source of the bleed.
  • Position client in high-Fowler's position with head turned to the affected side. If unable to turn the head to the side, turn the entire body.
  • Provide continuous suctioning.
  b. For internal hemorrhage:
  • Pack site with absorptive pressure dressing.
  • Position client to facilitate drainage from the airway.
  • Provide continuous suctioning.
  • If a tracheostomy is in place, inflate cuff.
	18. These measures aim to facilitate drainage, prevent aspiration, and suppress the hemorrhage (Cummings, 1993).

▼ Related Physician-Prescribed Interventions

Medications. Chemotherapy; also refer to the General Surgery Care Plan

Intravenous Therapy. Refer to the General Surgery Care Plan

Laboratory Studies. Arterial blood gas analysis; CBC with differential; also refer to the General Surgery Care Plan

Diagnostic Studies. Pulmonary function studies, chest X-ray film

Therapies. Oxygen with humidification, speech therapy, donor site care, respiratory therapy, physical therapy, psychiatric or social work counseling, nasogastric intubation, CT scan, irrigations, Doppler scanning, bradytherapy, external-beam radiotherapy, interstitial implantation, hyperbaric oxygen

Documentation

Flow records
  Vital signs
  Intake and output
  Wound site and drainage tube assessment
  Progressive notes

Nursing Diagnoses

High Risk for Impaired Physical Mobility: Shoulder, Head, Related to Removal of Muscles, Nerves, Flap Graft Reconstruction, Trauma Secondary to Surgery

Focus Assessment Criteria	Clinical Significance

1. Ability to perform ADLs: feeding, bathing, etc; also fine motor hand skill and vision
 	
2. Head and neck movements (passive and active)
  a. Flexion
  b. Extension
  c. Rotation
  d. Lateral turning
 	
3. Shoulder movements
  a. Flexion
  b. Extension
  c. Internal rotation
  d. External rotation
  e. Scapular elevation
	1–3. Assessing function identifies limitations and guides realistic goal setting. Documentation of baseline functional levels preoperatively enables comparison with postoperative findings to track progress toward goals.

4. Factors that impair mobility:
  a. Arthritis
  b. Previous injuries
  c. Previous surgeries
  d. Vertebral deformities
  e. Peripheral vascular disease
  f. Pain
	4. Passive and active muscle movements are necessary to maintain skin integrity, range of motion, and adequate circulation and to prevent contractures. Preoperative and postoperative physical conditions may impede client's ability to follow through on his or her exercise program.

5. Recent work history before surgery including amount of physical lifting required	5. Residual deficits from surgery may impair client's ability to return to the same work situation, particularly if cranial nerve XI was sacrificed. Vocational rehabilitation may be considered.

Goal

The client will demonstrate measures to prevent complications of decreased mobility.

Indicators

- State limitations on shoulder and head mobility and surgical factors that influence mobility postoperatively.
- Demonstrate optimal head and shoulder mobility postoperatively.

Interventions	Rationales
1. Consult with physician regarding an exercise program.	1. Physician determines when the exercise program should be initiated and recommends a program based on the extent of tissue

(continues on page 861)

Interventions continued	Rationales continued
	excision and reconstruction and progression of healing. Generally exercise is initiated after drains are removed, the suture line is intact, and postoperative edema resolves.
2. Teach client to do the following: a. Maintain good posture at all times; pull shoulders back frequently. b. Avoid sitting for prolonged periods. c. Avoid putting pressure on the arm of the operative side; use other arm to lift, pull, and press. d. When reclining, lie in the supine position (avoid lying on the operative side); place the involved arm to the side of the body with the elbow bent and support arm with pillows. e. Avoid lifting or carrying objects weighing more than 3 lb with the involved arm until approved by physician. f. Avoid injury to the involved side.	2. Positioning and activity instructions are the following. a. Good posture is essential to prevent chest muscles from tightening and pulling against weaker muscles on the back of the shoulder (e.g., rhomboids and levator). b. Prolonged sitting tires the muscles that provide good posture. c. These measures decrease stress on the remaining neuromuscular structures. d. Maintaining neutral alignment helps to prevent contractures. e. This restriction can prevent strain and pain in the involved arm. f. Minor injuries to the involved arm can compromise circulation and lymph drainage.
3. Provide pain medication as ordered before client begins prescribed exercises.	3. Pain can make client reluctant to perform prescribed exercises. Adequate pain relief can increase compliance with the therapeutic regimen.
4. Consult with physical therapy as appropriate.	4. Physical therapist can suggest specific exercises to strengthen remaining musculature and increase support and stability of shoulder joint.

 Documentation

Teaching flow records
Progress notes
  Client teaching
  Therapeutic exercises performed

High Risk for Disturbed Self-Concept Related to Change in Appearance

Focus Assessment Criteria	Clinical Significance
1. Past and present coping strategies 2. Ability to visualize the operative area	1–5. This assessment information helps nurse to evaluate current response and

(continues on page 862)

Focus Assessment Criteria continued	Clinical Significance continued
3. Ability to express feelings about the surgery 4. Ability to share feelings and concerns with family and others 5. Participation in self-care	measure progress. Discussions can identify misinformation and fears. Participation in self-care indicates an attempt to cope positively with the changes.
6. Exposure to others who have undergone radical neck dissection	6. Communicating with others who have undergone a neck dissection and resolved some of their negative reactions to the body-image changes can help to squelch client's misconceptions and facilitate client's own adjustment.
7. Support from family/significant others	7. Acceptance by family/significant others may be one of the first steps in moving the individual forward to a "reasonable quality of life" (Sigler et al., 1996).

Goal

The client will communicate feelings about the surgery and its outcome.

Indicators

• Acknowledge changes in body structure and function.
• Participate in self-care.

Interventions	Rationales

1. Identify clients at high risk for unsuccessful adjustment (Shipes, 1986):
  a. Previous history of psychiatric problems
  b. Poor ego strength
  c. Unrealistic expectations concerning surgery
  d. Exhibition of too much or too little concern in the preoperative period
  e. Ineffective problem-solving ability
  f. Difficulty learning new skills
  g. Lack of motivation
  h. External focus of control
  i. Poor health
  j. Unsatisfactory preoperative sex life
  k. Lack of effective support systems
  l. Unstable economic status
  m. Rejection of counseling
	1. Successful adjustment to appearance changes is influenced by factors such as these:
	  • Previous coping success
	  • Achievement of developmental tasks before surgery
	  • Extent to which the change interferes with goal-directed activity
	  • Sense of control
	  • Realistic perception of the change by the client and others (Shipes, 1986).

2. Contact client frequently and treat him or her with warm, positive regard.	2. Frequent contact by caregiver indicates acceptance and may facilitate trust. Client may be hesitant to approach staff because of a negative self-concept.

(continues on page 863)

Interventions continued	**Rationales** continued
3. Incorporate emotional support into technical care teaching sessions (e.g., wound care, bathing).	3. This encourages resolution of emotional issues while teaching technical skills.
4. Encourage client to look at the operative site.	4. Accepting the reality of the body change is the first step in successful adjustment to it.
5. Encourage client to verbalize feelings about surgery and perceptions of life style impacts. Validate his or her perceptions and reassure that the responses are normal and appropriate.	5. Sharing concerns and ventilating feelings provide an opportunity for nurse to correct any misinformation. Validating client's perceptions increases self-awareness.
6. Encourage client to participate in self-care. Give feedback and reinforce positive techniques and progress.	6. Participation in self-care is a sign of successful adjustment. Participation in self-care facilitates acceptance of body changes by providing client with some control over his or her environment. For many patients it can provide the first sense of control over their well-being since diagnosis (Dropkin, 1981).
7. Have client demonstrate proper wound care and teach procedure to a support person.	7. Successful return demonstration and ability to teach the skill to others indicate mastery.
8. Encourage support persons to become involved with wound care and to provide emotional support.	8. Support persons' acceptance is a critical factor in the client's own acceptance and adjustment.
9. Encourage the client to identify and verbalize personal strengths and positive self-attributes and to verbalize intent to resume normal activities as soon as possible.	9. Evidence of positive self-concept and desire to pursue goals and life style reflect successful adjustment.
10. Provide information about measures to help improve appearance: a. Wearing clothes with high collars, e.g., turtleneck sweaters b. Wearing ascots or scarves c. Wearing clothing with shoulder padding d. Wearing accessories that draw attention away from the neck, e.g., hats	10. Improving appearance can boost self-confidence and aid successful adjustment.
11. Refer a client at high risk for unsuccessful adjustment for professional counseling.	11. Follow-up therapy may be indicated to assist with effective adjustment.

Documentation

Progress notes
   Present emotional status
   Interventions
   Response to interventions

Risk for Imbalanced Nutrition Related to Swallowing Difficulties, Decreased Salivation, and Decreased Sense of Smell and Taste

Focus Assessment Criteria	Clinical Significance
1. Ability to swallow food and liquid 2. Ability to cough 3. Gag and swallowing reflexes	1. A thorough evaluation is indicated by a speech and swallowing specialist. Postoperative edema can cause swallowing problems. Removal of the epiglottis causes chronic aspiration risk (Bildstein & Blendowski, 1997).

Goal

The client will use methods to increase intake and maintain weight.

Indicators

• Demonstrate methods to improve swallowing.
• Relate reasons for decreased sense of taste and smell.
• Name resources available after discharge.

Interventions	Rationales
1. Administer tube feedings as prescribed. Refer to Enteral Nutrition Care Plan for additional interventions.	
2. Consult with speech or swallowing therapist for a thorough evaluation. Prepare for a video fluoroscopy and a modified "cookie" swallow barium.	2. A thorough evaluation is needed to determine mobility of tongue and pharynx.

3. Explain the affects of surgery on eating and nutrition:
  a. Loss of sense of smell
 	
  b. Decreased sense of taste
 	
  c. Swallowing
 	
  d. Decreased salivation
	3.
	
	  a. A permanent tracheostomy prevents air from passing over receptors in the nasal passages—a process necessary for smell.
	  b. Receptors in the tongue are bypassed, which decreases sense of taste.
	  c. Surgery can damage any of the cranial nerves needed for swallowing (e.g., trigeminal, facial, glossopharyngeal, vagus, spinal accessory, hypoglossal).
	  d. Surgical trauma to salivary glands can reduce salivation.

(continues on page 865)

Interventions continued	Rationales continued
4. Advise how these changes will affect nutrition: a. Food choices b. Time required to eat c. Social eating (e.g., restaurants)	4. a. Foods easier to swallow are selected regardless of their nutritional value. b. The time required to eat is longer (e.g., 10 to 15 minutes more). c. Social talking and eating are not easy.
5. Explain what foods are reported to improve enjoyment (fish, vegetables, pasta, potatoes, milk) and what foods are less enjoyed (red meat, bitter foods, breads, sweets, cheese).	5. Postlaryngectomy clients reported these food preferences (Lennie et al., 2001).
6. Advise that these alterations do not occur in enzyme; any that do may diminish over time.	6. In one study, 89% of participants rated their sense of smell as less affected and 63% reported a diminished sense of taste (Lennie et al., 2001).
7. Provide written instructions about how to improve eating and nutritional status. a. Chew food thoroughly. b. Provide enough time to eat. c. Drink fluids while eating. d. Add more spices to food. e. Supplement meals with protein drinks.	7. Postoperatively, the client and family will be overwhelmed, so information retention will be limited. a. This will help to prevent aspiration. b. The person must alternate breathing, chewing, and talking. c. This will moisten foods and help swallowing. d. This will enhance taste. e. Supplements will provide proteins, vitamins, and minerals
8. Encourage client after discharge to access information and join a support group such as the International Association of Laryngectomies (www.larynegectomies.inuk.com) and Web Whispers (www.webwhispers.org).	8. Clients reported that they were unprepared for changes when they were home (Lennie et al., 2001).

High Risk for Ineffective Therapeutic Regimen Management Related to Insufficient Knowledge of Wound Care, Signs and Symptoms of Complications, Exercises, and Follow-up Care

Focus Assessment Criteria	Clinical Significance
1. Readiness and ability to learn and retain information	1. A client or family failing to achieve learning goals requires a referral for assistance postdischarge.

Goals

The goals for this diagnosis represent those associated with discharge planning. Refer to the discharge criteria.

Interventions	Rationales
1. Teach wound care measures. (Refer to the General Surgery Care Plan for specific interventions.)	1.
2. Explain the normal functions of neuro-muscular structures and how they have been disrupted by surgery.	2. Client's understanding of the impairment can encourage compliance with post-operative instructions.
3. Discuss the importance of complying with the prescribed exercise regimen. Reinforce teaching and provide written instructions.	3. The postoperative exercise program aims to strengthen the levator scapulae and rhomboid muscles to compensate for loss of the trapezius. If these muscles are not strengthened, the pectoralis muscle will pull the shoulder forward and down and cause pain. Explanations and written instructions can encourage compliance (Sigler et al., 1996).

4. Instruct client to report the following promptly:
  a. Increased temperature
  b. New or increasing pain
  c. Change in amount, consistency, or color of drainage
  d. Leakage of food or fluid from incision line
	4. Early detection of complications enables prompt intervention to reduce their severity. Increased temperature, pain, and a change in drainage typically point to infection. Peri-incisional erythema with leakage of aurulent drainage, food, or other fluids indicates a fistula (Sigler et al., 1996).

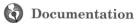 Documentation

Discharge summary record
   Client and family teaching
   Outcome achievement or status

NEPHRECTOMY

Nephrectomy is the removal of the kidney (simple nephrectomy) and possibly the surrounding peri-nephritic fat, Gerota's fascia, and lymph nodes (radial nephrectomy). Nephrectomy is used to treat renal cancer, massive trauma to the kidney, polycystic kidney disease, and renal failure. It is also used to gather kidneys for donation. Laparoscopic techniques are used for partial nephrectomies (nephron-sparing nephrectomy).

Time Frame
Preoperative and postoperative periods

DIAGNOSTIC CLUSTER

Preoperative Period

Collaborative Problems	Refer to
▲ PC: Hemorrhage/Shock	
▲ PC: Paralytic Ileus	
▲ PC: Renal Insufficiency	
△ PC: Pyelonephritis	
△ PC: Pneumothorax Secondary to Thoracic Approach	Thoracic Surgery

Nursing Diagnoses	Refer to
▲ High Risk for Ineffective Therapeutic Regimen Management related to insufficient knowledge of hydration requirements, nephrostomy care, and signs and symptoms of complications	
△ Acute Pain related to distention of renal capsule and incision	General Surgery
▲ High Risk for Ineffective Respiratory Function related to pain on breathing and coughing secondary to location of incision	General Surgery

Related Care Plan

General Surgery Generic Care Plan
Cancer (Initial Diagnosis)

▲ This diagnosis was reported to be monitored for or managed frequently (75%–100%).
△ This diagnosis was reported to be monitored for or managed often (50%–74%).

Discharge Criteria

Before discharge, the client and family will

1. Demonstrate nephrostomy tube care.
2. State measures for at-home wound care.
3. Share feelings regarding loss of kidney.
4. State signs and symptoms that must be reported to a health care professional.

Postoperative: Collaborative Problems

Potential Complication: Hemorrhage/Shock

Potential Complication: Paralytic Ileus

Potential Complication: Renal Insufficiency

Potential Complication: Pyelonephritis

Nursing Goal

The nurse will detect early signs and symptoms of (a) hemorrhage/shock, (b) paralytic ileus, (c) renal insufficiency (partial nephrectomy), and (d) pyelonephritis (partial nephrectomy) and will collaboratively intervene to stabilize client.

Indicators
- Calm, oriented, alert (a)
- Pulse 60–100 beats/min (a)
- Respirations 16–20 breaths/min (a)
- BP > 90/60, < 140/90 mm Hg (a)
- No chills (d)
- Temperature 98.5–99°F (d)
- Urine specific gravity 1.005–1.030 (c, d)
- Urine output >30 mL/hr (a, c, d)
- Full peripheral pulses (a)
- Capillary refill < 3 seconds (a)
- Dry warm skin (a)
- Pinkish, brownish or olive skin tones (a)
- Hemoglobin (a)
  - Male 13–18 gm/dL
  - Female 12–16 gm/dL
- Hematocrit (a)
  - Male 42–50%
  - Female 40–48%
- Bowel sounds present all quadrants (b)
- No abdominal distention (b)
- White blood cells 5,000–10,000/cu mm (d)
- Urine sodium 130–200 mEq/24h (c)
- Blood urea nitrogen 10–20 mg/dL (c)
- Potassium 3.8–5 mEq/L (c)
- Serum sodium 135–145 mEq/L (c)
- Phosphorus 2.5–4.5 mg/dL (c)
- Creatinine clearance 100–150 mL of blood cleared per mm (c)
- No costovertebral angle (CDA) tenderness (d)
- Urine negative-bacteria (d)
- No c/o dysuria or frequency (d)
- No bladder distention (d)

Interventions	Rationales

1. Monitor for signs and symptoms of hemorrhage/shock every hour for the first 24 hours then every 4 hours.
  a. Increasing pulse rate with normal or slightly decreased blood pressure
  b. Decreased oxygen saturation (pulse oximetry) <94%
  c. Urine output <30 mL/hr
  d. Restlessness, agitation, change in mentation
  e. Increasing respiratory rate
  f. Diminished peripheral pulses
  g. Cool, pale, or cyanotic skin
  h. Thirst
	1. Because the renal capsule is very vascular, massive blood loss can occur. The compensatory response to decreased circulatory volume is to increase blood oxygen by increasing heart and respiratory rates and decreasing circulation to extremities (manifested by decreased pulses and cool skin). Diminished cerebral oxygenation can cause changes in mentation. Decreased oxygen to kidneys results in decreased urine output (Gillenwater, Grayhack, Howards, & Duckett, 1996).

2. Monitor fluid status hourly.
  a. Intake (parenteral, oral)
  b. Output and loss (urinary, drainage, vomiting)
  c. Weigh daily at same time in same clothes if needed.
	2. Fluid loss due to surgery and nothing-by-mouth (NPO) status can disrupt fluid balance in some clients. Stress can produce sodium and water retention.
	    Accurate daily assessment of body weight is more accurate to measure fluid loss than intake and output because it accounts for the water loss during fever, diaphoresis, and respiration (Karlowitz, 1995).

3. Monitor surgical site for bleeding, dehiscence, and evisceration.	3. Frequent monitoring enables early detection of complications. Hypotension and vasospasm during surgery can cause temporary hemostasis and can result in delayed bleeding (Griffin, 1990).
4. Teach client to splint the incision site with a pillow when coughing.	4. Splinting reduces stress on suture lines by equalizing the pressure across the incision site.

5. Monitor for signs and symptoms of paralytic ileus.
  a. Decreased or absent bowel sounds
  b. Abdominal distention
  c. Abdominal discomfort
6. Do not initiate fluids until bowel sounds are present. Begin with small amounts. Note client's response and the type and amount of emesis if any.
	5,6. Reflex paralysis of intestinal peristalsis and manipulation of the colon to gain access make this client at high risk for ileus. The depressive effects of narcotics and anesthetics on peristalsis can also cause paralytic ileus. Ileus can occur between the third and fifth postoperative day. Pain can be localized, sharp, and intermittent (Gillenwater et al., 1996).

7. Monitor for early signs and symptoms of renal insufficiency.	7. Renal insufficiency can result from edema caused by surgical manipulation (partial nephrectomy) or a nonpatent nephrostomy tube.

(continues on page 870)

Interventions continued	**Rationales** continued
a. Sustained elevated urine specific gravity b. Elevated urine sodium level c. Sustained insufficient urine output (<30 mL/hr) d. Elevated blood pressure e. Elevated BUN and serum creatinine, potassium, phosphorus, and ammonia; decreased creatinine clearance	a,b. Ability of renal tubules to reabsorb electrolytes results in increased urine sodium levels and urine specific gravity. c,d. Decreased glomerular filtration rate eventually leads to insufficient urine output and increased renin production, resulting in elevated blood pressure in an attempt to increase renal blood flow. e. These changes result from decreased excretion of urea and creatinine in urine.
8. Monitor client for signs and symptoms of infection. a. Chills and fever b. Costovertebral angle (CVA) pain (a dull, constant backache below the 12th rib) c. Leukocytosis d. Bacteria and pus in urine e. Dysuria and frequency	8. Microorganisms can be introduced into the body during surgery or through incision. Urinary tract infections can be caused by urinary stasis (e.g., from a non-patent nephrostomy tube) or irritation of tissue by calculi. a. Endogenous pyrogens are released and they reset the hypothalamic set point to febrile levels. The body temperature is sensed as "too cool;" shivering and vasoconstriction result to generate and consume heat. Core temperature rises to new level of the set point, resulting in fever. WBCs are released to destroy some pathogens. Wound redness, tenderness, and edema result from lymphocyte migration to the area (Karlowitz, 1995). b. CVA pain results from distention of the renal capsule. c. Leukocytosis reflects an increase in WBCs to fight infection through phagocytosis. d. Bacteria and pus in urine indicate a urinary tract infection. e. Bacteria irritate bladder tissue, causing spasms and frequency.
9. Monitor for signs of urinary retention. a. Bladder distention b. Urine overflow (30–60 mL of urine every 15 to 30 minutes)	9. Trauma to the detrusor muscle and injury to the pelvic nerves during surgery can inhibit bladder function. Anxiety and pain can cause spasms of the reflex sphincters. Bladder neck edema can also cause retention. Sedatives and narcotics can affect the central nervous system and the effectiveness of smooth muscles (Gillenwater et al., 1996).
10. Instruct client to report bladder discomfort or inability to void.	10. Overdistention of the bladder can aggravate a person's ability to empty the bladder (Gillenwater et al., 1996).

Related Physician-Prescribed Interventions

Refer to the Care Plan for the surgical client.

Documentation

Flow records
  Vital signs
  Circulatory status
  Intake (oral, parenteral)
  Output (urinary, drainage tubes)
  Bowel function (bowel sounds, defecation pattern, abdominal distention)
  Wound status (color, drainage)

Postoperative: Nursing Diagnosis

High Risk for Ineffective Therapeutic Regimen Management Related to Insufficient Knowledge of Hydration Requirements, Nephrostomy Care, and Signs and Symptoms of Complications

Focus Assessment Criteria	Clinical Significance
1. Readiness and ability to learn and retain information	1. A client or family failing to achieve learning goals requires a referral for assistance postdischarge.

Goals

The goals for this diagnosis represent those associated with discharge planning. Refer to the discharge criteria.

Interventions	Rationales
1. Explain the need to maintain optimal hydration.	1. Optimal hydration reduces urinary stasis, decreasing risk of infection and calculi formation.
2. Teach and have client perform a return demonstration of nephrostomy care measures including these: a. Aseptic technique b. Skin care c. Tube stabilization	2. Proper techniques can reduce risk of infection. Movement of the tube can cause dislodgement or tissue trauma.
3. Teach client to use pillows to support back when on side.	3. Certain positions will decrease tension on the incisional area.
4. Explain why the pain is severe and other discomforts. Teach client to avoid lifting more than 10 lbs for 6 weeks.	4. The client's position and the incision's size cause severe pain. The client's position on the OR table will cause muscular aches and pains (Early & Poquette, 2000).

(continues on page 872)

Interventions continued	Rationales continued

5. Teach client to report the following:
   a. Decreased urine output
   b. Fever or malaise
   c. Purulent, cloudy drainage from or around the tube
	5. Early detection enables prompt intervention to prevent serious complications such as renal insufficiency and infection (Lancaster, 1995).

6. Refer client and family to a home health agency for follow-up care.	6. Home care nurse evaluates client's ability for home care and provides periodic assessment of renal function and development of infection.

Documentation

Discharge summary record
   Client and family teaching
   Outcome achievement or status
   Referrals

RADICAL PROSTATECTOMY

Radical prostatectomy is the surgical removal of the prostate gland, ejaculatory ducts, seminal vesicles, and sometimes the lymph nodes for cancer of the prostate confined to the prostate. The surgical approach can be via a perineal, suprapubic, or retropubic incision. Another procedure, transperitoneal laparoscopic radial prostatectomy, has the benefit of decreased hospital stay and less postoperative pain (Queen, 2001).

 Time Frame

Preoperative and postoperative periods

⊙⊙ DIAGNOSTIC CLUSTER

Preoperative Period

Nursing Diagnoses

▲ Anxiety related to upcoming surgery and insufficient knowledge of routine and post-operative activities

Postoperative Period

Collaborative Problems

▲ PC: Hemorrhage
▲ PC: Clot Formation
△ PC: Thrombophlebitis

Nursing Diagnoses

▲ Grieving related to potential loss of body function and perceived effects on life style (refer to Cancer: Initial Diagnosis Care Plan)
  Acute Pain related to bladder spasms; clot retention; and back, leg, and incisional pain
△ High Risk for Ineffective Sexuality Patterns related to fear of impotence resulting from surgical intervention
▲ High Risk for Ineffective Therapeutic Regimen Management related to insufficient knowledge of fluid restrictions, catheter care, activity restrictions, urinary control, and signs and symptoms of complications

Related Care Plan

General Surgery Generic Care Plan

▲ This diagnosis was reported to be monitored for or managed frequently (75%—100%).
△ This diagnosis was reported to be monitored for or managed often (50%—74%).

Discharge Criteria

Before discharge, the client and family will

1. Identify the need for increased oral fluid intake.
2. Demonstrate care of the indwelling (Foley) catheter.
3. Explain wound care at home.
4. Verbalize necessary precautions for activity and urination.
5. State the signs and symptoms that must be reported to a health care professional.
6. Verbalize an intent to share feelings and concerns related to sexual function with significant others.

Preoperative: Nursing Diagnosis

Anxiety Related to Upcoming Surgery and Insufficient Knowledge of Routine and Postoperative Activities

Focus Assessment Criteria	Clinical Significance
1. Understanding the surgical procedure and related preoperative and postoperative routines	1. Assessing client's knowledge level guides nurse in planning appropriate teaching strategies.
2. Readiness and ability to learn and retain information	2. Anxiety can interfere with learning.

Goal

The client will state the reasons for activity restrictions, indwelling catheterization, and increased fluid intake.

Interventions	Rationales

1. Reinforce physician's explanation of the scheduled surgery and answer any questions.
2. Explain expected postoperative procedures such as the following:
  a. Indwelling (Foley) catheterization in hospital and at home
  b. Continuous and manual irrigation
  c. IV infusions
  d. Drains
3. Explain expected activity restrictions and activities to prevent complications.
  a. Bed rest for first postoperative day
  b. Progressive ambulation beginning on first postoperative day
  c. Avoiding activities that put strain on bladder area
  d. Coughing and deep breathing exercises
	1–3. Client's understanding can help to reduce anxiety related to fear of the unknown. Preoperative education has been shown to reduce anxiety and also helps to improve compliance (Redman & Thomas, 1992). Immobilization on the operating room table for several hours will increase risk for pneumonia and venous stasis.

4. Explain that transient hematuria is normal in the immediate postoperative period.	4. Preparing client for postoperative hematuria prevents him from being shocked at its appearance.
5. Explain the need for increased fluid intake.	5. Dilute urine deters clot formation.
6. Provide teaching aids (e.g., pamphlets or video tapes) as available.	6. A multisensory approach to teaching enhances learning and retention (Redman & Thomas, 1992).

(continues on page 875)

Interventions continued	Rationales continued
7. Encourage client to share fears.	7. Clients are extremely anxious with major concerns regarding sexual competence and urinary control (Butler, Downe-Wambolt, Marsh, Bell, Jarvi, 2000).
8. Elicit what the surgeon has explained regarding effects of surgery on sexual function.	8. Nurse should not assume that client understands the ramifications of surgery just because he asks no questions. Many clients are reluctant to discuss sexual concerns. Privacy may encourage sharing.

Documentation

Discharge summary record
   Client teaching
   Outcome achievement or status

Postoperative: Collaborative Problems

Potential Complication: Hemorrhage

Potential Complication: Clot Formation

Potential Complication: Thrombophlebitis

Nursing Goal

The nurse will detect early signs and symptoms of (a) hemorrhage, (b) clot formation, (c) urinary retention, and (d) thrombophlebitis and will collaborative intervene to stabilize client.

Indicators

- Calm, oriented, alert (a)
- Pulse 60–100 beats/min (a)
- Respirations 16–20 breaths/min (a)
- BP > 90/60, < 140–90 mm Hg (a)
- Temperature (d)
- Urine output > 30 mL/hr (a, d)
- Pink or clear red urine (first 24 hr) (a, d)
- Amber→pink urine after 24 hours (a, d)
- Clots in urine (a, b, c)
- Warm, dry skin (a)
- Pinkish, brownish, or olive skin tones (a)
- Hemoglobin (a)
  ○ Male 13–18 gm/dL
  ○ Female 12–16 gm/dL
- Hematocrit (a)
  ○ Male 42–50%
  ○ Female 40–48%
- Continuous flowing bladder irrigation (b, c)
- No bladder distension (c)
- Positive Homans' sign (calf pain when foot is flexed upward) (d)
- No c/o calf tenderness, warmth or redness (d)
- No leg edema (d)

Interventions	Rationales

1. Monitor for signs and symptoms of hemorrhage:
  a. Abnormal urine characteristics, e.g., highly viscous, clots, bright red or burgundy color
  b. Increased pulse rate
  c. Urine output <30 mL/hr
  d. Restlessness, agitation
  e. Cool, pale, or cyanotic skin
  f. Hemoglobin and hematocrit values
	1. The prostrate gland is highly vascular, receiving its blood supply from the internal iliac artery. Elderly clients and those who have had prolonged urinary retention are vulnerable to rapid changes in bladder contents and fluid volume. During the first 24 hours after surgery, urine should be pink or clear red, gradually becoming amber to pink-tinged by the fourth day. Bright red urine with clots indicates arterial bleeding. Burgundy-colored urine indicates venous bleeding, which usually resolves spontaneously. Clots are expected; their absence may point to blood dyscrasias. Hemoglobin and hematocrit values decline if significant postoperative bleeding occurs (Kantaff et al., 2001).

2. Monitor dressings, catheters, and drains that vary depending on the type of surgery performed.
  a. Suprapubic approach:
    • Urethral catheter
    • Suprapubic tube
    • Abdominal drain
  b. Retropubic approach:
    • Urethral catheter
    • Abdominal drain
  c. Perineal approach:
    • Urethral catheter
    • Perineal drain
	2. Heavy venous bleeding is expected the first 24 hours for all approaches except the perineal approach. Blood loss can occur from the catheter or incision (Kantaff et al., 2001).

3. Instruct client to do the following:
  a. Avoid straining for bowel elimination.
  b. Do not sit in a firm, upright chair.
  c. Recline slightly on the toilet.
	3. Increased pressure on the rectum can trigger bleeding and perforated rectal tissue.

4. Provide bladder irrigation as ordered.
  a. Continuous (closed)
  b. Manual: Using a bulb syringe, irrigate the catheter with 30 to 60 mL normal saline solution every 3 to 4 hours as needed.
	4. Continuous bladder irrigation with normal saline dilutes blood in the urine to prevent clot formation. Manual irrigation provides the negative pressure needed to remove obstructive clots or tissue particles.

5. Ensure adequate fluid intake (oral, parenteral).	5. Optimal hydration dilutes urine to prevent clot formation.
6. Monitor for signs and symptoms of thrombophlebitis.	6. Initiation of the stress response during surgery results in hypercoagulability by

(continues on page 877)

Interventions continued	Rationales continued
a. Positive Homans' sign (pain on dorsiflexion of the foot resulting from insufficient circulation) b. Calf tenderness, unusual warmth, or redness c. Low-grade fever d. Extremity edema	inhibiting the fibrinolytic system. Pain, malignant disease, systemic infection, and cigarette smoking also cause hypercoagulability (Caswell, 1993).
7. Ambulate as soon as possible with at least 5 minutes of walking per hour. Avoid chair sitting with legs dependent.	7. Walking contracts leg muscles, stimulates the venous pump, and reduces stasis (Carroll, 1993).
8. Ensure that client uses sequential compression device as prescribed followed by antiembolic stockings.	8. These stockings reduce venous stasis by applying a graded degree of compression to ankle and calf (Carroll, 1993).

◥ Related Physician-Prescribed Interventions

Medications. Antispasmodics (oxybutynin, belladonna); analgesics; antibiotics

Intravenous Therapy. Refer to the General Surgery Care Plan Appendix II, prostatic fluid, cytology, urine cytology

Laboratory Studies. CBC, PTT, BC, magnesium, electrolytes, prostate-specific antigen (PSA), urine culture, serum prostatic acid phosphatase level

Diagnostic Studies. Cystourethroscopy, bone scans, prostatic biopsy, transrectal ultrasound, CT, flow cytometry, MRI (abdomen, pelvis), voiding cystourethrogram

Therapies. Indwelling catheterization, wound drains, catheter traction, bladder irrigation (manual or continuous), radiotherapy, sitz baths, endocrine manipulation, sequential compression stocking device, chemotherapy, nasogastric tube

Documentation

Flow records
  Vital signs
  Intake and output
  Urine (color, viscosity, presence of clots)
  Continuous irrigations
  Manual irrigations (times, amounts)

Postoperative: Nursing Diagnoses

Acute Pain Related to Bladder Spasms; Clot Retention; and Back, Leg, and Incisional Pain

Focus Assessment Criteria	Clinical Significance
1. Location, characteristics, and duration of pain	1. Postoperative pain may result from surgical manipulation, obstruction, or bladder spasms (Gray, 1992).

Goal

The client will report decreased pain after pain relief interventions.

Indicators

- Can do leg exercises.
- Increase activity progressively.

Interventions	Rationales
1. Monitor for intermittent suprapubic pain: bladder spasms, burning sensation at the tip of the penis.	1. Irritation from indwelling catheter can cause bladder spasms and pain in the penis.
2. Monitor for persistent suprapubic pain: bladder distention with sensations of fullness and tightness, inability to void.	2. Catheter obstruction can cause urinary retention, leading to increased bladder spasms and increased risk of infection.
3. Monitor for lower back and leg pain. Provide gentle massage to the back and heat to the legs, if necessary.	3. During surgery, client lies in the lithotomy position that can stretch and aggravate muscles that normally may be underused.
4. Anchor catheter to leg with tape or a catheter leg strap.	4. Pressure from a dangling catheter can damage the urinary sphincter, resulting in urinary incontinence after catheter removal. Catheter movement also increases the likelihood of bladder spasms.
5. Monitor for testicular pain.	5. Clipping the vas deferens causes congestion of seminal fluid and blood. This congestion resolves over several weeks.
6. Administer medication as ordered for pain and spasms.	6. Antispasmodic medications, i.e., eyopiote and belladonna suppositories, prevent bladder spasms. Analgesic medication diminishes the incisional pain.
7. Encourage adequate oral fluid intake (at least 2,000 mL/day unless contraindicated).	7. Adequate hydration promotes dilute urine that helps to flush out clots.
8. Manually irrigate the indwelling catheter only when prescribed.	8. Each time the closed system is opened for manual irrigation, risk of bacterial contamination increases.

 Documentation

Medication administration record
   Type, dose, route of all medications
Progress notes
   Complaints of pain (type, site, duration)
   Unsatisfactory pain relief

High Risk for Ineffective Sexuality Patterns Related to Fear of Impotence Resulting from Surgical Intervention

Focus Assessment Criteria	Clinical Significance
1. Usual pattern of sexual functioning 2. Perceived effects of surgery on sexual functioning	1,2. Misconceptions related to inaccurate information can lead to undue anxiety and stress, which may result in decreased libido and psychological impotence.

Goals

The client will discuss his and his partner's feelings and concerns regarding the effects of surgery on sexuality and sexual functioning.

Indicators

- Verbalize an intention to discuss concerns with partner after discharge from hospital.
- Explain effects of surgery on sexual function and expected course of resolution.

Interventions	Rationales
1. Explain the effects of surgery on sexual function (orgasms, erections, fertility, ejaculations).	1. If one or both nerve bundles responsible for erections are spared, erections will return. Orgasms will occur without ejaculations. It may take up to 2 years for full function to return after wound healing and all edema from surgery subsides. Men older than 70 years probably will not regain erections; ejaculate will be reduced but will still contain sperm.
2. Use familiar terms when possible and explain unfamiliar terms.	2. Unfamiliar medical terminology may cause confusion and misunderstanding.
3. Explain that the surgeon's permission to resume sexual activity is needed. Clearly state cancer of prostate is not transmitted sexually.	3. Complete healing is needed to prevent bleeding and to resolve edema, which usually takes 6 weeks to 3 months.
4. Encourage client to ask the physician questions during hospitalization and follow-up visits.	4. An open dialogue with the physician is encouraged to clarify concerns and to provide access to specific explanations.
5. Encourage open communication between client and partner regarding limitations and alternative methods of pleasure.	5. Partners of men with prostate cancer clearly see themselves as partners in managing the effects of cancer on their partner's lives (Butler et al., 2000).

(continues on page 880)

Interventions continued	Rationales continued
6. Provide opportunities for partner to share concerns and questions.	6. Partners are crucial to the recovery process. They manage their own anxiety and also assist their partner in managing his (Maliski, Heilemann, & McCorkle, 2001).
7. Encourage client to continue to discuss concerns with significant others and professionals post-discharge.	
8. Determine the person's expectations of effects of surgery on urinary continence.	8. Damage to the muscle controlling the urethral sphincter or its nerve supply can cause incontinence. The retropubic approach can result in a lower rate of incontinence. About 50% of clients experience temporary urinary incontinence. The literature reports a 2% to 44.5% rate of incontinence (Sueppel, Kreder, & See, 2001).

 Documentation

Progress notes
 Usual sexual patterns
 Expressed concerns
Discharge summary record
 Client teaching
 Response to teaching

High Risk for Ineffective Therapeutic Regimen Management Related to Insufficient Knowledge of Fluid Restrictions, Catheter Care, Activity Restrictions, Urinary Control, and Signs and Symptoms of Complications

Focus Assessment Criteria	Clinical Significance
1. Readiness and ability to learn and retain information	1. A client or family failing to achieve learning goals requires a referral for assistance postdischarge.

Goals

The goals for this diagnosis represent those associated with discharge planning. Refer to the discharge criteria.

Interventions	Rationales
1. Reinforce the need for adequate oral fluid intake (at least 2,000 mL/day unless contraindicated).	1. Optimal hydration helps to reestablish bladder tone after catheter removal by stimulating voiding, diluting urine, and decreasing susceptibility to urinary tract infections and clot formation.

(continues on page 881)

Interventions continued	Rationales continued

2. Teach indwelling catheter care.
  a. Wash the urinary meatus with soap and water twice a day.
  b. Increase the frequency of cleansing if drainage is evident around catheter insertion site.
	2. The indwelling catheter provides a route for bacteria normally found on the urinary meatus to enter the urinary tract. These measures help to reduce risk of urinary tract infection.

3. Reinforce activity restrictions that may include the following:
  a. Avoid straining with bowel movements; increase intake of dietary fiber or take stool softeners if indicated.
  b. Do not use suppositories or enemas.
  c. Avoid sitting with legs dependent.
  d. Avoid heavy lifting and strenuous activity.
  e. Avoid sexual intercourse until physician advises otherwise (usually within 6 to 8 weeks after surgery).
	3. These restrictions are necessary to reduce the risk of internal bleeding.

4. Advise that client may do the following:
  a. Take long walks.
  b. Use stairs.
  c. Drive 3 weeks after surgery if power steering is used.
	4. These activities do not impede healing of surgical site.

5. Explain expectations for urinary control after catheter is removed.
  a. Dribbling, frequency, and urgency may occur initially but gradually subside over weeks.
 	
  b. Perineal exercises (tense buttocks, hold, and release):
    • Tighten and hold for the count of 10 seconds then relax for 10 seconds; repeat 10 times.
    • Do exercises frequently 6 to 12 times a day (10 at a time).
  c. Avoiding caffeine and alcohol can help to prevent problems.
  d. Transient hematuria is normal and should decrease with increased fluid intake.
  e. Wear a pants liner or diaper if needed initially.
	5.
	
	  a. Difficulty resuming normal voiding patterns may be related to bladder neck trauma, urinary tract infection, or catheter irritation. While the indwelling catheter is in place, constant urine drainage decreases muscle control and increases flaccidity.
	  b. Regular contracture of sphincter muscles will strengthen pelvic floor muscles and decrease incontinence in 4 to 6 weeks.
	
	  c. Caffeine acts as a mild diuretic, making it more difficult to control urine. Alcohol may increase burning on urination.

6. Review signs and symptoms of complications and the need to report them:	6. Early detection enables prompt intervention to minimize severity of complications.

(continues on page 882)

Interventions continued	**Rationales** continued
a. Inability to void for more than 6 hours	a. Inability to void may indicate clot or tissue blockage.
b. Fever, chills, flank pain	b. These symptoms may indicate urinary tract infection.
c. Increased hematuria	c. Increased hematuria points to bleeding or hemorrhage.
7. Refer to community services (e.g., home care, counseling) and sources for information (e.g., www.cancer-prostate.com).	

 Documentation

Discharge summary record
    Client teaching
    Outcome achievement or status
    Referrals if indicated

THORACIC SURGERY

A term encompassing various procedures involving a surgical opening into the chest cavity, thoracic surgery may be a pneumonectomy (removal of entire lung), lobectomy (removal of a lobe), segmentectomy (removal of a segment), wedge resection (removal of a lesion), sleeve resection with bronchoplastic reconstruction (partial removal of bronchus), or exploratory thoracotomy (diagnostic). Thoracic surgery usually is indicated for lung cancer but also may be indicated to repair a traumatized lung and to isolate tuberculosis, abscesses, bronchiectasis, blebs, and bulla caused by emphysema.

 Time Frame
Preoperative and postoperative periods

⊙⊙ DIAGNOSTIC CLUSTER

Preoperative Period

Nursing Diagnoses	**Refer to**
△ Anxiety related to impending surgery and insufficient knowledge of preoperative routines, intraoperative activities, and postoperative self-care activities	

Postoperative Period

Collaborative Problems

	Refer to
△ PC: Mediastinal Shift	
▲ PC: Subcutaneous Emphysema	
▲ PC: Acute Pulmonary Edema	
▲ PC: Dysrhythmias	
▲ PC: Respiratory Insufficiency	Coronary Artery Bypass Grafting
▲ PC: Pneumothorax, Hemothorax	Abdominal Aortic Aneurysm Resection
▲ PC: Pulmonary Embolism	Abdominal Aortic Aneurysm Resection
△ PC: Thrombophlebitis	Abdominal Aortic Aneurysm Resection

Nursing Diagnoses	**Refer to**
▲ Ineffective Airway Clearance related to increased secretions and diminished cough secondary to pain and fatigue	
▲ Impaired Physical Mobility related to restricted arm and shoulder movement secondary to pain and muscle dissection and imposed position restrictions	
▲ Acute Pain related to surgical incision, chest tube sites, and immobility secondary to lengthy surgery	

(continues on page 884)

Nursing Diagnoses continued	Refer to continued
Grieving related to loss of body part and its perceived effects on life style	Enucleation
Risk for Ineffective Therapeutic Regimen Management	
Related Care Plan General Surgery Generic Care Plan Mechanical Ventilation Cancer: Initial Diagnosis	

▲ This diagnosis was reported to be monitored for or managed frequently (75%–100%).
△ This diagnosis was reported to be monitored for or managed often (50%--74%).

Discharge Criteria

Before discharge, the client or family will

1. Describe wound care at home.
2. Relate the need to continue exercises at home.
3. Verbalize precautions for activities.
4. State signs and symptoms that must be reported to a health care professional.
5. Identify appropriate community resources and self-help groups.
6. Describe pain management at home.

Preoperative: Nursing Diagnoses

Anxiety Related to Impending Surgery and Insufficient Knowledge of Preoperative Routines, Intraoperative Activities, and Postoperative Self-care Activities

Focus Assessment Criteria	Clinical Significance
1. Anxiety level (mild, moderate, severe, panic) 2. Readiness and ability to learn and retain information 3. Past surgical and anesthetic experience 4. Emotional response and coping mechanisms used during previous stressful events or hospitalizations	1–4. Anxiety can interfere with learning. Assessing anxiety level guides nurse in planning appropriate teaching strategies (Redman & Thomas, 1992).

Goal

The client will

1. Verbalize knowledge of routines and care before, during, and after surgery.
2. Share concerns and fears and demonstrate evidence of physical and psychosocial preparation for surgery.

Interventions	Rationales
1. Provide information regarding what to expect before, during, and after surgery; use appropriate client education materials, booklets, video, one-on-one instruction. Explain the expected events such as the following: a. Presence of chest tubes, drainage tubes, and indwelling catheter	1. Preoperative education improves client's ability to participate postoperatively and decreases anxiety associated with the unknown. a. Drainage tubes remove liquids and gas from the surgical site (thoracic cavity, pleural space, mediastinal cavity). Chest tubes re-expand the lungs by reestablishing negative intrapleural pressures. Chest tubes are not indicated after a pneumonectomy because it is desirable that the space accumulates fluid (Thelan, Urden, Lough, & Stacy, 1998).
b. Need for oxygen therapy and oximetry monitoring c. Pain and available relief measures such as	b. Supplemental oxygen is indicated to compensate for impaired ventilation. c. Moderate to severe pain is expected; client should be aware of this possibility. Accurate expectations of pain lead to lower levels of anxiety (Johnson, 1973; Tarsitano, 1992).
• Patient-controlled analgesia (PCA)	• Clients who are able to self-medicate with small IV doses of opioids by a programmable infusion pump have demonstrated less pain, anxiety, increased satisfaction, and early recovery and discharge (Ferrante, Ostheimor, & Covino, 1990).
• Epidural analgesia	• Pain control in the form of epidural analgesia after thoracic surgery provides excellent pain relief, improved pulmonary function, and overall recovery (Agency for Health Care Policy and Research (AHCPR), 1992).
d. Location and extent of incision e. Progression from ICU/recovery room to stepdown unit and average length of stay postoperatively	d,e. Explaining what to expect can help to reduce fears associated with the unknown (Johnson, Rice, Fuller, & Endress, 1978).
2. Teach client postoperative respiratory exercises and routines including the following: a. Coughing and deep breathing b. "Huff breathing" • Take a deep diaphragmatic breath and exhale forcefully against the hand with a "huff." • Start with small huffs and progress to one strong huff. c. Positioning d. Incentive spirometry e. Chest physiotherapy Reinforce their importance. Refer to General Surgery Care Plan, Appendix II.	2. Surgery on the lung reduces surface area for oxygen exchange, and trauma to the tracheobronchial tree produces excessive secretions and a diminished cough reflex. Respiratory exercises including CPT, incentive spirometry, and positioning stimulate pulmonary expansion and assist in alveolar inflation (Thelan et al., 1998).

(continues on page 886)

Interventions continued	Rationales continued
3. Instruct client to refrain from smoking postoperatively.	3. Irritants from smoking increase pulmonary secretions.
4. Implement strategies to relieve anxiety such as distraction, relaxation, and emotional support if necessary.	4. Psychological interventions for surgery intended to offer emotional support and relieve anxiety are often more effective than purely informational approaches.

 Documentation

Teaching record
  Instructional method used
  Outcome achievement or status

Postoperative: Collaborative Problems

Potential Complication: Acute Pulmonary Edema

Potential Complication: Mediastinal Shift

Potential Complication: Subcutaneous Emphysema

Potential Complication: Dysrhythmias

Nursing Goal

The nurse will detect early signs and symptoms of (a) increased pneumothorax, (b) pulmonary edema, (c) mediastinal shift, (d) subcutaneous emphysema, and (e) dysrhythmias and collaboratively intervene to stabilize client.

Indicators

- Alert, calm, oriented (a, b, c, d)
- Respirations 16–20 beats/min (a, b, c)
- Symmetrical easy, rhythmic respirations (a, b, c)
- Warm, dry skin (a, b, c)
- Breath sounds all lobes (a, b, c)
- No crackles or wheezing (a, b, c)
- Usual color (pinkish, brownish or olive skin tones) (a, b, c)
- Capillary refill < 3 sec (a, b, c)
- Oxygen saturation (PaO_2) > 94% (a, b, c)
- pH 7.35–7.45 (a, b, c)
- Carbon dioxide ($PaCO_2$) 35–45 mm Hg (a, b, c)
- Pulse 60–100 beats/min (a, b, c)
- BP > 90/60, < 140/90 mm Hg (a, b, c)
- Peripheral pulses equal full (a, b, c)
- Pulmonary artery pressure 25/9 mmHg (a, b, c)
- Central venous pressure 0–8 mmHg (a, b, c)
- Normal EKG (e)
- Larynx/trachea midline (c)
- No neck vein distention (c)
- Minimal subcutaneous air (d)

Interventions	Rationales
1. Maintain a closed intact chest drainage system. Inspect hourly during first 24 hours.	1. Malfunction or disconnection of the chest drainage system will cause air to enter pleural system, resulting in pneumothorax.
2. Monitor for malfunction of system and report signs and symptoms immediately: • No fluctuation in water seal chamber • Respiratory distress (excessive bubbling in water seal chamber) • Subcutaneous air under skin (e.g., neck, chest, face)	2. Malfunction of the chest drainage system causes air accumulation in the pleural space, compromising respirations and forcing air into the subcutaneous tissue (subcutaneous emphysema).
3. If a tube disconnects, reattach or place end under water as the person exhales. Do not clamp tube. Notify surgeon and plan for a stat chest x-ray.	3. Exhalation prior to reconnection will force excess air from pleural space. Clamping the tube can cause a tension pneumothorax.
4. Assess chest tube insertion site every 2 hours: a. Evidence of bleeding b. Intact occlusive dressing c. Correct position of chest tubes	4. a. Recent bleeding can be detected early. b. An occlusive dressing is needed to prevent air from entering pleural space. c. Improper positioning of tubes can increase air and drainage in pleural space.
5. Position tubing with excess tubing coiled on bed. Drain fluid in coiled tubing in collection device.	5. Proper positioning will promote drainage. Coiling the tubing can prevent accidental disconnection.
6. Every 2 hours, turn off suction and observe fluctuation of water level during respirations (tidalling).	6. Tidalling indicates an air tight drainage system. When lung expansion is complete, tidalling is not present.
7. Document amount, consistency, and color of chest tube drainage every hour according to protocol. Notify surgeon if drainage increases.	7. Increased drainage can indicate bleeding: no drainage can indicate a non-patent tube that can cause an increase in intrapleural pressure.
8. Prior to removal of chest tubes (3 to 4 days post-op), assess for absence of chest tube drainage, no tidalling with respirations, and breath sounds in affected area.	8. These clinical findings indicate lung reexpansion.
9. Assist surgeon to remove tubes. a. Medicate prior (½ to 1 hour) to removal per order.	9. a. This will reduce the pain of removal.

(continues on page 888)

Interventions continued	**Rationales** continued
b. Position in high-Fowler's. c. Instruct client to take a deep breath and cough. d. Apply an occlusive dressing.	b–c. High-Fowler's position and a deep breath provide for maximum lung expansion and positive intrapleural pressure d. An occlusive dressing is needed to prevent air leaks and infection.

10. After tube removal, evaluate respiratory status:
  a. No distress
  b. Breath sounds present in all lobes
  c. Even chest movement
  d. Calm
  e. No dysrhythmias
	10. Complications after tube removal can be pneumothorax, hemothorax. or mediastinal shift. Early changes in respiratory or cardiac function can prevent serious complications.

11. Instruct client to use spirometer three to four times an hour.	11. Frequent use of spirometer increases lung volumes and prevents pneumonia.
12. Monitor vital signs, pulse oximetry, pulmonary artery catheter readings, and arterial blood gases according to protocol.	12. Careful monitoring can detect early signs and symptoms of hypoxia.
13. Monitor respiratory function (rate, rhythm, capillary refill, breath sounds, skin color).	13. Frequent respiratory assessments are needed to evaluate early signs and symptoms of atelectasis, pneumothorax, and hemothorax
14. Provide oxygen and position in semi-Fowlers or full-Fowlers.	14. Semi-Fowler position aids in lung expansion. Oxygen may be needed until lungs are fully reexpanded.

15. Monitor for signs of acute pulmonary edema.
  a. Severe dyspnea
  b. Tachycardia
  c. Adventitious breath sounds
  d. Persistent cough
  e. Productive cough of frothy sputum
  f. Cyanosis
	15. Circulatory overload can result from the reduced size of the pulmonary vascular bed caused by removal of pulmonary tissue and the yet-unexpanded lung postoperatively. Hypoxia produces increased capillary permeability, causing fluid to enter pulmonary tissue and triggering signs and symptoms.

16. Cautiously administer IV fluids.	16. Caution is needed to prevent circulatory overload.
17. Encourage and assist client to get adequate rest and conserve strength.	17. Rest reduces oxygen consumption and decreases hypoxia.

(continues on page 889)

Interventions continued	**Rationales** continued

18. Monitor for signs of mediastinal shift.
   a. Increased weak, irregular pulse rate
   b. Severe dyspnea cyanosis and hypoxia
   c. Increased restlessness and agitation
   d. Deviation of larynx or trachea from midline
   e. Shift in the point of apical impulse
   f. Hypotension
   g. Asymmetric chest excursion
   h. Neck vein distention
	18. Increased intrapleural pressure on the operative side from fluid and air accumulations or excessive negative pressure on the operative side from inadequate fluid accumulation provides a space for the contents of the mediastinum (heart, trachea, esophagus, pulmonary vessels) to shift. Constriction of vessels (aorta, vena cava) creates hypoxia and its resultant signs and symptoms (Thelan et al., 1998).

19. If signs and symptoms of a mediastinal shift occur, do the following:
   a. Position client in a semi-Fowler's position.
   b. Maintain oxygen therapy.
   c. Assist client to clear present chest tube or reinsert a new one.
	19.
	   a. Sitting upright reduces mediastinal shifting.
	   b. Oxygen therapy reduces hypoxia.
	   c. The treatment of choice is insertion of a thoracic chest tube to release elevated intrapleural pressure (Thelan et al., 1998).

20. Monitor status of subcutaneous emphysema.
 	
   a. Mark periphery of the emphysematous tissue with a skin-marking pencil; reevaluate frequently.
   b. Monitor for neck involvement.
	20. Subcutaneous emphysema can occur after thoracic surgery as air leaks out of incised pulmonary tissue.
	   a. Serial markings help nurse to evaluate the rate of progression.
	
	   b. Severe subcutaneous emphysema can indicate air leakage through the bronchial stump and can compress the trachea.

21. If subcutaneous emphysema worsens, check patency of chest drainage system and notify surgeon.	21. Some subcutaneous emphysema may be present. Severe manifestations need to be corrected.
22. Monitor for cardiac dysrhythmias. Report any changes immediately and initiate protocol.	22. Decreased oxygen to myocardium causes cardiac dysrhythmias.

❤ Related Physician-Prescribed Interventions

Medications. Bronchodilators, opioids, expectorants, local anesthetics, narcotic, nonsteroidal anti-inflammatory

Intravenous Therapy. Refer to the General Surgery Care Plan

Laboratory Studies. Arterial blood gas analysis; also refer to the General Surgery Care Plan

Diagnostic Studies. Chest x-ray film, pulmonary function studies, fiberoptic bronchoscopy, computed tomography (CT) scan, continuous pulse oximetry, sputum cytology, fine-needle aspiration, gallium scan, MRI, pulse oximetry, pulmonary artery pressure monitoring, central venous pressure monitoring, central venous pressure monitoring

Therapies. Intermittent positive-pressure breathing (IPPB) treatments, chest drainage system, patient-controlled analgesia, chest physiotherapy, epidural analgesia, antiembolism devices, chemotherapy, radiation

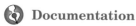 **Documentation**

Flow records
  Vital signs
  Intake and output records

Postoperative: Nursing Diagnoses

Ineffective Airway Clearance Related to Increased Secretions and Diminished Cough Secondary to Pain and Fatigue

Focus Assessment Criteria	Clinical Significance
1. Breath sounds (before and after coughing exercises)	1. Assessing breath sounds before then after coughing helps nurse to evaluate effectiveness of client's coughing effort.
2. Pain level	2. Pain can interfere with effective coughing.

Goal

The client will demonstrate adequate oxygen and ventilation.

Indicators

• Demonstrate effective coughing and increased air exchange.
• Explain rationale for interventions.

Interventions	Rationales
1. Teach client to sit as erect as possible; use pillows for support if needed.	1. Slouching and cramping positions of the thorax and abdomen interfere with air exchange.
2. Teach client the proper method of controlled coughing: a. Breathe deeply and slowly every 1 to 2 hours while sitting up as high as possible. b. Use diaphragmatic breathing. Hold breath for 3 to 5 seconds then slowly exhale as much as possible through the mouth. (The lower rib cage and abdomen should sink down.) c. Take a second breath, hold, and cough forcefully from the chest (not from the back of the mouth or throat) using two	2. Deep breathing dilates the airways, stimulates surfactant production, and expands the lung tissue surface; this improves respiratory gas exchange. Coughing loosens secretions and forces them into the bronchus to be expectorated or suctioned. In some clients, "huffing" breathing may be effective and is less painful.

(continues on page 891)

Interventions continued	**Rationales** continued
short, forceful coughs. Splint the chest with hands or pillow. Check any tube connections. d. If indicated, use the "huffing" breathing technique as taught preoperatively. e. Use spirometer three to four times per hour.	
3. Assess lung fields before and after coughing exercises.	3. Comparison assessments help to evaluate the effectiveness of coughing.
4. If breath sounds are moist-sounding, instruct client to rest briefly then repeat the exercises.	4. Rales indicate trapped secretions.
5. Assess the current analgesic regimen: a. Administer pain medication as needed. b. Assess its effectiveness: Is the client still in pain? If not, is he or she too lethargic? c. Note times when client seems to obtain the best pain relief with an optimal level of alertness and physical ability. This is the time to initiate breathing and coughing exercises.	5. Pain or fear of pain can inhibit participation in coughing and breathing exercises. Adequate pain relief is essential.
6. Provide emotional support: a. Stay with client for the entire coughing session. b. Explain the importance of coughing after pain relief is obtained. c. Reassure client that the suture lines are secure and that splinting by hand or pillow will minimize pain on movement.	6. Coughing exercises are fatiguing and painful. Emotional support provides encouragement; warm water can aid relaxation.
7. Maintain adequate hydration and humidity of inspired air.	7. These measures help to decrease viscosity of secretions. Tenacious secretions are difficult to mobilize and expectorate.
8. Move client out of bed to chair on postoperative day 1 and begin ambulation as soon as possible.	8. Early ambulation promotes aeration and can help to minimize pulmonary complications.
9. Provide motivation and plan strategies to avoid overexertion: a. Plan and bargain for adequate rest periods (e.g., "Work hard now, then I'll let you rest.").	9. The client's cooperation enhances the exercises' effectiveness.

(continues on page 892)

Interventions continued	Rationales continued
b. Vigorously coach and encourage coughing; use positive reinforcement. c. Plan coughing sessions for periods when client is alert and obtaining optimal pain relief. d. Allow for rest after coughing sessions and before meals.	
10. Evaluate the need for tracheobronchial suctioning.	10. Suctioning will be needed if client is unable to cough effectively (Thelan et al., 1998).

Documentation

Flow records
   Auscultation findings (before and after coughing exercises)
Progress notes
   Effectiveness of coughing
Teaching records
   Client teaching

Impaired Physical Mobility Related to Restricted Arm and Shoulder Movement Secondary to Pain and Muscle Dissection and Imposed Position Restrictions

Focus Assessment Criteria	Clinical Significance
1. ROM of arm and shoulder	1. Surgical resection reduces the ability to move arm and shoulder actively.
2. Tolerance to repositioning	2. Certain positions may compromise diaphragmatic movements.

Goal

The client will return or progress to preoperative arm and shoulder function.

Indicators

- Demonstrate knowledge of the need to maintain certain positions.
- Demonstrate ROM exercises.

Interventions	Rationales
1. Position client as indicated or prescribed: a. Supine position until consciousness is regained b. Semi-Fowler's position (30 to 45 degrees) thereafter	1. a. The supine position prevents aspiration. b. This position allows the diaphragm to resume its normal position, which reduces the effort of respiration (Thelan et al., 1998).

(continues on page 893)

Interventions continued	**Rationales** continued
2. Explain the need for frequent turning. Gently turn client from side to side every 1 to 2 hours unless contraindicated. Check with thoracic surgeon or institutional procedural manual.	2. Turning mobilizes drainage of secretions, promotes circulation, inhibits thrombus formation and aerates all parts of the remaining lung tissue. Lying on the operative side can be contraindicated following a wedge resection and pneumonectomy (Thelan et al., 1998).
3. Avoid extreme lateral turning following a pneumonectomy.	3. This can cause a mediastinal shift (refer to Potential Complication: Mediastinal Shift in this entry for more information).
4. Avoid traction on chest tubes during movement; check for kinks after repositioning.	4. Traction can cause dislodgment; kinks can inhibit drainage or negative pressure.
5. Explain the need for frequent exercises of arms, shoulders, and trunk even in the presence of some pain and discomfort.	5. The muscle groups transcended by a thoracotomy form the shoulder girdle and maintain the trunk's posture. Failure to perform exercises can result in muscle adhesions, contractures, and postural deformities.
6. Initiate passive ROM exercises on the operative arm and shoulder within 4 hours after recovery from anesthesia. Begin with two times every 4 hours for the first 24 hours; progress to 10 to 20 times every 2 hours.	6. Passive ROM exercises help to prevent ankylosis of shoulder and contractures of arm (Thelan et al., 1998).
7. Consult with physical therapist for active ROM exercises for client to perform starting 1 to 2 days after surgery: a. Hyperextending the arms to strengthen the latissimus dorsi b. Adducting and forward flexing the arms and shoulders to maintain shoulder girdle motion c. Adducting the scapula to strengthen the trapezius	7. Active ROM exercises help to prevent adhesions of two incised muscle layers.
8. Encourage use of the affected arm in ADLs and stress the need to continue exercises at home.	8. Regular use increases ROM and decreases contractures and shift (refer to Potential Complication: Mediastinal Shift in this entry for more information).

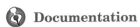 **Documentation**

Progress notes
    Limitations on performing activities
    Therapeutic exercises performed

Flow records
  Turning, positioning
Discharge summary record
  Client teaching
  Response to teaching

Acute Pain Related to Surgical Incision, Chest Tube Sites, and Immobility Secondary to Lengthy Surgery

Focus Assessment Criteria	Clinical Significance
1. Nature, location, quality, and intensity of pain. Use a rating scale to evaluate intensity.	1. A rating scale provides an objective means of evaluating pain.
2. Physical, physiologic, and behavioral signs of pain (i.e., restlessness; perspiration, elevated BP, heart rate, grimacing, and guarding)	2. Objective signs alert nurse to client's pain level.
3. Factors that influence pain tolerance (see Appendix II)	

Goal

The client will report satisfactory relief after pain relief interventions.

Indicators

- Verbalize or demonstrate behaviors that indicate improved level of comfort.
- Demonstrate knowledge of measures to decrease pain or cope appropriately with the pain.

Interventions	Rationales
1. Work with client, physician, and family to develop a pain management plan. To alleviate fears and clarify misconceptions, communicate openly about pain relief measures.	1. Collaboration and client involvement in the pain management plan help to minimize fears and feelings of loss of control.

2. Provide optimal pain relief with prescribed analgesia. See General Surgery Care Plan.
  a. Determine client's ability to tolerate epidural analgesia and ability to comply with PCA therapy. Consult physician if appropriate.
  b. Assess client's level of sedation, pain, and motor responses every 1 to 2 hours for 24 to 48 hours then every 40 hours for duration of pain therapy. Use pain scale (0 to 10).
  c. Assess client on a regular basis for the following signs and symptoms:
    • Respiratory depression
    • Motor blocks
	2. The proper administration rate optimizes the efficacy of pain medications.
	  a. Pain after thoracic surgery initially is best managed with epidural analgesia, with a change to PCA after 2 to 3 days (AHCPR, 1992).
	  b. Frequent assessment and use of pain scale will provide nurse with objective data that can be used to prevent potential complications and allow appropriate intervention.
	  c. There are multiple potential risks of epidural and PCA analgesia using opioids and local anesthetics listed.

(continues on page 895)

Interventions continued	Rationales continued
• Change in level of consciousness • Pruritus • Nausea and vomiting • Dysphoria • Urinary retention d. Keep intravenous naloxone at the bedside at all times.	d. Narcotics can depress the brain's respiratory center. IV naloxone can quickly reverse these symptoms.
2. Explain and assist client with noninvasive and nonpharmacologic pain relief measures (see General Surgery Care Plan).	2. Music, imagery, relaxation and other nonpharmacologic approaches have all shown effectiveness in reducing pain.
3. Provide a comfortable environment. Close door, pull curtains, dim lights, and so forth.	3. Privacy and a comfortable environment allow client to express pain in his or her own manner; this can help to reduce anxiety and pain.

Risk for Ineffective Therapeutic Regimen Management Related to Insufficient Knowledge of Activity Restrictions, Wound Care, Shoulder Exercises Signs and Symptoms of Complications and Follow-care

Focus Assessment	Clinical Significance
1. Readiness to learn and ability to learn and retain information	1. A client and/or family failing to achieve learning goals requires a referral for assistance post discharge.

Goals

The goals for this diagnosis represents those associated with the discharge planning. Refer to discharge criteria.

Interventions	Rationales
1. Explain restrictions a. Avoid heavy lifting or moving heavy items for 3 to 6 months. b. Avoid excessive fatigue. c. Avoid crowds and bronchial irritants (smoke, fumes, aerosol sprays).	1. a. Heavy lifting can increase tension on incision, which can prolong healing. b. Fatigue can prolong the healing process. c. Attempts should be made to prevent infection and irritations.
2. Practice breathing exercises and shoulder exercises (refer to Impaired Physical	2. These will prevent complications of contractures, pneumonia, and atelectasis.

(continues on page 896)

Interventions continued	Rationales continued
Mobility and Ineffective Airway Clearance for specifics). Provide written exercise instructions.	
3. Apply local/heat to intracostal region. Use analgesics as needed.	3. All attempts to relieve pain are needed to promote mobility and exercises.

4. Report to surgeon
  a. Chest pain
  b. Increasing shortness of breath
  c. Increasing fatigue
  d. Fever, chills
  e. Drainage from wound
  f. Increasing pain
	4. These signs and symptoms can indicate infection, bleeding and/or respiratory insufficiency.

5. Provide information on community resources (e.g., American Lung Association, American Cancer Association, smoking cessation programs, support groups, home health agencies, Meals-On-Wheels) and follow-up plan.	5. Client and/or family may need assistance after discharge.

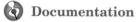 **Documentation**

Discharge summary record
    Client teaching
    Outcome achievement or status
    Referrals (e.g., PT)
Progress notes
    Exercises done

TOTAL JOINT REPLACEMENT (HIP, KNEE, SHOULDER)

Joint replacement (arthroplasty) is the surgical replacement of all or part of a joint. This surgery is indicated for irreversible damaged joints caused by degenerative or rheumatoid arthritis, fractures of hip or femoral neck with avascular necrosis, trauma, and congenital deformity.

For hip replacements, a ball and socket prosthesis is implanted with cement or uncemented. Uncemented prostheses have porous surfaces that allow the person's bone to grow into and stabilize the prosthesis.

For knee joint replacements, the prosthesis is a tricompartmental prosthesis with femoral, tibial, and patellar components. As with hip prostheses, the knee prosthesis can be cemented or uncemented.

 Time Frame

Preoperative and postoperative periods

⊙⊙ DIAGNOSTIC CLUSTER

Preoperative Period	**Refer to**
Nursing Diagnoses	
▲ Anxiety related to scheduled surgery and lack of knowledge of preoperative and postoperative routines, postoperative sensations, and use of assistive devices	Fractured Hip and Femur
Postoperative Period	
Collaborative Problems	
▲ PC: Hemorrhage/Hematoma Formation	
▲ PC: Dislocation/Subluxation of Joint	
▲ PC: Neurovascular Compromise	
▲ PC: Fat Emboli	Fractured Hip and Femur
▲ PC: Sepsis	Fractured Hip and Femur
▲ PC: Thromboemboli	Fractured Hip and Femur

Nursing Diagnoses	**Refer to**
▲ Impaired Physical Mobility related to pain, stiffness, fatigue, restrictive equipment, and prescribed activity restrictions	
▲ High Risk for Impaired Skin Integrity related to pressure and decreased mobility secondary to pain and temporary restrictions	

(continues on page 898)

Nursing Diagnoses continued	**Refer to** continued
△ High Risk for Ineffective Therapeutic Regimen Management related to insufficient knowledge of activity restrictions, use of assistive devices, signs of complications, and follow-up care	Amputation
▲ High Risk for Injury related to altered gait and use of assistive devices	Amputation

Related Care Plans

General Surgery Generic Care Plan
Anticoagulant Therapy

▲ This diagnosis was reported to be monitored for or managed frequently (75%–100%).
△ This diagnosis was reported to be monitored for or managed often (50%–74%).

Discharge Criteria

Before discharge, the client and family will

1. Describe activity restrictions.
2. Describe a plan for resuming ADLs.
3. Regain mobility while adhering to weightbearing restrictions.
4. State signs and symptoms that must be reported to a health care professional.

Postoperative: Collaborative Problems

Potential Complication: Hemorrhage

Potential Complication: Dislocation of Joint (Hip, Knee)

Potential Complication: Neurovascular Compromise

Nursing Goal

The nurse will detect early signs and symptoms of (a) hemorrhage/hematoma, (b) dislocation (hip, knee), and (c) neurovascular compromise and will collaboratively intervene to stabilize the client.

Indicators
- Alert, oriented, calm (a)
- Pulse 60–100 beats/min (a)
- Respirations 16–20 breaths/min (a)
- BP >90/60, <140/90 mm Hg (a)
- Capillary refill <3 sec (a, c)
- Peripheral pulses full, bilateral (a, c)
- Warm, dry skin, no blanching (a, c)
- Urine output >30 mL/hr (a)
- Hip in abduction or neutral rotation (b)
- Legs length even (b)
- Knee in neutral position (b)
- No c/o tingling, numbness (c)

- Ability to move toes (c)
- Oxygen saturation > 94% (a)
- Hemoglobin (a)
  - Male 13–18 gm/dL
  - Female 12–16 gm/dL
- Hematocrit (a)
  - Male 42–50%
  - Female 40–48%

If on anticoagulant therapy:
- Partial thromboplastin time 1.5 times control (a)
- Prothrombin time 1.5–2× normal (a)
- International Normalized Ratio (INR) 2–3 (a)

Interventions	Rationales
1. Identify individuals at high risk for complications: a. History of cardiac problems b. Poor nutritional status c. Obesity d. Diabetes mellitus e. History of DVT or PE f. Blood dyscrasias g. Deconditioned state h. Older adults	1. Wound healing is compromised by diabetes mellitus, inadequate nutrition, obesity, and impaired oxygen transport. Older adults are most vulnerable to postoperative complications and mortality.
2. Monitor drainage from suction device every hour.	2. The hip is a very vascular area, and the use of anticoagulants creates a high risk for bleeding. Expect 200 to 500 mL in the first 24 hours reducing to approximately 50 mL in 48 hours.
3. Maintain pressure dressing and ice to surgical area as ordered.	3. Pressure can reduce bleeding at site and reduce hematoma formation.
4. Monitor for early signs and symptoms of bleeding and hypoxia: • Increased pulse • Increased respirations • Decreased oxygen saturation < 94% • Urinary output > 30 mL hr	4. Early signs and symptoms of bleeding and hypoxia can prompt rapid interventions to prevent hemorrhage.
5. Monitor for hematoma: a. Increased pain at site b. Tense swelling in buttock and thigh	5. Bleeding into the surgical area can cause hematoma formation.
6. Notify surgeon if signs of symptoms of bleeding and hypoxia occur.	6. Client may need to return to OR for repair of bleeding vessels.

(continues on page 900)

Interventions continued	**Rationales** continued

7. Identify individuals at high risk for joint implant infection:
  a. Chronic urinary tract infections
  b. GI infection
  c. Dental infection or poor detention
	7. Joint implants can be infected through hematogenous route anytime postoperatively or postdischarge (Altizer, 1998).

8. Determine whether or not antiinflammatory medications have been discontinued 7 to 10 days preoperatively.	8. Platelet function is inhibited by antiinflammatory medications (Altizer, 1998).

9. Maintain correct positioning.
  a. Hip: Maintain hip in abduction, neutral rotation, or slight external rotation.
  b. Hip: Avoid hip flexion over 60 degrees.
  c. Knee: Keep knees apart at all times and slightly elevated from hip; avoid gatching bed under knee or placing pillows under knee (to prevent flexion contractures); pillows should be placed under calf.
	9. Specific positions are used to prevent prosthesis dislocation.

10. Assess for signs of joint (hip, knee) dislocation.
  a. Hip:
   • Acute groin pain in operative hip
   • Shortening of leg and in external rotation
  b. Hip, knee:
   • "Popping" sound heard by patient
   • Inability to move
   • Bulge at surgical site
	10. Until the surrounding muscles and joint capsule heal, joint dislocation may occur if positioning exceeds the limits of the prosthesis, such as when flexing or hyperextending the knee or abducting the hip more than 45 degrees.

11. Maintain bed rest as ordered. Keep affected joint in a neutral position with rolls, pillows, or specified devices.	11. Bed rest typically is ordered for 1 to 3 days after surgery to allow stabilization of the prosthesis.
12. Client may be turned toward either side unless contraindicated by physician. Always maintain abduction pillow when turning; limit use of Fowler's position.	12. If proper positioning is maintained including the abduction pillow, client may safely be turned toward operative and nonoperative sides. This promotes circulation and decreases the potential for pressure ulcer formation as a result of immobility. Prolonged Fowler's position can dislocate the prosthesis (Salmond, 1996).
13. Monitor for signs and symptoms of neurovascular compromise; compare findings with the unaffected limb.	13.

(continues on page 901)

Interventions continued	Rationales continued
a. Diminished or absent pedal pulses	a. Surgical trauma causes swelling and edema that can compromise circulation and compress nerves.
b. Capillary refill time >3 seconds	b. Prolonged capillary refill time points to diminished capillary perfusion.
c. Pallor, blanching, cyanosis, coolness of extremity	c. These signs may indicate compromised circulation.
d. Complaints of abnormal sensations (e.g., tingling and numbness)	d. These symptoms may result from nerve compression.
e. Increasing pain not controlled by medication	e. Tissue and nerve ischemia produces a deep, throbbing, unrelenting pain.
14. Instruct client to report numbness, tingling, coolness, or change in skin color.	14. Early detection of neurovascular compromise enables prompt intervention to prevent serious complications.
15. Use elastic stockings or sequential compression device as prescribed. Refer to Index—Thrombophlebitis for more interventions.	15. These aid in venous blood return and prevent stasis.

 Related Physician-Prescribed Interventions

Medications. Anticoagulants (e.g., low-molecular-weight heparin, warfarin)

Intravenous Therapy. Refer to the General Surgery Care Plan

Laboratory Studies. Coagulant studies (PT, PTT, INR); also refer to the General Surgery Care Plan, Appendix II

Diagnostic Studies. X-ray films, bone scans, MRI, CT scan

Therapies. Antiembolic hose, sequential compression devices, continuous passive motion machines, patient-controlled analgesia

 Documentation

Flow records
  Positioning
  Peripheral circulation status

Postoperative: Nursing Diagnoses

Impaired Physical Mobility Related to Pain, Stiffness, Fatigue, Restrictive Equipment, and Prescribed Activity Restrictions

Focus Assessment Criteria	Clinical Significance
1. Endurance level 2. Mobility	1,2. Pain and limited range of motion affect mobility. The client, particularly if elderly, may have a chronic disease that affects endurance.

Goal

The client will increase activity to a level consistent with abilities.

Indicators

- Demonstrate exercises.
- Report importance of continuing exercises at home.

Interventions	Rationales
1. Support an exercise program tailored to client's ability; consult with physical therapist. a. For hip: Quadriceps and gluteal settings, plantar flexion of foot, and leg lifts b. For knee: Quadriceps setting, isometrics, and leg lifts	1. Exercises are needed to improve circulation and strengthen muscle groups needed for ambulation.
2. Develop a plan for ROM exercise at regular intervals, increasing the use of involved extremity as ordered.	2. Active ROM increases muscle mass, tone, and strength and improves cardiac and respiratory functioning.
3. Collaborate with physical medicine and rehabilitation in teaching body mechanics and transfer techniques. Ensure proper body alignment.	3. Proper mechanics and alignment help to prevent dislocation of the prosthesis.
4. Encourage client's independence and reward progress. Include client in care planning and contracting.	4. Client's participation in decision-making about care increases self-esteem and can encourage compliance.
5. Schedule progressive and paced activities as appropriate. Consult with physical therapist for weightbearing regimen.	5. The amount of weightbearing depends on the type of prosthesis used and on client's condition and abilities.
6. Reinforce use of ambulatory aids as taught by physical therapy and supervise client ambulation as necessary.	6. Such devices must be used correctly and safely to ensure effectiveness and prevent injury.

 Documentation

Progress notes
  Activity level
  Response to activity

High Risk for Impaired Skin Integrity Related to Pressure and Decreased Mobility Secondary to Pain and Temporary Restrictions

Focus Assessment Criteria	Clinical Significance
1. Skin and circulation 2. Hydration and nutrition status 3. Ability to change positions	1–3. This assessment determines skin condition and identifies risk factors that contribute to pressure ulcer development.

Goal

The client will maintain intact skin.

Indicators

- Shift position every hour.
- Describe strategies to prevent pressure ulcers.

Interventions	Rationales
1. Use a pressure-relieving device (e.g., alternating mattress and heel protectors).	1. These and other devices can help to distribute pressure uniformly over skin surface.
2. Turn and reposition client every hour. Teach client ways to shift position in bed (e.g., lifting buttocks and legs) and to use overhead trapeze.	2. Frequent repositioning allows circulation to return to tissues where pressure has inhibited it.
3. Assess pressure points—shoulder blades, heels, elbow, sacrum, and hips—each shift.	3. Bony prominences are covered with minimal skin and subcutaneous fat and are more prone to skin breakdown from pressure.
4. Lightly massage bony prominences with lotion. Protect vulnerable areas with film dressings.	4. Light massage stimulates circulation. Film dressings provide more structure to prevent injury from shearing force.
5. Stress the importance of optimal nutritional intake and hydration.	5. Inadequate nutrition and hydration reduce circulation and increase tissue wasting.
6. Encourage ambulation as indicated.	6. Ambulation improves circulation and reduces pressure on vessels.
7. Avoid elevating head of bed more than 30 degrees and support feet with foot board.	7. These interventions prevent shear pressure that causes decreased capillary perfusion when feet are pinched as bony prominences slide across subcutaneous tissue.

 Documentation

Flow records
   Turning and repositioning
   Skin assessment

High Risk for Ineffective Therapeutic Regimen Management Related to Insufficient Knowledge of Activity Restrictions, Use of Assistive Devices, Signs of Complications, and Follow-up Care

Focus Assessment Criteria	Clinical Significance
1. Readiness and ability to learn and retain information	1. A client or family failing to achieve learning goals requires a referral for assistance post-discharge.

Goals

The goals for this diagnosis represent those associated with discharge planning. Refer to the discharge criteria.

Interventions	Rationales

1. Explain restrictions that typically include avoiding the following:
  a. Excessive bending and lifting
  b. Crossing the legs
  c. Jogging, jumping, and kneeling
	1. These activities can put great stress on the implant.

2. Explain the need to continue prescribed exercises at home.	2. Exercises increase muscle strength and joint mobility.
3. Teach wound care and assessment techniques.	3. Instructions are needed to prevent infection and to detect early signs of infection.
4. Reinforce and encourage the safe use of assistive devices and therapeutic aids. Request return demonstration of correct use.	4. Assistive devices may be needed. Return demonstration allows nurse to evaluate proper, safe use.
5. Explain the need to continue leg exercises (5 to 10 times an hour) and use of anti-embolic hose at home.	5. The risk of thrombophlebitis continues after discharge.

6. If continuous passive motion (CPM) will be used at home, teach client and family the following:
  a. Correct application and use of the CPM. Reinforce limited time of CPM to maintain motion.
  b. Signs and symptoms of potential complications:
    • Joint swelling, redness, tenderness
    • Unusual pain
    • Reappearance of drainage that previously had ceased
	6. Without properly learning CPM usage with daily reinforcement, client may not fully use the benefits of CPM and may predispose himself or herself for future postjoint arthroplasty complications (adhesions or decreased range of motion).

7. Initiate (CPM) for knee arthroplasty per protocol.
  a. Focus neurovascular assessment on extremity using CPM.
  b. Assess skin integrity of extremity in CPM (pressure points, heel, upper thigh, or elbow).
  c. Assess involved joint for increased drainage, swelling, tenderness, and condition of surgical incision.
	7. Passive motion has been shown to stimulate healing of articular cartilage and reduce potential for adhesion development. Continuous use is most effective to obtain and maintain desired degrees of flexion and extension (Salmond, 1996).
	  a–d. Thorough assessment of extremity using CPM is necessary to monitor for potential complications associated with CPM. As degrees of flexion are

(continues on page 905)

Interventions continued	Rationales continued
d. Assess level of pain while using CPM; intervene with appropriate analgesia.	increased on CPM, client may initially experience increased discomfort and may require analgesic intervention (Salmond, 1996).
8. Explain risk for infection: early, delayed, or late.	8. Early infection occurs during the first 3 months. Delayed infection occurs between 3 months and 1 year. Late infection occurs after 1 year.
9. Teach client to report signs and symptoms of complications. a. Increased temperature b. Red, swollen, draining incision c. Coolness of skin on affected limb or numbness d. Pain in calf or upper thigh	9. Early detection enables prompt interventions to prevent serious complications. a. Fever may indicate an infection or phlebitis. b. Incision changes may indicate infection. c. These signs indicate compromised circulation. d. Leg pain may point to thrombophlebitis.
10. If anticoagulants are prescribed, refer to the Anticoagulant Therapy Care Plan for specific interventions.	
11. Explain to client and family the importance of continuing therapy program at home for at least 6 to 12 months.	11. Clients with joint replacement should not be expected to regain full function for 6 to 12 months (Salmond, 1996).
12. Consult with community nursing service to prepare home and physical therapy environment for discharge.	12. Adaptations may be needed (e.g., commode, eliminate scatter rugs).

Documentation

Discharge summary record
   Client teaching
   Outcome achievement or status
Progress notes
   CPM usage
   Degree of flexion/extension

For a Clinical Pathway on Total Hip Replacement, visit http://connection.lww.com

UROSTOMY

Urinary diversions are performed to remove the bladder and divert urine from the ureters to a new exit site that is usually a stoma (opening in skin). This procedure is done for bladder tumors, pelvic tumors, birth defects, chronic infection causing renal damage, and intractable interstitial cystitis. The two types of urinary diversions are cutaneous and continent.

There are four types of continent urinary diversions: two involve the formation of a pouch in the ileum or small bowel. The third method modifies the Koch pouch to empty in the urethra, allowing for catheterization of the urethra. The fourth is a ureterosigmoidoscopy: the ureters are diverted into the sigmoid colon and urine flows out of the rectum.

In continent urinary diversion with an Indiana or Koch pouch, the ureters are diverted to a portion of the intestine, which creates a new reservoir (pouch) that holds at least 300 to 400 ml of urine. When a pouch is created, the urine is drained with a catheter. With cutaneous urinary diversion, an ileostomy bag is worn continuously. After the pouch heals, a catheter is inserted into the stoma to drain urine beginning every 2 hours and progressing to every 6 hours in 5 to 6 weeks.

 Time Frame

Preoperative and postoperative periods

 DIAGNOSTIC CLUSTER

Preoperative Period

Nursing Diagnoses

▲ Anxiety related to lack of knowledge of urostomy care and perceived negative effects on life style

Postoperative Period

Collaborative Problems

△ PC: Internal Urine Leakage
▲ PC: Urinary Tract Infection/Urinary Calculi/Peritonitis
▲ PC: Peristomal Ulceration/Herniation
▲ PC: Stomal Necrosis, Retraction, Prolapse, Stenosis, Obstruction

Nursing Diagnoses	Refer to
High Risk for Ineffective Sexuality Patterns related to erectile dysfunction (male) or inadequate vaginal lubrication (female)	
△ High Risk for Loneliness related to anxiety about possible odor and leakage from appliance	

(continues on page 907)

Nursing Diagnoses continued	Refer to continued
▲ High Risk for Ineffective Therapeutic Regimen Management related to insufficient knowledge of stoma pouching procedure, colostomy irrigation, peristomal skin care, perineal wound care, and incorporation of ostomy care into activity of daily living (ADL)	
△ High Risk for Ineffective Therapeutic Regimen Management related to insufficient knowledge of intermittent self-catheterization of continent urostomy	
△ High Risk for Disturbed Self-Concept related to effects of ostomy on body image	Ileostomy
High Risk for Ineffective Sexuality Patterns related to perceived negative impact of ostomy on sexual functioning and attractiveness	Ileostomy

Related Care Plan
General Surgery Generic Care Plan
Cancer: Initial Diagnosis

▲ This diagnosis was reported to be monitored for or managed frequently (75%–100%).
△ This diagnosis was reported to be monitored for or managed often (50%–74%).

Discharge Criteria

Before discharge, the client and family will

1. Describe routine ostomy care.
2. Demonstrate the proper stoma pouching procedure.
3. Identify measures to help maintain peristomal skin integrity.
4. Demonstrate intermittent self-catheterization.
5. State conditions of ostomy care at home: stoma, pouching, irrigation, skin care.
6. Discuss strategies for incorporating ostomy management into ADLs.
7. Verbalize precautions for medication use and fluid intake and prevention of UTI and stone formation.
8. State signs and symptoms that must be reported to a health care professional.
9. Verbalize an intent to share feelings and concerns related to ostomy with significant others.
10. Identify available community resources and self-help groups:
    a. Visiting nurse
    b. UOA
    c. Recovery of Male Potency; Help for Impotent Male
    d. American Cancer Foundation
    e. Community supplier of ostomy equipment
    f. Financial reimbursement for ostomy equipment

Preoperative Nursing Diagnoses

Anxiety Related to Lack of Knowledge of Urostomy Care and Perceived Negative Effects on Life Style

Focus Assessment Criteria	Clinical Significance
1. Understanding underlying disorder necessitating urinary diversion 2. Knowledge of structure and function of affected organs 3. Anticipated surgical procedure and stoma location 4. Previous exposure to a person with an ostomy 5. Familiarity with stoma pouching equipment 6. Emotional status, cognitive ability, memory, vision, manual dexterity 7. Life style, strengths, coping mechanisms, available support systems	1–7. Assessing client's knowledge of urinary diversion identifies learning needs and guides nurse in planning effective teaching strategies. Assessing client's emotional status, mental and physical abilities, and other relevant factors helps nurse to evaluate client's ability to accept, adjust to, and manage the ostomy and stoma.

Goal

The client will verbalize decreased anxiety related to fear of the unknown.

Indicators

- State reason for urostomy.
- Describe anatomic changes following urostomy surgery.
- Identify his or her own type of urostomy.

Interventions	Rationales
1. Identify and dispel any misinformation or misconceptions the client has regarding ostomy.	1. Replacing misinformation with facts can reduce anxiety (Schover, 1986).
2. Explain the normal anatomic structure and function of the genitourinary (GU) tract.	2. Knowledge increases confidence; confidence produces control and reduces anxiety.
3. Explain effects of client's particular disorder on affected organs.	3. Understanding the disorder can help the client accept the need for urostomy.
4. Use an anatomic diagram or model to show resultant altered route of elimination.	4. Understanding how urine elimination occurs after the diversion removal can help to allay anxiety related to altered body function.

(continues on page 909)

Interventions continued	Rationales continued
5. Describe appearance and anticipated location of stoma. Explain the following facts about the stoma: a. It will be the same color and moistness as oral mucous membrane. b. It will not hurt when touched because it has no sensory endings. c. It may bleed slightly when wiped; this is normal and not of concern. d. It will become smaller as the surgical area heals; color will remain the same. e. It may change in size depending on illness, hormone levels, and weight gain or loss.	5. Learning about expected events and sensations can help to reduce anxiety associated with the unknown and unexpected. Accurate descriptions of the stoma appearance help to ease shock at the first sight of it after ostomy surgery.
6. Discuss function of the stoma pouch. Explain that it serves as an external receptacle for storage of urine much as the bladder acts as an internal storage receptacle (Ewing, 1989; Lind & Hagan, 1997).	6. Understanding the purpose and need for a pouch encourages client to accept it and participate in ostomy management.
7. Encourage client to handle the stoma pouching equipment.	7. Many clients are relieved to see the actual size and material of a stoma pouch. Uninformed clients often envision large bags and complicated, difficult-to-manage equipment that can produce anxiety.

 Documentation

Progress notes
  Presence of dysfunctional anxiety
Teaching records
  Client teaching

Collaborative Problems

Potential Complication: Internal Urine Leakage

Potential Complication: Urinary Tract Infection/Urinary Calculi

Potential Complication: Peristomal Skin Ulceration

Potential Complication: Stomal Necrosis, Retraction, Prolapse, Stenosis, Obstruction

Nursing Goal

The nurse will detect early signs and symptoms of (a) internal urine leakage, (b) urinary tract infection/urinary calculi, peritonitis, (c) peristomal skin ulceration, and (d) stomal necrosis/retraction and will collaboratively intervene to stabilize client.

Indicators
- Temperature 98.5–99°F (a)
- Urinary output >30 mL/hr (a)
- Pulse 60–100 beats/min (b)
- BP >90/60, < 140/90 mm Hg (b)
- Respirations 16–20 breaths/min (b)
- Capillary refill < 3 sec (b)
- Oxygen saturation >94% (b)
- No sudden increase or decrease in drainage (a, b)
- Clear, light yellow urine (b)
- Urine pH 4.6–8.0 (b)
- No flank pain (b)
- No signs peristomal ulceration or herniation (d)
- No abdominal distension (d)
- No c/o nausea/vomiting (d)
- Stoma reducing in size with change in shape or color (d)

Interventions	Rationales
1. Monitor drainage amount and color every hour for first 24 hours from a. Incision b. Cecostomy catheter c. Urethral stents and bile catheters d. Stomal catheter e. Urethral catheter	1. A sudden decrease in urine flow may indicate obstruction (edema, mucus) or dehydration.
2. Irrigate cecostomy tube 2 to 3 times each day as prescribed.	2. Irrigation removes mucus to prevent blockage.
3. Report a sudden change in drainage (increased or decreased) or bleeding from stoma.	3. A change in drainage can indicate bleeding or infection (increased) or blockage (decreased).
4. Monitor every hour for the first 24 hours: a. Vital signs b. Capillary refill < 3 seconds c. Oxygen saturation (pulse oximetry) d. Urine output	4. Changes in vital signs (increased pulse, decreased BP, decreased urine output, decreased oxygen saturation, and increased capillary fill time) can indicate dehydration, bleeding, and/or hypoxia.
5. Monitor for signs of internal urine leakage. a. Abdominal distention with adynamic ileus b. Fever c. Elevated serum creatinine level d. Decreased urine output despite adequate hydration	5. Urine leakage either from the ureteroileal anastomosis or from the base of the conduit occurs in as many as 8% of clients with a urostomy. Leakage is confirmed through fluoroscopy. Small leaks may seal themselves with continuous drainage of the conduit via a stomal catheter.
6. Explain reason for cloudy urine.	6. Because the intestine produces mucus, mucus in the diversion will cause urine to appear cloudy (Early & Poquette, 2000).

(continues on page 911)

Interventions continued	Rationales continued

7. Monitor for signs and symptoms of urinary tract infection (Ewing, 1989).
   a. Fever
   b. Flank pain
   c. Malodorous, cloudy urine
   d. Alkaline urine pH
	7. Between 10% and 20% of clients with a urinary diversion develop pyelonephritis. The major cause is poor urine flow through the conduit, leading to urinary stasis and bacterial contamination through the stoma.

8. Consult with physician for a urine culture from a double lumen catheter specimen.	8. Cultures enable identification of the causative organism and guide pharmacological therapy.

9. Monitor for signs of peristomal ulceration or herniation.
   a. Decreased peristomal muscle tone
   b. Bulging beyond normal skin surface and musculature
   c. Persistent ulceration
	9. Early detection of ulcerations and herniation enables prompt intervention to prevent serious tissue damage.

10. Consult with clinical specialist or ostomy therapist regarding persistent ulceration.	10. Expert assistance may be needed for persistent skin problems.

11. Monitor for stomal necrosis, prolapse, retraction, stenosis, and obstruction. Assess the following:
   a. Color, size, and shape of stoma
 	
   b. Color and amount of urine from the urostomy or from each stent
 	
   c. Complaints of cramping abdominal pain, nausea and vomiting, abdominal distention
   d. Ostomy appliance and appliance belt fit
	11. Daily assessment is necessary to detect early changes in stoma condition.
	
	   a. Changes can indicate inflammation, retraction, prolapse, edema.
	   b. Changes can indicate bleeding or infection. Decreased output can indicate obstruction.
	   c. These complaints may indicate obstruction.
	
	   d. Improperly fitting appliance or belt can cause mechanical trauma to stoma.

✔ Related Physician-Prescribed Interventions

Medications. Refer to the General Surgery care plan.

Intravenous Therapy. Refer to the General Surgery care plan.

Laboratory Studies. Refer to the General Surgery care plan.

Diagnostic Studies. Intravenous pyelography, CT scan, cystoscopy, conduitogram, bone scan, endoscopy, flow cytometry, pouchogram

Therapies. Sitz baths, urinary diversion collection appliances

Documentation

Flow records
   Vital signs
   Intake and output
   Abdomen (girth, bowel sounds)
   Condition of peristomal area

Postoperative: Nursing Diagnoses

High Risk for Ineffective Sexuality Patterns Related to Erectile Dysfunction (Male) or Inadequate Vaginal Lubrication (Female)

Focus Assessment Criteria	Clinical Significance

1. Knowledge of the effects of surgery on sexual function:
  a. After radical cystectomy, penile sensation and the man's ability to reach orgasm remain intact. However, semen production ceases because the prostate, seminal vesicles, and proximal vas deferens are removed with the bladder.
  b. In women, satisfactory intercourse after radical cystectomy depends on vaginal preservation. Surgery typically involves removing the bladder, ovaries, fallopian tubes, uterus, cervix, and the anterior one-third to one-half of the vagina. The surgeon may rebuild the vagina; a common problem in a client with a rebuilt vagina is dyspareunia related to vaginal tightness and lack of lubrication.
	1. Assessing client's knowledge of possible effects on sexual function guides nurse in planning effective interventions.

Goal

The client will state the intent to discuss sexual concerns with partner after discharge.

Indicators
- Describe the possible effects of urostomy surgery on sexual function.
- Identify available community resources if necessary.

Interventions	Rationales

1. In men (Ofman, 1993)
  a. Suggest that sexual activity need not always culminate in vaginal intercourse and that orgasm can be reached through noncoital manual or oral stimulation. Remind client that sexual expression is not limited to intercourse but includes closeness, communication, touching, and giving and receiving pleasure.
  b. Explain the function of a penile prosthesis. Both semirigid and inflatable penile prostheses have a high rate of success.
  c. Suggest counseling with a certified sex therapist.
	1.
	  a. Alternative methods of sexual expression and gratification promote positive sexual function.
	
	  b. Penile implants provide the erection needed for intercourse and do not alter sensations or the ability to ejaculate.
	
	  c. Certain sexual problems require continuing therapy and the advanced knowledge of therapists.

(continues on page 913)

Interventions continued	Rationales continued

2. In women (Ofman, 1993)
  a. Suggest using a water-based vaginal lubricant for intercourse.
 	
  b. Teach client to perform Kegel exercises and instruct her to do them regularly.
 	
  c. Suggest that she sit astride her partner during intercourse.
	2.
	  a. Water-based lubricant can help to prevent dyspareunia related to inadequate vaginal lubrication.
	  b. Kegel exercises promote control of pubococcygeal muscles around the vaginal entrance; this can ease dyspareunia.
	  c. A woman on top can control the depth and rate of penetration; this can enhance vaginal lubrication and relaxation.

Documentation

Progress notes
  Interventions
  Response to interventions

High Risk for Loneliness Related to Anxiety About Possible Odor and Leakage from Appliance

Focus Assessment Criteria	Clinical Significance
1. Preoperative socialization pattern 2. Anticipated changes	1,2. A client at risk for social isolation must be assessed carefully; the suffering associated with isolation is not always visible. Feelings of rejection and repulsion are common.

Goal

The client will state the intent to reestablish preoperative socialization pattern.

Indicators
- Discuss methods to control odor and appliance leakage.
- State the intent to dialogue with other persons in the same situation.

Interventions	Rationales
1. Select an appropriate odorproof pouching system; explain to the client how it works.	1. Fear of accidents and odor can be reduced through effective management. Some pouches have charcoal filters to reduce urine odor.
2. Stress the need for good personal hygiene. 3. Teach client the care of a reusable appliance.	2,3. Proper hygiene and appliance care remove odoriferous retained urine.
4. Discuss methods for reducing odor.	4. Minimizing odor improves self-confidence and can permit more effective socialization.

(continues on page 914)

Interventions continued	Rationales continued
a. Avoid odor-producing foods such as asparagus and cabbage. b. Drink cranberry juice or use a liquid appliance deodorant. c. Empty or change the ostomy pouch regularly when one-third to one-half full.	Bacterial proliferation in retained urine increases odor over time. A full pouch also puts excessive pressure on seals, increasing the risk of leakage.
5. Encourage client to reestablish his or her preoperative socialization pattern. Help with measures such as progressively increasing client's socializing time in the hospital, role-playing possible situations that client feels may cause anxiety, and encouraging client to visualize and anticipate solutions to "worst-case scenarios" for social situations.	5. Encouraging and facilitating socialization helps to prevent isolation. Role-playing can help client identify and learn to cope with potential anxiety-causing situations in a nonthreatening environment.
6. Suggest that client meet with a person from the United Ostomy Association who can share similar experiences (Maklebust, 1985; Smith, 1992).	6. Others in a similar situation can provide a realistic appraisal of the situation and may provide information to answer client's unasked questions.

 Documentation

Progress notes
    Dialogues and interactions
Teaching record
    Client teaching

High Risk for Ineffective Therapeutic Regimen Management Related to Insufficient Knowledge of Stoma Pouching Procedure, Peristomal Skin Care, Perineal Wound Care and Incorporation of Ostomy Care into Activities of Daily Living (ADLs)

Focus Assessment Criteria	Clinical Significance
1. Type of urostomy	1. Urostomy care differs according to its type and concurrent therapies.
2. Knowledge of urostomy care: fluid intake, activity, hygiene, clothing, sexual expression, community resources, employment, travel, odor, skin care, appliances	2. Assessment identifies learning needs and guides nurse in planning effective teaching strategies.
3. Client's and support person's readiness and ability to learn and retain information	3. A family or client failing to achieve learning goals requires a referral for assistance post-discharge.

Goals

The goals for this diagnosis represent those associated with discharge planning. Refer to the discharge criteria.

Interventions	Rationales

1. Teach client the basic stoma pouching principles.
  a. Keeping peristomal skin clean and dry
 	
  b. Using a well-fitting antireflux appliance
 	
  c. Changing the pouch when the least amount of drainage is anticipated (usually on arising)
  d. Emptying the pouch when it is one-third to one-half full and changing routinely before a leak occurs
  e. Changing the pouch if pain or wetness occurs under the appliance
 	
  f. Observing condition of the stoma and peristomal skin during pouch changes
	1. Proper pouching techniques can prevent leakage and skin problems.
	  a. This ensures that appliance adheres to skin.
	  b. Proper fit protects surrounding skin surface from contact with drainage.
	  c. This prevents copious drainage from interfering with pouch changes.
	
	  d. A pouch filled more than halfway exerts increased pressure on the seal, which increases risk of leakage.
	  e. Pain or wetness may indicate that urine has undermined the skin barrier; prompt intervention is necessary to prevent skin breakdown.
	  f. Regular observation enables early detection of skin problems.

2. Teach client the procedure for preparing a stoma pouch.
  a. Select the appropriate stoma pouching system; avoid Karaya gum and pectin-based skin barriers.
    For urinary stomas, faceplates with convexity will lengthen wear time of the pouching system.
  b. Measure stoma carefully.
  c. Use appliance manufacturer's stoma measuring card if possible. If the card does not accommodate stoma size or shape, teach client to make a customized stoma pattern: Place clear plastic wrap from the skin barrier wafer over the stoma, trace the stoma with a marking pen, and cut a hole in the plastic to accommodate the stoma.
  d. Use this pattern to trace the opening onto the reverse side of a skin barrier wafer.
  e. Cut an opening in the center of the skin barrier slightly larger than the stoma (approximately 1/8 inch).
  f. Secure an appropriate antireflux pouch onto the skin barrier wafer (if using a two-piece appliance system). The pouch should have an antireflux valve to prevent urine from bathing the stoma.
	2. Preparing a new pouch beforehand ensures that the new pouch is ready to apply as soon as the used pouch is removed; this helps to minimize drainage on skin surface.

(continues on page 916)

Interventions continued	**Rationales** continued
3. Teach client the procedure for changing a disposable stoma pouch. a. Remove the old pouch by gently pushing the skin away from the paper tape and skin barrier wafer. b. Fold the old pouch over on itself and discard in a plastic bag. c. Hold gauze or toilet paper over the stoma. d. Cleanse peristomal skin with a wash cloth and warm tap water. e. Blot or pat skin dry. f. Apply new pouch to abdomen, carefully centering the hole in the skin barrier wafer over the stoma. Press on the wafer for a few minutes. g. Secure pouch by "picture framing" the wafer with four strips of hypoallergenic paper tape (if the wafer does not already have tape attached).	3. Correct pouch removal and attachment techniques minimize irritation and injury of peristomal skin and ensure a tight, reliable seal between the pouch and skin.
4. Teach client the procedure for emptying a stoma pouch. a. Put some toilet paper in toilet bowl and sit on toilet seat. b. Remove plug or turn valve to open pouch and carefully empty pouch contents into toilet.	4. Correct techniques can reduce spillage, soiling, and odor. Placing toilet paper in the bowl prevents water from splashing when pouch contents are emptied. Add a mucus dispersant to the pouch or straight drainage tubing if connected to a secondary receptacle.
5. Connect appliance to straight drainage when client is sleeping in bed.	5. Bacteria multiply rapidly as urine collects in the pouch. Bacterial contamination of the urinary tract can result from backflow of urine from a full pouch. Nighttime drainage systems hold large amounts of urine and drain urine away from the stoma.
6. Teach client strategies for preventing and managing peristomal skin problems. a. Shave peristomal skin with an electric razor rather than a blade; avoid using shaving cream, soap, and detergents except when showering. b. Evaluate all skin products for possible allergic reaction; patch-test all suspect products elsewhere on the abdomen. c. Do not change brands of skin barriers and adhesives casually; assess for allergic reaction before using a new brand.	6. A client with a stoma is at increased risk for peristomal skin breakdown. Factors that influence skin integrity include allergies; mechanical trauma; the underlying disease and its treatment (including medications); the quality of ostomy and peristomal skin care; availability of proper supplies; nutritional status; overall health status; hygiene; and activity level. When urine is allowed to remain in contact with skin for prolonged periods, it can result in maceration and hyperplasia of the epidermis.

(continues on page 917)

Interventions continued	**Rationales** continued
d. Avoid irritation from contact with urine; clean skin regularly. Cleanse urine encrustation on the stoma or peristomal skin with a 1:1 solution of vinegar and water. e. Avoid prolonged skin pressure, especially if client is fair-skinned or has thin, atrophic skin due to long-term corticosteroid therapy. f. Use corticosteroid creams sparingly and briefly; they can cause dryness and irritation. g. If bacterial or fungal infection is suspected, use a specific antibacterial or antifungal cream or powder. h. Use a liquid film barrier; avoid tincture of benzoin compound that can dry skin. i. Avoid aluminum paste and greasy ointments that can mask skin problems and interfere with pouch adherence. j. Protect the skin with barriers. k. Expect the stoma to shrink slightly over time. This necessitates remeasuring the stoma to ensure proper appliance fit.	

7. Promote measures to help client incorporate ostomy care into ADLs.
  a. Fluid management:
    • Drink 2 to 3 liters of fluids a day.
    • Consume cranberry juice, prune juice, plums, poultry, fish, whole grains.
    • Avoid excessive intake of milk, citrus fruits, and carbonized drinks.
  b. Working/traveling: Keep extra supplies at work. When traveling, carry supplies rather than pack them in a suitcase and risk losing them; keep in mind that pectin-based wafers melt in high environmental temperatures. Take a list of ostomy supplies when traveling.
  c. Exercise: The only limits involve contact sports during which trauma to the stoma may occur. Normal exercise is beneficial and may help to stimulate urine excretion.
  d. Wardrobe: Ostomy appliances are invisible under clothing. Any clothing worn preoperatively may be worn postoperatively. Dress comfortably.
  e. Bathing/showering/swimming: These activities may be done while wearing an ostomy appliance. "Picture-frame" the skin barrier with paper tape to seal the
	7. Successful incorporation of ostomy management into ADLs allows client to resume pre-urostomy life style and pursue goals and interests.
	  • Sufficient fluids flush urinary tract and prevent infection.
	  • These substances acidify urine and prevent bacteria growth.
	  • These substances create a more alkaline urine.

(continues on page 918)

Interventions continued	Rationales continued
edges and keep the barrier edge from getting wet. Showering may be done without an appliance and, in fact, is recommended on days of appliance changes.	

8. Teach measures to help prevent urinary calculi:
  a. Ensure optimal hydration.
  b. Avoid sulfa drugs and vitamin C supplements.
  c. Engage in regular physical activity.
	8. Inadequate hydration promotes urinary stasis and calculi formation. Certain drugs and inactivity can predispose to calculi formation (Gorshorn, 2000).

 Documentation

Discharge summary record
  Client and family teaching
  Outcome achievement or status

High Risk for Ineffective Therapeutic Regimen Management Related to Insufficient Knowledge of Intermittent Self-catheterization of Continent Urostomy

Focus Assessment Criteria	Clinical Significance
1. Readiness and ability to learn and retain information	1. A client or family failing to achieve learning goals requires a referral for assistance post-discharge.

Goals

The goals for this diagnosis represent those associated with discharge planning. Refer to the discharge criteria.

Interventions	Rationales
1. Explain the reasons for continuous drainage and frequent irrigations postoperatively.	1. Continuous drainage is needed to eliminate urine; irrigations help to keep the catheter from plugging with mucus.

2. Instruct client on how to perform intermittent self-catheterization (Early & Poquette, 2000) to drain pouch.
  a. Wash hands.
  b. Clean with cleanser of choice.
  c. Lubricate catheter.
  d. Insert catheter until urine flows.
	2. Proper technique is needed to prevent perforation and urinary stasis.

(continues on page 919)

Interventions continued	**Rationales** continued
e. When urine stops, move catheter in or pull out a little to drain more urine. f. Pinch catheter and remove. g. Place covering over stoma.	
3. Supervise client in self-catheterization.	3. Evaluation of skill performance is more accurate when observed.
4. Instruct client to notify physician immediately if he or she is unable to self-catheterize the stoma.	4. Inability to catheterize the stoma puts client at high risk for obstruction.
5. Provide a written catheterization schedule after collaborating with physician or advanced practice nurse (Early & Poquette, 2000). 　1st week—catheterization should be done every 2 hours during the day and every 3 hours at night. 　2nd week—catheterize every 3 hours during the day and every 4 hours at night. 　3rd week—catheterize every 4 hours during the day and every 5 hours at night. 　4th week—catheterize every 5 hours during the day and every 6 hours at night. 　5th week—catheterize every 6 hours during the day and not at all during the night.	5. This schedule will gradually increase the capacity for urine.
6. Teach irrigation of pouch: a. Irrigate daily for 2 months then only PRN if mucus increases. b. Use a 60 mL syringe or new poultry baster to instill normal saline. c. Normal saline can be made by mixing 2 teaspoons of salt in 1 quart of distilled water.	6. Irrigation of the pouch is needed to remove mucus to prevent blockage.
7. Observe client irrigating the pouch.	7. Direct observation is the best method to evaluate understanding.
8. Teach client to clean used catheters in warm soapy water; rinse with tap water. Air dry on a paper towel and store in a re-sealable plastic bag.	8. This procedure is clean, not sterile.

(continues on page 920)

Interventions continued	**Rationales** continued

9. If urinary reservoir is to skin or urethra, teach care of catheter.
  a. Flush with 60 ml normal saline every 4 hours during day.
  b. Shower with clear plastic covering on catheter or, if no drainage, remove bag and wash skin around drain.
  c. Empty bag when it is one-third to one-half full.
  d. Measure amount.
	9. Flushing prevents a plugged catheter.

10. If the continent urinary reservoir is to urethra, after the catheter is removed (usually in 3 weeks) instruct client how to self-catheterize.
  a. Wash hands.
  b. Sit on toilet or in front of toilet.
  c. Clean urethral opening; wash tip of penis or separate labia and wash with soap and water in a circular motion; start at urethra and move out.
  d. Lubricate catheter with water-soluble lubricant.
  e. Insert into urethra until urine flows; for male 6 to 8 inches, for female 1 to 1.5 inches then 1 inch further.
  f. Flush catheter with 60 ml of saline.
  g. Withdraw catheter slowly; pinch and remove.
  h. Assess if urine is cloudy, bloody, or foul smelling.
  i. Clean catheter as outlined in intervention 7.
	10. Self-catheterization is needed to drain urine.

11. Arrange for professional supervision of self-catheterization at surgeon's office or through home care.	11. Direct observation is needed to assure competency.
12. Advise client to call surgeon or advance practice nurse to report any changes or for questions.	12. After discharge, client will need assistance to manage problems and assess for complications.

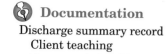 **Documentation**

Discharge summary record
  Client teaching
  Response to teaching
  Outcome achievement or status

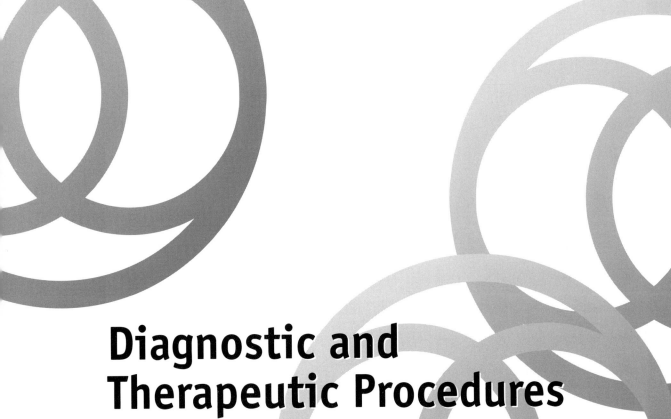

Diagnostic and Therapeutic Procedures

ANTICOAGULANT THERAPY

Anticoagulant therapy is treatment for a coagulation disorder (e.g., deep vein thrombosis, pulmonary embolism, atrial fibrillation, ischemic stroke) or prophylaxis for coagulation for people undergoing orthopedic surgery or receiving prosthetic cardiac valves.

Anticoagulants for therapy or prophylaxis include warfarin (Coumadin), heparin, low-molecular-weight heparin (Lovenox, Fragmin, Orgaran, Normiflo), all of which prevent clot extension and formation; antiplatelet agents (aspirin, Plavix, Ticlid) that interfere with platelet activity; and thrombolytic agents that dissolve existing thrombi (Arcangelo & Peterson, 2001). This care plan addresses the use of heparin and warfarin (Coumadin).

 Time Frame

Intratherapy

 DIAGNOSTIC CLUSTER

Collaborative Problems

Potential Complication:

▲ Hemorrhage

Nursing Diagnoses

△ High Risk for Ineffective Therapeutic Regimen Management related to insufficient knowledge of administration schedule, identification card/band, contraindications, risk factors, and signs and symptoms of bleeding

---

▲ This diagnosis was reported to be monitored for or managed frequently (75%–100%).
△ This diagnosis was reported to be monitored for or managed often (50%–74%).

Discharge Criteria

Before discharge, the client or family will

1. Describe proper medication use.
2. State indications for contacting a health care professional.
3. State an intent to wear Medic-Alert identification.
4. Identify the need for follow-up care.

Collaborative Problems

Potential Complication: Hemorrhage

Nursing Goal

The nurse will detect early signs and symptoms of hemorrhage and collaboratively stabilize client.

Indicators

- Clear, light-yellow urine
- No bruises or nosebleeds
- No change in stool color
- No bleeding gums

Interventions	Rationales
1. Monitor for signs and symptoms of bleeding: a. Bruises b. Nosebleeds c. Bleeding gums d. Hematuria e. Severe headaches f. Red or black stools	1. The prolonged clotting time caused by anticoagulant therapy can cause spontaneous bleeding anywhere in the body. Hematuria is a common early sign.
2. Reduce hematomas and bleeding at injection sites. a. Use small-gauge needles. b. Do not massage sites. c. Rotate sites. d. Use subcutaneous route. e. Apply steady pressure for 1 to 2 minutes.	2. These techniques will reduce trauma to tissues and avoid highly vascular areas (e.g., muscles).
3. Test stools daily for occult blood.	3. Signs of bleeding may be detected early.
4. Monitor lab results of activated partial thromboplastin time (aPTT) for heparin therapy and PT and INR for oral therapy. Report values over target therapeutic range.	4. Anticoagulant therapy will prolong both times. The therapeutic range goal for PT is 1.3 to 1.5 × control, or INR of 2.0 to 3.0 (Severson, Baldwin, & Dehoughery, 1997).
5. Carefully monitor older clients.	5. Older clients may be more susceptible to the effects of anticoagulants and may need a lower maintenance dose.
6. Report any signs of bleeding to prescribing practitioner.	6. The warfarin dose may be reduced or omitted and oral potassium given to reverse anticoagulant effects.

 Related Physician-Prescribed Interventions

Medications. Anticoagulant agents (dosage varies with daily coagulation test results)

Intravenous Therapy. For IV administration

Laboratory Studies. Activated partial thromboplastin time (aPTT), prothrombin time (PT), platelets, International Normalized Ratio (INR)

Documentation
Flow records
  Occult blood test results(urine and stool)
Progress notes
  Unusual complaints

Nursing Diagnosis

High Risk for Ineffective Therapeutic Regimen Management Related to Insufficient Knowledge of Administration Schedule, Identification Card/Band, Contraindications, and Signs and Symptoms of Bleeding

Focus Assessment Criteria	Clinical Significance
1. Knowledge of medication regimen	1. This assessment identifies client's learning needs and guides nurse in planning teaching strategies.
2. Readiness and ability to learn and retain information	2. A client or family failing to achieve learning goals requires a referral for assistance post-discharge.
3. Medication history for drugs that can potentiate or inhibit anticoagulant actions (Arcangelo & Peterson, 2001): a. Substances that can potentiate anticoagulant action include the following: • Alcohol • Allopurinol or probenecid * Amiodarone • Antibiotics • Chloral hydrate • Chloramphenicol • Cimetidine • Erythromycin • Fluconazole • Isoniazid • Metronidazole • Miconazole • Mineral oil • Nonsteroidal anti-inflammatory analgesics (NSAIAs) * Omeprazole • Tolbutamide (Orinase) • Piroxicam • Propafenone • Propranolol • Phenylbutazone • Salicylates * Sulfinpyrazone • Thyroid medications • Thrombolytics b. Substances that can inhibit anticoagulant action include the following: • Adrenal corticosteroids • Antacids • Barbiturates • Carbamazepine • Colestipol • Estrogens	3,4. Before initiation of therapy, nurse should identify any medications or conditions that can interfere with anticoagulant therapy.

(continues on page 926)

Focus Assessment Criteria continued	**Clinical Significance** continued

• Griseofulvin
• Nafcillin
• Oral contraceptives
• Rifampin
• Sucralfate
 	
4. Medical history for conditions that can increase or decrease PT time
  a. Conditions associated with increased PT time include the following:
    • Cachexia
    • Cancer
    • Collagen disease
    • Congestive heart failure
    • Diarrhea
    • Fever
    • Hepatic disorders
    • Malnutrition
    • Pancreatic disorders
    • Radiation therapy
    • Renal insufficiency
    • Thyrotoxicosis
    • Vitamin K deficiency
  b. Conditions associated with decreased PT time include the following:
    • Diabetes mellitus
    • Edema
    • Hereditary resistance to anticoagulants
    • Hypercholesterolemia
    • Hyperlipidemia
    • Hypothyroidism
    • Visceral carcinoma	

Goals

The goals for this diagnosis represent those associated with discharge planning. Refer to the discharge criteria.

Interventions	**Rationales**
1. Instruct client to take medication exactly as prescribed. Stress the importance of regular laboratory tests to monitor effects.	1. Adherence to the prescribed dosage schedule can prevent undermedication or overmedication.

2. If low-molecular-weight heparin (LMWH) is prescribed for home use:
  a. Review actions and dosing schedule.
  b. Teach subcutaneous injection technique to client or family member.
	2. LMWH is given subcutaneously and can be administered at home.

(continues on page 927)

Interventions continued	Rationales continued
c. Observe injection technique of client or family member.	
3. If warfarin is prescribed for home use: a. Review actions and dosing schedule. b. Advise client about the risk of Warfarin if client becomes pregnant.	3. Bleeding can occur if INR is prolonged or if another factor potentiates anticoagulant action. a. Understanding therapeutic goals can decrease adverse events. b. Warfarin causes fetal defects.
4. Instruct client and family to watch for and report signs and symptoms of bleeding immediately: a. Bruises b. Headaches c. Blood in stool or black stools d. Blood in urine e. Nosebleeds f. Bleeding gums g. Coughing or vomiting blood	4. Bleeding can occur if PT is prolonged or if another factor potentiates anticoagulant action.
5. Instruct client to avoid over-the-counter products that can affect coagulation: a. Alcohol b. Antacids c. Aspirin d. Nonsteroidal anti-inflammatory agents e. Vitamin C	5. Certain substances prolong coagulation by inhibiting anticoagulant metabolism (e.g., alcohol) or inhibiting procoagulant factors (e.g., aspirin and antacids).
6. Instruct client to avoid or limit intake of foods high in vitamin K, including the following: • Collard turnip greens • Broccoli, cauliflower, and brussel sprouts • Cabbage and lettuce • Asparagus and watercress • Beef liver and high-fat foods • Green tea, herbal tea, and coffee * Soy beans and olive oils * Beans * Dairy foods	6. Increased vitamin K (more than 500 mg per day) intake decreases anticoagulant action by promoting synthesis of vitamin K-dependent clotting factors. A balanced diet with some foods containing vitamin K will not interfere with therapy. Herbal and green teas should be avoided because they have large quantities of Vitamin K (> 1400 µg/m).
7. Advise client to try to avoid large fluctuations in dietary K intake but to have a consistent intake of dietary sources of Vitamin K.	

(continues on page 928)

Interventions continued	Rationales continued
8. Instruct client to alert all health care providers of his or her anticoagulant therapy before undergoing any procedures (e.g., dentist).	8. Precautions may be needed to prevent hemorrhage from routine medical procedures.
9. Instruct client to avoid potentially hazardous situations while on anticoagulant therapy (e.g., contact sports, use of razor, pregnancy).	9. Contact sports and razors put client at risk for bleeding from injury. Anticoagulants cross the placental barrier and can cause fatal fetal hemorrhage.
10. Encourage client to obtain and wear Medic-Alert identification if outpatient therapy is anticipated.	10. In an emergency, an ID alerts others that client is prone to bleeding.
11. Stress the importance of regular follow-up care and laboratory work.	11. Periodic laboratory blood work is needed to evaluate effects of therapy and risk of bleeding.

Documentation

Discharge summary record
  Client and family teaching
  Outcome achievement or status

CASTS

Casts are used to immobilize a fractured bone or dislocated joint, support injured tissues during the healing process, correct deformities, prevent movement of joints during healing, and provide traction force. Casting materials can be dehydrated gypsum that recrystallizes when reconstituted with water, fiberglass, and casting tape. The material used depends on the severity of the fracture's displacement. Plaster casts take 24 to 72 hours to dry; synthetic casts usually dry in 30 minutes.

 Time Frame

Intratherapy

 DIAGNOSTIC CLUSTER

Collaborative Problems

▲ PC: Compartmental Syndrome
▲ PC: Infection/Sepsis

Nursing Diagnoses

▲ High Risk for Impaired Skin Integrity related to pressure of cast on skin surface
▲ (Specify) Self-Care Deficit related to limitation of movement secondary to cast
▲ High Risk for Ineffective Therapeutic Regimen Management related to insufficient knowledge of cast care, signs and symptoms of complications, use of assistive devices, and hazards

---

▲ This diagnosis was reported to be monitored for or managed frequently (75%–100%).

Discharge Criteria

Before discharge, the client or family will

1. Describe precautions to take with the cast.
2. Identify how to monitor for signs and symptoms of complications.
3. Identify barriers in the home environment and relate strategies for overcoming these barriers.
4. Identify a plan to meet role responsibilities.

Collaborative Problems

Potential Complication: Compartmental Syndrome

Potential Complication: Infection

Nursing Goal

The nurse will monitor for early signs and symptoms of (a) compartmental syndrome and (b) infection/sepsis and will collaboratively intervene to stabilize client.

Indicators
- Alert, calm, oriented (b)
- Temperature 98.5–99°F (b)
- Heart rate 60–100 beats/min (b)

- Respirations 16–20 breaths/min (b)
- Deep relaxed respirations (b)
- Blood pressure >90/60, 140/90 mm Hg (b)
- Peripheral pulses—full, equal, strong (a)
- Sensation intact (a)
- No pain with passive dorsiflexion (calf and toes) (a)
- Mild edema (a)
- Pain relieved by analgesics (a)
- No tingling in legs (a)
- Can move legs (a)
- White blood cells 4,000–10,800 (b)
- Oxygen saturation 94%–100% (b)
- Capillary refill <3 sec (a)
- Blood urea nitrogen BUN 10–20 mg/dL (a)
- Creatinine 0.7–1.4 mg/dL (b)

Interventions	Rationales
1. Instruct client to report any changes however slight. Determine if these changes are new and different.	1. Neurovascular compromise often begins as minor sensations; early detection can enable prompt intervention to prevent serious complications (Bryant, 1998).
2. Monitor for signs and symptoms of compartmental syndrome. a. Deep, throbbing pain at fracture site b. Increasing pain with passive movement c. Decreased sensation to light touch d. Inability to distinguish between sharp and dull sensation in first web space of toes, sole, and dorsum and lateral aspect of foot e. Diminished or absent pedal pulses f. Increased edema and induration in extremity g. Increased capillary refill (toes or fingers) >3 seconds	2. These signs and symptoms are indicative of venous or arterial obstruction and nerve compression. Edema at the fracture site can compromise muscular vascular perfusion. Stretching damaged muscle causes pain. Sensory deficit is an early sign of nerve ischemia; the specific area of change indicates the affected compartment (Tumbarello, 2000).
3. Warn client not to mask pain with analgesics until the exact cause has been identified.	3. Identifying the location and nature of pain assists in differential diagnosis.
4. Investigate any complaints of pain or burning or an offensive odor from inside the cast. Smell the cast to check for odors.	4. These signs and symptoms may indicate that a pressure sore is forming or has become infected. Pathological tissue necrosis emits a musty, offensive odor that can easily be detected.
5. Feel cast surface to identify areas that are appreciably warmer than other areas ("hot spots"). Particularly evaluate areas over pressure points.	5. Often areas of tissue necrosis or infection cause the overlying area of the cast to feel warmer.

(continues on page 931)

Interventions continued	Rationales continued
6. If drainage is noted on cast, draw a mark around drainage area and record date and time on cast. Notify surgeon if drainage increases.	6. Marking the initial drainage will provide a baseline for comparison.
7. When moving client or body part, support plaster cast during hardening with palms of hands. Avoid pressure or sharp edges on cast.	7. Maximum hardness of plaster cast takes 24 to 72 hours depending on thickness. Careful hardening will prevent dents that can cause pressure on underlying tissue.

◤ Related Physician-Prescribed Interventions

Diagnostic Studies. X-ray films (preapplication and postapplication)

Therapies. Assistive devices, physical therapy, casts (plaster, non-plaster)

Documentation

Flow records
    Skin color (distal to injury)
    Pulses (distal to injury)
    Sensations (pain, paresthesias, paralysis)
    Odor (under cast)
    Temperature of cast surface
Progress notes
    Unusual complaints

Nursing Diagnoses

High Risk for Impaired Skin Integrity Related to Pressure of Cast on Skin Surface

Focus Assessment Criteria	Clinical Significance
1. Skin condition before cast application	1. Assessment of skin is required to identify any lesions or abnormalities that may be aggravated by the cast.
2. Fit and condition of cast	2. An improperly fitted or deteriorating cast can lead to problems with healing.
3. Skin under cast edges	3. Pressure from cast edges can cause skin abrasion or bruising.

Goal

The client will continue to have intact skin.

Indicators
- Relate instructions to prevent skin breakdown.
- Describe cast care and precautions.

Interventions	Rationales
1. Monitor common pressure sites in relationship to cast application: a. Leg: heel, malleoli, dorsal aspect of foot, head of fibula, and anterior surface of patella b. Arm: medial epicondyle of humerus, and ulnar styloid c. Plaster jackets or body spica casts: sacrum, anterior and superior iliac spines, and vertebral borders of scapulae To assess skin under the cast, pull skin taut and use a flashlight for illumination.	1. Prolonged pressure of cast on neuro-vascular structures and other body parts can cause necrosis, pressure sores, and nerve palsies (Bryant, 1998).
2. Inspect skin of uncasted body areas. Pad elbows and heels of unaffected extremities or the sacrum if applicable.	2. The heel on the unaffected side may become sore because client habitually pushes up in bed with the uninvolved leg. The elbows sometimes become sore because client braces himself or herself on elbows to see what is going on around him or her (Bryant, 1998).
3. Apply padding over bony prominences. (When between cast and skin surface, padding should fit smoothly without wrinkles.) Cover skin surface with stockinette or padding—usually both—before cast application.	3. Padding over bony prominences is essential to prevent pressure ulcers (Bryant, 1998).
4. Use proper technique in handling a wet or damp cast. Support cast with the open, flat palm of your hand at all times; avoid using fingertips.	4. Wrinkles or indentations caused by fingers produce pressure points on skin under the cast (Bryant, 1998).
5. Avoid rapid cast drying with excessive heat.	5. A cast should dry from the inside out. Too-rapid drying with excessive heat can cause the inner portions of the cast to remain damp and become moldy (Bryant, 1998).
6. Explain the intense heat sensation that can occur as the cast dries and the need to avoid covering a damp cast.	6. Covering the cast can precipitate increased heat that can cause skin damage.
7. After cast application, clean skin with a weak solution of vinegar on a cloth to remove excess plaster while it is still damp.	7. Unless removed, pieces of plaster can dry and get under the cast, causing skin damage.

(continues on page 933)

Interventions continued	**Rationales** continued
8. While plaster cast is drying, use soft pillows to support it properly; avoid contact with hard surfaces. (Place padding between cast and plastic-covered pillows.)	8. Plastic-covered pillows inhibit evaporation. A wet cast placed on a hard surface can become flattened over bony prominences; the resulting pressure causes decreased circulation to tissues enclosed in the cast (Bryant, 1998).

9. Keep cast edges smooth and away from skin surfaces.
  a. Petal the edges with moleskin or adhesive; place one side of the material on the inside surface of the cast (1 to 2 inches), then fold over to the outside surface of cast (1 to 2 inches).
  b. Bend cast edges slightly with a duck-billed cast bender.
  c. Elevate affected limb properly to prevent cast from pushing against skin surface.
	9. Rough or improperly bent plaster edges may cause damage to surrounding skin by friction. When an extremity is not elevated properly, cast edges press into skin and cause pain (Bryant, 1998).

10. Provide and teach correct skin and cast care.
  a. Bathe only accessible skin and massage it with emollient lotion. Massage skin underneath the cast.
  b. Inspect for loose plaster. Avoid using powder in cast.
  c. Inspect position of padding.
 	
  d. Avoid inserting any foreign object under cast.
	10.
	
	  a. Lotion or soap under cast creates a film and can irritate skin.
	
	  b. Loose plaster and powder irritate skin under the cast.
	  c. Padding that slips down must be pulled up and petaled.
	  d. Foreign objects can cause skin injury.

11. Using proper technique, turn a bed-ridden client every 2 to 4 hours. Turn toward the unaffected limb; enlist one or more experienced staff members to help. (Number of persons needed depends on client's size and weight and type of cast.)	11. Proper technique prevents damage to cast and injury to joints.

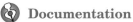 **Documentation**

Flow records
   Skin assessment
   Positioning
Discharge summary record
   Client teaching
      Outcome achievement or status

(Specify) Self-Care Deficit Related to Limitation of Movement Secondary to Cast

Focus Assessment Criteria	Clinical Significance
1. Ability to perform ADLs	1. This assessment determines need for and extent of assistance. Any injury requiring immobilization of a part interferes with client's ability to perform ADLs.
2. Available support system	2. Activities may need to be planned around availability of assistance.
3. Home environment	3. Assessment of home environment can identify any possible barriers and hazards.

Goals

The client will perform ADLs within the limitations of the cast. The client will perform muscle-strengthening exercises on a regular basis as permitted.

Indicators

• Demonstrate correct use of assistive devices.

Interventions	Rationales
1. Teach proper crutch-walking technique if indicated.	1. Proper technique is necessary to prevent injury.
2. Elevate a casted leg when client is not ambulatory. Elevate a casted arm with a sling when client is out of bed; teach client how to use the sling properly.	2. At rest, a dependent extremity develops venous pooling that causes pain and swelling. Elevation helps to prevent this problem.
3. Instruct client to use plastic bags to protect plaster cast during wet weather or while bathing.	3. Moisture weakens plaster casts. Moisture has no effect on fiberglass casts.
4. Teach client to use a blow dryer at home to dry small areas of a dampened cast.	4. Heat speeds drying.
5. Consult with physical therapist regarding actively exercising joints above and below the cast in the following ways: a. Raising a casted arm over head b. Moving each finger and thumb or toes c. Raising and lowering wrist d. Quadricep-setting: tightening and relaxing muscles	5. Exercise helps to prevent complications, promotes healing, and aids the rehabilitation process after cast removal. Moving frequently stimulates circulation and promotes venous return.

(continues on page 935)

Interventions continued	Rationales continued

e. Gluteal-setting
    f. Abdominal tightening
    g. Deep breathing
    h. Opening and closing hand	

6. Teach isometric exercises, starting with unaffected limb.	6. Isometric exercises produce muscle contraction without bending joints or moving limbs; they help to maintain muscle strength and mass.
7. Teach client to put unaffected joints through their full ROM four times daily.	7. Performing full ROM helps to maintain muscle tone and mobility.
8. Consult with a home health coordinator if indicated.	8. Referral can provide for needed services (e.g., transportation, housekeeping) after discharge.

 Documentation

Flow records
    Ability to perform ADLs

High Risk for Ineffective Therapeutic Regimen Management Related to Insufficient Knowledge of Cast Care, Signs and Symptoms of Complications, Use of Assistive Devices, and Hazards

Focus Assessment Criteria	Clinical Significance
1. Readiness and ability to learn and retain information	1. A client or family failing to achieve learning goals requires a referral for assistance postdischarge.

Goals

The goals for this diagnosis represent those associated with discharge planning. Refer to the discharge criteria.

Interventions	Rationales

1. Teach client and family to watch for and report the following symptoms:
    a. Severe pain
    b. Numbness or tingling
    c. Swelling
    d. Skin discoloration
    e. Paralysis or reduced movement
	1. Early detection of possible problems enables prompt intervention to prevent serious complications such as infection or impaired circulation (Slye, 1991).

(continues on page 936)

Interventions continued	Rationales continued
f. Cool, white toes or fingertips g. Foul odor, warm spots, soft areas, or cracks in the cast	
2. Instruct client never to insert objects down inside edges of cast.	2. Sharp objects used for scratching may cause breaks in skin continuity that provide an entry point for infectious microorganisms.
3. Teach client and family to handle a drying plaster cast with palms of hands only; using fingertips may cause indentations.	3. Cast indentations may lead to pressure sores.
4. Instruct client to keep cast uncovered until it is completely dry.	4. A damp, soiled cast can weaken and may cause skin irritation or promote bacteria growth.
5. Instruct client to avoid weightbearing or other stress on cast for at least 24 hours after application.	5. Covers restrict escape of heat, especially in a large cast, and prolong the drying process.
6. Instruct client to avoid getting plaster cast wet; teach how to protect cast from moisture.	6. Ultimate cast strength is obtained after cast is dry—within 48 to 72 hours depending on factors such as environmental temperature and humidity.
7. Encourage use of an orthopedic mattress or a mattress with a fracture board placed underneath.	7. A sagging or soft mattress tends to deform a green cast and may crack a dry cast.
8. Warn client against using cast braces or turnbuckles to lift a casted part.	8. These devices are not placed in casts to serve as handles. They may easily be broken, dislocated, or pulled out of casts.
9. Teach client what to expect with cast removal: a. Buzz of saw b. Vibrations c. Chalky dust d. Warmth on limbs as saw cuts; will not cut skin or burn e. Limb will be stiff f. Skin will be scaly	9. Explaining what the client can expect, why the procedures are done, and why certain sensations may occur can help to reduce fears associated with the unknown and unexpected (Christman & Kirchhoff, 1992).
10. Staff and client should use eye protection during cast removal use.	10. Cast particles can injure eyes.

(continues on page 937)

Interventions continued	Rationales continued
11. Apply a cold water enzyme wash (e.g., Woolite, Delicare) for 20 minutes then gently wash limb in warm water.	11. These solutions loosen dead cells and help to emulsify fatty and crusty lesions that can cause irritation (Elkin, Perry, & Potter, 2000).
12. Instruct client not to rub or scratch skin and to apply moisturizing skin lotion.	

 Documentation

Discharge summary record
   Client and family teaching
   Response to teaching
   Outcome achievement or status

CHEMOTHERAPY

This systemic cancer treatment modality aims to safely eradicate or control the growth of cancerous cells by producing maximum cancer cell death with minimum toxicity. Chemotherapy may be the sole treatment provided, as with leukemia, or it may be used in combination with surgery, radiation, or biologic response therapy. Chemotherapeutic agents may be given alone or in combination and may be administered either continuously or intermittently using various routes, techniques, and special equipment. Most agents affect proliferating cells and thus are most effective against rapidly dividing cancer cells. However, they also can damage rapidly dividing normal cells, such as blood cells and cells of the GI epithelium and hair follicles, producing adverse effects that require careful management (Tortorice, 2000).

 Time Frame

Pretherapy and intratherapy

DIAGNOSTIC CLUSTER

Collaborative Problems	Refer to
▲ PC: Anaphylactic Reaction	
△ PC: Cardiotoxicity	
▲ PC: Electrolyte Imbalance	
▲ PC: Extravasation of Vesicant Drugs	
△ PC: Hemorrhagic Cystitis	
▲ PC: Bone Marrow Depression	
▲ PC: Renal Insufficiency	
△ PC: Pulmonary Toxicity	
△ PC: Neurotoxicity	
PC: Renal Calculi	

Nursing Diagnoses	Refer to
▲ Anxiety related to prescribed chemotherapy, insufficient knowledge of chemotherapy, and self-care measures	
▲ Nausea related to gastrointestinal cell damage, stimulation of vomiting center, fear, and anxiety	
▲ Imbalanced Nutrition: Less Than Body Requirements, related to anorexia, taste changes, persistent nausea/vomiting, and increased metabolic rate	
▲ Impaired Oral Mucous Membrane related to dryness and epithelial cell damage secondary to chemotherapy	

(continues on page 939)

Nursing Diagnoses continued	**Refer to** continued
▲ Fatigue related to effects of anemia, malnutrition, persistent vomiting, and sleep pattern disturbance	Inflammatory Joint Disease
△ High Risk for Constipation related to autonomic nerve dysfunction secondary to *Vinca* alkaloid administration and inactivity	Immobility or Unconsciousness
▲ Diarrhea related to intestinal cell damage, inflammation, and increased intestinal mobility	Inflammatory Intestinal Disease
▲ High Risk for Impaired Skin Integrity related to persistent diarrhea, malnutrition, prolonged sedation, and fatigue	Immobility or Unconsciousness
△ Disturbed Self-Concept related to change in life style, role, alopecia, and weight loss or gain	Cancer (Initial Diagnosis)

▲ This diagnosis was reported to be monitored for or managed frequently (75%–100%).
△ This diagnosis was reported to be monitored for or managed often (50%–74%).

Discharge Planning

Before discharge, the client and family will

1. Explain treatment plan.
2. Describe signs and symptoms that must be reported to a health care professional.
3. Relate an intent to share feelings and concerns with significant others and health care professionals.
4. Identify available community resources.

Collaborative Problems

Potential Complication: Anaphylactic Reaction

Potential Complication: Cardiotoxicity

Potential Complication: Electrolyte Imbalance

Potential Complication: Extravasation of Vesicant Drugs

Potential Complication: Hemorrhagic Cystitis

Potential Complication: Bone Marrow Depression

Potential Complication: Renal Insufficiency

Potential Complication: Pulmonary Toxicity

Potential Complication: Neurotoxicity

Potential Complication: Renal Calculi

Nursing Goal

The nurse will detect early signs and symptoms of (a) anaphylactic reaction, (b) cardiotoxicity, (c) electrolyte imbalance, (d) extravasation of vesicant drugs, (e) hemorrhagic cystitis, (f) bone marrow depression, (g) renal insufficiency, (h) pulmonary toxicity, (i) neurotoxicity, and (j) renal calculi and collaboratively intervene to stabilize client.

Indicators

- Calm, alert, oriented (a, i)
- No complaints of urticaria or pruritus (a)
- No complaints of tightness in throat (a)
- No complaints of shortness of breath or wheezing (a, h)
- Temperature 98.5–99 °F (h)
- Pulse 60–100 beats/min (b, h)
- BP >90/160, <140/90 mm Hg (b, g)
- Normal sinus rhythm (b)
- Flat neck veins (b)
- Serum sodium 135–145 mEq/L (c, g)
- Serum potassium 3-8-5 mEq/L (c, g)
- Serum magnesium 1.3–2.4 mEq/L (c, g)
- Serum phosphorous 2.5–4.5 mEq/L (c, g)
- Serum calcium 8.5–10.5 mEq/L (c, g)
- Urine output > 30 ml/hour (c, g, j)
- Intact strength (c, i)
- Intact sensation (c, i)
- Stable gait (c, i)
- No seizures (c, i)
- No complaints of headache (c)
- No muscle cramps or twitching (c)
- No nausea or vomiting (c, j)
- Stools soft and formed (c, i)
- No swelling at IV site (d)
- No erythema or pain at IV site (d)
- No dysuria, frequency or urgency (e, j)
- Urine clear yellow (e, j)
- Urine specific gravity 1.005–1.030 (e, g)
- Urine sodium 130–2000 mEq/24h (g)
- White blood cells 4.800–10,000 cu mm (f)
- Red blood cells (f)
  - Male 4,600,000–6,200,000
  - Female 4,200,000–5,400,000 cu mm
- Platelet 100,000–400,000 cu mm (f)
- Monocytes 2–6% (f)
- Blood urea nitrogen 10–20 mg/dL (g)
- Serum creatinine 0.7–1.4 mg/dL (g)
- Skin color (pinkish, brownish, olive tones) (g)
- Serum pH 7.35–7.45 (h)
- Oxygen saturation (SAO_2) 94% (h)
- Carbon dioxide $(PACO_2)$ 34–45 mm/Hg (h)
- Normal chest x-ray (h)
- Normal pulmonary function tests (h)
- No complaints of flank or abdominal pain (j)

Interventions	Rationales
1. Inquire about previous drug reactions; record baseline vital signs and mental status before administering chemotherapy.	1. Any cytotoxic drug—including cisplatin, teniposide, nitrogen mustard, doxorubicin, bleomycin, methotrexate, L-asparaginase,

(continues on page 941)

Interventions continued	**Rationales** continued
a. Skin tests or test dose should be given when administering a drug known to have increased incidence of hypersensitivity.	and melphalan–can precipitate anaphylaxis. Release of histamine in an antigen—antibody reaction results in cutaneous symptoms (urticaria or pruritus) and systemic symptoms (laryngeal edema, bronchospasm, and dyspnea) (Porth, 2002).
2. Monitor for symptoms of anaphylactic reaction: a. Urticaria, pruritus b. Sensation of lump in throat c. Shortness of breath/wheezing	2. These assessment steps help to determine risk of complications and provide a baseline against which to compare subsequent findings.
3. If symptoms of anaphylaxis develop, discontinue chemotherapy and apply a tourniquet proximal to the injection site. Administer emergency drugs as ordered by physician (epinephrine, diphenhydramine, hydrocortisone) (Oncology Nurses Society, 1992).	3. Prompt discontinuation prevents possible serious response; tourniquet application retards drug absorption. Emergency drugs reduce histamine release, relieve edema and spasm, and prevent shock.
4. Monitor vital signs every 15 minutes until client is stable.	4. Careful monitoring can detect early signs of hypotension and shock.
5. Monitor for signs and symptoms of cardiotoxicity. Report promptly: a. Gradual increase in heart rate b. Increased shortness of breath c. Diminished breath sound, rales d. Decreased systolic blood pressure e. Presence of or increase in S3 or S4 gallop f. Peripheral edema g. Distended neck veins h. Arrhythmia 6. Assess for preexisting conditions (myocardial damage, radiation to mediastinum) (Camp-Sorrell, 2000).	5,6. Cardiotoxicity can be (1) acute, occurring soon after administration of chemotherapy; (2) subacute, associated with pericarditis and myocardial dysfunction that occur 4 to 5 weeks after treatment; and (3) cardiomyopathy, which occurs within months of treatment. Anthracyclines, such as doxorubicin and daunorubicin, are known for their potential to cause cardiotoxicity. In high doses, anthracyclines damage heart cells, causing loss of pumping ability and increased oxygen need. A QRS voltage change in an ECG may signal a life-threatening condition (Camp-Sorrell, 2000).
7. Monitor for electrolyte imbalances. a. Hyponatremia or hypernatremia	7. Chemotherapeutic agents often precipitate electrolyte imbalance (Camp-Sorrell, 2000). a. Hyponatremia is caused by secretion of antidiuretic hormone secondary to vincristine or cyclophosphamide therapy, excessive hydration, or decrease in peripheral blast count secondary to daunorubicin or cytosine therapy.

(continues on page 942)

Interventions continued	Rationales continued
	Hypernatremia may result from renal failure secondary to drug nephrotoxicity.
b. Hypokalemia or hyperkalemia	b. Hypokalemia may be due to intercellular shift, excessive diarrhea, or renal tubular injury. Hyperkalemia is caused by cell lysis and renal damage.
c. Hypomagnesemia	c. Hypomagnesemia can result from vomiting, diarrhea, or cisplatin therapy, which causes excretion of divalent ions.
d. Hypophosphatemia	d. Hypophosphatemia is associated with hypercalcemia, hypokalemia, and hypomagnesemia.
e. Hypocalcemia or hypercalcemia (refer to the Collaborative Problems section of the Chronic Renal Failure Care Plan for specific signs and symptoms of each electrolyte imbalance).	e. Hypercalcemia is secondary to hypophosphatemia, renal failure, or mithramycin therapy; hypocalcemia is secondary to hyperphosphatemia or renal failure.

8. Monitor and teach client and family to monitor for and report the following:
  a. Excessive fluid loss or gain
  b. Change in orientation or level of consciousness
  c. Changes in vital signs
  d. Weakness or ataxia
  e. Paresthesias
  f. Seizure activity
  g. Persistent headache
  h. Muscle cramps, twitching, or tetany
  i. Nausea and vomiting
  j. Diarrhea
	8. Electrolyte imbalances affect neurotransmission, muscle activity, and fluid balance.

9. Take steps to reduce extravasation of vesicant medications—agents that cause severe necrosis if they leak from blood vessels into tissue. Examples of vesicant medications are the following: amsacrine, bisantrene, dactinomycin, dacarbazine, daunomycin, daunorubicin, estramustine, maytansine, mithramycin, mitomycin, nitrogen mustard, pyrazofurin, vinblastine, vincristine, and vindesine.
  a. Preventive measures are as follows:
    • Avoid infusing vesicants over joints, bony prominences, tendons, neurovascular bundles, or the antecubital fossa (Goodman & Riley, 2000).
    • Avoid multiple punctures of the same vein within 24 hours.
    • Administer drug through a longterm venous catheter.
	9. Extravasation may occur secondary to improper placement, damaged vein, or obstructed venous drainage secondary to superior vena cava syndrome, edema, or tumor.

(continues on page 943)

Interventions continued	**Rationales** continued
• Do not administer drug if edema is present or blood return is absent. • If peripheral IV site is used, evaluate its status and if it is less than 24 hours old. • Observe peripheral infusion continuously. • Provide infusion through a central line and check every 1 to 2 hours. • Infuse vesicant before any other medication, even antiemetics.	• The venous integrity is greatest earlier in procedure.
10. Monitor during drug infusion. 　a. Assess patency of intravenous (IV) infusion line. 　b. Observe tissue at the IV site every 30 minutes for the following: 　　• Swelling (most common) 　　• Leakage 　　• Burning/pain (not always present) 　　• Inflammation 　　• Erythema (not seen initially) 　　• Hyperpigmentation 11. If extravasation occurs, take the following steps with gloves on: 　a. Stop administration of drug. 　b. Leave needle in place. 　c. Gently aspirate residual drug and blood in tubing or needle. 　d. Avoid applying direct pressure on site. 　e. Give antidote as ordered by physician or institutional policy. 　f. If plant alkaloid extravasation, apply warm compresses 15 to 20 minutes QID for 24 hours. 　g. If anthracycline extravasation, apply ice for 15 to 20 minutes every 3 to 4 hours for 24 to 48 hours. 　h. Monitor site: 　　• Elevate limb above heart for 48 hours. 　　• After 48 hours, encourage client to use limb normally. 　　* Outline area of extravasation with pen.	10,11. Detecting signs of extravasation early enables prompt intervention to prevent serious complications including tissue necrosis.
12. Monitor for erythema, pain, and indication every hour for 4 hours and then every 4 to 8 hours according to protocol. • For future intravenous sites, avoid sites that infuse vesicants over joints, bony prominences, tendons, neuro-	12. Extravasation can cause underlying tissue damage resulting in permanent damage. • This will reduce the concentration of drug at site. This will serve as a baseline for subsequent assessments.

(continues on page 944)

Interventions continued	**Rationales** continued
vascular bundles, and antecubital fossa (Goodman, 2000). • Avoid multiple punctures in the same vein within 24 hours.	Necrosis of tissue can occur. These sites if extravasated into can cause permanent damage or deformity. • Multiple punctures make the vessel more vulnerable to infiltration.
13. When administering cyclophosphamide, monitor for signs and symptoms of hemorrhagic cystitis. a. Dysuria b. Frequency c. Urgency d. Hematuria	13. Cyclophosphamide administration is associated with the development of hemorrhagic cystitis.
14. Administer cyclophosphamide early in the day.	14. Administration early in the day reduces the high drug concentration that can occur during the night secondary to reduced intake.
15. Teach client to do the following: a. Void every 2 hours. b. Increase fluid intake to 2,500 to 3,000 mL/day unless contraindicated.	15. Frequent voiding and optimal hydration reduce drug concentration in bladder.
16. Monitor for signs of bone marrow depression: a. Decreased WBC and RBC counts b. Decreased platelet count c. Decreased granulocyte count	16. Chemotherapy interferes with cell division of bone marrow stem cells that form blood cells. Granulocytes are mainly neutrophils that are the first line of defense against infection (Tortorice, 2000).
17. Explain risks of bleeding and infection. (Refer to the Corticosteroid Therapy Care Plan for strategies to reduce these risks.)	17. Decreased granulocytes impair the body's phagocytic defense against microorganisms. Platelets form a temporary plug to stop bleeding and activate clotting factors; decreased platelets can interfere with clotting. Chemotherapy-induced renal toxicity can occur (1) directly, as with cisplatin, methotrexate, and mitomycin, which can produce toxic effects on renal glomeruli and tubules, and (2) indirectly because of rapid tumor cell lysis, causing hyperuricemia and nephropathy (Camp-Sorrell, 2000).
18. Monitor for signs of renal insufficiency. a. Sustained elevated urine specific gravity b. Elevated urine sodium levels	18. Lung inflammation and fibrosis are associated with administration of bleomycin and nitrosoureas (e.g., carmustine and busulfan). The extent of fibrosis

(continues on page 945)

Interventions continued	**Rationales** continued
c. Sustained insufficient urine output (<30 mL/hr) d. Elevated blood pressure e. Hypomagnesemia or hypocalcemia f. Increasing BUN and serum creatinine, potassium, phosphorus, and ammonia, and decreased creatinine clearance	determines the severity of respiratory dysfunction (Camp-Sorrell, 2000).
19. Monitor for pulmonary toxicity (pneumonitis or fibrosis) when administering bleomycin and nitrosoureas; signs and symptoms include the following: a. Cough b. Fever c. Tachycardia d. Dyspnea e. Rales f. Weakness g. Cyanosis h. Abnormal arterial blood gas analysis i. Abnormal chest x-ray film j. Abnormal pulmonary function tests	
20. Instruct client to cough and do deep breathing every 2 hours.	20. These activities help to reduce retention of secretions and dilate alveoli.
21. Monitor for signs and symptoms of neurotoxicity when administering *Vinca* alkaloids and L-asparaginase, procarbazine, and intrathecal methotrexate. a. Paresthesias b. Gait disturbance c. Altered fine motor activity d. Constipation e. Lethargy f. Numbness g. Muscle weakness h. Foot or wrist drop i. Somnolence j. Disorientation k. Impotence l. Confusion	21. Chemotherapy may be toxic to the central nervous system because of meningeal irritation, encephalopathies, and hypothalamic release of antidiuretic hormone (Camp-Sorrell, 2000).
22. If dysfunction results from neurotoxicity, refer to the Immobility Care Plan for interventions to prevent complications.	22. Prompt intervention is necessary to prevent serious complications.
23. Monitor for signs and symptoms of renal calculi.	23. Renal calculi may result from chemotherapy because rapid cell lysis of tumor cells

(continues on page 946)

Interventions continued	Rationales continued
a. Flank pain b. Nausea and vomiting c. Abdominal pain	produces hyperuricemia. Pain is caused by pressure of calculi on the renal tubules. Afferent stimuli in renal capsule may cause pylorospasm of the smooth muscle of the enteric tract and adjacent structures.
24. Refer to the Urolithiasis Care Plan for specific interventions to reduce risk of renal calculi.	

 Related Physician-Prescribed Interventions

Medications. Antiemetics, anti-anxiety, dexamethasone, chemotherapeutic agents

Laboratory Studies. Complete blood count, urinalysis, electrolytes, BUN, serum albumin, pulmonary function test

Diagnostic Studies. Chest X-ray, pulse oximetry

Documentation

Flow records
    Vital signs
    Abnormal laboratory values (electrolytes, CBC, platelets, and BUN)
    Condition of injection sites
    Intake and output
    Urine specific gravity
    Client teaching
Progress notes
    Complaints of rashes or unusual sensations

Nursing Diagnoses

Anxiety Related to Prescribed Chemotherapy, Insufficient Knowledge of Chemotherapy, and Self-care Measures

Focus Assessment Criteria	Clinical Significance
1. Attitude and experiences with chemotherapy	1. Chemotherapy is poorly understood and feared by the general public. Personal experiences with friends and relatives influence the client's emotional response.
2. Knowledge of treatment plan 3. Knowledge of the effects and management of chemotherapy effects	2,3. Client's understanding of the chemotherapeutic regimen and side effects and their management enhances his or her sense of control and can reduce anxiety.
4. Knowledge of signs and symptoms of toxicity	4. This information enables client to detect problems early and promotes involvement in the care regimen.

Goal

The client will share feelings regarding scheduled chemotherapy.

Indicators

- Describe the anticipated effects of chemotherapy.
- Relate signs and symptoms of toxicity.
- Identify important self-care measures.

Interventions	Rationales
1. Encourage client to share feelings and beliefs regarding chemotherapy. Delay teaching if high levels of anxiety are present.	1. Verbalization can identify sources of client anxiety and allow nurse to correct mis-information. High anxiety impairs learning.
2. Reinforce physician's explanations of the chemotherapeutic regimen—the drugs, dosage schedules, and management of side effects.	
3. Explain the therapeutic effects of cytotoxic drugs; provide written information. (*Note:* Client education booklets are available from the National Cancer Institute and the American Cancer Society.)	

4. Explain the common side effects and toxicities of chemotherapy:
   a. Decreased WBC count
   b. Decreased platelet count
   c. Infection
   d. GI alterations
   e. Hair loss
   f. Fatigue
   g. Emotional responses
	4. Specific explanations provide information to help reduce anxiety associated with fear of the unknown and loss of control.

5. Discuss self-care measures to reduce risk of toxicities:
   a. Nutrition
   b. Hygiene
   c. Rest
   d. Activity
   e. Managing bowel elimination problems
   f. Managing hair loss
   g. Monitoring for infection
   h. Prioritizing activities
	5. Individuals who receive side-effect management report a higher degree of perceived effectiveness than those who did not receive this information (Dadd, 1983).

6. Refer also to the Cancer (Initial Diagnosis) Care Plan for additional information.	

🔁 Documentation

Discharge summary record or teaching record
  Client teaching
  Outcome achievement or status
Progress notes
  Dialogues

Nausea Related to Gastrointestinal Cell Damage, Stimulation of Vomiting Center, Fear, and Anxiety

Focus Assessment Criteria	Clinical Significance

1. Factors contributing to or promoting nausea and vomiting including
  a. Chemotherapeutic agents
  b. Antiemetic therapy
  c. Activity
  d. Fear and anxiety
  e. Food or fluid ingestion
  f. Changes in taste sensation
  g. Environmental conditions (e.g., odors)
  h. Family support
	1. Chemotherapy-induced nausea and vomiting result from physiological and psychological factors. Cytotoxic drugs damage GI cells, which can produce a vagal response. They also can stimulate the vomiting center in the brain. Anxiety and fear contribute to the problem. Chemotherapy effects can lead to marked disruption in self-care, requiring more family support (Camp-Sorrell, 2000).

2. Frequency and severity of vomiting episodes 3. Signs and symptoms of fluid and electrolyte imbalance	2,3. Severe or prolonged vomiting can cause fluid and electrolyte imbalances.

Indicators
- Report decreased nausea and vomiting.
- Report increasing ability to tolerate food and fluids.
- Describe what to avoid.

Interventions	Rationales
1. Promote a positive attitude about chemotherapy; reinforce its cancer cell-killing effects.	1. Frank discussions can increase motivation to reduce and tolerate nausea.
2. Explain possible reasons for nausea and vomiting.	2. Helping client to understand reasons for nausea and vomiting can reduce fear associated with the unexpected.
3. Explain the rationale for antiemetic agents; administer them before initiating chemotherapy and during the time chemotherapy drugs are most likely to cause nausea and vomiting.	3. Antiemetics are given before chemotherapy to reduce nausea.

(continues on page 949)

Interventions continued	**Rationales** continued
4. Infuse cytotoxic drugs slowly.	4. Slow infusion can decrease stimulation of the vomiting center.
5. Eat only lightly before therapy.	5. This will avoid gastric overstimulation.
6. Administer nightly emetic and cytotoxic drugs at night (during sleep if possible) or have client lie quietly for 2 hours after administration.	6. Activity stimulates the GI tract, which can increase nausea and vomiting.
7. If delayed nausea develops 3 to 4 days after treatment, consult with nurse or physician.	7. Delayed nausea is usually unresponsive to standard antiemetics. Antianxiety agents (e.g., lorazepam, are often as effective as dexamethasone).
8. If taste alterations occur, suggest that the client suck on hard candy during chemotherapy.	8. Hard candy can reduce the metallic or bitter taste that client may experience from chemotherapy.
9. Encourage client to eat small, frequent meals and to eat slowly. Cool, bland foods and liquids are usually well tolerated. Vary diet.	9. Intake of small amounts prevents gastric distention from stimulating vomiting.
10. Eliminate unpleasant sights and odors from the eating area.	10. Eliminating noxious stimuli can decrease stimulation of the vomiting center.

11. Instruct client to avoid the following:
 	
  a. Hot or cold liquids
 	
  b. Foods containing fat and fiber
 	
  c. Spicy foods
  d. Caffeine
	11. Certain foods increase peristalsis and provoke nausea and vomiting.
	  a. Cold liquids can induce cramping; hot liquids can stimulate peristalsis.
	  b. High-fat and high-fiber food and drinks increase peristalsis.
	  c. Caffeine stimulates intestinal motility.

12. Encourage client to rest in semi-Fowler's position after eating and to change position slowly.	12. Muscle relaxation can reduce peristalsis.

13. Teach stress reduction techniques such as these:
  a. Relaxation exercises
  b. Visual imagery
	13. These techniques reduce muscle tension and decrease client's focus on nausea.

Documentation

Flow records
  Intake and output
  Tolerance of intake

Imbalanced Nutrition: Less Than Body Requirements Related to Anorexia, Taste Changes, Persistent Nausea/Vomiting, and Increased Metabolic Rate

Focus Assessment Criteria	Clinical Significance
1. Actual weight versus ideal weight 2. History of weight loss 3. Dietary intake	1–3. A baseline is needed to assess quality and amount of intake and to monitor for negative nitrogen balance.

4. Reports of the following:
  a. Fatigue
  b. Anorexia
  c. Taste changes
  d. Nausea and vomiting
  e. Chemotherapy
  f. Stress and anxiety
  g. Mouth sores
	4. This assessment identifies factors that may be interfering with intake.

5. Laboratory findings: serum albumin and protein	5. Decreased protein intake results in decreased plasma proteins.

Indicators
• Maintain ideal weight with minimal further weight loss.
• Exhibit normal BUN and serum albumin and protein laboratory values.
• Describe strategies to increase nutritional intake.

Interventions	Rationales

1. Help client to identify reasons for inadequate nutrition and explain possible causes.
  a. Increased metabolic rate
  b. GI tract alterations
  c. Stimulation of vomiting
  d. Decreased appetite
  e. Taste changes
  f. Anxiety and fear
	1. Nutritional deficits associated with chemotherapy can have many causes. Cytotoxic drugs can stimulate the vomiting center in the brain. (See the nursing diagnosis Altered Comfort: Nausea/Vomiting in this entry for more information.) They also can alter GI cells, causing anorexia, taste changes, nausea and vomiting, and altered protein metabolism. Damage to the absorptive surface of the GI mucosa can lead to nutrient malabsorption. Chemotherapy-induced mucositis also inhibits intake and absorption of nutrients. Finally, anxiety and stress can inhibit appetite and lead to decreased intake (Camp-Sorrell, 2000).

(continues on page 951)

Interventions continued	**Rationales** continued
2. Stress the need to increase caloric intake.	2. Cytotoxic drugs raise the metabolic rate through destruction of rapidly proliferating cells. This factor, coupled with the body's increased nutritional needs resulting from GI damage or other factors, necessitates increased caloric intake to maintain adequate nutritional status (Goodman, 2000).
3. Encourage resting before meals.	3. Fatigue further decreases appetite.
4. Offer small, frequent meals (optimally six per day plus snacks).	4. Increased intra-abdominal pressure from fluid accumulation (ascites) compresses the GI tract and decreases capacity.
5. Restrict liquids with meals and avoid fluids 1 hour before and after meals.	5. Fluid restrictions at meals can help to prevent gastric overdistention and can enhance appetite.
6. Maintain good oral hygiene before and after eating.	6. Poor oral hygiene can result in foul odors or taste that diminish appetite.
7. Arrange to have foods with the greatest protein and caloric value served at times the client feels most like eating.	7. This strategy increases client's chance of consuming more protein and calories.
8. Teach techniques to reduce nausea. a. Avoid the smell of food preparation and other noxious stimuli. b. Loosen clothing before eating. c. Sit in fresh air. d. Avoid lying flat for at least 2 hours after eating. (A client who must rest should sit or recline with head elevated at least 4 inches higher than feet.)	8. Nausea can be reduced by controlling environmental conditions and promoting positions that minimize abdominal pressure.
9. Instruct client to limit foods and fluids high in fat.	9. Fatty foods are difficult to absorb.
10. Suggest dietary modifications such as these: a. Eating fish, chicken, eggs, and cheese if pork and beef taste bitter b. Eating meat for breakfast rather than later in the day c. Experimenting with different flavorings and seasonings	10. These measures can help to make food more palatable and encourage increased intake.

(continues on page 952)

Interventions continued	Rationales continued

11. Teach techniques to enhance protein and calorie content when preparing meals at home.
  a. Add powdered milk or egg to milk-shakes, gravies, sauces, puddings, cereals, meatballs, or milk to increase protein and calorie content.
  b. Add blenderized or baby foods to meat juices or soups.
  c. Use fortified milk (i.e., 1 cup instant non-fat milk added to 1 quart fresh milk).
  d. Use milk or half-and-half instead of water when making soups and sauces; soy formulas can also be used.
  e. Add cheese or diced meat whenever able.
  f. Add cream cheese or peanut butter to toast, crackers, celery sticks.
  g. Add extra butter or margarine to soups, sauces, vegetables.
  h. Use mayonnaise (100 cal/T) instead of salad dressing.
  i. Add sour cream or yogurt to vegetables or as dip.
  j. Use whipped cream (60 cal/T) as much as possible.
  k. Add raisins, dates, nuts, and brown sugar to hot or cold cereals.
  l. Have snacks readily available.
	11. These simple measures can increase the nutritional content of foods even when intake is limited.

12. Refer client to dietitian for further nutritional information.	12. Additional nutritional information can be acquired from an expert.
13. Give client copy of *Eating Hints,* a National Cancer Institute publication.	

 Documentation

Flow records
    Weight
    Intake (type and amount)
Progress notes
    Complaints of nausea and vomiting

Impaired Oral Mucous Membrane Related to Dryness and Epithelial Cell Damage Secondary to Chemotherapy

Focus Assessment Criteria	Clinical Significance
1. Oral mucosa for redness, swelling, dryness, lesions, ulcerations, viscous saliva, white patches, and hemorrhagic ulcerations	1–3. Cytotoxic drugs damage the rapidly dividing epithelial cells lining the oral mucosa. They also decrease WBC count.

(continues on page 953)

Focus Assessment Criteria continued	Clinical Significance continued
2. Difficulty swallowing 3. Pain or discomfort in oral mucosa 4. Smoking or alcoholism 5. Periodontal disease 6. Poor oral hygiene	As the nadir occurs, neutropenia increases risk of bacterial, fungal, or viral infection. Stomatitis leads to dryness, which further increases risk of infection. Difficulty swallowing inhibits oral fluid intake, which also enhances oral dryness and discomfort (Goodman, Hiderley, & Purl, 1997).

Indicators
- Relate the need for optimal oral hygiene.
- Report decreased discomfort.
- Describe how to prevent oral injury.

Interventions	Rationales
1. Explain the need for regular, meticulous oral hygiene. 2. Dental work should be done before chemotherapy begins.	1,2. Chemotherapy increases the mucosal cells' susceptibility to infection. Frequent oral hygiene removes microorganisms and reduces risk.

3. Instruct client to do the following:
  a. Perform oral care regimen after meals and before bedtime (and before breakfast if necessary).
  b. Avoid mouthwashes high in alcohol, lemon/glycerine swabs, and prolonged use of hydrogen peroxide.
  c. Use an oxidizing agent to loosen thick, tenacious mucus; gargle and expectorate. For example, use hydrogen peroxide and water ¼ strength (avoid prolonged use) or 1 T sodium bicarbonate mixed in 8 oz warm water (flavored with mouthwash, oil of wintergreen, etc. if desired).
  d. Rinse mouth with saline solution after gargling.
  e. Apply a lubricant to lips every 2 hours and as needed (e.g., lanolin, A & D ointment, petroleum jelly).
  f. Inspect mouth daily for lesions and inflammation; report any alterations.
	3. These practices can eliminate sources of microorganism growth and prevent mucosal drying and damage.

4. If client cannot tolerate brushing or swabbing, teach mouth irrigation. a. Use a baking soda solution (4 T in 1 liter warm water) in an enema bag (labeled for oral use only) with a soft irrigation catheter tip.	4. Brushing can further damage irritated mucosa. These measures enable maintenance of good hygiene in client who cannot brush.

(continues on page 954)

Interventions continued	Rationales continued
b. Place catheter in the mouth and slowly increase flow while standing over a basin or having someone hold a basin under chin. c. Remove dentures before irrigation; do not replace them if client has severe stomatitis. d. Perform irrigation every 2 hours or as needed.	
5. Teach precautionary measures. 　a. Breathe through nose rather than mouth. 　b. Consume cool, soothing liquids and semisolids such as gelatin. 　c. Avoid smoking. 　d. Avoid hot and spicy or acidic food and fluids. 　e. Omit flossing if excessive bleeding occurs.	5. These practices can reduce oral irritation.
6. Explain the importance of hydration and good nutrition.	6. Optimal nutritional status can increase healing ability.
7. Consult with physician for an oral pain relief solution (e.g., lidocaine [Xylocaine], diphenhydramine, and antimicrobial agents).	7. Medications may be needed to reduce pain and enable adequate nutritional intake.

 Documentation

Flow records
　Oral assessments
　Treatments

CORTICOSTEROID THERAPY

Corticosteroid is the generic name for commercial adrenocortical hormones and synthetic analogues. Corticosteroids are indicated as replacement therapy for adrenal insufficiency, for inflammation suppression, for control of allergic reactions, and for reducing the risk of graft rejection in transplantation. A client on long-term corticosteroid therapy has suppressed pituitary and adrenal functions. Some indications for corticosteroid therapy are severe autoimmune diseases, rheumatoid arthritis, severe asthma, cancer, multiple sclerosis, and psoriasis.

 Time Frame

Pretherapy and intratherapy

DIAGNOSTIC CLUSTER

Collaborative Problems

▲ PC: Steroid-Induced Diabetes
△ PC: Hypertension
△ PC: Osteoporosis
△ PC: Peptic Ulcer
△ PC: Thromboembolism
△ PC: Hypokalemia
* PC: Pseudotumor Cerebri
   PC: Hypocalcemia

Nursing Diagnoses

▲ High Risk for Excess Fluid Volume related to sodium and water retention
△ High Risk for Imbalanced Nutrition: More Than Body Requirements related to increased appetite
▲ High Risk for Infection related to immunosuppression
△ High Risk for Disturbed Body Image related to changes in appearance
△ High Risk for Ineffective Therapeutic Regimen Management related to insufficient knowledge of administration schedule, adverse reactions, signs and symptoms of complications, hazards of adrenal insufficiency, and potential causes of adrenal insufficiency

---

▲ This diagnosis was reported to be monitored for or managed frequently (75%–100%).
△ This diagnosis was reported to be monitored for or managed often (50%–74%).
* This diagnosis was not included in the validation study.

Discharge Criteria

Before discharge, the client or family will

1. Relate proper use of the medication.
2. Identify circumstances that require notification of a health care professional.
3. Relate dietary sodium restrictions.
4. Identify signs and symptoms of side effects and adverse reactions.
5. Describe practices that can reduce the side effects of corticosteroid therapy.
6. Verbalize the intent to seek ongoing follow-up care.
7. Verbalize the intent to wear Medic-alert identification.

Collaborative Problems

Potential Complication: Steroid-Induced Diabetes

Potential Complication: Hypertension

Potential Complication: Osteoporosis

Potential Complication: Peptic Ulcer Disease

Potential Complication: Thromboembolism

Potential Complication: Hypokalemia

Potential Complication: Pseudotumor Cerebri

Potential Complication: Hypocalcemia

Interventions	Rationales

1. Monitor for signs and symptoms of diabetes mellitus:
  a. Polyuria, polydipsia
  b. Glycosuria
  c. Proteinuria
	1. Excessive glucocorticoid level antagonizes insulin and promotes *glyconeogenesis,* resulting in hyperglycemia (Porth, 2002).

2. Monitor for hypertension.	2. Mineralocorticoids increase sodium reabsorption, with resulting fluid retention that can adversely affect persons with preexisting hypertension or CHF.

3. Monitor for signs and symptoms of osteoporosis especially in ribs and vertebrae.
  a. Pain
  b. Localized tenderness
 	
4. Monitor for hypocalcemia.
  a. Altered mental status
  b. Muscle cramps
  c. Numbness/tingling in fingers and toes
  d. ECG changes
  e. Seizures
	3,4. Corticosteroids oppose the effects of vitamin D, thus reducing calcium absorption and increasing urinary excretion of calcium. The release of growth hormone is inhibited, which decreases osteoblast function and thinning of epiphyseal plates (Porth, 2002).

5. Teach client about measures to reduce risk of pathologic fractures. (Refer to the Osteoporosis Care Plan in the index for more details.)	5. A client on long-term corticosteroid therapy—especially an older client—is at increased risk for fractures owing to loss of bone density.
6. Teach client the relationship of increased calcium and vitamin D intake and weightbearing exercise to reduced risk of osteoporosis.	6. Increase in vitamin D and calcium intake increases their availability to bone. Weightbearing exercise (e.g., walking) slows rate of calcium loss from bone.

(continues on page 957)

Interventions continued	Rationales continued

7. Monitor for signs and symptoms of peptic ulcer.
   a. Positive guaiac stool test
   b. Gastric pain
	7. Clients with cirrhosis, nephrotic syndrome, or connective tissue disorders receiving over 1 g of steroids or those taking potentially ulcerogenic medications concurrently are susceptible to peptic ulcers.

8. Teach client to take prescribed medication with food or milk.	8. Food or milk can help to neutralize gastric hydrochloric acid; this minimizes gastric upset.

9. Monitor for signs and symptoms of hypokalemia.
   a. Weakness
   b. Lethargy
   c. Serum potassium level <3.5 mEq/L
   d. Nausea and vomiting
   e. Characteristic ECG changes
	9. Excessive mineralocorticoids increase sodium retention and potassium excretion.

10. Monitor for pseudotumor cerebri.
   a. Headaches
   b. Visual changes
   c. Nausea
	10. This is a well-recognized complication of unknown pathophysiology manifested by intracranial hypertension and papilledema. It has been associated when therapy is decreased or the preparation changed, is self-limiting, and reverses when therapy is discontinued.

 Related Physician-Prescribed Interventions

Symptom-specific

Nursing Goal

The nurse will detect early signs and symptoms of (a) steroid-induced diabetes, (b) hypertension, (c) osteoporosis, (d) peptic ulcer, (e) thromboembolism, (f) hypokalemia, (g) pseudotumor cerebri, and (h) hypocalcemia and collaboratively intervene to stabilize client.

Indicators

- Alert, oriented (f, g, h)
- Urine output > 30mL/hr (a)
- Specific gravity 1.005–1.030 (a)
- Urine negative for protein (a)
- Urine negative for glucose (a)
- Stool negative blood (guaiac) (d)
- BP >90/60, <140/90 mm Hg (b)
- No c/o bone pain (c)
- No c/o muscle cramps (b)
- No c/o numbness/tingling in fingers or toes (h)
- Muscle strength—intact (f)
- No seizure activity (h)
- No c/o gastric pain (d)
- No c/o of headaches (g)
- No c/o visual changes (g)
- No c/o of nausea or vomiting (f, g)

- Normal sinus rhythm (EKG) (f, h)
- Serum potassium 3.8–5 mEq/L (f)
- Serum calcium 8.5–10.5 mg/dL (h)

 Documentation

Flow records
Vital signs
Urine glucose and other laboratory values
Pain and numbness in extremities
Gastric pain
Intake and output
Stool guaiac results

Nursing Diagnoses

High Risk for Excess Fluid Volume Related to Sodium and Water Retention

Focus Assessment Criteria	Clinical Significance
1. Current daily corticosteroid dosage 2. Recent weight gain 3. Presence and extent of edema 4. Dietary sodium intake 5. Blood pressure readings	1–5. These assessment data help nurse to identify risks factors and provide a baseline for reassessment for presence of edema.

Goal

The client will report no or minimal edema.

Indicators
- Relate causative factors of edema.
- State controllable factors for edema prevention.

Interventions	Rationales

1. Encourage client to decrease salt intake. Limit sodium to 6 gm a day. Teach client to take the following actions:
  a. Read food labels for sodium content. Review foods high in sodium: mineral water, club soda, crackers, snacks (chips, nuts, and pretzels), muffins, instant cooked foods (cereals, potato soup, sauces, entrees, and vegetables), granola, buttermilk, regular cheese, regular salad dressing, smoked or cured products, sauerkraut, tomato juice, V-8, olives, pickles, and certain seasonings (Ac' Cent, soy sauce, mustard, catsup, horseradish, steak sauces, and seasoned salt).
  b. Cook without salt and use spices (e.g., lemon, basil, tarragon, and mint) to add flavor.
	1. Corticosteroids contain both glucocorticoid and mineralocorticoid elements. The mineralocorticoid element promotes sodium reabsorption and potassium excretion from distal renal tubules. Resultant sodium retention expands extracellular fluid volume by preventing water excretion.

(continues on page 959)

Interventions continued	Rationales continued
c. Use vinegar in place of salt to flavor soups, stews, and so on (e.g., 2 to 3 teaspoons of vinegar to 4 to 6 quarts, according to taste). d. Foods low in sodium are poultry, pumpkin, turnips, egg yolks, cooked vegetables, fruits, grits, honey, jams, jellies, lean meats, potatoes, puffed wheat and rice, red kidney beans, lima beans, sherbet, and unsalted nuts.	
2. Identify strategies to decrease dependent edema. a. Changing positions frequently b. Avoiding constrictive clothing c. Elevating legs when sitting d. Wearing elastic support stockings	2. Edema develops as increased extracellular fluid enters interstitial spaces and the blood; this increases interstitial fluid and blood volume.
3. Teach the importance of a daily walking program.	3. Lymph flow is propelled by contracting skeletal muscles. Exercise increases muscle efficiency (Sieggreen, 1989).
4. Explain measures to protect skin from injury. a. Avoid walking barefoot. b. Break in new shoes slowly. c. Avoid contact sports. d. Prevent dry skin with lubricants.	4. Besides increased risk of skin injury due to edema, loss of perivascular collagen in the skin's small vessels makes them more susceptible to damage.

 Documentation

Flow records
  Weight
  Presence and degree of edema

High Risk for Imbalanced Nutrition: More Than Body Requirements Related to Increased Appetite

Focus Assessment Criteria	Clinical Significance
1. Current corticosteroid dosage 2. Knowledge of nutritional concepts 3. Current eating patterns	1–3. Weight gain associated with corticosteroid therapy is related to fluid retention and the drug's appetite-enhancing effects.
4. Willingness to comply with dietary modifications	4. The client's cooperation is essential to prevent weight gain or to promote weight loss.

Goal

The client will maintain present weight.

Indicators

- Relate factors that contribute to weight gain.
- Identify behaviors that remain under his or her control.

Interventions	Rationales

1. Increase client's awareness of actions that contribute to excessive food intake:
  a. Request that client write down all the food eaten in the past 24 hours.
  b. Instruct client to keep a diet diary for 1 week that specifies the following:
    • What, when, where, and why eaten
    • Whether he or she was doing anything else (e.g., watching television or cooking) while eating
    • Emotions before eating
    • Others present (e.g., snacking with spouse and children)
  c. Review diet diary to point out patterns (e.g., time, place, emotions, foods, and persons) that affect food intake.
  d. Review high- and low-calorie food items.
	1. The ability to lose weight while on corticosteroid therapy likely depends on limiting sodium intake and maintaining a reasonable caloric intake.

2. Teach client behavior modification techniques to decrease caloric intake.
  a. Eat only at a specific spot at home (e.g., the kitchen table).
  b. Do not eat while performing other activities.
  c. Drink an 8-oz glass of water immediately before a meal.
  d. Decrease second helpings, fatty foods, sweets, and alcohol.
  e. Prepare small portions that are just enough for one meal; discard leftovers.
  f. Use small plates to make portions look bigger.
  g. Never eat from another person's plate.
  h. Eat slowly and chew food thoroughly.
  i. Put down utensils and wait 15 seconds between bites.
  j. Eat low-calorie snacks that must be chewed to satisfy oral needs (e.g., carrots, celery, and apples).
  k. Decrease liquid calories by drinking low-sodium diet soda or water.
  l. Plan eating splurges (save a number of calories each day and have a treat once a week) but eat only a small amount of "splurge" foods.
	2. These measures can help to control caloric intake. Often obesity is promoted by an inappropriate response to external cues—most often, stressors. This response triggers an ineffective coping mechanism in which client eats in response to stress rather than physiologic hunger.

(continues on page 961)

Interventions continued	Rationales continued

3. Instruct client to increase activity level to burn calories; encourage her or his to do the following:
   a. Use stairs instead of elevators.
   b. Park at the farthest point in parking lots and walk to buildings.
   c. Plan a daily walking program with a progressive increase in distance and pace.
     Urge client to consult with physician before beginning any exercise program.
	3. Increased activity can promote weight loss. Keep in mind, however, that the client's ability to exercise may be limited by the pathological condition that necessitates corticosteroid therapy as well as by the drug's adverse effects (e.g., osteoporosis or muscle wasting).

4. Refer to care plan on Obesity in index for more information.	

Documentation
Flow records
  Weight
  Intake
  Activity level

High Risk for Infection Related to Immunosuppression

Focus Assessment Criteria	Clinical Significance
1. Current corticosteroid dosage 2. Changes in overall health status (e.g., fatigue and decreased appetite) 3. Evidence of infection with opportunistic organisms	1–3. Glucocorticoids cause atrophy of thymus and decrease number of lymphocytes, plasma cells, and eosinophils. The rate of conversion of lymphocytes into antibodies is decreased. These effects limit the body's usual protective mechanism and cause delayed wound healing.

Goal
The client will be infection free or report early signs or symptoms.

Indicators
- Relate risk factors associated with potential for infection.
- Practice appropriate precautions to prevent infection.

Interventions	Rationales
1. Explain the increased risk of infection; stress the importance of reporting promptly any change in status.	1. High doses of 50 mg or more of prednisone for more than 2 weeks may increase opportunistic infections. Corticosteroids can mask

(continues on page 962)

Interventions continued	Rationales continued
	the usual signs and symptoms of infection such as fever and increased WBC count; this necessitates increased vigilance for subtle changes.
2. Instruct client to avoid persons with infections and large crowds in close quarters.	2. These precautions can help to limit exposure to infectious microorganisms.
3. Explain the vulnerability of skin and risk for injury.	3. Glucocorticoids promote mobilization of fatty acids from adipose tissue, resulting in thin fragile skin.

 Documentation

Flow records
 Temperature
Progress notes
 Change in health status

High Risk for Disturbed Body Image Related to Changes in Appearance

Focus Assessment Criteria	Clinical Significance
1. Signs of iatrogenic Cushing's syndrome, including the following: a. Redistribution of subcutaneous fat (central obesity, moon face, or buffalo hump) b. Alopecia c. Hirsutism d. Fluid retention e. Skin changes (purpura, acne, or petechiae) f. Extremity muscle wasting	1. Excessive corticosteroid levels can cause virilism, protein tissue wasting, some matrix wasting, and abnormal fat distribution.
2. Response to appearance changes	2. This assessment can provide a starting point to begin dialogue.

Goal

The client will demonstrate movement toward reconstruction of an altered body image.

Indicators
• Relate factors contributing to disturbed body image.
• Describe changes related to corticosteroid therapy.

 Documentation

Progress notes
Interactions

Interventions	Rationales
1. Explain that appearance changes are drug-induced and will diminish or resolve with discontinuation or dosage reduction.	1. This explanation can reduce the fear of permanent appearance changes and help to preserve positive self-concept.
2. Encourage client to express feelings about appearance changes.	2. Sharing concerns promotes trust and enables clarification of misconceptions.
3. Promote social interaction.	3. Social isolation can promote fear and unrealistic perceptions.
4. Refer to Disturbed Body Image in index for additional interventions.	

High Risk for Ineffective Therapeutic Regimen Management Related to Insufficient Knowledge of Administration Schedule, Adverse Reactions, Signs and Symptoms of Complications, Hazards of Adrenal Insufficiency, and Potential Causes of Adrenal Insufficiency

Focus Assessment Criteria	Clinical Significance
1. Knowledge of corticosteroid therapy	1. Assessing knowledge level identifies client's learning needs and guides nurse in planning effective teaching strategies.
2. Readiness and ability to learn and retain information	2. A client or family failing to achieve learning goals requires a referral for assistance post-discharge.

Goals

The goals for this diagnosis represent those associated with discharge planning. Refer to the discharge criteria.

Interventions	Rationales
1. Instruct client to take drug dose exactly as prescribed in the morning; keeping in mind these considerations: a. Do not discontinue administration because of adverse effects; if unable to tolerate oral medication, contact physician for instructions.	1. Abrupt cessation of medication after 2 weeks of therapy may precipitate an adrenal crisis. Early morning doses stimulate the body's natural peak excretion. Taking the medication in the morning can reduce hyperactivity at bedtime.

(continues on page 964)

Interventions continued	**Rationales** continued
b. If possible, take daily dose in the morning. c. Take the daily B$_{12}$ dose before 4 PM.	
2. Provide written instructions on dosage schedule if appropriate.	2. A printed schedule may help to improve compliance and avoid under or over dosing.

3. Teach client to watch for and report serious adverse effects such as the following:
   a. Altered mood such as euphoria or even psychosis
   b. Increased susceptibility to skin injury
   c. Weight gain
   d. Increase in BP
   e. Excessive thirst, urination
   f. Severe edema
   g. Change in vision, eye pain
   h. Weakness
   i. Leg pain
   j. Change in stool color
   k. Change in appetite
   l. Rash
	3. The client's vigilance can aid early detection of serious side effects such as hypokalemia, cataracts, diabetes, mellitus, thromboembolism, and peptic ulcer.

4. Teach client to recognize and report signs and symptoms of adrenal insufficiency.
   a. Hypoglycemia
   b. Nausea and vomiting
   c. Diarrhea
   d. Decreased mental acuity
   e. Fatigue, weakness, and malaise
   f. Hyponatremia
   g. Orthostatic hypotension
   h. Palpitations
   i. Decreased appetite
   j. Weight loss
	4. Corticosteroid therapy inhibits pituitary function, resulting in inhibited adrenal function. Early detection enables prompt intervention to prevent serious complications.

5. Encourage client scheduled for long-term corticosteroid therapy to obtain and wear Medic-alert identification.	5. A visible identification bracelet or necklace can aid early detection of adrenal insufficiency.
6. Inform client that he or she should notify physician about a possible increase in corticosteroid dosage before undergoing invasive procedures or vaccinations or when experiencing infection.	6. Additional stress normally triggers an increased adrenal response; however, corticosteroid therapy interferes with adrenal function, possibly necessitating increased corticosteroid dosage to maintain homeostasis. When vaccinated for a disease, a client whose immune system is compromised can get the disease.

(continues on page 965)

Interventions continued	**Rationales** continued

7. Teach client that corticosteroids can increase or decrease the effectiveness of certain medications. Other medications can influence the effectiveness of corticosteroids. Instruct client to consult with pharmacist before taking a medication.
  a. Medications affected are digitalis products, salicylates, amphotericin B, diuretics, potassium supplements, ritodrine, somatrem, vaccines, and immunizations.
  b. Medications that affect corticosteroid affects are antacids, mitotane, oral contraceptives, liver-enzyme–inducing agents, phenobarbital, rifampin, phenytoin, and aminoglutethimide.
	7. The chemical effects of corticosteroids on the body can influence the effects of other chemicals.

8. Teach client to have regular eye examinations.	8. Systemic corticosteroid use can cause posterior subcapsular cataracts and increased intraocular pressure (glaucoma).

9. Advise client to
  a. Start smoking cessation program.
  b. Limit alcohol intake.
  c. Engage in weight bearing exercises for 30 to 60 minutes per day.
	9. These measures increase the effectiveness of corticosteroids.

10. Discuss the addition of calcium 1500 mg with Vitamin D 800 mg a day.	10. Corticosteroid therapy inhibits calcium mobilization and causes decreased calcium levels.
11. Advise client of the effects on triglycerides levels and the need for follow-up lipid profiles.	11. Corticosteroids promote glyconeogenesis, which raises blood glucose and triglyceride levels.
12. Advise client to wear a medical-alert bracelet.	12. Abrupt cessation of corticosteroids can precipitate an adrenal crisis.
13. Encourage client to keep regular follow-up appointments.	13. Because of the seriousness of adverse effects, careful monitoring is needed.

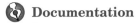 **Documentation**

Discharge summary record
Client teaching
Outcome achievement or status

ENTERAL NUTRITION

Enteral nutrition is the administration of an elemental liquid diet (calories, minerals, and vitamins) to the GI tract through a nasogastric, nasojejunostomy gastric, or jejunostomy tube. Enteral nutrition can include both oral supplements and tube-feeding techniques. The person with a functioning intestine but who is unable to eat sufficient calories is a candidate (Pace et al., 1997). Enteral nutrition is not recommended in persons experiencing severe diarrhea, intensive chemotherapy, immediate postoperative stress period, severe acute pancreatitis, shock, ileus, intestinal obstruction, or high-output external fistulas or when the client or legal guardian does not desire aggressive nutritional support (if in accordance with agency policy and existing law).

 Time Frame

Preprocedure and postprocedure

 DIAGNOSTIC CLUSTER

Collaborative Problems

▲ PC: Hypoglycemia/Hyperglycemia
▲ PC: Hypervolemia
△ PC: Hypertonic Dehydration
▲ PC: Electrolyte Imbalances
△ PC: Mucosal Erosion

Nursing Diagnoses

▲ High Risk for Infection related to gastrostomy incision and enzymatic action of gastric juices on skin
▲ Impaired Comfort: Cramping, Distention, Nausea, Vomiting related to type of formula, administration rate, route, or formula temperature
▲ Diarrhea related to adverse response to formula, rate, or temperature
▲ Risk for Aspiration related to position of tube and client
△ High Risk for Disturbed Self-Concept related to inability to taste or swallow food and fluids
△ High Risk for Ineffective Therapeutic Regimen Management related to lack of knowledge of nutritional indications/requirements, home care, and signs and symptoms of complications

---

▲ This diagnosis was reported to be monitored for or managed frequently (75%–100%).
△ This diagnosis was reported to be monitored for or managed often (50%–74%).

Discharge Criteria

Before discharge, the client or family will

1. Identify therapeutic indications and nutritional requirements.
2. Demonstrate tube feeding administration and management.
3. Discuss strategies for incorporating enteral management into ADLs.
4. State signs and symptoms that must be reported to a health care professional.

Collaborative Problems

Potential Complication: Hypoglycemia or Hyperglycemia

Potential Complication: Hypervolemia

Potential Complication: Hypertonic Dehydration

Potential Complication: Electrolyte and Trace Mineral Imbalance

Potential Complication: Mucosal Erosion

Nursing Goal
The nurse will detect early signs and symptoms of (a) hypoglycemia/hyperglycemia, (b) hypervolemia, (c) hypertonic dehydration, (d) electrolyte imbalances, and mucosal erosion and will collaboratively intervene to stabilize client.

Indicators
- Alert, oriented, calm (a)
- Pulse 60–100 beats/min (a, b)
- Respirations easy, rhythmic 16–20 breaths/min (b)
- Respiratory, no rales or wheezing (b)
- BP >90/60, <140/90 mm Hg (b)
- No complaints of dizziness (a)
- Intact muscle strength (a)
- Warm, dry skin (a)
- Urine output 730 mL/hr (a)
- Urine specific gravity 1.005–1.030 (c)
- Serum potassium 3.8–5 mEq/L (c, d)
- Serum sodium 135–145 mEq/L (c, d)
- Serum osmolality 280–300 mOsm/kg H_2O (c, d)
- No peripheral edema (b)
- Moist mucous membranes (oral) (c)
- Intact mucosa at tube exit site (d)
- No complaints of fatigue (a)
- No complaints of nausea (a)

Interventions	Rationales
1. Monitor for symptoms of hypoglycemia after completion of tube feeding. a. Tachycardia b. Diaphoresis c. Confusion d. Dizziness e. Generalized weakness	1. Sudden cessation of enteral feedings in a physiologically stressed client may trigger a hypoglycemic reaction.
2. Monitor for symptoms of hyperglycemia during formula administration. a. Thirst b. Increased urination c. Fatigue d. Generalized weakness e. Increased respirations f. Increased pulse g. Nausea	2. Hyperglycemia most commonly occurs in clients with inadequate insulin reserves. Enteral formulas with a higher fat percentage are less likely to contribute to hyperglycemic reaction.

(continues on page 968)

Interventions continued	**Rationales** continued

3. Monitor for signs and symptoms of over-hydration during formula administration.
  a. Tachycardia
  b. Elevated blood pressure
  c. Pulmonary edema
  d. Shortness of breath
  e. Peripheral edema
	3. Hypervolemia usually is associated with the high water and sodium contents of the enteral formula. This complication most often occurs as feeding is initiated or re-introduced in a client with compromised cardiac, renal, or hepatic function.

4. Monitor for signs and symptoms of hypertonic dehydration during formula administration.
  a. Dry mucous membranes
  b. Thirst
  b. Decreased serum
  c. Serum sodium decreased
  d. Circulatory overload (increased BP, increased respirations)
  e. Decreasing urine output
  f. Concentrated urine
	4. Hypertonic dehydration most often results when a formula of high osmolarity and protein content is administered to a client unable to recognize or respond to thirst. It causes circulatory overload and cellular dehydration.

5. Monitor tube exit and entrance sites for
  a. Mucosal erosion
  b. Pain and tenderness
  c. Bleeding
  d. Ulceration
 	
6. Take steps to reduce tube irritation.
  a. Tape tubes securely without causing pressure or tension.
  b. Prepare skin prior to taping with a skin protective agent.
  c. Use small-bore silicone tubes for enteral feedings administered by the naso-gastric route.
	5,6. External pressure or tension on delicate structures can produce mucosal erosion. Prolonged use of large-bore polyvinyl chloride (PVC) catheters has been linked to nasal cartilage destruction.

 Related Physician-Prescribed Interventions

Medications. Formula (frequency and dilution)

Intravenous Therapy. Not applicable

Laboratory Studies. Serum prealbumin, electrolytes, serum glucose, serum transferrin

Diagnostic Studies. Radiogram (verification)

Therapies. Dependent on the type of tube used, weights

Documentation

Flow records
  Vital signs
  Intake and output
  Urine specific gravity
  Serum glucose
  Tube site condition

Nursing Diagnoses

High Risk for Infection Related to Gastrostomy Incision and Enzymatic Action of Gastric Juices on Skin

Focus Assessment Criteria	Clinical Significance
1. Temperature 2. Gastrostomy incision and tube insertion site 3. Drainage characteristics 4. Complaints of discomfort	1–5. Leaking of gastric or intestinal digestive juices to skin surface can cause subsequent excoriation and ulceration. The gastrostomy tube provides an entry site for microorganisms.

Goal

The client will

1. Describe measures for infection prevention.
2. Report any discomfort around the gastrostomy site.

Interventions	Rationales
1. Cleanse incision and tube insertion site regularly following standard protocol.	1. Cleaning removes microorganisms and reduces risk of infection.
2. Protect skin around the external feeding tube with a protective barrier film. Apply a loose dressing cover and change it when moist. For excessive drainage, protect skin with an adhesive barrier square and ostomy pouch to capture drainage; change the barrier when nonadherent or soiled.	2. The catheter can irritate skin and mucosa. Gastric juices can cause severe skin breakdown.
3. For a temporary gastrostomy or jejunostomy tube, anchor tube to an external surface to minimize tube migration and retraction.	3. Movement can cause tissue trauma and create entry points for opportunistic microorganisms.
4. Teach client to promptly report discomfort around incision or tube.	4. Early detection and reporting enables prompt intervention to prevent serious inflammation.
5. If skin problems persist, consult clinical nurse specialist or enterostomal therapist for assistance.	5. The expertise of a skin care specialist may be needed.

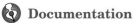 **Documentation**

Flow records
    Vital signs
    Drainage (characteristics, amount)
    Site condition

Impaired Comfort: Cramping, Distention, Nausea, Vomiting Related to Type of Formula, Administration Rate, Route, or Formula Temperature

Focus Assessment Criteria	Clinical Significance
1. History of lactose or fat intolerance 2. Residual contents (gastric feedings only) 3. Complaints of cramping, nausea, vomiting, and abdominal distention	1–3. A high-osmolarity formula administered rapidly can cause retention, nausea, and vomiting. These complications also may occur after administration to a client with formula/delivery intolerance.
4. Complaints of foul formula odor	4. The odor of enteral formula seems to provoke nausea and vomiting in some clients.
5. Consider route of enteral feeding before determining appropriate regimen.	5. Consideration of feeding route and client LOC will assist in determining whether the intermittent or continuous regimen is utilized. Intermittent is routinely suggested for stomach feeding, whereas jejunal feedings adapt well to a continuous delivery mode (Pace et al., 1997).

Goal

The client will tolerate enteral feedings without episodes of cramping, distention, nausea, or vomiting.

Interventions	Rationales
1. Review enteral product information for formula characteristics (i.e., lactose, osmolarity, calories, and fiber). Consult with nutritional expert.	1. Many current enteral products have a significantly lower osmolarity and are now lactose free. Specialty formulas (i.e., specific for renal or liver conditions) tend to have higher osmolarities because of their increased calorie-to-milliliter ratio.
2. Initiate feedings slowly; gradually increase rate based on tolerance. Begin with an isotonic, lactose-free formula or alternately dilute other types of feedings with water to decrease osmolarity. 3. Instill formula at room temperature directly from the can whenever possible.	2,3. The feeding regimen itself may cause problems. For example, a bolus feeding of high osmolarity at cold temperature can provoke gastric and digestive problems. Uncontrolled feedings by jejunal route are particularly prone to these complications because the feeding is not processed in the stomach before it reaches the intestines.
4. Discard unused portions or store in a tightly sealed container. 5. For continuous feeding, fill container with enough formula for a 4-hour feeding. Do not overfill or allow formula to stand for a longer period.	4,5. Extended exposure of a feeding to room temperature promotes microorganism growth.

(continues on page 971)

Interventions continued	Rationales continued
6. For intermittent feeding, instill formula gradually over a 15- to 45-minute period. Do not administer as a bolus or at a rapid rate.	6. Slow administration can reduce cramping, nausea, and vomiting.

Documentation

Flow records
  Intake and output
Progress notes
  Unusual events or problems

Diarrhea Related to Adverse Response to Formula Rate or Temperature

Focus Assessment Criteria	Clinical Significance
1. Bowel pattern before initiation of enteral feedings 2. Current bowel pattern: amount, nature, and consistency 3. Elimination pattern in relation to feedings 4. Formula characteristics (osmolarity, lactose, fiber, and protein) content and feeding regimen (amount, rate, times)	1–4. Diarrhea results from altered intestinal absorptive capacity. Severe malnutrition and protein depletion can precipitate this reaction because of impaired ability of the osmotic transport mechanism to transfer nutrients to the intestinal capillary network.

Goal

The client will demonstrate a tolerable, consistent bowel pattern with no episodes of diarrhea.

Interventions	Rationales
1. Initiate feedings slowly; progress gradually as tolerated. Begin with an isotonic, lactose-free, fiber-enriched supplement.	1. Diminished intestinal absorption must be compensated for through gradual, progressive introduction of enteral supplements.
2. Instill formula at room temperature directly from the can when possible.	2. Administering cold formula can cause cramping and possibly lead to elimination problems.
3. Discard unused portions or store in a tightly sealed container.	3. These precautions can minimize growth of microorganisms.

(continues on page 972)

Interventions continued	Rationales continued
4. For continuous feeding, fill container with enough formula for a 4-hour feeding. Do not overfill or allow formula to stand for a longer period.	4. Each type of formula has an individual shelf-life after opening. Formula should be protected from environmental contaminants to prevent bacterial growth and possible resultant diarrhea. Jejunal intestinal feedings are particularly sensitive to diarrhea because they lack hydrochloric acid.
5. For intermittent feeding, instill formula gradually over a 15- to 45-minute period. Do not administer as a bolus or at a rapid rate.	5. Intermittent feedings simulate a normal feeding regimen and allow for stomach digestion and emptying. Intermittent stomach feedings also allow for unencumbered physical care between feedings.
6. Consult with physician for antidiarrheal medications as necessary.	6. Medications may be needed to control severe diarrhea.

 Documentation

Flow records
   Intake and output

High Risk for Aspiration Related to Position of Tube and Client

Focus Assessment Criteria	Clinical Significance
1. Vital signs 2. Breath sounds 3. Position of tube 4. History of aspiration, swallowing difficulty 5. Abdominal distention, bloating and bowel sounds	1–5. Aspiration pneumonia is a potential complication for all tube-fed clients. Most commonly, it is marked by sudden onset of respiratory distress or failure following an episode of vomiting. Sometimes the presence of aspiration is insidious and occurs without overt evidence of vomiting. This type of aspiration occurs most commonly in a client with impaired mentation, glottic stenosis, swallowing difficulty, or tracheostomy.

Goal

The client will digest feedings without aspiration.

Interventions	Rationales
1. Elevate head of the bed 30 to 45 degrees during feedings and for 1 hour afterward.	1. Upper body elevation can prevent reflux through use of gravity.

(continues on page 973)

Interventions continued	Rationales continued
2. For a nasogastric or nasojejunal tube, verify proper tube placement by air auscultation. 3. For a tube positioned gastrically, verify placement by aspirating for residual contents.	2,3. Proper tube position must be verified before feeding to prevent introducing formula into the respiratory tract.
4. Administer a scheduled intermittent tube feeding only if residual contents are <150 mL. When a high residual is identified, return it to the stomach. Administer continuous feeding only if residual contents are not >20% of the hourly administration rate. Delay feeding if it is intermittent; stop it for 1 hour if it is continuous. Recheck the residual in 1 hour; if it is still high, notify physician. A different rate, method, route, or formula change may be indicated.	4. Administering feedings in the presence of excessive residual contents increases risks of reflux and aspiration (Pace et al., 1997).
5. Regulate intermittent gastric feedings to allow gastric emptying between feedings. 6. Regulate continuous feedings to allow periods of rest so client can ambulate unencumbered by feeding apparatus.	5,6. Such regulation is necessary to prevent overfeeding and increased risk of reflux and aspiration. Gastric feedings should be administered intermittently when the potential for aspiration is high. Continuous feedings increase the risk of aspiration because the stomach contains a constant supply of formula (Pace et al., 1997).
7. When assessing for aspiration, to distinguish gastric secretions in tracheal contents, test the aspirate for glucose. If the concentration is >150 mg/dL, the client has probably aspirated the enteral feeding.	7. Normal tracheal secretions do not contain glucose unless the feeding supplement has entered the respiratory tract (Metheny, 1993).
8. Flush feeding tube with water after completion of feeding.	8. Flushing is necessary to remove formula that can provide a medium for microorganism growth.

 Documentation

Flow records
  Vital signs
  Breath sounds
  Intake and output
Progress notes
  Unusual complaints

High Risk for Disturbed Self-Concept Related to Inability to Taste or Swallow Food and Fluids

Focus Assessment Criteria	Clinical Significance
1. Feelings and concerns related to inability to ingest food orally	1. Food and eating have many social and cultural implications besides nutritional intake. Prolonged or permanent NPO status can interfere with socialization and create isolation.

Goals

The client will

1. Share feelings related to lack of oral ingestion.
2. Verbalize the necessity of continued enteral feedings.

Interventions	Rationales
1. Encourage client to verbalize concerns related to lack of oral ingestion.	1. Sharing helps to identify and clarify client's concerns and problems; this guides nurse in planning effective interventions.
2. Explore possible alternatives to oral ingestion or substitute diversional activities.	2. Substituting activities for meals may help to reduce the sense of loss related to lack of oral intake.
3. Provide regular feedback on progress and positive reinforcement on appearance and weight gain.	3. Feedback and reinforcement promote self-esteem and encourage continued compliance.
4. Arrange for visits from others on enteral nutrition if feasible.	4. Sharing with others in the same situation allows opportunities for mutual validation and support.
5. If permitted, allow the client to taste—but not swallow–desired foods.	5. Placing food in the mouth without swallowing may help to satisfy client's need to taste and smell food.

⊛ Documentation

Progress notes
  Dialogues

High Risk for Ineffective Therapeutic Regimen Management Related to Lack of Knowledge of Nutritional Indications/Requirements, Home Care, and Signs and Symptoms of Complications

Focus Assessment Criteria	Clinical Significance
1. Understanding therapeutic indications and requirements	1. Assessment establishes a baseline for teaching.
2. Available support persons to assist with home therapy	2. Assistance is often needed for at-home treatment.
3. Readiness and ability to learn and retain information	3. Client or family failing to achieve learning goals requires a referral for assistance postdischarge.

Goals

The goals for this diagnosis represent those associated with discharge planning. Refer to the discharge criteria.

Interventions	Rationales
1. Explain rationale for and aspects of enteral nutrition therapy. Discuss client's specific nutritional requirements and specific indications for therapy.	1. Explaining the need for optimal nutrition and the advantages of enteral feedings can reduce misconceptions and encourage compliance.
2. Explain rationale for continued diagnostic tests (e.g., routine weighing, intake and output measurements, urine tests, and serum evaluation)	2. Careful monitoring is needed to evaluate the effectiveness and safety of enteral therapy and enable early detection of problems or complications.
3. Review potential problems and complications such as these: a. Vomiting b. Improper tube placement c. Aspiration	3. Client's and family's understanding of potential complications enables them to detect and report signs and symptoms soon after they develop.
4. Refer client to a home care agency for follow-up home visits.	4. A home health agency can provide ongoing assistance and support.
5. Teach client to do enteral tube care and maintenance. In certain cases, nasogastric tube insertion may be taught.	5. Some clients and families can be taught insertion of gastric feeding tubes. Tubes positioned to feed specific areas of the GI tract are generally more complex and require radiologic confirmation.

(continues on page 976)

Interventions continued	**Rationales** continued
6. Teach client aspects of the enteral feeding regimen; cover these elements: a. Handwashing b. Work surface preparation c. Formula preparation d. Administration procedure e. Completion of feeding f. Dressing changes and skin protection measures g. Equipment operation and care	6. Certain knowledge is needed for proper administration and prevention of complications.
7. Have client or support person perform return demonstration of selected care measures.	7. Return demonstration lets nurse evaluate client's and family's abilities to perform feedings safely.
8. Explain measures to prevent aspiration. (Refer to the nursing diagnosis Potential for Aspiration in this entry for more information)	8. Aspiration is a potential complication of all types of tube feedings.
9. Teach other self-care measures including these: a. Use tap water to irrigate feeding tube before and after instilling formula. b. Chew gum if indicated. c. Brush teeth and use mouthwash three to four times a day. d. Review client medications and teach proper administration to ensure correct dosing and absorption. Medications should not be added to formula container. e. Mark tube when it is in the correct position.	9. a. Irrigation allows evaluation of tube patency, clears tubes, and ensures delivery of a full dose of formula. b. Gum can help to keep the mouth moist. c. Frequent mouth care can maintain moist mucous membranes and remove microorganisms. d. Medications added directly to the formula container can alter dosages, block the feeding tube, or decrease medication effectiveness. e. Markings provide a visible cue of a tube position change.
10. Provide client with a written list of required equipment and supplies and sources for these items.	10. Advance planning can prevent shortages and improper substitutions.

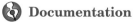 **Documentation**

Discharge summary record
  Client and family teaching
  Outcome achievement or status
  Referrals if indicated

HEMODIALYSIS

Hemodialysis is the removal of metabolic wastes and excess electrolytes and fluids from the blood to treat acute or chronic kidney disease. The procedure uses the principles of diffusion, osmosis, and filtration. Blood is pumped into an artificial kidney through a semipermeable, cellophane-like membrane surrounded by a flow of dialysate, which is a solution composed of water, glucose, sodium, chloride, potassium, calcium, and acetate or bicarbonate. The amounts of these constituents vary depending on the amount of water, waste products, or electrolytes to be removed.

Time Frame
Pretherapy, intratherapy, and post-therapy

DIAGNOSTIC CLUSTER

Collaborative Problems	Refer to
▲ PC: Electrolyte Imbalance (Potassium, Sodium)	
* PC: Hemolysis	
△ PC: Dialysis Disequilibrium Syndrome	
▲ PC: Clotting	
▲ PC: Air Embolism	
▲ PC: Pyrogen Reaction	
▲ PC: Fluid Imbalances	Peritoneal Dialysis
▲ PC: Anemia	Chronic Kidney Disease

Nursing Diagnoses	Refer to
▲ High Risk for Infection Transmission related to frequent contacts with blood and high risk of hepatitis B and C	
△ Powerlessness related to need for treatments to live despite effects on life style	Chronic Kidney Disease
△ Interrupted Family Processes related to the disruption in role responsibilities caused by the treatment schedule	Chronic Kidney Disease

Related Care Plans

Chronic Kidney Disease or Acute Kidney Failure

External Arteriovenous Shunting

▲ This diagnosis was reported to be monitored for or managed frequently (75%–100%).
△ This diagnosis was reported to be monitored for or managed often (50%–74%).
* This diagnosis was not included in the validation study.

Discharge Criteria

Before discharge, the client and or family will

1. Describe the purpose of hemodialysis.
2. Discuss feelings and concerns regarding the effects of long-term therapy on self and family.
3. State signs and symptoms that must be reported to a health care professional.

Collaborative Problems

Potential Complication: Electrolyte Imbalance (Potassium, Sodium)

Potential Complication: Hemolysis

Potential Complication: Dialysis Disequilibrium Syndrome

Potential Complication: Clotting

Potential Complication: Air Embolism

Potential Complication: Fluid Imbalances

Potential Complication: Anemia

Nursing Goal

The nurse will monitor to detect early signs and symptoms of (a) electrolyte imbalance, (b) hemolysis, (c) dialysis disequilibrium syndrome, (d) clotting, (e) air embolism, (f) fluid imbalances, and (g) anemia, and will intervene collaboratively to stabilize the client.

Indicators

- Alert, oriented, calm (c)
- Skin warm, dry, usual color (e)
- No or minimal edema (f)
- B/P > 90–60, < 140/90 mm Hg (c, e)
- Pulse pressure (40 mm Hg difference in systolic or diastolic) (c, e)
- Pulse 60–100 beats/min (c, e)
- Respirations 16–20 breaths/min (e)
- Respirations relaxed, rhythmic (e)
- No rales or wheezing (e)
- No weight change (f)
- No headache (c)
- No chest pain (e)
- No change in vision (e)
- No c/o of nausea/vomiting (c)
- No seizures (c)
- Serum potassium 3.5–5 mEq/L (a)
- Hemoglobin (g)
    - Male 13.5–17.5 g/dL
    - Female 13–16 g/dL
- Hematocrit (g)
    - Male 40%–54%
    - Female 37%–47%
- Serum sodium 135–148 mm/dL (a)
- Serum creatinine 0.6–1.2 mg/dL (a)
- Blood urea nitrogen 7–18 mg/dL (a)
- Intact access site (d)
- Intact connections (d)
- No burning at site (b)
- No blood in venous line (b)

Interventions	Rationales
1. Assess the following:	1. Predialysis assessment and documentation of client's status are mandatory before initiation of the hemodialysis procedure to establish a baseline and to identify problems.
a. Skin (color, turgor, temperature, moisture, and edema)	a. Skin assessment can provide data to evaluate circulation, level of hydration, fluid retention, and uremia.
b. Blood pressure (lying and sitting)	b. Low blood pressure may indicate intolerance to transmembrane pressure, hypovolemia, or the effects of antihypertensive medication given predialysis. High blood pressure may indicate overhydration, increased renin production, or dietary and fluid indiscretion.
c. Apical pulse (rhythm and rate)	c. Cardiac assessment evaluates the heart's ability to compensate for changes in fluid volume.
d. Respirations (rate, effort, and abnormal sounds)	d. Respiratory assessment evaluates compensatory ability of the system and presence of infection.
e. Weight (gain or loss)	e. Predialysis weight indicating gain or loss may necessitate a need to reevaluate dry weight.
f. Vascular access (site and patency)	f. The vascular access site is assessed for signs of infection or abnormal drainage. Patency is evaluated by assessment of bruits and thrills.
g. Pretreatment BUN, serum creatinine, sodium, and potassium levels	g. Pretreatment serum levels are used as a baseline for evaluation of the effectiveness of the dialysis (Brundage, 1992).
2. Assess the client's complaints of the following symptoms: a. Chest pain b. Shortness of breath c. Cramps d. Headache e. Dizziness f. Blurred vision g. Nausea and vomiting h. Change in mentation or speech.	2. These assessment data help to determine if there has been a change in the client's condition since last treatment or if a change in treatment is indicated. When a client presents with problems predialysis, underlying etiology needs to be determined before initiation of treatment.
3. Check the dialysis machine set-up for the following: a. Evidence of air in line b. Secure connections c. Armed air detector d. Poor connection or crack around the hub of the vascular needles e. Fluid in normal saline bag f. Arterial needle site collapse, allowing air to enter around the needle	3. Careful checking can detect air or leaks.

(continues on page 980)

Interventions continued	**Rationales** continued
4. Intradialysis—monitor for signs and symptoms of potassium and sodium imbalance. (Refer to the Peritoneal Dialysis Care Plan for more information.)	4. Dialysate fluid composition and rates of inflow and outflow determine electrolyte imbalances.
5. Do not leave the client unattended at any time during dialysis.	5. A complication such as hemorrhage, transfusion reaction, or clotting can become serious quickly if not detected and treated promptly. Early detection can prevent substantial blood loss.
6. Alternate puncture sites with every treatment and question the client regarding pain in the area of access.	6. Repeated needle punctures at the same site can cause an aneurysm.
7. Apply pinpoint pressure to fistula sticks postdialysis to control bleeding. When cannulating a new shunt, maintain pressure for 20 minutes, then apply pressure dressings after bleeding is controlled.	7. These measures can help to prevent exsanguination from access site.
8. Check the shunt dressing every 2 hours for bleeding or disconnection.	8. Bleeding can be a sign of disconnected or clotted shunt tubing.
9. Monitor for manifestations of hemolysis: a. Bright red blood in venous line b. Burning at the circulatory return site c. Pink- to red-tinged dialysate	9. Rupture of red blood cells can result from the hypotonic dialysate, high dialysate temperature, or chloramines, nitrates, copper, zinc, or formaldehyde in the dialysate.
10. Monitor for seizure activity.	10. Hypotension caused by rapid fluid loss can precipitate a seizure.
11. Monitor for signs and symptoms of dialysis/disequilibrium syndrome: a. Headache b. Nausea c. Vomiting d. Restlessness e. Hypertension f. Increased pulse pressures g. Altered sensorium h. Convulsions i. Coma	11. As a result of hemodialysis, the concentration of BUN is reduced more rapidly than the urea nitrogen level in cerebrospinal fluid and brain tissue because of the slow transport of urea across the blood-brain barrier. Urea acts as an osmotic agent, drawing water from the plasma and extracellular fluid into the cerebral cells and producing cerebral edema. Other factors, such as rapid pH changes and electrolyte shifts, also can cause cerebral edema (Brundage, 1992).

(continues on page 981)

Interventions continued	**Rationales** continued

12. Monitor for clotting:
  a. Observe for clot formation in kidney and drip chambers.
  b. Monitor pressure readings every 15 minutes.
  c. Observe for clots when aspirating fistula needles, arteriovenous shunt, or subclavian catheter.
	12. Blood contacting the nonvascular surface of the extracorporeal circuit activates the normal clotting mechanism. During dialysis, fibrin formation within the venous trap and a gradual increase in the circuit's venous pressure (resulting from clotting in the venous trap or needle) may indicate inadequate heparinization. Clot formation elevates blood pressure readings (Lancaster, 1997).

13. Monitor for signs and symptoms of air embolism:
  a. Cyanosis
  b. Shortness of breath
  c. Chest pain
  d. Visual changes: diplopia, "seeing stars," and blindness
  e. Anxiety
  f. Persistent cough
	13. As little as 10 mL of air introduced into the venous circulation is clinically significant. Large air bubbles are changed to foam as they enter the heart. Foam can decrease the volume of blood entering the lungs, decreasing left heart blood flow and cardiac output. Entry of air into the respiratory circulatory system causes a profound negative response.

14. If signs and symptoms of air embolism occur, take these steps:
  a. Clamp the venous line and stop the blood pump.
  b. Position client on his or her left side with feet elevated for 30 minutes.
	14.
	
	  a. Clamping the line and stopping the pump can halt infusion of air.
	
	  b. This prevents air from going to the head and traps air in the right atrium and in the right ventricle away from the pulmonic valve.

 Related Physician-Prescribed Interventions

Medications. Refer to the Chronic Kidney Disease Care Plan.

Laboratory Studies. Refer to the Chronic Kidney Disease Care Plan.

Diagnostic Studies. Refer to the Chronic Kidney Disease Care Plan.

Therapies. Dialysate solution

Documentation
Flow records
  Vital signs
  Weight
  Vascular access site
  Dialysis (time, solution)
Progress notes
  Predialysis complaints
  Intradialysis complaints

Nursing Diagnoses

High Risk for Infection Transmission Related to Frequent Contacts with Blood and People at High Risk for Hepatitis B and C

Focus Assessment Criteria	Clinical Significance
1. Monitor laboratory results regarding hepatitis surveillance as recommended by the U.S. Centers for Disease Control and Prevention. 2. Assess for signs and symptoms of hepatitis. 3. Elicit history of exposure to hepatitis.	1–3. Clients and personnel are at high risk for HBV/HCV because of many contacts with blood or blood products.:

Goal

The client will relate the risks of hepatitis B transmission.

Indicators
- Have antibodies to HBV.
- Take precautions to prevent transmission of HBV.

Interventions	Rationales

1. Observe strict isolation procedure.
  a. Wear an isolation gown and mask during dialysis treatment.
  b. Dialysis should be performed in client's private room or a dialysis unit isolation area.
  c. All blood or dialysis effluent spills must be cleaned up immediately with antimicrobial soap and water.
  d. Observe isolation disposal procedure for all needles, syringes, and effluent.
  e. Do not permit staff and other personnel or visitors to eat or drink anything within the dialysis treatment area.
  f. Ensure that all specimens for laboratory analysis are labeled "Isolation" and placed in bags also labeled "Isolation."
  g. Use special disposable thermometers to assess temperature.
  h. Avoid contact with other dialysis clients, if staffing level permits. If contact is necessary, change isolation gowns and wash hands carefully.
  i. Avoid any skin contact with the client's blood.
  j. Follow isolation procedure for waste and linen disposal per institutional protocol.
  k. Follow the recommended sterilization procedure for the hemodialysis machine after use.
	1. HBV/HCV is found in the blood, saliva, semen, and vaginal secretions. Transmission is usually through blood (percutaneous or permucosal). Regularly practicing certain precautions provides protection (Lancaster, 1997).

(continues on page 983)

Interventions continued	Rationales continued
2. Administer immunizations, as appropriate, following facility policies.	2. High-risk clients and others should be immunized.
3. Explain that there is no prophylaxis for HCV and that it can go unnoticed for years.	3. Only 10% of people report an acute illness.
4. Minimize use of anticoagulants in clients with liver disease. 5. Collaborate with physician and/or advanced practice nurse to adjust medications with potential hepatotoxicity, including immuno-suppressants. 6. Reinforce to client and family the serious nature of HBV/HCV, precautions, and risks.	4–6. Reiterating the seriousness of HBV/HCV and its possible sequelae may encourage compliance with instructions and precautions.

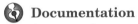 **Documentation**

Teaching record
    Client and family teaching
Flow records
    Monthly HBV screening results

LONG-TERM VENOUS ACCESS DEVICES

Long-term venous access devices (VADs) are used for clients who have a need for frequent venous access to deliver chemotherapy, intravenous fluids, and blood products. They also provide access for blood samples.

There are four groups of central venous access devices: nontunneled (percutaneous) central catheters; peripherally inserted central catheters; tunneled catheters (e.g., Groshong, Hickman-Broviac); and implanted ports. These devices can last weeks, months, or years. Percutaneous central catheters have the shortest duration.

 Time Frame

Preprocedure and postprocedure

⊗ DIAGNOSTIC CLUSTER

Collaborative Problems

▲ PC: Hemorrhage
△ PC: Embolism/Thrombosis
▲ PC: Sepsis
  PC: Phlebitis (site)
  PC: Extravasation (site)

Nursing Diagnoses

▲ Anxiety related to upcoming insertion of catheter/port and insufficient knowledge of procedure
△ High Risk for Ineffective Therapeutic Regimen Management related to insufficient knowledge of home care, signs and symptoms of complications, and community resources
▲ High Risk for Infection related to catheter's direct access to bloodstream (Refer to Total Parenteral Nutrition)

Related Care Plans

Cancer: Initial Diagnosis
Chemotherapy

▲ This diagnosis was reported to be monitored for or managed frequently (75%–100%).
△ This diagnosis was reported to be monitored for or managed often (50%–74%).

Discharge Criteria

Before discharge, the client and or family will

1. Demonstrate procedure and discuss conditions of catheter care and administration at home.
2. Discuss strategies for incorporating catheter management in activities of daily living (ADLs).
3. Verbalize necessary precautions.
4. State signs and symptoms that must be reported to a health care professional.
5. Identify available community resources.

Collaborative Problems

Potential Complication: Hemorrhage

Potential Complication: Embolism/Thrombosis

Potential Complication: Sepsis

Potential Complication: Phlebitis (site)

Potential Complication: Extravasation (site)

Nursing Goal

The nurse will monitor for early signs and symptoms of (a) hemorrhage, (b) embolism/thrombosis, (c) sepsis, (d) phlebitis (site), and (e) extravasation and collaboratively intervene to stabilize the client.

Indicators

- Calm, alert, oriented (b, c)
- Warm, dry, skin (a, c)
- B/P >90/60, <140/90 mm Hg (a, b, c)
- Pulse 60–100 beats/min (a, b, c)
- Respirations 16–20 breaths/min (a, b, c)
- Respirations easy, rhythmic (a, b, c)
- Temperature 98.5–99°F (c, d)
- Urine output > 30mL/hr (a, c)
- Urine negative for bacteria, WBC (c)
- Negative blood culture (c)
- Intact insertion site (d, e)
- Patient catheter with blood return (d, e)
- No swelling, tenderness, drainage at site (d, e)
- No c/o of stinging, pain, or burning at insertion site (d, e)

Interventions	Rationales
1. Follow agency protocols for insertion, maintenance and management of local complications. If chemotherapeutic agents are administered, refer to chemotherapy care plan.	1. Institutional policies will specifically outline monitoring and interventions for catheter care and local complications (e.g., phlebitis, extravasation [leakage of chemotherapeutic or other caustic agents into surrounding tissues]).

2. Monitor for signs and symptoms of hemorrhage.
  a. Hypotension
  b. Tachycardia
  c. Evidence of bleeding
	2. Hemorrhage is a serious surgical complication of long-term venous access catheter placement. It can occur within several hours of insertion—after blood pressure returns to preinsertion levels and puts increased pressure on a newly formed clot. It also can develop later, secondary to vascular erosion due to infection.

3. Monitor for signs and symptoms of embolism. Report changes to physician and advanced nurse practitioner.
  a. Anxiety, restlessness
  b. Altered level of consciousness
	3. A client with a long-term VAD is at increased risk for embolism. Accidental leakage of air from catheter can occlude a major pulmonary artery; obstruction of blood flow to the alveoli decreases alveolar perfusion,

(continues on page 986)

Interventions continued	**Rationales** continued
c. SOB d. Tachycardia	shunts air to patent alveoli, and leads to bronchial constriction and possible collapse of pulmonary tissue.

4. Monitor for signs and symptoms of hematoma.
   a. Tenderness and swelling at insertion site
   b. Discoloration at insertion site
	4. Long-term VAD placement can cause soft tissue injury resulting in rupture of small vessels. As blood collects at insertion site, hematoma forms.

5. Monitor for signs of sepsis. Report changes to physicians or advanced nurse practitioners.
   a. Temperature >101°F or <98.6°F
   b. Decreased urine output
   c. Tachycardia, tachypnea
   d. Pale, cool skin
   e. WBCs and bacteria in urine
   f. Positive blood culture
	5. The invasive nature of a VAD puts client at risk for opportunistic infection and septicemia. If the VAD is used to instill chemotherapy, the possibility of chemotherapy-induced leukopenia further increases risk. Sepsis causes massive vasodilatation and resultant hypovolemia, leading to tissue hypoxia and decreased renal and cardiac function. The body's compensatory response increases respiratory and heart rates in an attempt to correct hypoxia and acidosis.

6. Monitor for phlebitis:
   a. Redness or streak of red at insertion site
   b. Purulent drainage at insertion site
   c. Tenderness
   d. Elevated temperature
   e. Elevated WBC
	6. Phlebitis is inflammation of a vein from chemical or mechanical infiltration. The incidence of phlebitis increases with the length of time the IV line is in place.

7. Monitor for catheter displacement, damage, infiltration, extravasation, and obstruction.
   a. Superior vena cava syndrome (facial edema, distention of thoracic and neck veins)
   b. Swelling, redness, tenderness or drainage from insertion site (extravasation)
   c. Leakage of fluid from catheter
   d. Inaccurate infusion rate
   e. Inability to infuse or draw blood
   f. Bulging of catheter during infusion
	7. Catheters can malfunction, obstruct, or displace from misuse or defects.

8. If signs of skin infection are assessed, remove needle from the port and do not reaccess until infection is cleared.	8. To prevent systematic infections, treatment is required before nurse reaccesses.

◤ Related Physician-Prescribed Interventions

Refer to the care plan for the underlying condition necessitating VAD use (e.g., Cancer: Initial Diagnosis).

Documentation
Flow records
Vital signs
Respiratory assessment
Catheter site/patency assessment

Nursing Diagnoses

Anxiety Related to Upcoming Insertion of Catheter/Port and Insufficient Knowledge of Procedure

Focus Assessment Criteria	Clinical Significance
1. Knowledge of procedure 2. Knowledge of therapy	1,2. Knowledge about therapy and its effects enhances client's sense of control and can reduce anxiety associated with fear of the unknown. Assessing client's knowledge level guides nurse in planning effective teaching strategies to address learning needs.
3. Anxiety level (mild, moderate, severe, or panic)	3. Extreme anxiety can interfere with client's coping ability. Modifiable factors that contribute to extreme anxiety include inaccurate or incomplete information about the threatening event.

Goal

The client will report decreased anxiety after explanations.

Indicators
- Share feelings regarding scheduled catheter insertion.
- Relate what to expect during insertion.

Interventions	Rationales
1. Reinforce physician's explanation of surgical diagnostic procedure. Notify physician if additional explanations are indicated.	1. The physician is legally responsible for explanations for an informed consent; the nurse is legally responsible for clarifying information, evaluating patient's understanding, and notifying physician if more information is necessary.
2. Provide an opportunity for client to share fears and beliefs regarding chemotherapy. Delay teaching if high levels of anxiety are present.	2. Sharing helps nurse to identify sources of anxiety and correct misinformation. High anxiety prevents retention of information.
3. Explain what to expect. a. Preprocedure (e.g., site preparation and draping)	3. Perception of an event is gained through all senses. Providing sensory information along with procedural information gives

(continues on page 988)

Interventions continued	Rationales continued
b. During insertion (e.g., positioning and sensations)	client more data to use to accurately interpret and master the event.

4. Instruct client on how he or she can assist during the procedure.
  a. Communicate any sensations felt to physician.
  b. Following physician's instructions (e.g., holding breath and lying still during insertion; coughing, deep breathing, and exercising legs postprocedure).
	4. Eliciting client's cooperation with the procedure can help to improve compliance and reduce risk of complications.

5. Explain that nursing staff monitor the following at frequent intervals:
  a. Blood pressure
  b. Pulse rate and rhythm
  c. Condition of catheter insertion site
  d. Condition of limb distal to insertion site.
  Also, explain that a chest x-ray film will be obtained.
	5. Instructions about specific procedures can help to reduce anxiety associated with the unknown and the unexpected.

6. Instruct client about the need to immobilize the limb used for the procedure for the prescribed length of time.	6. Immobilization helps to reduce complications of hemorrhage or thrombosis.
7. Refer to the Cancer: Initial Diagnosis Care Plan for additional specific strategies to reduce anxiety.	

 Documentation

Teaching record
Client teaching
Outcome achievement or status

High Risk for Ineffective Therapeutic Regimen Management Related to Insufficient Knowledge of Home Care, Signs and Symptoms of Complications, and Community Resources

Focus Assessment Criteria	Clinical Significance
1. Knowledge of the procedure and perception of why it is needed	1. Assessing knowledge level identifies client's learning needs and guides nurse in planning effective teaching strategies.
2. Available support systems to assist with home therapy	2. Successful home management often hinges on availability of needed support systems.

(continues on page 989)

Focus Assessment Criteria continued	**Clinical Significance** continued
3. Readiness and ability to learn and retain information	3. A client or family failing to achieve learning goals requires a referral for assistance post-discharge.

Goals

The goals for this diagnosis represent those associated with discharge planning. Refer to the discharge criteria.

Interventions	**Rationales**
1. Reinforce physician's explanation of the catheterization procedure, including line placement; incorporate individually oriented media when possible.	1. Explanations can reduce misconceptions and increase participation.
2. Explain advantages and disadvantages of atrial catheters and vascular access ports. a. Atrial catheters (open and closed)—advantages: • Provide unlimited venous access • Eliminate need for painful needle sticks • Can be used for continuous infusion in both hospital and home • Carry a reduced risk of extravasation • Cause little discomfort b. Atrial catheters (open and closed)—disadvantages: • Require dressing changes • Require heparin (open) or saline (closed) flushes • Require cap changes (usually weekly) c. PICC lines are silastic or polyurethane catheters that are placed antecubitally and advanced to a large central vein: • PICC advantages include the following: PICC lines are less expensive and easier to insert. They are placed by specially trained nurses and can be inserted at the bedside or in the home setting. There is less risk for air embolism because insertion site is well below the heart.	2. Discussing different devices can help client to better understand how the decision was made about which type to use. Knowing the logic behind the decision may encourage compliance. a. Open catheter method provides a catheter at the skin surface for medication administration. Single- and double-lumen catheters are available. Double-lumen catheters provide greater flexibility with treatment (e.g., chemotherapy and total parenteral nutrition [TPN] can be administered simultaneously). Both the open and closed catheters require surgical insertion.

(continues on page 990)

Interventions continued	**Rationales** continued
No possibility of pneumothorax exists (Lucas, 1992; Masoorli and Angeles, 1990). • PICC disadvantages include the following: Phlebitis incidence is higher than with other VADs. Smaller lumen does not lend itself to blood sampling. If blood aspiration is done, it must be done slowly with a syringe to prevent catheter collapse. Catheter is easily displaced because it is held in place with steristrips (arm exercise contra-indicated). Catheter may be easily ruptured if irrigated with high pressure. Catheter requires daily heparin flushes (Lucas, 1992; Masoorli and Angeles, 1990). d. Vascular access ports—advantage: • Free client from most responsibility for routine dressing changes and flushing e. Vascular access ports—disadvantages: • Require needle sticks through the skin to gain access • Allow a limited number of accesses, depending on needle size (typically 1000–2000) • Require surgery to implant and remove	e. Vascular access ports consist of a chamber with a septum attached to a catheter. Chamber and catheter are surgically implanted under the skin. Drugs and fluids are administered by injecting a non-coring needle through the skin and into the chamber. Fluid flows through the needle into the chamber and through the catheter into the right atrium.
3. Explain reasons for continued assessment procedures and diagnostic tests (e.g., daily weights, intake and output monitoring, and urine and serum evaluations)	3. The client's understanding that careful monitoring is needed to assess status and to detect problems early promotes cooperation with procedures.
4. Explain aseptic technique; obtain return demonstration of handwashing and preparation of work surface.	4. Understanding enables compliance with measures to prevent infection.
5. Explain home care measures and discuss roles and expectations of all concerned—client, family members, visiting nurse, and others as appropriate.	5. Expectations should be clear to prevent misunderstanding.

(continues on page 991)

Interventions continued	**Rationales** continued
6. Teach manipulation of syringe and needle and method of drawing up solution. Obtain return demonstrations from client and family members to demonstrate understanding and mastery.	6. These skills are needed for home management.

7. Teach catheter care according to protocols; obtain return demonstrations of care measures as necessary. Provide written material for the following:
  a. Dressing change
  b. Site care
  c. Emergency measures
  d. Catheter irrigation (Kelly, Dumenko, McGregor, & McHutcheon, 1992)
  e. Changing injection cap
  f. Catheter repair
	7. Understanding protocols and techniques for home care is critical to prevent infection and clotting and to manage problems or emergencies.

8. Discuss strategies for keeping the home environment safe and conductive to good care.
  a. Store supplies in a clean, dry place.
  b. Do not tell others that syringes are stored in the home.
  c. Use a shoebox with a small hole in the top for discarding used syringes.
  d. Tape and discard the box when filled.
  e. Keep clean syringes, the used syringe box, and heparin out of reach and sight of children and confused adults.
  f. Perform catheter care in a clean area where a sink is available for hand washing.
  g. Thoroughly clean the work area before laying out supplies.
	8. These measures help to reduce risk of injury and infection transmission.

9. Explain signs and symptoms of VAD complications.
 	
  a. Fever
  b. Tenderness, swelling, and drainage at site
  c. VAD occlusion
  d. Inability to infuse
 	
  e. Facial edema and distended neck veins
 	
  f. Phlebitis management
	9. Understanding signs and symptoms of complications enables early detection and reporting to a health care professional for timely intervention.
	  a,b. Fever and changes at the insertion site may indicate infection.
	
	  c,d. Inaccurate infusion rate or inability to infuse points to obstruction or catheter damage.
	  e. Facial edema and neck vein distention may indicate superior vena caval syndrome.
	  f. Phlebitis has been observed in 12.5% to 23% patients with PICC lines (Lucas, 1992).

(continues on page 992)

Interventions continued	Rationales continued
10. Provide a list of required equipment and supplies.	10. Planning can prevent shortages and improper substitutions.
11. Instruct client or family about whom to call with questions day or night (e.g., nurses' station or physician).	11. Questions are likely to arise after discharge.

 Documentation

Discharge summary record
Client and family teaching
Outcome achievement or status

MECHANICAL VENTILATION

Mechanical ventilation is indicated for a variety of clinical conditions that lead to an inadequate ventilation or oxygenation. Negative pressure ventilators, such as the iron lung, are rarely used today. Positive pressure ventilators are either pressure, time, or volume cycled. These ventilators force air into the lungs during inspiration, generating positive alveolar pressure. Exhalation is passive. For continuous use, endotracheal intubation or tracheostomy is required. Conditions that necessitate continuous mechanical ventilation include central nervous system disorders that compromise the respiratory center in the medulla; musculoskeletal conditions that limit chest expansion; neuromuscular disorders; heart failure; respiratory disorders; and upper airway obstruction.

Time Frame
During acute therapy in facility

DIAGNOSTIC CLUSTER

Collaborative Problems

▲ PC: Respiratory Insufficiency
▲ PC: Atelectasis
△ PC: Oxygen Toxicity
△ PC: Decreased Cardiac Output
△ PC: GI Bleeding

Nursing Diagnoses	**Refer to**
△ High Risk for Dysfunctional Weaning Response related to weaning attempts, respiratory muscle fatigue secondary to mechanical ventilation, increased work of breathing, supine position, protein-calorie malnutrition, inactivity, and fatigue	
△ Disuse Syndrome	Immobility or Unconsciousness
△ Fear related to the nature of the situation, uncertain prognosis of ventilator dependence, or weaning	Chronic Obstructive Pulmonary Disease
▲ Impaired Verbal Communication related to effects of intubation on ability to speak	Tracheostomy
▲ High Risk for Infection related to disruption of skin layer secondary to tracheostomy	Tracheostomy

(continues on page 994)

Nursing Diagnoses continued	Refer to continued
▲ High Risk for Ineffective Airway Clearance related to increased secretions secondary to tracheostomy, obstruction of inner cannula, or displacement of tracheostomy tube	Tracheostomy
△ Powerlessness related to dependency on respirator, inability to talk, and loss of mobility	Chronic Obstructive Pulmonary Disease

▲ This diagnosis was reported to be monitored for or managed frequently (75%–100%).
△ This diagnosis was reported to be monitored for or managed often (50%–74%).

Discharge Criteria

Because mechanical ventilation in this care plan is discontinued before discharge, no discharge criteria are applicable.

Collaborative Problems

Potential Complication: Respiratory Insufficiency

Potential Complication: Atelectasis

Potential Complication: Oxygen Toxicity

Potential Complication: Decreased Cardiac Output

Potential Complication: GI Bleeding

Nursing Goal

The nurse will monitor for early signs and symptoms of (a) respiratory insufficiency, (b) atelectasis, (c) pneumothorax, (d) oxygen toxicity, (e) decreased cardiac output, (f) GI bleeding and will collaboratively intervene to stabilize the client.

Indicators
- Alert, calm, oriented (a, b, c, d)
- Respiratory rate 16–20 breaths/min (a, c, d)
- Respirations easy, rhythmic (a, c, d)
- Symmetrical chest movements (a, c)
- Pulse 60–100 beats/min (a, c)
- BP >90/60, <140/90 mm Hg (a, c)
- Temperature 98.5–99°F (b)
- Oxygen saturation (SaO_2) > 94% (a, c)
- Carbon dioxide ($PaCO_2$) 35–45 mm Hg (a, c)
- Arterial pH 7.35–7.45 (a, c)
- Warm, dry skin (a)
- No change in usual skin color (a, b)
- No c/o of numbness, tingling in extremities (d)
- No c/o of substernal distress (d)
- Stool negative for occult blood (f)
- Gastric pH > 4 (f)

Interventions	Rationales
1. Follow agency protocols for management and documentation of ventilator (settings, maintenance). Consult with respiratory therapist.	1. The type of ventilator used will have specific nursing responsibilities.

2. Monitor respiratory status:
  a. Respiratory rate
  b. Breath sounds
  c. Chest movements symmetry
  d. Pulse oximetry
  e. Arterial blood gases
  f. Peripheral pulses
  g. Capillary refill
  h. Nasal flaring
  i. Tracheal tug
  j. Intractable cough
  k. Use of accessory muscles
  l. Air leaks
	2. These criteria will serve to determine the effectiveness of mechanical ventilation. Asymmetrical chest movements can indicate improper tube placement, atelectasis, or pneumothorax.

3. Monitor for signs of respiratory insufficiency.
  a. Increased respiratory rate
  b. Labored respirations
  c. Restlessness, agitation, confusion
  d. Increased pulse and B/P
  d. Decreased SaO_2; increased $PaCO_2$
	3. Respiratory insufficiency can result from airway obstruction, ventilator problems, atelectasis, bronchospasm, or pneumothorax.

4. Monitor for signs of atelectasis.
  a. Marked dyspnea
  b. Anxiety
  c. Cyanosis
  d. Tachycardia
	4. Atelectasis can result from bronchial obstruction due to a mucous plug or from upward diaphragmatic displacement due to increased intra-abdominal pressure. Resulting signs and symptoms reflect decreased alveolar exchange and circulating oxygen.

5. Monitor for pneumothorax:
  a. Sudden decrease in oxygen saturation
  b. Sudden onset of respiratory distress
  c. Limited lung movement
	5. Excessive positive pressure from ventilator can cause trauma to alveoli and result in pneumothorax.

6. Initiate emergency measures (e.g., chest tube insertion).	6. Pneumothorax can be a life-threatening event.
7. Maintain a patent airway; suction as needed. Advise client to take deep breaths every hour during sign mechanism.	7. Airway obstruction causes respiratory insufficiency. An intubated client who has ineffective cough reflex or fatigue is dependent on suctioning to remove secretions.

(continues on page 996)

Interventions continued	Rationales continued
8. Maintain proper cuff inflation of tracheostomy. Refer to Tracheostomy care plan.	8. Underinflation allows aspiration of gastric or respiratory secretions. Over-inflation can cause tracheal tissue compression, resulting in ulceration.

9. Monitor for signs and symptoms of oxygen toxicity.
  a. Substernal distress
  b. Paresthesias in extremities
  c. Progressive dyspnea
  d. Restlessness
	9. Oxygen toxicity, resulting from prolonged administration of excessive oxygen concentrations, leads to decreased surfactant secretion causing decreased lung compliance and colloid degeneration causing hyaline membrane formation in the lung lining and the development of pulmonary edema.

10. Monitor for signs of decreased cardiac output.
  a. Dysrhythmias
  b. Diminished peripheral pulses
  c. Altered vital signs
  d. Cold, clammy skin
  e. Dyspnea
  f. Decreased urine output
	10. Positive-pressure ventilation increases intrathoracic pressure, which can reduce venous return and cardiac output. The resulting signs reflect decreased venous return and hypoxemia.

11. Monitor for GI bleeding:
 	
  a. Stool positive for occult blood
 	
  b. Acid gastric pH
	11. Profound stimulation of the vagus nerve causes hypersecretion of gastric secretions and possible ulcer formation.
	  a. Microscopic bleeding can be detected.
	  b. The pH of stomach is 2. To prevent ulcer formation, pH is maintained above 4.

Related Physician-Prescribed Interventions

Medications. Bronchodilators, short-acting hypnotics, antacids, H_2 blockers

Intravenous Therapy. Total parenteral nutrition, fluid/electrolyte replacement

Laboratory Studies. Arterial blood gases, serum electrolytes, albumin, blood urea nitrogen, CBC, creatinine

Diagnostic Studies. Chest x-ray film, pulse oximetry

Therapies. Type and operation of ventilator (volume, pressure, rate, control mode, percentage of oxygen), positive end-expiratory pressure; type and size of endotracheal/tracheostomy tube; enteral feeding

Documentation

Flow records
  Vital signs
  Respiratory assessment
  Cuff pressure
  Proximal inspiratory pressure (PIP)

Nursing Diagnoses

High Risk for Dysfunctional Weaning Response Related to Weaning Attempts, Respiratory Muscle Fatigue Secondary to Mechanical Ventilation, Increased Work of Breathing, Supine Position, Protein-calorie Malnutrition, Inactivity, and Fatigue

Focus Assessment Criteria	Clinical Significance

1. Respiratory function
2. Laboratory studies:
  a. Hemoglobin and hematocrit
  b. ABG analysis
  c. Serum protein and electrolytes
3. Intake (oral and parenteral)
4. Urine output
5. GI function (bowel sounds, bowel movements)
6. Daily weights
7. Sleep (quality and quantity)
8. Activity level
	1–8. Continuous assessment is needed to detect factors that could impair weaning.

9. Weaning parameters	

Goal

The client will achieve progressive weaning goals.

Indicators
• Demonstrate required protein and calorie intake.
• Participate in activities to reduce inactivity.
• Demonstrate required fluid intake.

Interventions	Rationales
1. Remove secretions as necessary.	1. A tube partially obstructed with secretions increases resistance to flow, which increases the work of breathing.
2. Promote chest expansion.	2. Any impediment to chest expansion increases the work of breathing.

3. Assess for tube-related causes of resistance to flow such as these:
  a. Too-small endotracheal tracheostomy tube
  b. Too-long endotracheal tracheostomy tube
  c. Inflated cuff
  d. T-piece weaning
	3. An endotracheal tube's caliber and length influence resistance to flow. If risk of aspiration is minimal, a deflated cuff reduces resistance. Continuous positive airway pressure decreases the work of breathing as compared to T-piece weaning. For every 1-mm decrease in the endotracheal tube diameter, the work of breathing increases 34% to 152% (Porth, 2000).

(continues on page 998)

Interventions continued	Rationales continued
4. Assess for dyspnea.	4. Dyspnea interferes with successful weaning. A weaning schedule that reduces tidal volume slowly and increases endurance is recommended.
5. Position client upright, sitting, or in bed with legs dangling.	5. An upright position maximizes diaphragm excursion, increasing lung volume and gas exchange.
6. Plan adequate rest periods before and after activity and during weaning efforts.	6. Respiratory muscle fatigue can result from prolonged artificial ventilation, increased work of breathing, and reduction in energy reserves. a. Rest periods help to replenish energy expended in activity. b. Alternating weaning with rest periods on mechanical ventilation rests fatigued muscles.
7. Take precautions to prevent infection. a. Change tubing every 24 to 48 hours. b. Remove lines early. c. Reduce endogenous organisms through frequent handwashing, careful housekeeping, universal precautions, and other measures. d. Remove Foley catheter early.	7. A client on long-term ventilation is at increased risk of infection owing to altered defense mechanisms and microorganisms on equipment and in the environment.
8. Promote optimal nutrition. a. Consult nutritionist to calculate specific protein and calorie needs. b. Weigh client daily.	8. Malnutrition has a negative effect on respiratory function that depends on adequate muscle function and uses energy continuously. A malnourished client has a decreased response to hypoxia, expiratory muscle weakness, reduced muscle endurance, decrease surfactant, impaired immune responses, and fluid imbalances from electrolyte changes. a. Nurse may need assistance to calculate client's specific nutritional requirements according to metabolic demands. Caloric intake should be 1.4 to 1.6 times the energy expenditure. Underfeeding can increase risk of pulmonary complications; overfeeding can increase metabolic rate and carbon dioxide production. b. Actual weight on a properly calibrated scale can provide a reflection of overall nutritional status. Weekly weight loss of 1% to 2% of total body weight is significant.

(continues on page 999)

Interventions continued	**Rationales** continued
c. Monitor laboratory study results: • Serum albumin and transferrin • CBC • Creatinine index d. Maintain adequate hydration.	c. Laboratory data can provide information on nutritional status especially when weight fluctuates with fluid retention or loss. d. This reduces viscosity of secretions decreasing airway resistance.
9. Consult with physician regarding enteral or parenteral nutrition as appropriate.	9. In most cases, a client with an artificial airway is unable to meet his or her nutritional needs solely through oral ingestion. When supplemental feeding is required, the enteral route is preferred over the parenteral route because of the parenteral route's greater risk of catheter-related sepsis. Enteral feeding decreases the chances of GI bleeding.
10. Take steps to prevent constipation. a. Ensure adequate fluid and fiber intake. b. Establish a regular time for defecation and promote a close-to-normal (semi-squatting) position on the bedpan, commode, or toilet.	10. Abdominal distention from gas, ileus, or constipation prevents adequate diaphragm function.
11. Promote optimal activity. a. Encourage active or perform passive ROM exercises as the client's ability permits. b. Provide a wheelchair for a client with a portable ventilator. c. Consult physical therapy. d. Consult occupational therapist.	11. Inactivity decreases respiratory muscle size and strength; this interferes with optimal respiratory effort. c. Exercise promotes respiratory muscle strength, chest mobility, and muscle tone. d. Client should participate as much as possible with self-care needs.
12. Institute measures to ensure uninterrupted rapid-eye-movement (REM) sleep (4 to 5 cycles of 70 to 100 minutes). a. Reduce noise. b. Teach relaxation techniques. c. Consult with physician for a short-acting hypnotic agent if needed.	12. Deprivation of REM sleep frequently occurs in the hospital. Prolonged inadequate REM sleep results in sluggish thought processes and anxiety.
13. Take steps to reduce pain to tolerable levels (e.g., analgesics or nonpharmacologic pain relief measures such as relaxation, distraction, and guided imagery).	13. Pain can contribute to anxiety, inhibit chest excursion on respiration, and restrict coughing.

(continues on page 1000)

Interventions continued	**Rationales** continued

14. Consult with physician to delay weaning if any of these factors occurs:
  a. Irreversible underlying disease
  b. Metabolic alkalosis or acidosis
  c. Multisystem failure
  d. Clinical instability
  e. Protein-calorie malnutrition
 	
  f. Decreased maximal inspiratory pressure (MIP) during weaning
  g. Rapid, shallow breathing during weaning
	14.
	
	a–d. A client who is not improving or is not clinically stable does not have the reserves to accommodate successfully to weaning.
	e. A malnourished client is unable to produce sufficient energy supplies to allow weaning.
	f,g. A decrease in MIP or rapid, shallow breathing in response to weaning indicates poor respiratory muscle strength.

15. Before weaning, discuss the process with client and family.	15. Adequate preparation is needed to reduce fears. Emphasizing the client's improvement, explain the procedure and provide constant supervision to improve motivation and decrease anxiety.

16. Before, during, and after weaning attempts, assess the following factors:
  a. Vital capacity
  b. Inspiratory force
  c. Vital signs
  d. Arterial blood gas values or SaO_2
	16. The client's ventilator capacities and perfusion serve as criteria for evaluating whether or not to progress weaning.

 Documentation

Flow records
  Vital signs
  Ventilator settings
  Type of tube (inflation)
  Respiratory assessment
  Intake and output
  Bowel sounds
  Rest and activity patterns
  Suctioning provided
  Pre-, intra-, and postweaning assessments
  Client teaching
Progress notes
  Psychological status

PACEMAKER INSERTION (PERMANENT)

A pacemaker is an electrical device implanted to help maintain normal cardiac rate and sometimes rhythm in the presence of sinoatrial atrioventricular (SA AV) node conduction disturbances (e.g., any bradycardia such as heart block, junctional rhythm, atrial fibrillation with a slow ventricular response, or asystole) and certain tachyarrhythmias. In the implantation procedure, a bipolar or unipolar electrode is inserted through the subclavian vein into the right atrium or right ventricle under fluoroscopy. Permanent pacemakers have a pulse generator implanted in a subcutaneous pouch in the upper right or left chest. Pacemaker generators also can be placed in a subcutaneous pouch in the abdomen with the pacemaker wires placed in the epicardial surface of the heart. This is done in conjunction with open-heart surgery or via a thoracotomy approach. The pulse generator houses the batteries, which eventually become depleted. When this occurs, the old generator is removed and a new one is implanted.

The Inter-Society Commission for Heart Disease has a code system for pacemakers to provide a method of communicating about their functions. The code system has five letters but usually only three are used, except with permanent pacemakers. The code system is as follows:

1st letter—chamber being paced
  A-Atrium V-Ventricle D-Dural (both)
2nd letter—chamber being sensed
  A-Atrium V-Ventricle D-Dual O-Off
3rd letter—type of response by pacemaker to sensory
  I-Inhibited (pacemaker will not function when the person's heart beats)
  O-None
4th letter—ability of generator to be programmed
  O-None
  P-Simple programmability
  M-Multi-programmability
  C-Telemetry ability
  P-Ability of rate to change with activity
5th letter—ability of generator to defibrillate
  P-Antitachycardia pacing
  S-Shock
  D-Antitachycardia processing and shock
  O-None

 Time Frame

Preprocedure and postprocedure

 DIAGNOSTIC CLUSTER

Preprocedure Period

Nursing Diagnoses

▲ Anxiety related to impending pacemaker insertion and prognosis

Postprocedure Period

Collaborative Problems

* PC: Perforation of the Right Ventricle
▲ PC: Cardiac Dysrhythmias

(continues on page 1002)

DIAGNOSTIC CLUSTER continued

∗ PC: Pneumothorax
▲ PC: Pacemaker Malfunction (failure to sense, failure to fire, or failure to capture)
∗ PC: Infection
△ PC: Necrosis over Pulse Generator

Nursing Diagnoses

△ Impaired Physical Mobility related to incisional site pain, activity restrictions, and fear of lead displacement
△ Disturbed Self-Concept related to perceived loss of health and dependence on pacemaker
△ High Risk for Ineffective Therapeutic Regimen Management related to insufficient knowledge of activity restrictions, precautions, signs and symptoms of complications, and follow-up care

▲ This diagnosis was reported to be monitored for or managed frequently (75%–100%).
△ This diagnosis was reported to be monitored for or managed often (50%–74%).
∗ This diagnosis was not included in the validation study.

Discharge Criteria

Before discharge, the client or family will

1. Demonstrate accuracy in counting a pulse.
2. Verbalize precautions to take with regard to the pacemaker.
3. State signs and symptoms that must be reported to a health care professional.
4. Verbalize an intent to share feelings and concerns related to the pacemaker with significant others.
5. Demonstrate site care.
6. Relate activity restrictions.

Preprocedure: Nursing Diagnoses

Anxiety Related to Impending Pacemaker Insertion and Prognosis

Focus Assessment Criteria	Clinical Significance
1. Understanding symptoms, the need for a pacemaker, and preprocedure and postprocedure care measures	1. Assessment is needed to determine if additional information is needed.
2. Method of implantation (transvenous [endocardial] versus surgical [epicardial])	2. Preprocedure and postprocedure nursing care varies depending on the implantation method. (Refer to Thoracic Surgery or Coronary Artery Bypass Grafting Care Plan.)

Goal

The client will

1. Verbalize the goal of pacemaker implantation as treatment, not cure.
2. Verbalize accurate information about the procedure and postprocedure care.

Interventions	Rationales
1. Reinforce physician's explanation of the surgical procedure.	1. If anxiety impedes client's ability to assimilate information, repeated exposure to this or any other information may be helpful.
2. Assess client's understanding and notify physician if additional explanations are needed.	2. The physician is legally responsible for explaining the surgery to client and family; the nurse for determining the level of client understanding and notifying physician if they require additional explanations.
3. Have client recall symptoms leading to the present point. Explain that symptoms are the manifestation of a heart-rhythm disturbance.	3. Recognition of symptoms as a manifestation of an underlying problem helps client to understand and accept the need for a pacemaker.
4. Show client a pulse generator if available. Explain its functions (see description of letter codes)	4. Handling actual equipment provides visual and tactile information and helps client better understand the device and its operation.
5. If client is on cardiac monitor preprocedure, avoid placing ECG electrodes over potential incision sites on upper right or left chest.	5. Pulling off electrodes can cause potential skin breakdown and lead to possible infection postprocedure.
6. Describe preprocedural routine (as appropriate for client) of blood tests, ECG, chest x-ray film, and food and fluid restrictions.	6–9. Explaining what to expect may help to reduce client's anxiety related to fear of the unknown and unexpected and may enhance his or her sense of control over the situation.
7. Explain that client will be awake during insertion, but that a sedative will be given to aid relaxation and a local anesthetic will be given to numb incisional area.	
8. Explain physical appearance of catheterization laboratory or operating room, wherever the procedure will be done.	

9. Instruct client concerning pacemaker insertion and associated sensations; cover the following:
  a. Time of procedure
  b. Approximate length of procedure
  c. Attachment of telemetry leads to monitor cardiac rate and rhythm
  d. Insertion of intravenous lines to provide direct IV access if needed	

(continues on page 1004)

Interventions continued	**Rationales** continued

e. Preparation of skin with a cold solution where incision is to be made
   f. Injection of local anesthetic into entire area where generator will be placed; explain that initial injection may burn slightly
   g. Expected sensations of pressure and pulling during lead insertion, with no sensation after insertion is complete
   h. The need to notify nurse or physician of pain experienced during procedure
   i. Positioning x-ray machine over the body and loud clicking sounds from x-ray machine
   j. Possibility of palpitations during assessment of lead placement
   k. Creation of a small pocket underneath skin and closure with sutures (internal or external depending on physician preference)
   l. Return to recovery room or unit on telemetry
   m. Likelihood that he or she will notice the pulse generator under the skin for about 2 months; at this point conscious awareness of the implant should diminish and edema should be gone
   n. When client will be able to see family and other support persons post-procedure	

10. Instruct client on postprocedure routine; cover these factors:
   a. Frequent monitoring of blood pressure, pulse and temperature, pulse oximetry
   b. Telemetry ECG
   c. Frequent assessment of insertion site
   d. Presence of pressure dressing over incision for about 24 to 48 hours after procedure
	10. The client's understanding that careful monitoring is necessary to evaluate her or his response to the pacemaker can ease anxiety and encourage cooperation.
	
	   d. The pressure dressing is to prevent bleeding into pacemaker pocket.

11. Instruct client not to use affected arm while transferring from or to the bed or pushing herself or himself up in bed for the first 24 to 48 hours. A sling may be applied to affected arm to help restrict movement.	11. Movement restrictions aim to prevent displacement of leads.
12. Instruct client to report the following immediately:	12. Early detection enables prompt intervention to reduce the severity of complications.

(continues on page 1005)

Interventions continued	Rationales continued
a. Pain at insertion site	a. Pain at site may indicate compression from hemorrhage or edema.
b. Palpitations	b. Palpitations can indicate failure of pacemaker to control heart rate.
c. Dizziness	c. Dizziness may result from decreased cardiac output with resultant cerebral hypoxia resulting from pacemaker failure.
d. Hiccups or chest muscle twitching	d. Hiccups or chest muscle twitching may point to perforation of ventricle and stimulation of diaphragm or intercostal muscle by the lead.
13. Provide written materials that reinforce teaching.	13. Client and family can retain and refer to written materials after discharge. Such materials also can provide information to support persons not accompanying the client for teaching.
14. If possible, arrange for client to talk with a person who has successfully gone through pacemaker implantation.	14. A person who has had a pacemaker implanted successfully can provide a role model for the client and promote a relaxed, healthy attitude toward the procedure.
15. Refer client to clinical nurse specialist, social worker, or clergy if anxiety is dysfunctional.	15. For some clients, referrals may be necessary for intensive interventions and consultation.

 Documentation

Teaching record
Client teaching
Outcome achievement or status
Progress notes
Unusual responses
Referrals if indicated

Postprocedure: Collaborative Problems

Potential Complication: Perforation of the Right Ventricle

Potential Complication: Cardiac Dysrhythmias

Potential Complication: Pneumothorax

Potential Complication: Pacemaker Malfunction (failure to sense, failure to fire, or failure to capture)

Potential Complication: Infection

Potential Complication: Necrosis over Pulse Generator

Nursing Goal

The nurse will detect early signs and symptoms of (a) perforation of the right ventricle, (b) cardiac dys-rhythmias, (c) pneumothorax, (d) pacemaker malfunction, (e) infection (site), and (f) necrosis over pulse generator and will collaboratively intervene to stabilize the client.

Indicators

- Calm, alert oriented (a, c)
- BP >90/60, <140/90 mm Hg (a)
- Pulse 60–100 beats/min (a, b)
- Respirations 16–20 breaths/min (a, c)
- Respirations relaxed, rhythmic (a, c)
- Symmetrical chest movements (c)
- Breath sounds in all lobes (c)
- Flat neck veins (a)
- No c/o of chest pain (a, c)
- Stable pulse pressure (approximately 40 mm/Hg difference between diastolic and systolic pressure) (a, c)
- EKG—normal sinus rhythm implantation (b)
- Intact wound (site) (e, f)
- Minimal drainage or bleeding (e, f)
- Oxygen saturation (SaO_2) > 94% (a, b, c)
- Carbon dioxide ($PaCO_2$) 35–45 mm Hg (a, b, c)
- Arterial pH 7.35–7.45 (a, b, c)

Interventions	Rationales

1. Monitor for signs of perforation of right ventricle.
  a. Distended neck veins
  b. Hepatic engorgement
  c. Narrow pulse pressure
  d. Decreased blood pressure
 	
2. Initiate emergency measures for cardiac arrest.
	1,2. Perforation of right ventricle into left ventricle or pericardium results in decreased cardiac output, circulatory congestion (particularly in hepatic and neck areas), and shock.

3. Monitor for dysrhythmias.	3. Rhythm disturbances are common for 48 to 72 hours after implantation owing to myocardial irritability and injury from lead insertion.

4. Monitor for signs and symptoms of pneumothorax.
  a. Shortness of breath
  b. Decreased or absent breath sounds
  c. Sudden stabbing chest pain
  d. Asymmetric chest movement
  e. Decreased arterial oxygen saturation
  f. Increased arterial carbon dioxide
	4. Placement of any catheter into the subclavian vein can potentially cause puncture of the lung on the affected side.

5. Monitor for electromagnetic interference marked by onset of prepacemaker symptoms when near a source of electromagnetic interference (e.g., TENS units,	5. Electromagnetic interference can inhibit pacemaker function or cause it to revert to a fixed mode of pacing (Woods & Froelicher, 1995).

(continues on page 1007)

Interventions continued	Rationales continued
electromagnets, MRI scanners or lithotripsy) or by intermittent failure to pace with an artifact absent. If it occurs, move client away from source of interference.	
6. Monitor for sensing problems.	6.
a. Monitor for undersensing (failure to sense). The pacemaker is not sensitive enough to the heart's own electrical signals and will pace as though there were no intrinsic signals.	a. The danger of undersensing is that the pacemaker may deliver an unnecessary stimulus during ventricular repolarization (T-wave on the ECG) because it cannot sense intrinsic beats properly. Ventricular repolarization is the most vulnerable phase of the cardiac cycle and any electrical stimulus during this time can cause ventricular tachycardia or ventricular fibrillation.
b. Monitor for oversensing. Pacemaker is too aware of the heart's intrinsic electrical signals or of other electrical signals such as skeletal muscle electrical signals. In this case, pacemaker will not pace if it senses these "false" electrical signals.	b. The danger of oversensing is that the pacemaker may interpret an inappropriate electrical signal as a QRS complex and will not pace when it should, thus reducing cardiac output and causing potential hemodynamic compromise.
7. Monitor for failure to fire. Pacemaker fails to deliver a stimulus, so there will be no pacer spike and no ventricular depolarization (no pacemaker spike and no QRS complex on the ECG).	7. Fractured lead wires, circuitry failure, or faulty lead connections can cause pacemaker to fail to fire. This can lead to slow heart rates, decreased cardiac output, and potential hemodynamic compromise.
8. Monitor for failure to capture. Pacemaker will deliver a stimulus at the appropriate pacing interval but it will not be followed by a ventricular depolarization (there will be a pacemaker spike at the appropriate time but no QRS complex on the ECG).	8. Failure to capture may be caused by lead displacement (lead is no longer in contact with endocardial surface) or by high thresholds of the myocardium from fibrosis or ischemia at the lead tip. This can lead to slow heart rates, decreased cardiac output, and potential hemodynamic compromise (Guzzetta, 1992).
9. Monitor for pacemaker-mediated tachycardia with dual chamber pacemakers (DDD). This tachycardia is marked by sustained ventricular upper-rate limit pacing caused by loss of AV synchrony and retrograde conduction from ventricle to atrium.	9. Sustained upper rate ventricular pacing may cause hemodynamic compromise in some persons or feelings of palpitations.

(continues on page 1008)

Interventions continued	Rationales continued
10. Monitor for diaphragmatic or phrenic nerve pacing—diaphragmatic contractions or hiccups at the pacemaker rate with pacemaker artifact.	10. Lead placement near diaphragmatic portion of the right ventricle or tip of the atrial lead may be too close to the phrenic nerve, leading to stimulation of these nerves.
11. Monitor for chest muscle stimulation around the pulse generator; if it occurs, verify that client is not moving the pulse generator.	11. Chest muscle stimulation may result from high pacemaker output, high current density, lead fracture, flipped pulse generator, or low threshold to muscle pacing.
12. Monitor the pulse generator implantation site for the following: a. Hemorrhage b. Signs and symptoms of infection c. Skin inflammation or necrosis over and around pulse generator	12. The surgical implantation and the presence of a foreign body increase risk of hemorrhage, necrosis, and infection. Careful monitoring can help to ensure early detection of problems. Antibiotics are prescribed preprocedure and postprocedure prophylactically.

 Related Physician-Prescribed Interventions

Medications. Antibiotics (preprocedure and postprocedure)

Intravenous Therapy. Intravenous line for direct venous access

Laboratory Studies. Electrolytes, arterial blood gases

Diagnostic Studies. ECG, electrophysiology studies, chest x-ray film

Therapies. Pacemaker setting, site care, pulse counting, activity restrictions, pulse oximetry

 Documentation
Flow records
Vital signs
Rhythm strips
Wound and dressing status
Unusual symptoms

Postprocedure: Nursing Diagnoses

Impaired Physical Mobility Related to Incisional Site Pain, Activity Restrictions, and Fear of Lead Displacement

Focus Assessment Criteria	Clinical Significance
1. ROM of affected extremity 2. Pain at incision site	1,2. Pain and activity restrictions serve as signals to client to immobilize the affected extremity.
3. Understanding activity restrictions, fears regarding movement	3. Fear of lead displacement may magnify the significance of these signals to such a degree that client inappropriately immobilizes the arm.

Goal

The client will demonstrate the ability to perform ADLs.

Indicators

- Demonstrate the ability to maintain arm restriction limitations.
- Verbalize prescribed restrictions.

Interventions	Rationales
1. Explain the need to remain on bed rest for up to 24 hours post procedure (or as prescribed)	1. Bed rest is prescribed to allow fibrosis to occur around the pacemaker and electrodes; this helps to prevent dislodgement.
2. Medicate with prescribed analgesics before client engages in any activity.	2. Judicious use of pain medication keeps pain signals from discouraging use of affected arm.
3. Explain that incision and subcutaneous pocket should feel sore for 3 to 4 weeks but discomfort eventually disappears.	3. Understanding that discomfort is temporary encourages client to accept the pacemaker and participate in activity.
4. Explain that affected arm and shoulder should not be moved in an overzealous manner (i.e., over the head) for 48 hours or as prescribed. Encourage client to perform active ROM (except for overzealous movements) in affected arm following physician's instructions.	4. Overzealous arm movements may potentially cause lead dislodgement, but regular active ROM exercise maintains joint function and prevents muscle contractures.
5. Encourage early and complete participation in ADLs.	5. Self-care increases independence and a sense of well-being.
6. Reinforce physician-prescribed postoperative activity restrictions; these may include no driving, no lifting, no golfing, no bowling, etc., for 4 to 6 weeks after surgery.	6. Activity restrictions allow continued fibrosis around pacemaker and electrodes to provide increased stabilization.
7. Provide written information on activity instructions and restrictions.	7. Written materials can serve as a valuable resource for postdischarge care at home.

🖋 Documentation

Discharge summary record
Level of activity
Client teaching
Outcome achievement or status
Referrals if indicated

Disturbed Self-Concept Related to Perceived Loss of Health and Dependence on Pacemaker

Focus Assessment Criteria	Clinical Significance
1. Accuracy of client's perceptions regarding pacemaker	1. Pacemaker implantation can cause a sense of loss, which can negatively affect self-concept.
2. Client's self-concept before pacemaker implantation	2. Acceptance of pacemaker can be affected by many factors; however, a person's ability to adjust depends on his or her ability to identify personal strengths still present, compensate for what is lost, and view himself or herself as a unique person.
3. Length of preoperative illness	3. A client with longstanding symptoms before pacemaker implantation generally adjusts better than one with an acute preoperative illness.
4. Availability of support	4. A strong support system can greatly aid the client's adjustment.

Goal

The client will participate in self care.

Indicators

- Verbalize an intent to follow the prescribed medical regimen.
- Verbalize recognition that despite the physical loss, he or she remains much the same person.

Interventions	Rationales
1. Identify and correct any misinformation client may have regarding pacemakers.	1. Incorrect assumptions can cause doubt and uncertainty and contribute to poor self-concept. Many times, client and family have information related to old pacemakers. Today's pacemakers can be self-adjusting (versus fixed rate) and require less frequent battery changes (e.g., 5 to 10 years).
2. Encourage client to share feelings and concerns about living with a pacemaker.	2. Sharing gives nurse the opportunity to identify and clarify misconceptions and address areas of concern.
3. Assist client in distinguishing areas of life in which he or she is not dependent on others.	3. This measure emphasizes areas for control and self-determination in learning to accept the pacemaker and altered body image.
4. Help client to identify personal strengths that might aid coping.	4. Discussing strengths encourages client to de-emphasize the disability.

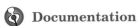 **Documentation**
Progress notes
Emotional status
Dialogues

High Risk for Ineffective Therapeutic Regimen Management Related to Insufficient Knowledge of Activity Restrictions, Precautions, Signs and Symptoms of Complications, and Follow-up Care

Focus Assessment Criteria	Clinical Significance
1. Readiness and ability to learn and retain information	1. A client or family failing to achieve learning goals requires a referral for assistance postdischarge.

Goals

The goals for this diagnosis represent those associated with discharge planning. Refer to the discharge criteria.

Interventions	Rationales
1. Review postprocedural routine as needed.	1. Reviewing enables nurse to evaluate whether or not client needs additional teaching.
2. Instruct on incisional care including the following: a. Wound cleansing b. Suture removal if present (usually after 7 days) c. Expected swelling for 2 to 4 weeks d. Recognizing signs and symptoms of infection e. For a woman, wearing a brassiere for support with a gauze pad over the pulse generator to decrease rubbing over the suture line	2. Proper incision care helps to prevent infection and other complications.
3. Instruct client on home care measures. a. Keep affected arm immobile for 24 to 48 hours postprocedure. b. Continue taking prescribed cardiac medication until otherwise instructed by physician.	3. Understanding home care enables client to comply with the regimen. a. Arm movement could cause traction on the lead and possible lead displacement. b. Pacemaker implantation does not preclude the need for medication.
4. Teach client and family to watch for and promptly report the following: a. Redness, swelling, warmth, drainage, or pain at the surgical wound, or temperature greater than 101°F	4. Early detection enables prompt treatment to prevent serious complications. a. These signs and symptoms point to wound infection.

(continues on page 1012)

Interventions continued	**Rationales** continued
b. Join stiffness, pain, and muscle weakness in affected arm	b. Joint stiffness, pain, and muscle weakness may indicate neurovascular compression.
c. Light-headedness, fainting, dizzy spells, or chronic fatigue	c. Light-headedness, fainting, dizzy spells, or chronic fatigue may result from cerebral hypoxia owing to insufficient cardiac output secondary to pacemaker malfunction.
d. Very rapid or very slow pulse	d. Pulse changes may indicate pacemaker failure.
e. Chronic hiccups or chest muscle twitching	e. Chronic hiccups or chest muscle twitching may indicate lead displacement and electrical stimulation of diaphragm or intercostal muscles.
f. Swollen ankles or hands	f. Swelling ankles or hands may indicate congestive heart failure related to insufficient cardiac output.
5. Instruct client to check with physician before engaging in the following activities: a. Driving b. Lifting anything weighing more than 25 lb c. Using an ax by lifting it over the head and dropping it to cut d. Participating in contact sports or sports such as golf or bowling e. Using an air hammer f. Firing a rifle from the affected side g. Serving overhead-style when playing tennis h. Diving head first into water	5. These activities could potentially damage either the pulse generator or leads.
6. Reassure that pacemaker should not interfere with sexual activity.	6. Specifically discussing sexual activity can reduce fears and let client share concerns.
7. Instruct client to carry a pacemaker identification card at all times. (He or she will receive a temporary card before going home; pacemaker manufacturer will mail a permanent card later.) Encourage client to apply for a Medic-Alert bracelet.	7. A pacemaker identification card and Medic-Alert bracelet provide important information to caregivers in emergency situations.
8. Instruct client to notify physicians, nurses, and dentists about his or her pacemaker so that prophylactic antibiotics may be given before invasive procedures if needed.	8. Because the pulse generator increases tissue susceptibility to infection, prophylactic therapy is indicated before many invasive procedures.
9. Instruct client to avoid strong electromagnetic fields including magnetic resonance	9. Electromagnetic fields can interfere with pacemaker function. A clients with any

(continues on page 1013)

Interventions continued	**Rationales** continued
imaging equipment, arc welding equipment, high-intensity power lines, dental ultrasonic cleaners, drills, internal combustion engines, and poorly shielded microwave ovens (older microwave ovens). a. Instruct client to avoid leaning over open hood of a running car engine.	anxiety about using a microwave oven should stand about 6 feet away from oven when it is operating. a. Anything that revolves at high revolutions can cause an electromagnetic field; therefore, this could lead to pacemaker malfunction.
10. Warn that pacemaker triggers magnetic detection alarms such as those found at airports. Instruct client to carry pacemaker identification card to verify pacemaker placement with airport security personnel.	10. This information allows client to inform airport security personnel at detectors to avoid misunderstanding and embarrassment.
11. Emphasize the necessity of long-term follow-up care; reinforce physician's instructions.	11. Regular follow-up care is essential for ongoing evaluation.
12. Explain that the battery is not lifelong and replacement might be necessary (average battery life is 5 to 10 years).	12. Understanding the need for battery replacement assists with coping should replacement be needed.
13. Teach pulse-taking if appropriate and instruct client to notify physician if pulse rate falls below pacemaker set rate.	13. Pulse taking may help to enhance client's sense of control over the situation (although some studies show that clients can become anxious about pulse counting).
14. Instruct client on functions of pacemaker (refer to codes in beginning of this care plan). Advise client to carry a card or wear an ID bracelet indicating pacemaker and functions in codes.	14. Pacemakers have varied options. In an emergency the specific options need to be known.
15. Explain the importance of seeking medical care or advice (phone) if shock function occurs.	15. Further evaluation may be needed.
16. Provide written instructional materials at discharge.	16. Written information reinforces teaching and serves as a resource at home.
17. Provide client with names and phone numbers of persons to call should questions or an emergency arise (day or night).	17. This can help to reassure client that direct access for assistance is always available.

(continues on page 1014)

Interventions continued	**Rationales** continued
18. Explain transtelephonic follow-up care, a system in which client uses a transmitter at home to have the pacemaker checked over the telephone.	18. Knowing what to expect after discharge may decrease client's anxiety. Transtelephone monitoring provides reassurance to client that the pacemaker is working properly and can determine the need for battery replacement. It does not preclude the need for physician follow-up visits.

 Documentation

Discharge summary record
Client and family teaching
Outcome achievement or status

PERITONEAL DIALYSIS

Peritoneal dialysis—the repetitive instillation and drainage of dialysis solution into and from the peritoneal cavity—uses the processes of osmosis, ultrafiltration, and diffusion to remove wastes, toxins, and fluid from the blood. The procedure is indicated for acute or chronic kidney disease and severe fluid or electrolyte imbalances unresponsive to other treatments.

Numerous techniques for instillation and drainage of dialysis fluid have been developed. These methods are both manual and automated. Therapy can be continuous or intermittent.

Continuous therapies include continuous ambulatory peritoneal dialysis (CAPD) and continuous cycling peritoneal dialysis (CCPD). CAPD is most commonly used and provides dialysate inflow with the disposable bag and tubing remaining connected, folded, and secured to the torso during dwell time. Exchanges are done four times per day with 2.0 to 2.5 liters. CCPD uses an automated cycler to perform exchanges during sleep and the abdomen is left full during the day.

Intermittent peritoneal dialysis (IPD) consists of treatment periods with dwell time and alternates with periods of peritoneal cavity draining. Intermittent techniques use multiple short dwell exchanges three or four times a week. Automated intermittent exchanges may occur with repeated small (tidal peritoneal dialysis) or at night (nightly intermittent peritoneal dialysis). Manual IPD also may be done in hospitals for a prescribed number of cycles and length of time based on client requirements. Manual peritoneal dialysis requires careful control of dialysate instillation (2 liters), dwell time, and outflow.

 Time Frame
Pretherapy and intratherapy

 DIAGNOSTIC CLUSTER

Collaborative Problems

▲ PC: Fluid Imbalance
▲ PC: Electrolyte Imbalances
▲ PC: Uremia
△ PC: Hemorrhage
△ PC: Hyperglycemia
△ PC: Bladder/Bowel Perforation
▲ PC: Inflow/Outflow Problems

Nursing Diagnoses	Refer to
▲ High Risk for Infection related to access to peritoneal cavity	
△ High Risk for Ineffective Breathing Pattern related to immobility, pressure, and pain	

(continues on page 1016)

Nursing Diagnoses continued	**Refer to** continued
△ Acute Pain related to catheter insertion, instillation of dialysis solution, outflow, suction, and chemical irritation of peritoneum	
△ High Risk for Ineffective Therapeutic Regimen Management related to insufficient knowledge of rationale of treatment, medications, home dialysis procedure, signs and symptoms of complications, community resources, and follow-up care	
△ Imbalanced Nutrition: Less Than Body Requirements related to anorexia	Chronic Kidney Disease
△ Interrupted Family Processes related to the effects of interruptions of the treatment schedule on role responsibilities	Chronic Kidney Disease
△ Powerlessness related to chronic illness and the need for continuous treatment	Chronic Kidney Disease

▲ This diagnosis was reported to be monitored for or managed frequently (75%–100%).
△ This diagnosis was reported to be monitored for or managed often (50%–74%)

Discharge Criteria

Before discharge, the client or family will

1. Be able to demonstrate home peritoneal dialysis procedures if appropriate.
2. State signs and symptoms of infection.
3. Discuss the expected effects of long-term dialysis on the client and family.
4. State signs and symptoms that must be reported to a health care professional.

Collaborative Problems

Potential Complication: Fluid Imbalances

Potential Complication: Electrolyte Imbalances

Potential Complication: Uremia

Potential Complication: Hemorrhage

Potential Complication: Hyperglycemia

Potential Complication: Bladder or Bowel Perforation

Potential Complication: Inflow or Outflow Problems

Nursing Goal

The nurse will detect early signs and symptoms of (a) fluid imbalances, (b) electrolyte imbalances, (c) uremia, (d) hemorrhage, (e) hyperglycemia, (f) bladder or bowel perforation, and (g) inflow or outflow problems and will intervene collaboratively to stabilize the client.

Indicators

- Alert, oriented, calm (a, b, c)
- Skin warm, dry, usual color, no lesions (a, c, d, e)
- No or minimal edema (a)
- B/P > 90/60, < 140/90 mm Hg (a, b, d)
- Pulse pressure (40 mm Hg difference in systolic or diastolic) (a, b, d)
- Pulse 60–100 beats/min (a, b, d)
- Respirations 16–20 breaths/min (a)
- Respirations relaxed, rhythmic (a)
- No rales or wheezing (a)
- No weight change (a)
- Flat neck veins (a)
- No headache (b)
- Bowel sounds present (b)
- No chest pain (c)
- No abdominal pain (b, e)
- Intact reflexes (b)
- No change in vision (c)
- No c/o of nausea/vomiting (c)
- Intact muscle strength (b, c)
- No seizures (b)
- Serum potassium 3.5–5 mEq/L (b, c)
- Fasting blood glucose 70–110 mg/dL (e)
- Hemoglobin (d)
  - Male 13.5–17.5 g/dL
  - Female 13–16 g/dL
- Hematocrit (d)
  - Male 40%–54%
  - Female 37%–47%
- Serum sodium 135–148 mm/dL (c)
- Serum creatinine 0.6–1.2 mg/dL (c)
- Blood urea nitrogen 7–18 mg/dL (c)
- Patent inflow and outflow (g)
- Intact connections, no kinks (g)
- No urinary urgency (f)
- No glucose in urine (e, f)
- No bowel urgency (f)
- No diarrhea (c, f)
- No fecal material in dialysate (f)

Interventions	Rationales
1. Monitor for signs and symptoms of hypervolemia. a. Edema b. Dyspnea or tachypnea c. Rales or frothy secretions d. Rapid, bounding pulse e. Hypertension f. Jugular vein distention g. S₃ heart sounds	1. Hypervolemia may occur if dialysate does not drain freely or if excess IV or oral fluids have been infused or injected (Graham-Macaluso, 1991). Excess fluid greater than 5% of body weight is needed to produce edema. Fluid in lungs produces signs and symptoms of hypoxia. Increasing flow rate will increase fluid removal with little change in clearance of solutes.
2. Monitor for signs and symptoms of hypovolemia: a. Dry skin and mucous membranes b. Poor skin turgor	2. Hypovolemia may occur from excessive or too-rapid removal of dialysate fluid, inadequate salt and fluid intake, increased insensible loss, or overuse of hypertonic

(continues on page 1018)

Interventions continued	**Rationales** continued

c. Thirst
    d. Tachycardia
    e. Tachypnea
    f. Hypotension with orthostatic changes
    g. Narrowed pulse pressure
    h. Altered level of consciousness
	solution. Decreasing dextrose concentration to 1.5% may remove solutes without fluid (Smith, 1992).

3. Monitor intake and output.	3. Urine output varies depending on renal status.
4. Enforce fluid restrictions as ordered.	4. Physician may restrict fluid intake to insensible losses or the previous day's urine output.
5. Weigh daily or before and after each dialysis treatment.	5. Daily weights help to evaluate fluid balance.
6. Add medications to dialysate as ordered.	6. Heparin commonly is added to decrease fibrin clots in the catheter. Potassium is added to prevent hypokalemia.
7. Monitor peritoneal dialysis inflow, dwell time, and outflow.	7. *Inflow* (usually taking less than 15 minutes) is the infusion of dialysis solution by gravity into the peritoneal cavity. *Dwell time* (0 to 20 minutes) is the length of time that the dialysis solution remains in the peritoneal cavity, which determines the amount of diffusion and osmosis that occurs. *Outflow* (usually less than 20 minutes) is the emptying of the peritoneal cavity by gravity.

8. Monitor for signs and symptoms of hypernatremia with fluid overload:
    a. Thirst
    b. Agitation
    c. Convulsions
	8. Dialysate solution > 4.25% or rapid outflow can cause hypernatremia (Persons, 1987).

9. Monitor for signs and symptoms of hyponatremia:
    a. Lethargy or coma
    b. Weakness
    c. Abdominal pain
    d. Muscle twitching or convulsions
	9. Hyponatremia results from the dilutional effects of hypervolemia. Extracellular volume decrease lowers blood pressure and leads to hypoxia.

10. Monitor for signs and symptoms of hyperkalemia:	10. Prolonged dwell time can increase potassium fluctuations that can affect neuro-

(continues on page 1019)

Interventions continued	**Rationales** continued
a. Weakness or paralysis b. Muscle irritability c. Paresthesias d. Nausea, vomiting, abdominal cramping, or diarrhea e. Irregular pulse	muscular transmission, reduce action of GI smooth muscles, and impair electrical conduction of the heart. Infusing dialysate with a lower potassium than that of the plasma can decrease overall potassium.
11. Monitor for signs and symptoms of hypokalemia: a. Weakness or paralysis b. Decreased or absent tendon reflexes c. Hypoventilation d. Polyuria e. Hypotension f. Paralytic ileus	11. Hypokalemia impairs neuromuscular transmission and reduces action of respiratory muscles and GI smooth muscles. The kidneys become less sensitive to the effects of antidiuretic hormone and thus excrete large quantities of dilute urine.
12. Monitor for signs and symptoms of uremia: a. Skin and mucous membrane lesions b. Pericardial friction rub c. Pleural friction rub d. GI disturbances e. Peripheral neuropathy f. Vision changes g. Central nervous system impairment h. Tachypnea i. Musculoskeletal changes	12. A multisystem syndrome, uremia is a manifestation of end-stage renal disease resulting from waste products of protein metabolism including urea, creatinine, and uric acid. To increase removal of wastes, the number of exchanges can be increased.
13. Monitor for vessel perforation and hemorrhage marked by increasingly bloody dialysate return.	13. Perforation of a blood vessel during catheter insertion can cause bloody dialysate, urine, or stool, or bleeding at insertion site.
14. Explain procedure and expected sensations and provide support during temporary catheter insertion.	14. Explanations encourage client to avoid sudden movement during catheter insertion.
15. If bleeding persists, apply a pressure dressing and carefully monitor vital signs.	15. Pressure may stop bleeding.
16. Monitor for signs and symptoms of hyperglycemia: a. Elevated or depressed blood glucose level b. Polyuria c. Polyphagia d. Polydipsia e. Abdominal pain f. Diaphoresis	16. The amount of dextrose absorbed from the dialysate varies with dextrose concentration and number of cycles. In two cycles of 1.5% solution, 41 kcal are absorbed. After dialysis is complete, hypoglycemia may occur because of increased insulin production during instillation of high dextrose concentrations.

(continues on page 1020)

Interventions continued	**Rationales** continued

17. Monitor for signs and symptoms of bladder or bowel perforation:
  a. Fecal material in dialysate
  b. Complaints of urgency
  c. Increased urine output with high glucose concentrations
  d. Complaints of pressure in the sensation to defecate
  e. Watery diarrhea
	17. Catheter insertion may perforate bowel or bladder, allowing dialysate to infuse into bowel or bladder.

18. Have client empty bladder and bowel before insertion of peritoneal dialysis catheter.	18. Emptying bladder and bowel decreases risk of perforation during catheter insertion.
19. Monitor drug levels during dialysis to maintain therapeutic treatment (Smith, 1992).	19. Drugs may be added to the dialysate.

20. If inflow or outflow problems occur, do the following:
  a. Increase height of the dialysate bag and lower the bed.
 	
  b. Reposition client and instruct him or her to cough.
  c. Check for kinks and closed clamps.
  d. Remove a nontransparent dressing to check for catheter obstruction.
  e. Check dressing for wetness. Dialysate leaking from exit site presents as a clear fluid testing strongly for glucose.
  f. Assess abdominal pain on outflow.
 	
  g. Assess amount of dialysate return. Notify physician if >50% of inflow is retained (Smith, 1992).
  h. Ascertain if heparin has been added to dialysate.
  i. If ordered, irrigate with heparinized saline (Golper, Burkart, & Piraino, 1997).
  j. If ordered, irrigate with fibrinolytic agents.
  k. Assess for constipation.
	20. These measures can enhance the effectiveness of dialysis and prevent complications.
	  a. Raising the bag and lowering the bed can help to maximize gravity drainage.
	  b. Repositioning and coughing may help to clear a blocked or kinked catheter.
	
	  d. Dressing can obscure an external obstruction or kink.
	  e. Leakage at site may be from poor insertion technique or delayed healing and infection.
	
	  f. Abdominal pain may result from excessive suction on abdominal viscera or incorrect catheter position.
	  g. If catheter does not drain, omentum may be obstructing or fibrin may have formed in the catheter.
	  h,i. Heparin can help to prevent catheter blockage from fibrin or blood clots.
	
	  j. Fibrinolytic agents may be effective in removing blockage.
	  k. Constipation may lead to shifting of catheter position, drainage failure, and catheter loss.

21. Calculate inflow and outflow volume at the end of each dialysis cycle. Report discrepancies in accordance with hospital protocol.	21. Accurate inflow and outflow records determine fluid loss or retention by client.

Related Physician-Prescribed Interventions

Medications. Heparinized saline, fibrinolytic agents

Laboratory Studies. Refer to either the Acute Kidney Failure or Chronic Kidney Disease Care Plan.

Therapies. Dialysate solution, dwell time, number of cycles

 Documentation

Flow records
   Vital signs
   Intake and output
   Weight and medications
   Dialysate color
   Abdominal girth
   Serum glucose
   Urine specific gravity
   Other laboratory values
Progress notes
   Changes in status
   Inflow or outflow problems
   Interventions

Nursing Diagnoses

High Risk for Infection Related to Access to Peritoneal Cavity

Focus Assessment Criteria	Clinical Significance

1. Catheter site for redness, inflammation, purulent drainage, tenderness, warmth, and leaks
 	
2.
  a. Assess exit site and sinus tract for evidence of infection or irritation.
  b. Palpate catheter tunnel for firmness and tenderness.
  c. Observe symptoms of systemic infection.
 	
3. Signs and symptoms of systemic infection:
  a. Fever
  b. Chills
  c. Diaphoresis
  d. Nausea and vomiting
  e. Abdominal pain and rebound tenderness
  f. Malaise
  g. Tachycardia
  h. Hypotension
  i. Increased WBC
	1,2,3. Catheterization and instillation of dialysate entail an increased risk of local and systemic infections. An exit site infection is an inflammation of the site with purulent drainage.

Goal

The client will be infection free at catheter site and will not develop peritonitis or a systemic infection.

Indicators
- Temperature 98.5–99°F
- No edema or drainage at site

Interventions	Rationales
1. Ensure use of sterile technique when setting up equipment.	1–5. Aseptic technique reduces microorganisms and helps prevent their introduction into the system.
2. Ensure complete skin preparation before catheter insertion.	
3. Use sterile technique when assisting with catheter insertion or removal and when performing dialysis. Wear gloves to examine exit site.	
4. Apply masks to all staff and the client during catheter insertion, removal, and dressing changes.	
5. Minimize catheter movement at exit site (Stein, 1990).	
6. Warm dialysate solution in a dedicated peritoneal dialysis microwave oven for the institution's recommended time frame. Agitate bag before infusing.	6. Because microwave ovens vary in rate, consistency, and method of heating, each institution needs to establish its own time frame (Armstrong & Zalatan, 1992).
7. Determine that dialysate is between 36.5°C to 37.5°C (97.7 to 99.5°F) before infusing.	7. External temperature may be measured by folding the bag over an electronic thermometer (Armstrong & Zalatan, 1992).
8. When performing manual peritoneal dialysis, prevent contamination of spikes when changing dialysate bags.	8. Peritoneal dialysate may be done manually with a manifold setup or by an automatic cycler (Smith, 1992). Use of bags allows the peritoneal dialysis system to remain closed except when spiking.
9. Monitor dialysate return for color and clarity. Obtain culture of any drainage.	9–13. Turbidity may indicate infection (Smith, 1992).
10. Perform routine exit site care using aseptic technique.	
11. Increase frequency of exit site care as needed.	
12. Change cleansing agent for exit site care as indicated.	
13. Teach alternative methods of exit site care.	

 Documentation

Progress notes
   Signs and symptoms of infection
Flow records
   Dressing changes

High Risk for Ineffective Breathing Pattern Related to Immobility, Pressure, and Pain

Focus Assessment Criteria	Clinical Significance

1. Indicators of respiratory status
  a. Respiratory rate and rhythm
  b. Abdominal girth
  c. Pain
  d. Dyspnea
  e. Cough
  f. Pleural friction rub
  g. Secretions
  h. Breath sounds
 	
2. Assess degree of back pain.
 	
3. Assess degree of abdominal fullness.
 	
4. Assess degree of shoulder pain and sequence of events leading to discomfort.
	1–4. Hypoventilation may result from increased pressure on the diaphragm as a result of dialysate instillation and position during cycle. Pulmonary edema, pleuritis, infection, or uremic lung also may contribute to respiratory distress.

Goal
The client will demonstrate optimal respiratory function.

Indicators
- By bilateral breath sounds
- Arterial blood gases

Interventions	Rationales
1. Encourage regular coughing and deep breathing exercises.	1. These exercises promote lung expansion.
2. Evaluate effect of smaller dialysate solution volumes on adequacy and initiate if appropriate. 3. If client experiences respiratory distress, immediately stop inflow or begin outflow. 4. Evaluate potential for PD modality change to cycling therapy. 5. Support physical therapy, exercise, and weight loss program as indicated. 6. Administer analgesics as indicated.	2–6. Stopping flow reduces pressure on the diaphragm, possibly relieving distress.

 Documentation
Progress notes
  Abnormal respiratory status

Acute Pain Related to Catheter Insertion, Instillation of Dialysis Solution, Outflow Suction, and Chemical Irritation of Peritoneum

Focus Assessment Criteria	Clinical Significance
1. Pain: Location, intensity, duration, quality, onset, precipitating factors.	1–5. Constant abdominal distention and chemical irritation of the peritoneum contribute to abdominal pain or cramping during dialysis.
2. Evaluate for peritonitis, exit site, or tunnel infection.	
3. Assess dialysis solution temperature, dextrose concentration, and additives.	
4. Observe for rate-related or "jet-effect" discomfort during fill or drain.	
5. Observe for pain/cramping at end of drain cycle.	

Goal

The client will be as comfortable as possible during peritoneal dialysis.

Indicators

* No pressure or pain during the procedure
* Reports measures used that reduced pain

Interventions	Rationales
1. Instruct client to report excessive pain on catheter insertion or dialysate instillation. Have client describe pain's severity on a scale of 0 to 10 (0 = no pain; 10 = most severe pain).	1. Pain on catheter insertion calls for catheter repositioning; pain during dialysate instillation may result from various factors including too-rapid inflow rate, cool dialysate temperature, and complications of treatment.
2. Position client to minimize pain while maintaining good air exchange and free-flowing dialysate.	2. Certain positions can reduce abdominal discomfort during instillation.
3. Drain effluent to assess for cloudy or bloody fluid. Initiate protocol for peritonitis if indicated.	3. Lidocaine may be used as an intraperitoneal analgesic (Smith, 1992).
4. As necessary, use nonpharmacological pain relief techniques such as distraction, massage, guided imagery, and relaxation exercises.	4. Nonpharmacological pain relief techniques can offer effective, safe alternatives to medication in some clients.
5. Check temperature of dialysate before and during instillation.	5. A too-cool dialysate temperature can cause abdominal cramps; too warm a temperature can cause tissue damage.

(continues on page 1025)

Interventions continued	Rationales continued
6. If client reports extreme pain during dialysis, decrease inflow rate and consult with physician to decrease temporarily the amount of dialysate instilled (Clochesy, Breu, Cardin, Rudy, & Whittaker, 1993).	6. A slower installation rate reduces intra-abdominal pressure and may decrease pain. A decrease in volume reduces degree of abdominal distention, especially on initiation of dialysis.
7. Investigate carefully any client reports of pain in the shoulder blades.	7. Referred pain to the shoulders may be from diaphragmatic irritation or from air infused on insertion (Smith, 1992).

✥ Documentation

Progress notes
  Pain
  Relief measures instituted
  Client's response

High Risk for Ineffective Therapeutic Regimen Management Related to Insufficient Knowledge of Rationale of Treatment, Medications, Home Dialysis Procedure, Signs and Symptoms of Complications, Community Resources, and Follow-up Care

Focus Assessment Criteria	Clinical Significance
1. Readiness and ability to learn and retain information	1. A client or family failing to achieve learning goals requires a referral for assistance postdischarge.

Goals

The goals for this diagnosis represent those associated with discharge planning. Refer to the discharge criteria.

Interventions	Rationales
1. Reinforce physician's explanations of renal disease and of peritoneal dialysis procedure and its effects. 2. Discuss all prescribed medications, covering purpose, dosage, and side effects.	1,2. Client's understanding can help to increase compliance and tolerance of treatment.

3. As appropriate, teach client the following and ask client to perform return demonstrations so nurse can evaluate client's ability to do procedures safely and effectively:
  a. Aseptic technique
  b. Catheter care and insertion
	3. Many clients can perform home peritoneal dialysis without assistance. Proper technique can help to prevent infection and inflow and outflow problems (Graham-Macaluso, 1991; Stein, 1990).

(continues on page 1026)

Interventions continued	Rationales continued
c. Dialysate preparation d. Positioning during treatment e. Instilling additives to dialysate f. Inflow and outflow procedure	
4. Discuss how to manage inflow pain by ensuring proper temperature and flow rate of dialysate.	4. Cold dialysate, too-rapid inflow, acid dialysate, and stretching of diaphragm can cause inflow pain.
5. Teach client to maintain adequate protein and calorie intake.	5. Low serum albumin levels are known to be associated with an increased risk of death (Herrman, 1992).
6. Teach client to prevent constipation through adequate diet, fluid intake, and physical activity.	6. Constipation or bowel distention impedes dialysate outflow. Large protein losses occur with peritoneal dialysis (Clochesy et al., 1993).
7. Teach client to watch for and promptly report: a. Unresolved pain from inflow b. Outflow failure c. Low-grade fever, cloudy outflow, malaise, and catheter site changes (redness, inflammation, drainage, tenderness, warmth, and leaks). d. Signs of fluid/electrolyte imbalance (see PC: Fluid Imbalance, PC: Electrolyte Imbalances for specific signs and symptoms of various imbalances) e. Abdominal pain, stool changes, constipation	7. Early detection of complications enables prompt intervention to minimize their seriousness (Logston-Boggs & Wooldridge-King, 1993). a. This finding can indicate intra-peritoneal infection. b. This finding may result from catheter obstruction, peritonitis, dislodged catheter, or a full colon. c. These signs can point to infection. d. Dialysis alters fluid and electrolyte levels possibly resulting in imbalance. e. Bowel distention impedes outflow.
8. Provide information on where to purchase necessary supplies.	8. Knowledge of sources of supplies can prevent incorrect substitutions.
9. Teach client to record the following: a. Vital signs and weight before and after dialysis b. Percent of dialysate and amount of inflow c. Amount of outflow d. Number of exchanges required	9. Accurate records aid in evaluating effectiveness of treatment.

(continues on page 1027)

Interventions continued	Rationales continued
e. Medications taken f. Problems g. Urine output and number and character of stools	
10. Initiate referral to a home health agency for necessary follow-up.	10. The initial home care visit is needed to evaluate client's suitability for home dialysis and takes into account factors such as physical condition, ability, environment, financial needs, and support system. Subsequent visits are indicated to assess client for signs of infection, improper procedures, and complications (e.g., electrolyte, fluid, and nutritional imbalances).
11. Provide information on available community resources and self-help groups (e.g., National Kidney Foundation).	11. Access to resources and self-help groups may ease difficulties of home dialysis and help to minimize its effects on home life.

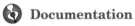 **Documentation**

Discharge summary record
　Client and family teaching
　Outcome achievement or status
　Referrals if indicated

RADIATION THERAPY

Radiation therapy is the use of high-energy ionizing radiation to destroy cancer cells. It also can serve as palliative treatment to relieve pain, prevent fracture, or mobilize a client following cord compression. When used in cancer treatment, radiation therapy aims to kill maximum cancer cells while causing minimal damage to normal tissue.

The ionizing radiation can be delivered in two ways. In *external beam radiation (teletherapy),* a radioactive source or electromagnetic energy from a machine placed at some distance from the target site delivers the treatment. The distance is advantageous because the dose is relatively uniform across a given volume and allows for dose-shaping or modifying devices to be interposed between the source and the client. In *internal therapy (brachytherapy),* the radioactive sources are placed directly into the tumor or tumor bed. A high dose is near the sources in the tumor bed and a much lower dose in the normal tissues. Combination teletherapy and brachytherapy is used in the treatment of many neoplasms. *Radiation sensitizers* are compounds that enhance the damaging effects of ionizing radiation. *Radioprotector* compounds protect cells and tissues from the damaging effects of radiation. A *radiolabeled antibody* is an antibody with a radioactive substance attached to its molecular structure that binds the antibody and radioisotope.

Tissues with a rapid rate of cellular division are more sensitive to the effects of radiation therapy. Some examples of radiosensitive tissues include bone marrow, epithelial cells lining the GI and GU tracts, gonad, and hair follicles. Radioresistant tissues with a slow generation time, such as muscles, tendons, and nerves, have a less dramatic response. The response of tissues to radiation is divided into three specific time periods: *acute, subacute,* and *chronic.* Acute response period is the first 6 months after exposure to radiation. Subacute response period occurs 6 months to 1 year after exposure, and late or chronic response occurs 1 to 5 years longer after exposure to radiation.

General side effects include fatigue, anorexia, and skin alterations. The remaining side effects depend on the site treated (refer to site-specific chart) (Hilderley, 2000).

Site	Acute Effects	Late Effects

Head and neck	Eye
	  Dryness
	  Itching
		Eye
		  Cataracts
		  Optic nerve
		  Keratitis
		  Glaucoma
		  Retinal hemorrhage
		  Sicca

	Other
	  Mucositis
	  Xerostomia
	  Dysphagia
	  Taste alterations
	  Pharyngitis
		Other
		  Xerostomia or dental caries
		  Osteoradionecrosis
		  Taste changes
		  Trismus
		  Soft tissue edema
		  Subcutaneous fistula
		  Flap necrosis
		  Hypothyroidism

Chest	Esophagus
	  Esophagitis
		Esophagus
		  Stricture
		  Fistula

	Lung
	  Pneumonitis
		Lung
		  Pneumonitis

(continues on page 1029)

	Dysphagia		Fibrosis
	Dyspnea		Alveolar type II pneumocytes
	Breast		Heart
	Breast Edema		Coronary artery disease
	Lymphedema		Pericarditis
Abdomen	Stomach		Stomach
	Retching		Atrophy
	Nausea		Ulcer
	Vomiting		Liver
	Indigestion		Hepatitis
			Cirrhosis
Pelvis	Bowel		Bowel
	Diarrhea		Adhesions
			Enteritis
			Proctitis
	Bladder		Bladder
	Cystitis		Contracted bladder
	Dysuria		Cystitis
	Urinary frequency/urgency		
	Hematuria		
	Urinary incontinence		
	Urinary retention		
	Vagina		Vagina
	Vaginal discharge		Fibrosis
	Amenorrhea		Loss of lubrication
	Vaginal dryness		Gonadal effects
	Dyspareunia		Impotence
			Loss of fertility
			Ovary—menstrual irregularity or cessation
			Testis—oligospermia; aspermia
			Genetic effects
			Alopecia
Brain and central nervous system			
	Cerebral edema		
	Motor deficits		
	Nausea/vomiting		
	Neurologic deficits		
	Sensory deficits		

(Adapted from Brunner, D., Iwamoto, R., Keane, K., & Strohl, R. [1992]. *Manual for radiation oncology nursing practice and education.* Pittsburgh, PA: Oncology Nursing Society.)

 Time Frame
Pretherapy and intratherapy

 DIAGNOSTIC CLUSTER

Collaborative Problems	**Refer to**
▲ PC: Myelosuppression (Infection, Bleeding)	
PC: Malabsorption	
PC: Pleural Effusion	
PC: Cerebral Edema	
△ PC: Cystitis, Urethritis, and Tenesmus	
△ PC: Mucositis, Esophagitis, Pneumonitis	
△ PC: Myelitis and Parotitis	
△ PC: Fluid and Electrolyte Imbalance	Renal Failure

(continues on page 1030)

Nursing Diagnoses continued	Refer to continued
▲ Anxiety related to prescribed radiation therapy and insufficient knowledge of treatments and self-care measures	
△ High Risk for Impaired Oral Mucous Membrane related to dry mouth or inadequate oral hygiene	
▲ Impaired Skin Integrity related to effects of radiation on epithelial and basal cells and effects of diarrhea on perineal area	
△ Impaired Comfort related to stimulation of the vomiting center and damage to the gastrointestinal mucosa cells secondary to radiation	Gastroenteritis
▲ Fatigue related to systemic effects of radiation therapy	
Impaired Comfort related to damage to sebaceous and sweat glands secondary to radiation	Inflammatory Joint Disease Cirrhosis
▲ Imbalanced Nutrition: Less Than Body Requirements related to decreased oral intake, reduced salivation, mouth discomfort, dysphasia, nausea/ vomiting, increased metabolic rate, and diarrhea	Chemotherapy
△ Disturbed Self-Concept related to alopecia, skin changes, weight loss, sterility, and changes in role, relationships and life styles	Cancer: Initial Diagnosis
△ Grieving related to changes in life style, role, finances, functional capacity, body image, and health losses	Cancer: Initial Diagnosis
△ Interrupted Family Processes related to imposed changes in family roles, relationships, and responsibilities	Cancer: Initial Diagnosis

▲ This diagnosis was reported to be monitored for or managed frequently (75%–100%).
△ This diagnosis was reported to be monitored for or managed often (50%–74%).

Discharge Criteria

Before discharge, the client or family will

1. Relate skin care, oral care, and rest requirements
2. State the intent to discuss fears and concerns with a trusted friend.
3. Relate signs and symptoms that must be reported to a health care professional.

Collaborative Problems

Potential Complication: Myelosuppression (Infection, Bleeding)

Potential Complication: Malabsorption

Potential Complication: Pleural Effusion

Potential Complication: Cerebral Edema

Potential Complication: Cystitis, Urethritis, and Tenesmus

Potential Complication: Mucositis, Esophagitis, Pneumonitis

Potential Complication: Myelitis and Parotitis

Nursing Goal

The nurse will monitor to detect early signs and symptoms of (a) myelosuppression (infection, bleeding); (b) malabsorption; (c) pleural effusion; (d) cerebral edema; (e) mucositis (esophagitis, pneumonitis); (f) cystitis, urethritis, and tenesmus; and (g) myelitis and parotitis and collaboratively intervene to stabilize client.

Indicators
- Calm, alert oriented (a, c, d)
- Temperature 98.5–99°F (a, c, d)
- Pulse 60–100 beats/min (a, c, d)
- Stable pulse pressure (approximately 40 mm Hg difference between diastolic and systolic pressures) (d)
- BP > 90/60, <140/90 mm Hg (a, c, d)
- Respirations 16–20 breaths/min (a, c, d, e)
- No rales or wheezing (a, c, d, e)
- Respirations relaxed, rhythmic (a, c, e)
- Breath sound in all lobes (a, d)
- Clear sputum (a, d)
- No abdominal pain (b)
- No chest pain (c)
- No rectal, abnormal vaginal, or nasal bleeding (a)
- No prolonged bleeding after invasive procedure (e.g., IV, IM) (a)
- No evidence of petechiae or ecchymoses (pinpoint or more diffuse bleeding under skin) (a, b)
- Clear, yellow urine (a)
- Urine output > 30 mL/hr (a)
- Urine specific gravity 1.005–1.030 (e)
- Sensation intact (b)
- Strength intact (d)
- Range of motion intact (d)
- No change in vision (d)
- Pupils equal and reactive to light (d)
- Pinkish or brownish oral mucous membranes (e)
- Oral mucous membranes intact (e)
- No swallowing difficulties (e)
- Stable weight (b, e)
- No nausea and vomiting (d)
- No change in urge to void or defecate (f)
- No edema in parotid glands (g)
- White blood count 4,800–10,000/cu mm (a)

- Red blood count (a)
  - Male 4,600,000–6,200,000/cu mm
  - Female 4,200,000–5,400,000/cu mm
- Platelet count 100,000–400,000/cu mm (a)
- Hemoglobin (a, b)
  - Male 13–18 g/dL
  - Female 12–16 g/dL
- Hematocrit (a, b)
  - Male 42%–50%
  - Female 40%–48%
- Serum iron 50–160 µg/dL (b)
- Vitamin B_6 3.6–1.8 mg/ml (b)
- Folic acid 2.5–20 ng/mL (b)
- Prothrombin time 9.5–12 (b)
- INR 1.0 (b)
- No change at radiation site (f)
- No change in bowel function (b)
- Normal chest x-ray (c)

Interventions	Rationales
1. Monitor for signs of myelosuppression. a. Decreased WBC and RBC counts b. Decreased platelet count	1. Myelosuppression (bone marrow depression) occurs when large volumes of active bone marrow are irradiated (e.g. pelvis, brain, chest, long bones). The results are decreased production of WBCs and platelet cells. RBCs are less affected because of their longer life span (Hilderley, 2000).
2. Monitor for signs and symptoms of spontaneous or excessive bleeding. a. Petechiae, ecchymoses, or hematomas b. Bleeding from nose or gums c. Prolonged bleeding from invasive procedures d. Hemoptysis e. Hematuria f. Vaginal bleeding g. Rectal bleeding h. Change in vital signs i. Change in neurologic status j. Change in respiratory status	2. Platelets are most important for hemostasis or the formation of a hemostatic mechanical plug. They also facilitate the action of clotting factors of the intrinsic system when needed. Platelets are required for lysis of the fibrin clot and vessel repair. When platelet levels are decreased, clotting is impaired and uncontrolled bleeding can occur (Gobel, 2000).
3. Instruct client to a. Use soft toothbrushes. b. Use electric razors. c. Avoid injections. d. Avoid medications that interfere with hemostasis/platelet function. e. Avoid venipuncture. If necessary, avoid prolonged tourniquet use. Apply direct pressure 3 to 5 minutes after. f. Avoid forceful coughing, sneezing, nose blowing. g. Avoid straining during defecation.	3. Clients with diminished clotting ability and at risk for infection are taught methods to prevent trauma, which can initiate bleeding or be a site for infection (Gobel, 2000).

(continues on page 1033)

Interventions continued	**Rationales** continued

4. Monitor for signs and symptoms of infection:
  a. Fever
  b. Redness/swelling at site
  c. Pus formation
  d. Pain/discomfort
	4. Lymphocytes provide long-term protection against various microorganisms. They produce antibodies that neutralize foreign proteins and facilitate phagocytosis (Ellerhorst-Ryan, 2000).

5. Explain risks of bleeding and infection. (Refer to the Corticosteroid Therapy Care Plan for strategies to reduce the risk of infection.)	5. Refer to rationales 2 and 4

6. Monitor for signs and symptoms of malabsorption.
  a. Diarrhea
  b. Steatorrhea
  c. Abdominal pain
  d. Iron deficiency anemia
  e. Easy bleeding or bruising
  f. Paresthesias
  g. Skin and vision changes
  h. Weight loss
  i. Abnormal laboratory study results: vitamin B_{12}, folic acid, hemoglobin, hematocrit, electrolytes, and prothrombin time and International Normalized Ratio (INR)
	6. Radiation damage to the small intestine results in shortening of intestinal villi and loss of absorptive surface. Radiation doses >5,000 rads to the pelvis or abdomen can denude intestinal mucosa, impairing absorption of amino acids, carbohydrates, fats, fat-soluble vitamins (A, E, D, K), folic acid, vitamin B, and iron (Foltz, 2000).

7. Monitor for signs and symptoms of pleural effusion.
  a. Dyspnea
  b. Cough
  c. Chest pain
  d. Tachycardia
  e. Tachypnea
  f. Bulging of intercostal spaces
  g. Decreased breath sounds
  h. Abnormal chest x-ray film
	7. High-dose radiation therapy to the lungs can cause lung inflammation (pneumonitis) and changes in membrane transfer capability, leading to fluid leakage into the interpleural space (Hilderley, 2000).

8. Monitor for signs and symptoms of cerebral edema.
  a. Restlessness, irritability, memory loss
  b. Somnolence
  c. Headache
  d. Vomiting
  e. Seizure activity
  f. Increased systolic blood pressure with widening pulse pressure
  g. Bradycardia
  h. Depressed respirations
  i. Weakness
	8. Radiation therapy administered to treat radiosensitive brain tumors such as medulloblastomas or metastatic brain tumors can cause cerebral edema. Effects mimic those of increased intracranial pressure (Hilderley, 2000).

(continues on page 1034)

Interventions continued	**Rationales** continued

j. Hemiparesis
    k. Vision changes
    l. Abnormal pupillary response to light	

9. Monitor for signs and symptoms of mucositis.
    a. White patches on oral mucosa
    b. Reddened, swollen mucous membranes
    c. Ulcerated, bleeding lesions
	9. Radiation therapy commonly causes tissue inflammation; higher doses generally produce more damage. Severe mucositis may necessitate interruption of radiation therapy (Hilderley, 2000).

10. Instruct client to do the following:
    a. Perform diphenhydramine (Benadryl) mouth irrigations every 4 hours.
    b. Avoid alcohol, smoking, and spicy or acidic foods.
    c. Avoid very hot or cold liquids and foods.
	10. These agents can help to reduce or ease pain of local inflammation. Alcohol, smoking, hydrogen peroxide, spicy or acidic foods, and very hot or cold foods and liquids can irritate mucosa (Hilderley, 2000).

11. Monitor for signs and symptoms of pneumonitis.
    a. Shortness of breath
    b. Hemoptysis
    c. Dry cough
 	
12. Monitor for signs and symptoms of esophagitis.
    a. Difficulty swallowing
    b. Sore throat
    c. Nausea and vomiting
	11,12. Radiation to the chest or back can cause pneumonitis or esophagitis (Hilderley, 2000).

13. Monitor for signs and symptoms of cystitis urethritis.
    a. Urinary urgency and frequency
    b. Hematuria
    c. Dysuria
    d. Negative urine cultures
	13. Irradiation of the pelvic area can cause cystitis or urethritis. Symptoms mimic those of urinary tract or bladder infection except with negative urine cultures (Hilderley, 2000).

14. Monitor for tenesmus. a. Persistent sensation of need to void or defecate	14. Radiation to the anal or urinary sphincter area can cause mucositis of sites (Hilderley, 2000).

15. Monitor for signs and symptoms of myelitis.
    a. Paresthesias in back or extremities
    b. Shocklike sensation on neck flexion
 	
16. Monitor for signs and symptoms of parotitis.
    a. Painful, swollen parotid glands
	15,16. Radiation therapy to head and neck can cause myelitis or parotitis. These problems usually are transient, not serious, and resolve spontaneously (Hilderley, 2000).

Related Physician-Prescribed Interventions

Depend on cancer site, stage, and extent

Documentation

Flow records
Intake and output
Abnormal laboratory values
Assessments (skin, oral, respiratory, neurologic)
Stool for occult blood
Daily weights

Nursing Diagnoses

Anxiety Related to Prescribed Radiation Therapy and Insufficient Knowledge of Treatment and Self-care Measures

Focus Assessment Criteria	Clinical Significance

1. Understanding radiation principles:
  a. External therapy
  b. Internal therapy
  c. Radiosensitizers
 	
2. Understanding treatment plan:
  a. Consultation
  b. Simulation (planning phase)
  c. Treatment phase
  d. Follow-up phase
 	
3. Understanding expected side effects of treatment:
  a. Description
  b. Duration
  c. Site specific
 	
4. Understanding self-care measures to minimize side effects and promote health
 	
5. Misconceptions and concerns about radiation therapy
	1–5. Many clients and their families poorly understand and fear radiation therapy. Most often, their fears are based on assumptions about early types of radiation therapy that often were crude and caused unfavorable outcomes. In contrast, current technology enables very precise and effective radiation treatment. Through careful assessment and thorough teaching, nurse can help to clear up misconceptions, which reduces fear and anxiety (Hilderley, 2000).

Goal

The client will report less anxiety after teaching.

Indicators

• Verbalize rationale for radiation treatment and treatment plan.
• Identify expected side effects and their management.
• Describe self-care measures to reduce fatigue, promote nutrition, manage skin problems, and prevent infection and bleeding.

Interventions	Rationales
1. Encourage client to share fears and beliefs regarding radiation. Delay teaching if client is experiencing severe anxiety.	1. Sharing enables nurse to identify sources of client anxiety and to correct misinformation. Severe anxiety prevents retention of learning.

(continues on page 1036)

Interventions continued	Rationales continued
2. Review general principles of radiation therapy as necessary. Provide written materials such as a client education booklet from the National Cancer Institute.	2. A client undergoing radiation therapy is likely to have many questions about the treatment and its effects. Reinforcing information provided by physician and radiologist and answering questions can help to reduce client's anxiety related to lack of knowledge (Hilderley, 2000).
3. Reinforce physician's explanation of the treatment plan; cover the following items: a. Area to be irradiated b. Treatment schedule c. Dose to be administered d. Simulation to compute dose and delivery of radiation e. Markings and tattoos f. Shielding of vital organs	3. This information can help to reduce client's anxiety associated with fear of the unknown and the unexpected.
4. Explain the fatigue that accompanies radiation therapy.	4. Several contributing factors can contribute to fatigue: recent surgery, chemotherapy, pain, malnourishment, medications, frequency of treatments, tumor burden, anemia, and respiratory compromise (Hilderley, 2000).
5. Refer to Fatigue in index for additional interventions.	
6. Explain skin reactions and precautions. (Refer to Impaired Skin Integrity in this care plan.)	
7. Explain site-specific radiation side effects. a. Neck: • Mucositis • Dry mouth • Altered taste • Dental problems • Hoarseness • Dysphagia b. Head: • Headache • Alopecia • Nausea and vomiting c. Chest and back: • Pneumonitis • Esophagitis d. Abdomen and pelvis: • Nausea and vomiting • Cystitis • Tenesmus • Diarrhea • Abdominal cramps	7. Understanding what to expect can decrease anxiety related to fear of the unknown and the unexpected and can help client to recognize and report adverse effects.

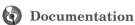 **Documentation**
Progress notes
Anxiety level
Client teaching
Outcome achievement or status

High Risk for Impaired Oral Mucous Membrane Related to Dry Mouth or Inadequate Oral Hygiene

Focus Assessment Criteria	Clinical Significance
1. Understanding possible effects of radiation on oral cavity: a. Mucositis b. Stomatitis c. Dental caries or tooth loss d. Pharyngitis e. Taste alteration f. Xerostomia	1. Radiation therapy to the head and neck increase the acidity of saliva, which can lead to destruction of tooth enamel and increased risk of tooth decay. Radiation therapy also can damage the periodontal membrane resulting in alveolar absorption of radiation and eventual tooth loss. Decreased WBC counts, secondary to radiation therapy, further increase risks of mucositis and stomatitis (Hilderley, 2000).
2. Understanding necessary oral hygiene measures 3. Assess oral cavity before treatment for any of the following: a. Loose teeth b. Dental caries c. Gingivitis d. Infection	2,3. Inadequate oral hygiene or preexisting dental problems increases risk of infection and other complications.

Goal
The client will maintain intact oral mucosa.

Indicators
- Describe the possible effects of radiation on the oral cavity.
- Explain proper techniques for oral care.

Interventions	Rationales
1. Explain signs and symptoms of mucositis and stomatitis.	1. Client's understanding can help to ensure early detection and prompt intervention to minimize problems.
2. Stress the need to have caries filled and bad or loose teeth extracted before initiation of radiation therapy to the head and neck.	2. Preexisting dental problems increase risk of radiation-induced infection.
3. Emphasize the need for regular oral hygiene during and after therapy. Instruct client to do the following:	3. Proper oral hygiene eliminates microorganisms and reduces risk of infection.

(continues on page 1038)

Interventions continued	Rationales continued
a. Brush with fluoridated toothpaste after meals. b. Use a soft-bristle toothbrush. c. Rinse mouth with topical fluoride solution after each brushing. d. Use a molded dental carrier and fluoride gel daily.	
4. If gingival tissue becomes inflamed, suggest an oral rinse.	4. Rinsing removes debris and microorganisms without causing trauma to mucosal tissue.
5. Teach client to avoid the following: a. Commercial mouthwashes b. Very hot foods/drinks c. Alcoholic beverages d. Tobacco e. Highly seasoned foods f. Acidic foods (grapefruit, tomatoes, and oranges)	5. These substances are irritating to oral mucosa and can increase inflammation (Hilderley, 2000).
6. Explain the need for dental examinations during and after course of treatment.	6. Increased risk of dental caries and gum disease persists for months to years after completion of radiation therapy. Long-term follow-up dental care decreases the risk.

 Documentation

Flow records
   Mouth assessment
   Oral care
Teaching record
   Client teaching
   Outcome achievement or status

Impaired Skin Integrity Related to Effects of Radiation on Epithelial and Basal Cells and Effects of Diarrhea on Perineal Area

Focus Assessment Criteria	Clinical Significance
1. Skin in irradiated area(s)	1. Radiation therapy causes skin reactions ranging from mild erythema to weeping desquamation that leaves skin tissue (epidermal and basal layers) raw and irritated. Severity of reaction depends on the dose, depth, and area of irradiation. Moist areas such as axillae tend to develop more severe reactions. Healing usually occurs within a few weeks after treatment completion. Some clients experience long-term fibro-

(continues on page 1039)

Focus Assessment Criteria continued	Clinical Significance continued
	sclerotic changes in the subcutaneous layer; this gives the affected area a taut, shiny appearance (Hilderley, 2000).
2. Nutritional status	2. Malnutrition and anemia commonly are associated with radiation therapy and can cause increased skin fragility. Combined with decreased mobility, this skin change can predispose client to pressure ulcers.
3. Bowel patterns and perineal area	3. Radiation-induced diarrhea does occur with radiation of abdomen and pelvis. It exposes the rectal and perineal areas to irritants that promote skin breakdown (Hilderley, 2000).

Goal

The client will demonstrate healing of tissue.

Indicators

- Relate strategies to reduce skin damage.
- Relate importance of good nutrition.

Interventions	Rationales
1. Explain the effects of radiation on skin (e.g., redness, tanning, peeling, itching, hair loss, decreased perspiration), and monitor skin in the irradiated area(s).	1. Radiation damages epithelial, sebaceous, and hair follicle cells, causing localized skin reactions. Understanding the reason for these effects can promote compliance with protective and preventive measures (Hilderley, 2000).
2. Explain the need for optimal nutritional intake; provide instruction.	2. During radiation treatments, the body must build and repair tissue and protect itself from infection. This process requires increased intake of protein, carbohydrates, vitamins, and minerals (Hilderley, 2000).
3. Teach client the precautions to protect skin integrity: a. Do not wash treated area until therapist allows. b. If tattoos are used for skin markings, wash irradiated skin with a mild soap and tepid water; do not remove markings.	3. These measures can help to maintain skin integrity. a. Moisture enhances skin reactions. b. To reduce irritation, harsh soaps and hot water should be avoided. The tattoo must remain to guide evaluation and subsequent therapy if necessary.

(continues on page 1040)

Interventions continued	Rationales continued
c. Avoid harsh soap, ointments, creams, cosmetics, and deodorants on treated skin unless approved by health care professionals.	c. Harsh substances may increase skin's vulnerability to damage.
d. Avoid exposure of radiated skin to sun, chlorinated pools, wind, and shaving.	d. This exposure can cause additional damage.
e. Wear loose-fitting cotton clothing over treated skin.	e. Loose-fitting cotton clothing can minimize irritation and injury to the epithelial surface.
f. Apply a thin layer of vitamin A and D ointment for dry skin if needed.	f. Vitamin A and D ointment can prevent or treat dry skin.
g. Apply cool air to the affected area; avoid heat lamps and warmth.	g. Coldness reduces irritating sensory stimulation (e.g., pruritus) and prevents moist desquamation.
h. Use an electric razor only—no blades—to shave irradiated area.	h. An electric razor can protect sensitive skin from razor cuts.
i. If moist desquamation is present, shower or irrigate the area frequently; use a moist wound healing dressing.	i. Showering or irrigation and moist wound dressings can help to debride the area and aid healing.
4. Instruct client to report any skin changes promptly.	4. Early detection of moist desquamation with shedding of surface epithelium enables prompt intervention to prevent severe skin damage and subsequent fibrosis.
5. Teach client to keep rectal and perineal areas clean and to apply protective ointment after each cleaning.	5. Good hygiene and application of non-water-soluble ointments reduce erosion of acidic excreta on perineal area.
6. After skin is completely healed, teach client precautions in sun. a. Use no. 15 sun block. b. Increase exposure time very slowly. c. Discontinue sun exposure if redness occurs. d. Protect treated skin with hats, long sleeves.	6. Radiation will temporarily deter the protective capacity of the epidermis, so specific precautions are required (Hilderley, 2000).

 Documentation

Flow records
  Skin assessments
Teaching record
  Client teaching
  Outcome achievement or status

TOTAL PARENTERAL NUTRITION

Total parenteral nutrition (TPN) involves IV administration of an elemental diet (dextrose, amino acids, and lipids) in a hypertonic solution to a client who cannot ingest or assimilate sufficient calories or who has increased metabolic needs that oral ingestion cannot meet. Total nutritional admixture (TNA) system combines IV lipids with the base TPN solution. This admixture is often referred to as three-in-one solution because it contains dextrose, amino acid, and lipids. TPN solutions that contain more than 10% dextrose may be infused only in a central line. Indications for TPN include cancer, chronic nausea and vomiting of any etiology, anorexia nervosa, massive burns, and GI disorders such as inflammatory bowel disease and bowel obstruction.

 Time Frame
Intratherapy

⊗ DIAGNOSTIC CLUSTER

Collaborative Problems

△ PC: Pneumothorax, Hemothorax, or Hydrothorax
△ PC: Air Embolism
▲ PC: Sepsis
▲ PC: Hyperglycemia
▲ PC: Metabolic

Nursing Diagnoses

▲ High Risk for Infection related to catheter's direct access to bloodstream
* High Risk for Disturbed Self-Concept related to inability to ingest food
* High Risk for Activity Intolerance related to deconditioning
△ High Risk for Ineffective Therapeutic Regimen Management related to insufficient knowledge of home care, signs and symptoms of complications, catheter care, and follow-up care (laboratory studies)

▲ This diagnosis was reported to be monitored for or managed frequently (75%–100%).
△ This diagnosis was reported to be monitored for or managed often (50%–74%).
* This diagnosis was not included in the validation study.

Discharge Criteria

Before discharge, the client or family will

1. Demonstrate proper catheter care and TPN administration at home.
2. Discuss strategies for incorporating TPN management into ADLs.
3. Verbalize precautions for medication use.
4. Relate causes, prevention, and treatment of hypoglycemia and hyperglycemia.
5. State signs and symptoms that must be reported to a health care professional.

Collaborative Problems

Potential Complication: Pneumothorax, Hemothorax, or Hydrothorax

Potential Complication: Air Embolism

Potential Complication: Sepsis

Potential Complication: Hyperglycemia

Potential Complication: Metabolic

Nursing Goal

The nurse will detect early signs and symptoms of (a) pneumothorax, hemothorax, and hydrothorax; (b) air embolism; (c) sepsis; (d) hyperglycemia; and (e) metabolic complications and will intervene collaboratively to stabilize the client.

Indicators

- Alert, calm, oriented (a, b, c, d, e)
- Respirations 16–20 breaths/min (a, b, e)
- Respirations relaxed, rhythmic (a, b, e)
- Pulse 60–100 beats/min (a, b, e)
- BP > 90/60, < 140/90 mm Hg (a, b, e)
- Temperature 98.5–99°F (c)
- Flat neck veins (b)
- Skin usual color, dry, warm (a, b, e)
- No c/o of chest pain (a, b)
- Urine output > 30 mL/hr (d, e)
- Specific gravity 1.005–1.030 (d, e)
- Urine negative for glucose (d, e)
- Negative blood cultures (c)
- Intact insertion site (c)
- No drainage at insertion site (c)
- No or minimal weight loss (d)
- Phosphorous 3.0–4.5 mg/dL (e)
- Calcium 8.5–10.5 mg/dL (e)
- Aspartate transaminase (AST) 7–21 u/L (e)
- Alanine transaminase (ALT) 5–35 u/L (e)
- Sodium 135–145 mEq/L (e)
- Magnesium 1.5–2.5 mEq/L (e)
- Potassium 3.5–5.0 mEq/L (e)
- Total cholesterol < 200 mg/dL (e)
- Triglycerides (e)
  - Male 40–160 mg/dL
  - Female 35–135 mg/dL
- Blood glucose < 140 mg/dL (e)
- Prealbumin 3–7 (e)
- Serum ammonia 20–120 µg/dL (e)
- Blood urea nitrogen 5–25 mg/dL (e)
- Creatinine 0.7–1.4 mg/dL (e)
- Oxygen saturation (SaO_2) > 94% (e)
- Carbon dioxide ($PaCO_2$) 35–45 mm/Hg (e)
- Arterial pH 7.35–7.45 (e)
- White blood count 4,800–10,000 cu mm (c)

Interventions	Rationales
1. Monitor for signs and symptoms of pneumothorax, hemothorax, and hydrothorax: a. Acute chest pain b. Dyspnea	1. Pneumothorax, which is the most common complication of subclavian catheter placement, can result from puncture or laceration of the pleura or lung. In most cases the air leak is self-limiting and pneumothorax resolves spontaneously;

(continues on page 1043)

Interventions continued	**Rationales** continued
	some cases require aggressive intervention. The less common complications—hemothorax and hydrothorax—can occur from perforation of a great vessel during catheter insertion. It commonly is diagnosed when the physician cannot obtain a free flow of blood in the syringe.
2. During cannulation of subclavian catheter procedure, maintain client in Trendelenburg's position with head turned to the side.	2. Trendelenburg's position before and during subclavian catheter insertion provides maximum vein distention and minimizes risk of complications.
3. Assist with radiography after cannula placement.	3. A chest x-ray film confirms catheter placement and helps rule out complications.
4. Monitor for signs and symptoms of air embolism during dressing and IV tubing changes and on accidental separation of IV connections. a. Acute, sharp chest pain b. Dyspnea c. Cyanosis d. Tachycardia e. Neck vein distention f. Hypotension	4. Air embolism can occur with IV tubing changes, with accidental tubing separations, and during catheter insertion and disconnection. (For example, client can aspirate as much as 200 mL of air from a deep breath during subclavian line disconnection.) Entry of air into circulatory system can block blood flow and cause cardiac arrest.
5. Secure proximal catheter connection with a Luer-locking IV set and tape all connections.	5. These precautions can help to prevent accidental disconnection.
6. Instruct client to perform Valsalva's maneuver during IV tubing disconnections.	6. Valsalva's maneuver with breath holding minimizes air aspiration and reduces risk of embolism.
7. Explain potential problems with tubing separation and instruct client to crimp tubing near entry site if it occurs.	7. Immediate action can prevent air embolism.
8. Monitor for signs and symptoms of sepsis or catheter-related infection. a. Fever b. Chills c. Altered mental status d. Increased WBC count e. Sudden glucose intolerance f. Local signs of infection at insertion site g. Positive blood cultures	8. The high glucose concentration of the TPN solution and frequent catheter manipulation put client at high risk for infection.

(continues on page 1044)

Interventions continued	**Rationales** continued
9. Monitor for signs and symptoms of hyperglycemia. a. Kussmaul's respirations b. Polyuria c. Low urine specific gravity d. Glycosuria e. Mental status changes (e.g., lethargy or disorientation) f. Elevated serum glucose g. Weight change	9. Osmotic diuresis can result from inability to compensate for rapid instillation of high-glucose solution. The subsequent rise in serum glucose causes fluid shifts to the vascular compartment in an attempt to dilute the hyperosmolar glucose concentration. Increased fluid volume along with the exogenous source is lost rapidly in urine. If unrecognized and untreated, this condition can progress rapidly to nonketotic hyperglycemic coma (Goff, 1997).

10. Monitor for metabolic complications related to CHO content of TPN (Goff, 1997).
a. Hyperglycemia (increased blood sugar glycosuria)
b. Hypoglycemia
c. Hyperglycemic hyperosmolar, nonketotic dehydration (HHNKD)
  • Increased blood glucose
  • Increased urine output
  • Increased serum sodium
  • Changes in mental status
	10.
	a. The high CHO content of TPN makes hyperglycemia the most common metabolic complication.
	b. Abrupt discontinuation of TPN can cause hypoglycemia.
	c. HHNKD is a risk with rapid infusion to those with mild diabetes, renal insufficiency, or congestive heart failure.

11. Monitor blood glucose level every 2 hours during and after discontinuation of TPN. Report changes and early signs and symptoms of HHNKD.	11. Fluctuations in blood glucose level need to be detected early.
12. Monitor for metabolic complications related to protein content of TPN (Goff, 1997). a. Increased BUN b. Increased creatinine c. Increased serum ammonia d. Increased AST e. Increased ALT f. Change in mental status	12. The protein content in TPN can cause amino acid imbalance and azotemia (increased BUN and creatinine). The amount of protein produces increased urea that a compromised kidney (e.g., older adult, pre-existing renal insufficiency) cannot excrete. People with hepatic insufficiency cannot metabolize certain amino acids: this causes increased ammonia levels and hepatic encephalopathy.
13. Monitor for metabolic complications related to lipid content especially triglyceride level.	13. Clients who cannot metabolize more lipids experience hypertriglyceridemia. Rapid infusion can precipitate this condition.
14. Monitor for gallbladder dysfunction commonly shown by dyspepsia.	14. For unknown reasons, some clients develop gallstones or sludge in gallbladder as early as 3 weeks after treatment begins (Goff, 1997).

(continues on page 1045)

Interventions continued	Rationales continued
15. Monitor for metabolic acidosis: a. Hyperkalemia b. Decreased thiamin levels c. Decreased biotin levels d. Decreased pH e. Decreased or normal $PaCO_2$ f. Headache, confusion g. Decreased BP h. Cold, clammy skin i. Increased respiratory rate and depth	15. Metabolic acidosis is produced by loss of bicarbonate or excess of acid in extra-cellular fluid caused by excessive GI or renal losses, inadequate acetate in solution, impaired renal function, and inadequate thiamin and biotin intake (Goff, 1997).

◤ Related Physician-Prescribed Interventions

Intravenous Therapy. Nutritional solution; additives (e.g., insulin)

Laboratory Studies. Serum albumin; prealbumin; thyroxine-binding prealbumin; CBC; electrolytes; liver enzymes; serum transferrin; amino acid profile; glucose, BUN, and PT; 24-hour creatinine excretion; arterial blood gases

Diagnostic Studies. Chest x-ray film

Therapies. Daily weights; anthropometric measurements; catheter site care

Documentation

Flow records
   Vital signs
   Intake and output
   Weight
   Serum glucose
   Urine specific gravity
   Catheter site
Progress notes
   Unusual complaints

Nursing Diagnoses

High Risk for Infection Related to the Catheter's Direct Access to Bloodstream

Focus Assessment Criteria	Clinical Significance
1. Vital signs at least every shift	1. TPN catheter provides a route for micro-organism invasion of the bloodstream.
2. Local signs of infection at catheter insertion site	2. Catheter irritation can lead to infection.
3. Serum WBC count	3. Elevated WBC count indicates active infection.

Goal

The client will continue to be free of infection.

Indicators
- Verbalize understanding of precautions for catheter care.
- Report any need for additional dressing changes.

Interventions	Rationales
1. Use aseptic technique and follow appropriate protocols when changing catheter dressings, IV tubing, and solutions. Change insertion site dressing when wet, soiled, or nonocclusive.	1. Aseptic technique can prevent contamination.
2. Avoid administering other IV solutions piggybacked into the TPN/TNA line unless otherwise ordered.	2. Risk of bacterial contamination increases with additional IV junctions, stopcocks, and ports. To minimize risk, TPN/TNA line should be used exclusively for that purpose unless otherwise ordered.
3. Discontinue lipid emulsions and change infusion tubing immediately after infusion.	3. Lipid emulsions and IV tubes should be discontinued promptly because of microbial contamination.
4. Secure proximal IV connections with a Luer-locking set if possible.	4. This precaution can help to prevent disconnection and subsequent contamination.
5. Securely tape all IV connections.	5. Securing with tape helps to prevent tissue trauma resulting from catheter manipulation.
6. Teach client the following: a. The importance of proper catheter care b. The need to notify nurse when dressing becomes soiled or nonadherent c. How to crimp tubing to stop flow should it become accidentally disconnected	6. Client's understanding of care and precautions can improve compliance and reduce risk of complications.

 Documentation

Flow records
  Dressing and tubing changes
  Condition of IV insertion site

High Risk for Disturbed Self-Concept Related to Inability to Ingest Food

Focus Assessment Criteria	Clinical Significance
1. Feelings and concerns related to inability to ingest food orally.	1. Food and eating have many social and cultural implications besides nutritional intake. Prolonged or permanent NPO status can interfere with socialization and create isolation.

Goal

The client will participate in self-care and grooming activities.

Indicators

- Share feelings related to lack of oral ingestion.
- Verbalize the necessity of continued TPN therapy.

Interventions	Rationales
1. Encourage client to verbalize concerns related to lack of oral ingestion.	1. Sharing helps to identify and clarify client's concerns and problems; this guides nurse in planning effective interventions.
2. Explore possible alternatives to oral ingestion or substitute diversional activities.	2. Substituting activities for meals may help to reduce sense of loss related to lack of oral intake.
3. Provide regular feedback on progress and positive reinforcement on appearance and weight gain.	3. Feedback and reinforcement promote self-esteem and encourage continued compliance.
4. Arrange for visits from others on parenteral nutrition if feasible.	4. Sharing with others in the same situation allows mutual validation and support.
5. If permitted, allow client to taste—but not swallow—desired foods.	5. Placing food in mouth without swallowing may help to satisfy the client's need to taste and smell food.

 Documentation

Progress notes
  Dialogues

High Risk for Activity Intolerance Related to Deconditioning

Focus Assessment Criteria	Clinical Significance
1. Muscle strength, ROM, gait, and balance before and throughout TPN/TNA therapy	1. TPN/TNA therapy without activity leads to inappropriate nutrient use and steady loss of muscle strength and joint ROM.

Goal

The client will maintain current activity level and make progress toward improved conditioning.

Indicators

- Verbalize the need for participation in progressive activity.
- Demonstrate correct performance of isometric and ROM exercises.

Interventions	Rationales
1. Initiate an appropriate activity and exercise regimen that may include the following: a. Active or passive ROM b. Isometric exercises c. Chair-setting d. Trapeze use e. Progressive ambulation	1. Progressive activity or exercise promotes metabolism of TPN/TNA solution into muscle rather than into fat and promotes muscle strengthening.
2. Advance activity according to improved tolerance.	2. Excessive activity beyond limits of tolerance can cause activity intolerance and hypoxia.
3. Emphasize importance of activity during TPN/TNA therapy, and discuss exercises that client can perform without assistance (e.g., walking).	3. Client's understanding can promote compliance with the activity and exercise program.

 Documentation

Progress notes
   Activity level
   Exercises performed

High Risk for Ineffective Therapeutic Regimen Management Related to Insufficient Knowledge of Home Care, Signs and Symptoms of Complications, Catheter Care, and Follow-up Care (Laboratory Studies)

Focus Assessment Criteria	Clinical Significance
1. Understanding of the TPN/TNA procedure and reasons why it is indicated	1. Identifying learning needs guides nurse in planning effective teaching strategies.
2. Available support persons to assist with TPN/TNA therapy at home if applicable	2. Client may need assistance with home TPN/TNA management.
3. Readiness and ability to learn and retain information	3. A client or family failing to achieve learning goals requires a referral for assistance post-discharge.

Goal

The goals for this diagnosis represent those associated with discharge planning. Refer to the discharge criteria.

Interventions	Rationales
1. Reinforce teaching about TPN/TNA and the infusion and catheter insertion procedures.	1. Client's understanding can reduce misconceptions and encourage participation in care.
2. Encourage client and family to ask questions and express concerns about TPN/TNA therapy.	2. Sharing concerns and questions identifies learning needs and misconceptions; this allows nurse to address problem areas.
3. Using understandable terms, explain nutritional constituents of TPN/TNA solution and how solution meets nutritional needs.	3. Understanding TPN/TNA constituents and their purpose can encourage compliance with therapy.
4. Discuss reasons for continued diagnostic tests: daily weights, urinalysis, and laboratory tests.	4. Ongoing monitoring is needed to evaluate therapy and nutritional status.
5. Teach and evaluate learning with return demonstration. a. Aseptic technique b. Preparation and storage of TPN/TNA solution c. Preparation of tubing for infusion d. Use of pump e. Discontinuation of infusion f. Heparinization of the catheter g. Catheter care h. Dressing changes	5. Many clients and families can perform home TPN/TNA without outside assistance. Proper technique is mandatory to prevent infection and air in infusion line.
6. Teach about hyperglycemia. a. Signs and symptoms: nausea, weakness, thirst, headaches, elevated blood glucose level b. Prevention: maintain prescribed rate; avoid increasing rate to "catch up" c. Treatment: consult with physician for possible insulin supplement	6. Because TPN/TNA solution contains high glucose concentrations, sudden changes in rate can increase blood glucose levels.
7. Teach about hypoglycemia. a. Signs and symptoms: sweating, pallor, palpitations, nausea, headache, shaking feeling, hunger, blurred vision b. Prevention: avoid stopping TPN/TNA too abruptly; slow TPN/TNA rate gradually to allow the body to decrease insulin production c. Treatment: glass of orange juice, teaspoon of honey	7. During TPN/TNA infusion, the body produces insulin in response to high glucose concentrations. Too much insulin in TPN/TNA or too-rapid discontinuation of TPN/TNA can produce hypoglycemia.

(continues on page 1050)

Interventions continued	**Rationales** continued
8. Teach client or family to report the following: a. Fever, malaise b. Redness or purulent drainage at catheter insertion site c. Unstable blood glucose level	8. Early detection of complications enables prompt intervention to minimize their seriousness.
9. Teach client to keep records of these things: a. Weight b. Temperature c. Amount and infusion rate of TPN/TNA d. Serum glucose level (if advised to monitor) e. Any problems f. Oral intake	9. Accurate records aid in evaluating the safety and effectiveness of TPN/TNA therapy.
10. Refer to a home health agency for follow-up care.	10. The initial home care visit evaluates suitability for home TPN/TNA by considering client's ability, environment, financial needs, and support system. Subsequent visits are needed to assess client's nutritional status, blood glucose levels, laboratory results, insertion site, and catheter patency.
11. Provide a list of required equipment, supplies, and available sources.	11. Planning can prevent shortages and improper substitutions.

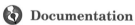 **Documentation**

Discharge summary record
   Client and family teaching
   Outcome achievement or status
   Referrals if indicated

American Association of Legal Nurse Consultants (ALNC) (Greater Detroit Chapter) (2001). Sexual assault: The victim and evidence collection, Journal of legal nurse consultants, 12(3), 20–21.

Adinolfi, A. (2001). Assessment and treatment of HIV-related fatigue. Journal of Association of Nurses in AIDS Care, 12 (Suppl.), 33–39.

Agency for Health Care Policy and Research (AHCPR). (1992). Acute pain management: Operative or medical procedures and trauma (AHCPR Publication No. 92-0022). AHCPR, Public Health Service, U.S. Department of Health and Human Services.

Agency for Health Care Policy and Research (AHCPR). (1992). Pressure ulcers in adults: Prediction and prevention: Clinical practice guideline (No. 3, Publication No. 92-0047). Rockville, MD: AHCPR, Public Health Service, U.S. Department of Health and Human Services.

Agency for Health Care Policy and Research (AHCPR). (1992). Preventing pressure ulcers: A patient's guide (Publication No. 92-0048). Rockville, MD: AHCPR, Public Health Service, U.S. Department of Health and Human Services.

Agency for Health Care Policy and Research (AHCPR). (1994). Evaluation and management of early HIV infection. Clinical Practice Guideline, 7. Washington, DC: AHCPR, Public Health Service, U.S. Department of Health and Human Services.

Agency for Health Care Policy and Research (AHCPR). (1994). Treatment of pressure ulcers (Publication No. 95-0652). Rockville, MD: AHCPR, Public Health Service, U.S. Department of Health and Human Services.

Agency for Health Care Policy and Research (AHCPR) Acute Pain Management Guideline Panel. (1991). Acute pain management: Operative or medical procedures and trauma. Rockville, MD: AHCPR, Public Health Service, U.S. Department of Health and Human Services.

Agency for Health Care Policy and Research (AHCPR) Acute Pain Management Guideline Panel. (1992). Acute pain management in adults: Operative procedures: Quick reference guide for clinicians (Publication No. 92-0019). Rockville, MD: AHCPR, Public Health Service, U.S. Department of Health and Human Services.

Agency for Health Care Policy and Research (AHCPR) Cataract Management Guideline Panel. (1993). Cataract in adults: Management of functional impairment (Clinical Practice Guideline No. 4, AHCPR Publication No. 93-0524). Rockville, MD: AHCPR, Public Health Service, U.S. Department of Health and Human Services.

Agency for Health Care Policy and Research (AHCPR) Panel for Urinary Incontinence in Adults. (1992, March). Urinary incontinence in adults: Clinical guidelines (AHCPR Publication No. 92-0038). Rockville, MD: AHCPR, Public Health Services, U.S. Department of Health and Human Services.

Albano, S., & Wallace, D. (2001). Managing fatigue in patients with SLE. The Journal of Musculoskeletal Medicine, 18(1), 149–152.

Albiar, E. (1992). Hydroxyapatite implants—A new trend in enucleation and orbital reconstructive surgery. Insight, 1, 25–28.

Alexander, T., Hiduke, R., & Stevens, K. (1999). Rehabilitation nursing procedures manual (2nd ed.). Chicago: Rehabilitation Institute of Chicago.

Alfaro, R. (1989). Applying nursing diagnosis and nursing process: A step-by-step guide (2nd ed.). Philadelphia: J.B. Lippincott.

Alfaro-LeFevre, R. (1998). Applying nursing process/A step by step guide (4th ed.). Philadelphia: Lippincott-Raven.

Alfaro-Lefevre, R. (2002). Applying nursing process: A step-by-step guide (5th ed.). Philadelphia: Lippincott Williams & Wilkins.

Allen, J., & Oberle, K. (1993). Follow-up of day-surgery cataract patients. Journal of Ophthalmic Nursing and Technology, 5, 211–216.

Allman, R. M., Walker, J. M., Hart, M. K., Laprade, C. A., Noel, L. B., & Smith, C. R. (1987). Air fluidized beds or conventional therapy for pressure ulcers. Annals of Internal Medicine, 107, 641–648.

Allman, R. M., et al. (1995). Pressure ulcer risk factors among hospitalized patients with activity limitation. Journal of the American Medical Association, 273(1995), 865–870.

Alpers, D., Greenberg, J., & Sodeman, W. (1990). Gastroenteritis treatment tips. Patient Care, 24(6), 18–31.

Alt, H. L. (1992). Psychiatric aspects of asthma. Chest, 101(6), 4045–4066.

Altizer, L. L. (1998). Degenerative disorder. In A. B. Maher, S. W. Salmond, & T. A. Pellino. Orthopedic nursing (2nd ed.). Philadelphia: W.B. Saunders.

American College of Cardiology and American Heart Association. (1999). Guidelines for the management of patients with acute myocardial infarction, 28(5), 1328–1428.

American College of Chest Physicians/Society of Critical Care Medicine (ACCP-SCCM) Consensus Conference Committee. (1992). American College of Chest Physicians/Society of Critical Care Medicine Consensus Conference: Definitions for sepsis and organ failure and guidelines for the use of innovative therapies in sepsis. Critical Care Medicines, 20, 6.

American Diabetes Association. (1994). Consensus statement self-monitoring of blood glucose. Diabetes Care, 17(1), 81–86.

American Diabetes Association. (1994). Diabetes translation: A blueprint for the future. Diabetes Care, 17, (Suppl. 1), 1–66.

American Diabetes Association. (1994). Medical management of type II diabetes (4th ed.). Alexandria, VA: American Diabetes Association.

American Diabetes Association. (1995). Intensive diabetes management. Alexandria, VA: American Diabetes Association.

American Diabetes Association. (1996). The health professional's guide to diabetes and exercise. Alexandria, VA: American Diabetes Association.

American Diabetes Association. (1997). Clinical practice recommendations. Diabetes Care, 20, (Suppl. 1), 1–70.

American Diabetes Association. (1997). Diabetes medical nutrition therapy: A professional guide to management and nutrition education resources. Alexandria, VA: American Diabetes Association.

American Diabetes Association. (1997). Direct & indirect costs of diabetes in the US. Alexandria, VA: American Diabetes Association.

American Heart Association. (1989). 1989 stroke facts. Dallas: American Heart Association.

American Heart Association. (1993). Heart and stroke fact statistics. Dallas: American Heart Association.

American Journal of Kidney Diseases Clinical Practice Guidelines. (1997). PD Adequacy, 30(3), Supp. (2). Philadelphia: W.B. Saunders.

American Nurses Association. (1991). Standards of clinical practice. Washington, DC: American Nurses Association.

American Nurses Association. (1992). Case management by nurses. Washington, DC: American Nurses Association.

Anders, R., & Ornellas, E. M. (1997). Acute management of patients with hip fracture: A research literature review. Orthopedic Nursing, 16(2), 31–47.

Anders, R., & Ornellas, E. (1997). Acute management of patients with hip fractures: A research literature review. Orthopedic Nursing, 16(2), 31–46.

Anderson, E. D. (1986). The cirrhotic process in the alcoholic. Critical Care Quarterly, 8(4), 74–78.

Anderson, S. (1992). Guillain-Barré syndrome: Giving the client control. Journal of Neuroscience Nursing, 24(3), 158–162.

Annon, J. S. (1976). The PLISS T model: A proposed conceptual scheme for the behavioral treatment of sexual problems. Journal of Sexual Education and Therapy, 2, 211–215.

Arcangelo, V., & Peterson, A. (2001). Pharmacotherapeutics for advanced practice. Philadelphia: Lippincott Williams & Wilkins.

Armstrong, S., & Zalatan, S. J. (1992). Microwave warming of peritoneal dialysis fluid. ANNA (American Nephrology Nurses' Association) Journal, 19(6), 535–540.

August, D. A. (2000). Clinical guidelines: An evidence-based tool to lead nutrition practice into the new millennium. Nutrition in Clinical Practice, 15(2), 211–212.

Auth, P. C. (1997). Assessment and treatment of arterial ulcers. Physician Assistant, 21(3), 64, 67–70, 79.

Babel, K. (1997). Substance Abuse: Treating acute alcohol withdrawal. The American Journal of Nursing, 97(1), 22–23.

Bades, B. (1995). Indices to include in wound healing assessment. Advances in Wound Care, 8, 25–33.

Badger, T., Braden, & Michel, M. (2001). Depression burden, Self-help. Interventions and side effects experience in women receiving treatment for breast cancer. Oncology Nursing Forum, 28(3), 567–574.

Baer, C., & Lancaster, L. (1992). Acute renal failure. Critical Care Nursing Quarterly, 14(4), 1–21.

Bagley, S. M. C. (1996). Nutritional needs of the acutely ill with acute wounds. Critical Care Nursing Clinics of North America, 8(2), 159–167.

Ballas, S., & Delengowski, A. (1993). Pain measurement in hospitalized adults with sickle cell painful episodes. Annals of Clinical and Laboratory Science, 23(5), 358–361.

Bandura, A. (1982). Self-efficacy mechanisms in human agency. American Psychology, 37(3), 122–147.

Bangsberg, D. R., Hecht, F. M., Charlebois, E. D. Zolopa, A. R., Holodniy, M., Sheiner, L., Bamberger, J. D., Chesney, M. A., & Moss, A. (2000). Adherence to protease inhibitors, HIV-1 viral load, and development of drug resistance in an indigent population. AIDS, 14, 357–366.

Banks, P. A. (1997). Practice guidelines in acute pancreatitis. American Journal of Gastroenterology, 92, 377–386.

Barn, R., Fey, J., Raboy, S., Laler, H., Borgen, Temple, K., & Vanzer, J. (2002). Eighteen sensations after breast cancer surgery: A comparison of sentinel lymph node biopsy and axillary lymph node dissection. Oncology Nursing Forum, 29(4), 651–659.

Barsevick, A. M., Much, J., & Sweeney, C. (2000). Psychosocial responses of cancer. In S. L. Groenwald, M. H. Frogge, M. Goodman, & C. Yarbro. Cancer nursing: Principles and practice (5th ed.). Boston: Jones and Bartlett.

Bartlett, J. G., & Finkbeiner, A. K. (2002). The guide to living with HIV infection (6th ed.). Baltimore: The Johns Hopkins University Press.

Bauldoff, G., Hoffman, L. Sciurba, F., & Zullo, T. (1996). Home based upper arm exercises training for patients with chronic obstructive pulmonary disease. Heart and Lung, 25(4), 288–294.

Baxendale, L. (1992). Pathophysiology of coronary artery disease. Nursing Clinics of North America, 27(1), 143–151.

Belec, R. H. (1992). Quality of life: Perceptions of long-term survivorships of bone marrow transplantation. Oncology Nursing Forum, 19(1), 31–37.

Ben-Zacharia, A. (2001). Palliative care in patients with multiple sclerosis. Neurologic Clinics, 19(4), 801–827.

Bernstein, A. D. et al. (1997). The NASPE/BPEC generic pacemaker code. PACE, 10(4), 794–99.

Bertino, L. (1989). Stress management with SCI clients. Rehabilitation Nursing, 14(3), 127–129.

Best Practice. (2001). Smoking cessation interventions and strategies. Glensdale, CA: CINHAL Information Services.

Bildstein, C. Y. & Blendowski, C. (1997). Head & neck malignancies. In S. L. Groenwald, M. H. Frogge, M. Goodman, & C. H. Yarbro (Eds.). Cancer nursing: Principles and practice (4th ed.). Boston: Jones and Bartlett.

Billas, A. (1990). Lower respiratory tract infections. Primary Care, 17(4), 811–824.

Bilodeau, B. A., & Degner L. F. (1996). Information needs, sources of information and decisional roles in women with breast cancer. Oncology Nursing Forum, 23(4), 691–696.

Blackburn, G., Miller, D., & Chun, S. (1997). Pharmaceutical treatment of obesity. Nursing Clinics of North America, 32(4), 831–848.

Blackburn, K., & Neaton, M. E. (1997). Redesigning the care of carotid endarterectomy patients. Journal of Vascular Nursing, 15(1), 8–12.

Blackman, P. G. (2000). A review of chronic compartment syndrome in the lower leg. Medicine & Science in Sports & Exercise, 32–35, 4–10.

Blackwell, J. (2002). Identification, evaluation and treatment of overweight and obese adults. Journal of the American Academy of Nurse Practitioners, 14(5), 196–198.

Blair, S. (2001). Epilepsy: Working through loss and grief. Epilepsy USA Staff. *Epilepsy Foundation.org*.

Blevins, D., & Lubkin, J. (1995). Compliance impact. In: J. Lubkin (Ed.), Chronic illness: Impact and interventions (3rd ed.). Boston: Jones and Bartlett.

Blom, E. D. (2000). Current status of voice restoration following total laryngectomy. Oncology 14(6), 915–929.

Booth, R. (1997). Hepatitis C. Professional Nurse, 12(4), 287–390.

Botes, H., Mistiaeu, P., Duyhouner, E., & Groenewegen, I. (1998). The problem of elderly patients at home after ophthalmic treatment. Journal of Ophthalmic Nursing and Technology, 17(2), 59–65.

Botoman, V. A., Bonner, G., & Botoman, D. (1998). Management of inflammatory bowel disease. American Family Physician, 57(1), 57–68.

Bower, C. (1993). Patient outcomes and nursing diagnosis: Expanding the value of critical paths (workshop). Pasadena, CA, September 1993.

Braden, C. J. (1990). A test of the self-help model: Learned response to chronic illness experience. Nursing Research, 39(1), 42–47.

Braverman, K., Dworkin, H., & MacIndoe, J. (1997). Thyroid disease: When to screen, when to treat. Thyroid Disease, 31(6), 19–43.

Breslin, E. (1992). Dyspnea-limited response in chronic obstructive pulmonary disease: Reduced unsupported arm activities. Rehabilitation Nursing, 17(1), 13–20.

Bridges, E. J. (1992). Transition form ventilatory support: Knowing when the patient is ready to wean. Critical Care Nursing Quarterly, 15(1), 14–20.

Briones, T. L. (1992). Pressure support ventilation: New ventilatory techniques. Critical Care Nurse, 12(4), 51–56.

Broadhead, W. E., Kaplan, B. H., & James, S. A. (1983). The epidemiologic evidence for a relationship between social support and health. American Journal of Epidemiology, 117, 521–537.

Brockapp, J., & Taban, H. (1993). The nurse case manager in acute care settings. Journal of Nursing Administration, 23(10), 53–61.

Brown, A. (1991). Acute pancreatitis: Pathology, nursing diagnoses and collaborative problems. Focus on Critical Care, 18(2), 121–130.

Brown, M. A., & Powell-Cope, G. (1991). AIDS family caregiving transitions through uncertainty. Nursing Research, 40(6), 338–345.

Brown, R. (1993). Community-acquired pneumonia: Diagnosis and therapy of older adults. Geriatrics, 48(2), 43–44, 46–50.

Brundage, D. (1992). Renal disorders. St. Louis: Mosby-Year Book.

Brunner, D., Iwamoto, R., Keane, K. & Strohl, R. (Eds.). (1992). Manual for radiation oncology nursing practice and education. Pittsburgh, PA: Oncology Nursing Society.

Bryant, G. G. (1998). Modalities for immobilization. In A. B. Maher, S. W. Salmond, & T. A. Pellino. Orthopedic nursing (2nd Ed.). Philadelphia: W. B. Saunders.

Buchanan, J. D. (2001). A 72-year old man with chest pain and hypotension. Physician Assistant, 25(4), 20–30.

Bulechek, G., & McCloskey, J. (1989). Nursing interventions: Treatments for potential nursing diagnoses. In M. Carroll-Johnson (Ed.), Classification of nursing diagnosis: Proceedings of the eighth national conference. Philadelphia: J. B. Lippincott.

Bullock, B., & Henze, R. (2000). Focus on pathophysiology. Philadelphia: Lippincott Williams & Wilkins.

Burckhardt, C. S. (1987). Coping strategies of the chronically ill. Nursing Clinics of North America, 22(3), 543–549.

Burckhardt, P. (1992). Treatment of osteoporosis. Current Opinion in Rheumatology, 4, 402–409.

Burgess, W., & Raglands, E. (1983). Community health nursing: Philosophy, process, practice. Norwalk, CT: Appleton-Century-Crofts.

Burkart, J. M., & Nolph, K. D. (1996). Peritoneal dialysis. In Brenner and Rector's the kidney (5th ed., Vol. II). Philadelphia: W. B. Saunders.

Burke, J. (1989). Maintaining adequate nutrition in the head and neck patient undergoing radiation therapy. Journal of the Society of Otorhinolaryngology Head-Neck Nurses, 7(1), 8–12.

Burke, L., & Murphy, J. (1995). Charting by exception (2nd ed.) New York: John Wiley & Sons.

Burrage, R. L. (1999). Arthritis. In J. T. Stone, J. F. Wyman, & S. A. Salisbury (Eds.), Clinical gerontological nursing. A guide to advanced practice (pp. 469–487). Philadelphia: W.B. Saunders Company.

Burrows-Hudson, S. (1999). ANNA Standards and guidelines of clinical practice for nephrology nursing. Pitman, NJ: Jennett.

Burton, G., Hodgkin, J., Ward, J., Hess, J., Pilbeam, C., & Tietsort, L. (1997). Respiratory care: A guide to clinical practice (4th ed.). Philadelphia: Lippincott Williams & Wilkins.

Butler, D., Turkal, N., & Seidl, J. (1992). Amputation: Preoperative psychological preparation. Journal of American Board of Family Practice, 5(1), 69–73.

Butler, L., Downe-Wambolt, B., Marsh, S., Bell, D., & Jarvi, K. (2000). Behind the scenes: Partners' perceptions of quality of life post radical prostatectomy. Urologic Nursing, 20(4), 254–258.

Bushkin, E. (1993). Signposts of survivorship. Oncology Nursing Forum, 20(6), 869–875.

Byrne, B. (2002). Deep vein thrombosis prophylaxis. Journal of Vascular Nursing, 20(2), 53–59.

Calkins, M. E. (1996). Pathophysiology of congestive heart failure in ESRD. Anna Journal, 23(5), 457–463.

Campbell, S. M., & Cope, F. (1990). Dietary modification in HIV disease. Ross Laboratories. Camp-Sorrell, D. (2000). Chemotherapy: Toxicity management. In S. L. Groenwald, M. H., Frogge, M. Goodman, & C. H. Yarbro. Comprehensive cancer nursing review (5th ed.). Boston: Jones and Bartlett.

Caregaro, L., Alberino, F., Amodio, P., Merkel, C., Bolognesi, M., Angeli, C., & Gattu, A. (1996). Malfunction in alcoholic and virus related cirrhosis. American Journal of Clinical Nutrition, 63(4), 602–609.

Carhson, E. (1998). Irritable bowel syndrome. Nurse Practitioner, 23(1), 82–84, 86–91.

Carpenito, L. J. (1983). Nursing diagnosis: Application to clinical practice. Philadelphia: J. B. Lippincott.

Carpenito, L. J. (1987). Nursing diagnosis: Application to clinical practice (2nd ed.). Philadelphia: J. B. Lippincott.

Carpenito, L. J. (1987). Nursing interventions as indicators for differentiating diagnoses. MINDA News, 3(2), 2–3.

Carpenito, L. J. (1992). Nursing diagnosis: Application to clinical practice (4th ed.). Philadelphia: J. B. Lippincott.

Carpenito, L. J. (1995). Nursing care plans and documentation (2nd ed.). Philadelphia: Lippincott.

Carpenito, L. J. (1997). Nursing diagnosis: Application to clinical practice (7th ed.). Philadelphia: J. B. Lippincott.

Carpenito, L. J. (1999). Nursing diagnosis: Application to clinical practice (8th ed.). Philadelphia: J. B. Lippincott.

Carpenito, L. J., & Duespohl, T. A. (1985). A guide to effective clinical instruction (2nd ed.). Rockville, MD: Aspen Systems Corp.

Carpenito-Moyet, L. J. (2002). Nursing diagnosis: Application to clinical practice (9th Ed.). Philadelphia: Lippincott Williams & Wilkins.

Carpenito-Moyet, L. J. (2004). Nursing diagnosis: Application to clinical practice (10th ed.). Philadelphia: Lippincott Williams & Wilkins.

Carroll, P. (1993). Deep venous thrombosis: Implications for orthopedic nursing. Orthopedic Nursing, 12(3), 33–41.

Carosella, C. (1995). Who's afraid of the dark? New York: Harper Collins.

Carrougher, G. J. (1998). Burn care and therapy. St. Louis: Mosby.

Carscadden, J. S. (1993). On the cutting edge: A guide for working with people who self injure. London, Ontario: Self-published.

Carson, V., & Green, H. (1992). Spiritual well being: A predictor of hardiness in patients with acquired immunodeficiency syndrome. Journal of Professional Nursing, 8(4), 209–220.

Casey, K. (1997). Malnutrition associated with HIV/AIDS. Part two: Assessment and interventions. Journal of the Association of Nurses in AIDS Care, 8(5), 39–48.

Caswell, D. (1993). Thromboembolic phenomena. Critical Care Nursing Clinics of North America, 5(3), 489–497.

Centers for Disease Control (2000). Guidelines for prevention of transmission of HIV and hepatitis B virus to health care and public safety workers. MMWR 49, 7–11.

Chapman, D., & Goodman, M. (2000). Breast cancer. In S. L. Groenwald, M. H. Frogge, M. Goodman, & C. Yarbro (Eds.), Cancer nursing: Principles and practice (5th ed.). Boston: Jones & Bartlett.

Cheskin, L., & Lacy, B. (2003). Selected gastrointestinal problems: Bleeding, diarrhea, abdominal pain. In L. R. Barker, J. Burton, & P. D. Aieve (Eds.), Principles of ambulatory medicine (6th ed.). Philadelphia: Lippincott Williams & Wilkins.

Chorzempa, A. & Tabloski, P. (2001). Post myocardial infarction treatment in the older adult. Nurse Practitioner 26 (3) 39–40.

Christman, N., & Kirchhoff, K. (1992). Preparatory sensory information. In G. Bulecheck & J. McCloskey (Eds.), Nursing interventions. Philadelphia: W. B. Saunders.

Chulay, M. (1992). Airway and ventilatory management. In B. M. Dossey, C. E. Guzzetta, & C. V. Kenner (Eds.). Critical care nursing: Body-mind-spirit (3rd ed.). Philadelphia: J. B. Lippincott.

Chung, C., Cackovic, M., & Kerstein, M. D. (1996). Leg ulcers in patients with sickle-cell disease: Advances in wound care. Journal for prevention and healing, 9(5)(1), 46–50.

Cimprich, B. (1992). Attentional fatigue following breast cancer surgery. Research in Nursing and Health, 15, 199–207.

Clanet, M. (2000). The management of multiple sclerosis patients. Current Opinion in Neurology, 13(3), 263–270.

Clement-Stone, S., Eigigasti, D. G., & McGuire, S. L. (2001). Comprehensive family and community health nursing (6th ed.). St. Louis: Mosby-Year Book.

Clinical Evidence. June 2002. Secondary prevention of ischemic cardiac events. Issue 7, pp. 19, 20.

Clochesy, J. M., Breu, C., Cardin, S., Rudy, E. B., & Whittaker, A. A. (1993). Critical care nursing. Philadelphia: W. B. Saunders.

Coe, M., et al. (1988). Concerns of clients and spouses regarding ostomy surgery. Journal of Enterostomal Therapy, 15(6), 232–239.

Cohen, E. (1996). Nurse case management in the 21st century. St. Louis: Mosby-Year Book.

Cohen, E. & Merritt, (1992). Sleep promotion. In G. Bulechek & J. McCloskey (Eds.), Nursing interventions (2nd ed.). Philadelphia: W. B. Saunders.

Cohen, F., & Lazarus, R. S. (1983). Coping and adaptation in health and illness. In D. Mechanic (Ed.), Handbook of health, health care, and health professions. New York: Free Press.

Cohen, F., & Merritt, S. (1992). Sleep promotion. In G. Bulechek, & J. McCloskey (Eds.), Nursing interventions: Essential nursing treatments (3rd ed.). Philadelphia: W. B. Saunders.

Compton, P. (1989). Drug abuse: A self care deficit. Journal of Psychosocial Nursing & Mental Health Services, 27(3), 22–26.

Consortium for Spinal Cord Medicine. (1997, Feb.) Clinical practice guidelines. Treatment of autonomic depreflexia.

Consortium for Spinal Cord Medicine. (2000). Clinical practice guidelines. Pressure ulcer & prevention & treatment following SCI, 1–77.

Core curriculum for orthopaedic nursing (4th Ed). (NAUN) 2001.

Core Curriculum for Orthopaedic Nursing (NAON) (4th Ed.) 2001.

Crewe, R. A. (1987). Problems of rubber ring nursing cushions and a clinical survey of alternative cushions for ill patients. Care Science Practice, 5(2), 9–11.

Cronin, C. & Maklebust, J. (1989). Case-managed care: Capitalizing on the CNS. Nursing Management, 20(3), 39–39, 42–47.

Crosby, L. J. (1988). Stress factors, emotional stress and rheumatoid arthritis disease activity. Journal of Advanced Nursing, 13(4), 452–461.

Cummings, C. (Ed.). (1993). Otolaryngology—Head and neck surgery (2nd ed., Vols. 2 & 3). St. Louis: Mosby-Year Book.

Cunningham, S. (1992). The epidemiologic basis of coronary disease prevention. Nursing Clinics of North America, 27(1), 153–170.

Cushing, M. (1988). Nursing jurisprudence. Norwalk, CT: Appleton & Lange.

Cutler, M. (1997). Administration of Epoetin alfa. ANNA Journal, 24(4), 459–465.

Dadd, M. (1983). Self care for side effects. In Cancer chemotherapy: An assessment of nursing interventions. Part II. Cancer Nursing, 6, 63–66.

Dahl, J., & Penque, S. (2000). The effects of an advanced practice nurse-directed heart failure program. The Nurse Practitioner, 25(3) 61–77.

Dahlen, R., & Roberts, S. (1996). Congestive heart failure: Preventing complications. DCCN, 15(5), 226–242.

Damianos, A., & McGarrity, T. (1997). Treatment strategies for Helicobacter pylori infection. American Family Physician, 55(8), 2765–2774.

Davis, R. (1993). Phantom sensation, phantom pain, and stump pain. Archives of Physical Medicine and Rehabilitation, 74(1), 79–91.

Davidson, J. K. (1998). Clinical diabetes mellitus: A problem-oriented approach (3rd ed.). New York: Thieme.

DeBaun, B. (1998). Prevention of infection in the orthopedic surgery patient. Nursing Clinics of North America, 33(4), 671–684.

Decker, S., Schultz, R., & Wood, D. (1989). Determinants of well-being in primary caregivers of spinal cord injured persons. Rehabilitation Nursing, 14(1), 6–8.

DeGrott, L. J., et al. (Eds.) (1995). Endocrinology (3rd ed.). Philadelphia: W. B. Saunders.

Derstine, J., & Hargreve, S. D. (2001). Comprehensive rehabilitation nursing. Philadelphia: W. B. Saunders.

DeVita, V. T., Hellman, S., & Rosenberg, S. A. (2001). Cancer: Principles and practice or oncology (6th ed.). Philadelphia: Lippincott Williams & Wilkins.

DeVito, A. (1990). Dyspnea during hospitalization for acute phase of illness as recalled by patients with chronic obstructive pulmonary disease. Heart & Lung, 19(2), 186–191.

DeVivo, M., Black, K., & Stover, S. (1993). Causes of death during the first 12 years after spinal cord injury. Archives of Physical Medicine and Rehabilitation, 74, 248–254.

Dewey, R., Delley, R., & Shulman, L. (2002). A better life for patients with Parkinson's disease. Patient Care, 36(7).

Diabetes Control and Complication Trial Research Group. (1993). The effect of intensive treatment of diabetes on the development and progression of long-term complications in insulin-dependent diabetes mellitus. New England Journal of Medicine, 329(14), 977–986.

Dickson, A. C., Dodd, M. J., Carrier, V., et al. (1985). Comparison of a cancer-specific locus of control and the multidimensional health locus of control scales in chemotherapy. Oncology Nursing Forum, 12(3), 49–54.

DiSaisa, P. J. & Walker, J. L. (1994). Perioperative care. In J. R. Scott, P. J. DiSaisa, C. B. Hammond, & W. N. Spellacy (Eds.). Danforth's obstetrics and gynecology (7th ed.). Philadelphia: J. B. Lippincott.

Dolin, R. Masur, H., and Saag, M. (2003). AIDS Therapy (2nd ed). Philadelphia: Churchill Livingston.

Doughty, D. B. (1992). Principles of wound healing and wound management. In R. B. Bryant (Ed.), Acute and chronic wounds: Nursing management. St. Louis: Mosby-Year Book.

Dracup, K. (1996). Heart failure secondary to left ventricular systolic dysfunction: Therapeutic advances and treatment recommendation. American Journal of Primary Healthcare, 21(9), 56, 58, 61.

Dudas, S. (1993). Altered body image and sexuality. In S. L. Groenwald, M. H. Frogge, M. Goodman, & C. Yarbro (Eds.). Cancer nursing: Principles and practice (3rd ed.). Boston: Jones and Bartlett.

Dudek, S. (2001). Nutritional handbook for nursing practice (4th ed.). Philadelphia: Lippincott Williams & Wilkins.

Dunkin, M. A. (2000). Juvenile rheumatoid arthritis. Arthritis Today, 14(1), 32–33.

Dyck, S. (1991). Surgical instrumentation as a palliative treatment for spinal cord compression. Oncology Nursing Forum, 18(3), 515–521.

Early, L. M., & Poquette, R. (2000). Bladder and kidney cancer. In S. L. Groenwald, M. H. Frogge, M. Goodman, & C. H. Yarbro (Eds.), Cancer nursing: Principles and practice (5th ed.). Boston: Jones and Bartlett.

Edelber, H. (2002). Assessing mobility and preventing falls in older patients. Patient Care, Jan. 30, 2002; 18–29.

Edelman, C., & Mandle, C. (1998). Health promotion throughout the lifespan. St. Louis: Mosby.

Edwards, R., Abullarade, C., & Turnbull, N. (1996). Nursing management and following of the postoperative vascular patient in a clinic setting. Journal of Vascular Nursing, 14(3), 62–67.

Eftychiou, V. (1996). Clinical diagnoses and management of the patient with deep venous thromboembolism and acute pulmonary embolism. Nurse Practitioner, 21(3), 50, 50–69, 52, 58, 61, 62, 64, 67.

Eisenberg, P. (1990). Monitoring gastric pH to prevent stress ulcer syndrome. Focus on Critical Care, 17(4), 316–322.

Eisenhaurer, L., Nichols, L., Spencer, R., & Bergan, F. (1997). Clinical pharmacology and nursing management (5th ed.). Philadelphia: J. B. Lippincott.

Elkin, M. K., Perry, A. G., & Potter, P. A. (2000). Nursing interventions and clinical skills (2nd Ed.). St. Louis: Mosby.

Ellerhorst-Ryan, J. M. (2000). Infection. In S. Groenwald, M. Frogge, M. Goodman, & C. Yarbro (Eds.). Cancer nursing: Principles and practice. (5th ed.). Boston: Jones and Bartlett.

Elliott, T. & Frank, R. G. (1996). Depression following spinal cord injury. Archives of Physical Medicine and Rehabilitation, 77(8), 816–823.

Ellis, C., & Saddler, D. A. (2000). Colorectal cancer. In T. Yamada, D. H. Alpers, C. Owyang, D. W. Powell, & F. E. Silverstein (Eds.), Textbook of gastroenterology (3rd Ed). Philadelphia: Lippincott Williams & Wilkins.

Ellis, C. T., & Saddler, A. (2000). Colorectal cancer. In C. Yarbro, M. H. Frogge, M. Goodman, & S. Groenwald (Eds.), Cancer nursing (5th ed.). Boston: Jones and Bartlett.

Emma, L. (1992) Chronic arterial occlusive disease. Journal of Cardiovascular Nursing, 7(1), 14–24.

Eslinger, P. (2002). Empathy and social-emotional factors in recovery from stroke. Current Opinion in Neurology, 15(1), 91–97.

Estey, A., Jeremy, P., & Jones, M. (1990). Developing printed materials for patients with visual deficiencies. Journal of Ophthalmic Nursing and Technology, 6, 247–249.

Ewing, G. (1989). The nursing preparation of stoma patients for self-care. Journal of Advanced Nursing, 14, 411–420.

Ewing, J. A. (1984). Detecting alcoholism: The CAGE questionnaire. Journal of American Medical Association, 252, 1905–1907.

Feather, B. L., & Wainstock, J. M. (1989). Perceptions of postmastectomy patients: I. The relationships between social support and network providers. Cancer Nursing, 12(5), 293–300, 301–309.

Feldhaus, K. (2002). A 21st century challenge: Improving the care of the sexual assault victim, 39(6), 653–655.

Felton, G. (1992). Preoperative teaching. In G. Bulechek & J. McClosky. Nursing interventions: Treatments for nursing diagnoses (2nd ed.). Philadelphia: W. B. Saunders.

Ferrans C., & Powers, M. (1993). Quality of life of hemodialysis patients. ANNA, 20(5), 575–581.

Ferrante, F. M., Ostheimor, G. W., & Covino, B. G. (1990). Patient controlled analgesia. Chicago: Blackwell.

Ferrell, B. R., Rhiner, M., Cohen, M. Z., & Grant, M. (1991). Pain as a metaphor for illness. Part 1: Impact of cancer pain on family caregivers. Oncology Nursing Forum, 18(8), 1303–1309.

Ferrell, J., & Boyle, J. (1992). Bereavement experiences: Caring for a partner with AIDS. Journal of Community Health Nursing, 9(3), 127–135.

Feste, C. (1987). The physician within: The wellness series. Minnetonka, MN: Diabetes Centers.

Fife, B. L. (1985). A model for predicting the adaptation of families to medical crisis: An analysis of role integration. Image: The Journal of Nursing Scholarship, 18(4), 108–112.

Fishbach, F. T. (1991). Documenting care communication: The nursing process and documentation standards. Philadelphia: F. A. Davis.

Flaherty, A. M. (2000). Oncologic emergencies. In C. Yarbro, M. Frogge, M. Goodman, S. Groewald. Cancer Nursing: Principles and Practice (5th ed). Boston: Jones & Bartlett.

Flaherty, M., & O'Brien, M. (1992). Family styles of coping in end stage renal disease. ANNA, 19(4), 345–349.

Flanagan, L. (1974). One strong voice. Kansas City, MO: American Nurses Association.

Flaskerud, J., & Ungrarski, P. (1999). HIV/AIDS: A guide to nursing care (3rd ed.). Philadelphia: W. B. Saunders.

Fleming, D. R. (1994). Accuracy of blood glucose monitoring for patients: What it is and how to achieve it. The Diabetes Educator, 20(6), 495–500.

Fleming, D. R., Jacober, S. J., Vandenberg, M. A., Fitzgerald, J. T., & Grunberger, G. (1997). The safety of injecting insulin through clothing. Diabetes Care, 20(3), 244–247.

Folcarelli, P. H. & Carleton, P. F. (1997). Vascular disease. In S. A. Price & L. M. Wilson (Eds.). Pathophysiology: Clinical concepts of disease processes (5th ed.). St. Louis: Mosby-Year Book.

Foltz, A. (2000). Nutritional disturbances. In S. Groenwald, M. Frogge, M. Goodman & C. Yarbro (Eds.). Cancer nursing: Principles and practice (5th ed.). Boston: Jones and Bartlett.

Franklyn, J., & Sheppard, M. (1990). Thyroxine replacement treatment and osteoporosis. British Medical Journal, 300, 693–694.

Freund, K. (1995). Osteoporosis. In P. L. Carr, K. Freund, & S. Somani. The medical care of women. Philadelphia: W. B. Saunders.

Friedman-Campbell, M., & Hart, C. (1984). Theoretical strategies and nursing interventions to promote psychological adaptation to spinal cord injuries and disability. Journal of Neurosurgical Nursing, 16(6), 335–342.

Fryback, P. B., & Reinert, B. R. (1997). Alternative therapies and control for health in cancer and AIDS. Clinical Nurse Specialist 11(2), 64–9.

Fujita, T. (1992). Vitamin D in the treatment of osteoporosis. Society for Experimental Biology and Medicine, 199, 394–399.

Gainotti, G. (2001). Relationship between depression after stroke, antidepressant therapy, and functional recovery. Journal of Neurology, Neurosurgery, and Psychiatry, 71(2), 258–261.

Galica, L. A. (1997). Parenteral nutrition. Nursing Clinics of North America, 32(4), 705–717.

Galis, A. (1996). Sexual issues for the person with an ostomy. Journal of Wound, Ostomy, and Continence Nursing, 23(1), 33–37.

Gammon, J., & Mulholland, C. (1996). Effect of preparatory information prior to elective total hip replacement in psychological coping outcomes. Journal of Advanced Nursing, 24(2), 303–308.

Gawlinski, A. (1989). Nursing care after AMI: A comprehensive review. Critical Care Nurse Quarterly, 12(2), 64–70.

Gift, A., Moore, T., & Soeken, K. (1992). Relaxation to reduce dyspnea and anxiety in COPD patients. Nursing Research, 41(4), 342–346.

Gil, K., Carson, J., Sedway, J., Porter, L., Schaeffer, J., & Orringer, E. (2000). Follow-up of coping skills training in adults with sickle cell disease. Health Psychology, 19(1), 85–90.

Gillenwater, J. Y., Grayhack, J. T., Howards, S. S., & Duckett, J. W. (1996). Adult and pediatric urology (3rd ed.). St. Louis: Mosby-Year Book.

Glaser, V. (Ed). (1997). Rheumatoid arthritis: What's new in treatment. Patient Care, 31(5), 81, 93, 96, 99.

Glaser, V. (1999). Multiple sclerosis. Patient Care, October 15, 1999.

Glaser, V. (2000). Topics in geriatrics: Effective approaches to depression in older patients. Patient Care, 17, 65–80.

Gloves, T. L. (2000). How drug resistant microorganisms affect nursing. Orthopaedic Nursing, 19(2), 19–27.

Gobel, B. H. (2000). Bleeding disorder. In S. Groenwald, M. Frogge, M. Goodman & C. Yarbro (Eds.). Cancer nursing: Principles and practice (5th ed.). Boston: Jones and Bartlett.

Goff, K. (1997). Metabolic monitoring in nutrition support. Nursing Clinics of North America, 32(4), 741–753.

Goldblum, K. (1992). Knowledge deficit in the ophthalmic patient. Nursing Clinics of North America, 3, 715–725.

Golper, T. A., Burkart, J. M., & Piraino, B. (1997). Peritoneal dialysis. In Diseases of the kidney (6th ed., Vol. III). Boston: Little, Brown and Company.

Goodman, M. (2000). Chemotherapy: Principles of administration. In S. L. Groenwald, M. H. Frogge, M. Goodman, & C. H. Yarbro. Comprehensive cancer nursing review (5th ed.). Boston: Jones and Bartlett.

Goodman, M. (2000). Chemotherapy principles of administration. In S. Groenwald, M. H. Frogge, M. Goodman, & C. H. Yarbro (Eds.), Cancer nursing: Principles & practice (5th ed.). Boston: Jones and Bartlett.

Goodman, M., Hilderley, L. J., & Purl, S. (1997). Integumentary and mucous membrane alternatives. In S. L. Groenwald, M. H. Frogge, M. Goodman, & C. H. Yarbro. Comprehensive cancer nursing review (4th ed.). Boston: Jones and Bartlett.

Gordon, P. A., Norton, J., Gurra, J., & Perdue, S. T. (1997). Position of chest tubes: Effects on pressure and drainage. American Journal of Critical Care, 6(1), 33–38.

Goroll, A., & Mulley, A. (2000). Primary care medicine: Office evaluation and management of the adult patient (4th ed.). Philadelphia: Lippincott Williams & Wilkins.

Goshorn, J. (2000). Management of patients with urinary and renal dysfunction. In S. Smeltzer and B. Bare (Eds.), Brunner & Suddarth's textbook of medical-surgical nursing (9th ed.). Philadelphia: Lippincott Williams & Wilkins.

Graham-Macaluso, M. M. (1991). Complications of peritoneal dialysis: Nursing care plans to document teaching. ANNA Journal, 18(5), 479–483.

Grainger R. (1990). Anxiety interrupters. American Journal of Nursing, 90(2), 14–15.

Henderson, V., & Nite, G. (1960). Principles and practice of nursing (5th ed.). New York: Macmillan.

Greenfield, E. (1998). Integumentary disorders. In M. Kinney, S. B. Dunbar, Brooks-Brunn, N. Molter & J. Vitello Cicciu. AACN clinical reference for critical care nursing (4th ed.). St. Louis: Mosby-Year Book.

Greenfield, L. J. (1997). Surgery: Scientific principles and practice (2nd ed.) Philadelphia: J. B. Lippincott.

Griffin-Broan, J. (2000). Diagnostic evaluation, classification, and staging. In C. Yarks, M. H. Frogge, M. Goodman, & S. Groenwald (Eds.), Cancer nursing (5th ed.). Boston: Jones and Bartlett.

Groenwald, S. L., Frogge, M., Goodman, M., & Yarbro, C. (2000). Cancer nursing: Principles and practice (5th ed.). New York: Jones and Bartlett.

Gulliver, M. (2000). Middle ear dysfunction following laryngectomy. Journal of Speech-Language Pathology and Audiology, 24(1), 19–25.

Guthrie, D. W., & Guthrie, R. A. (1997). Nursing management of diabetes mellitus: A guide to the pattern approach (4th ed.). New York: Springer.

Hager, C., A., & Brnich, N. (1998). Fat embolism syndrome. A complication of orthopedic trauma. Orthopaedic Nursing, 17(2), 41–46, 58.

Hahn, K. (1989). Sexuality and COPD. Rehabilitation Nursing, 14(4), 191–195.

Hailey, B. J. (1988). The mastectomy experience: Patients' perspectives. Women's Health, 14(1), 75–88.

Hall, B. (1990). The struggle of the diagnosed terminally ill person to maintain hope. Nursing Science Quarterly, 3, 177–184.

Hall, C. M. (1997). Wound dressings: Use and selection. Geriatric Nursing, 18(6), 266–267.

Hall, G. R. (1994). Caring for people with Alzheimer's disease using the conceptual model of progressively lowered stress threshold in the clinic setting. Nursing Clinics of North America, 29, 129–141.

Hamburg, D. A., & Adams, J. E. (1953). A perspective on coping behaviors. Archives of General Psychiatry, 17, 1–20.

Hammond, M. (2000). Physical medicine and rehabilitation. Topics in Spinal Cord Injury, Feb.

Hanhan, U. (2001). Status epilepticus. Pediatric Clinics of North America, 48(3), 683–694.

Hardy, E. M., & Ritlenberry, K. (1994). Myasthenia gravis: Anoverivieca. Orthopedic Nursing, 13(6), 37–42.

Harris, L. (2000). Head and neck malignancies. In C. Yarbro, M. Frogge, M. Goodman, & S. Groenwald (Eds.), Cancer nursing: Principles and practice (5th ed.). Boston: Jones and Bartlett.

Harris, L. H., & Gore, S. (1996). Sickle cell disease: Care throughout the life span. Journal of National Black Nurses' Association, 8(1), 33–44.

Hart, B. P. (1993). Vascular consequences of smoking and benefits of smoking cessation. Journal of Vascular Nursing, 11(2), 48–51.

Hart, L., Freel, M., & Milde, F. (1990). Fatigue. Nursing Clinics of North America, 25(4), 967–976.

Hartshorn, J. (1996). Seizures and the elderly: Critical care. Nursing Clinics of North America, 8(1), 71–79.

Hassey Dow, K., & Hilderley, L. (1992). Nursing care in radiation oncology. Philadelphia: W. B. Saunders.

Hayes, C. (2002). Identifying important issues for people with Parkinson's disease. British Journal of Nursing, 11(2), 91–97.

Heinrich, L. (1987). Care of the female rape victim. Nurse Practitioner, 12(11), 9–27.

Held, & Warmkessel, J. (2000). Prostate cancer. In S. Groenwald, M. Frogge, M. Goodman, & C. Yarbro (Eds.), Cancer nursing (5th ed.). Boston: Jones and Bartlett.

Helt, J. (1991). Foot care and footwear to prevent amputation. Journal of Vascular Nursing, 9(4), 2–8.

Helton, M., Gordon, S., & Nunnery, S. (1980). The correlation between sleep deprivation and intensive care unit syndrome. Heart & Lung, 9(5), 464–468.

Herrmann, F. R., et al. (1992). Serum albumin level on admission a predictor of death, length of stay and readmission. Archives of Internal Medicine, 152, 125–136.

Hertzer, N. R. (1995). Postoperative management and complications following carotid endarterectomy. In R. B. Rutherford (Ed.). Vascular surgery (4th ed., Vol. 2). Philadelphia: W. B. Saunders.

Hickey, J. (1997). The clinical practice of neurological and neurosurgical nursing (4th ed.). Lippincott Williams & Wilkins.

Hickey, J. U. (2002). Clinical practice of neurological nursing (5th ed.). Philadelphia: Lippincott Williams & Wilkins.

Hickey, J. V. (2001). The clinical practice of neurological and neurosurgical nursing (5th ed.). Philadelphia: Lippincott Williams & Wilkins.

Hickey, J., & Minton, M. (1999). Neuroscience nursing for a new millennium. The Nursing Clinics of North America, 34(3), 731–734.

Hilderley, L. (2000). Radiotherapy. In S. Groenwald, M. Frogge, M. Goodman, & C. Yarbro (Eds.). Cancer nursing: Principles and practice (5th ed.). Boston: Jones and Bartlett.

Hileman, J. W., Lackey, N. R., & Hassanein, R. S. (1992). Identifying the needs of home caregivers of patients with cancer. Oncology Nursing Forum, 19(5), 771–777.

Hill, A., Nioen, C. A., Krussen, C., & McGreath, S. W. (1995). British Journal of Therapy and Rehabilitation, 2(11), 593–598.

Hinojosa, R. J. & Layman, A. S. (1996). Breast reconstruction through tissue expansion. Plastic Surgery Nursing, 16(3), 139–145, 176–178.

Hodges, L., & Rapp, C. (1990). New drugs for Parkinson's disease. Journal of Neuroscience Nursing, 22(4), 254–257.

Hoebler, L. (1997). Colon and rectal cancer. In S. L. Groenwald, M. H. Frogge, M. Goodman, & C. Yarbro (Eds.). Cancer nursing: Principles and practice (4th ed.). Boston: Jones and Bartlett.

Hollaway, G. A. (1996). Arterial ulcers. Assessment and diagnosis. Ostomy/Wound Management, 42(3), 46–48, 50–51.

Holloway, R. (2000). Pramipexole vs levodopa as initial treatment for Parkinson's disease. A randomized controlled trial. Journal of American Medical Association, 284, 1931–1938.

Holmes, S. B. (1998). Autoimmune and inflammatory disease. In A. B. Maher, S. W. Salmond, & T. Pellino, Orthopedic nursing (2nd Ed.). Philadelphia: W. B. Saunders.

Hoskins, C. N., Baker, S., Sherman, D., Bohlander, J., Bookbinder, M., Budin, W., Ekstrom, D., Knauer, C., & Maislin, G. (1996). Social support and patterns of adjustment to breast cancer. Scholarly Inquiry for Nursing Practice, 10(2), 99–123.

Hoskins, L. (2000). Stress and adaptation. In S. Smeltzer & B. Bare, Brunner & Suddarth's textbook of medical-surgical nursing (9th ed.). Philadelphia: Lippincott Williams & Wilkins.

House, J. S. (1981). Work stress and social support. Reading, MA: Addison-Wesley.

Hoyt, M. J., & Stacts, J. A. (1991). Wasting and malnutrition in patients with HIV/AIDS. Journal of American Nurses in AIDS Care, 2(3), 16–26.

Hubner, C. (1987). Exercise therapy and smoking cessation for intermittent claudication. Journal of Cardiovascular Nursing, 1(2), 50–58.

Hughes, K. (1993). Psychological and functional status of breast cancer patients. Cancer Nursing, 16(3), 222–229.

Hull, M. M. (1992). Coping strategies of family caregivers in hospice home care. Oncology Nursing Forum, 19(8), 1179–1187.

Hunt, A. (1998). Metabolic complications. In A. B. Maher, S. Salmond, & T. Pellino. Orthopedic nursing (2nd Ed.). Philadelphia: W. B. Saunders.

Hunter, M., & King, D. (2001). COPD: Management of acute exacerbations and chronic stable disease. American Family Physician, 64(4), 603–612.

Hurwitz, A. (1989). The benefit of a home exercise regimen for ambulatory Parkinson's disease patients. Journal of Neuroscience Nursing, 21(3), 180–184.

International Standards of Neurological Classification. ASIA Scale. Atlanta, GA 2000.

Irvine, E. J., Feagan, B., Rochon, J., Archambault, A., Fedorak, R. N., Groll, A., et al. (1994). Quality of life: A valid and reliable measure of therapeutic efficacy in the treatment of inflammatory bowel disease. Gastroenterology, 106, 287–296.

Jablonski, R. (2000). Discovering asthma in the older adult. The Nurse Practitioner, 25(1), 14, m24–525,29–32+.

Jackson, D. (1995). Latex allergy and anaphylaxis: What to do. Journal of Intravenous Nursing, 18, 33–52.

Jassak, P. F. (1992). Families: An essential element in the care of the patient with cancer. Oncology Nursing Forum, 19(6), 871–876.

Jenkins, T. (2002). Sickle cell anemia in pediatric intensive care unit. AACN Clinical Issues, 13(2), 154–168.

Joaquin, J. M. (1993). Update: Guidelines for treating hypertension. American Journal of Nursing, 93(3), 42–49.

Johnson, A. P. (1988). The elderly and COPD. Journal of Gerontology Nursing, 14(12), 20–24.

Johnson, B. (1997). Psychiatric mental health nursing (4th ed.). Philadelphia: Lippincott.

Johnson, C. L. (1987). The role of physical therapy. In J. A. Bosuick (Ed.), The art and science of burn care. Maryland: Aspen Publishers.

Johnson, J. E. (1978). Sensory information, instruction in a coping strategy, and recovery from surgery. Research in Nursing and Health, 1, 14–17.

Johnson, J. E., Rice, V., Fuller, S., & Endress, P. (1978). Sensory information instruction in coping strategy and recovery from surgery. Research in Nursing and Health, 1(1), 4–17.

Johnson, R. (1993). Total shoulder arthroplasty. Orthopedic Nursing, 12(1), 14–22.

Johnson, R. A., & Justin, R. (1988). Documenting patients' end of life decisions. Nurse Practitioner, 13(6), 41.

Joint Commission on Accreditation of Healthcare Organizations (JCAHO). (1994). Accreditation manual for hospitals.

Kalb, R. C. & Scheinberg, L. C. (1992). Multiple sclerosis and the family. New York: Demos.

Kane, K. K. (1983). Carotid artery rupture in advanced head and neck cancer patients. Oncology Nursing Forum, 10(1), 14–18.

Kannel, W. B., D'Agostino, R. B., & Belanger, A. L. (1987). Fibrinogen, cigarette smoking and risk of cardiovascular disease: Insights from the Framingham Study. American Heart Journal, 13, 1006–1010.

Kantaff, P., Carroll, P., D'Amico, A., Isaacs, J., Ross, R., & Schertt. (2001). Prostate cancer: Principles and practice. Philadelphia: Lippincott Williams & Wilkins.

Kaplan, P. W., & Fisher, R. S. (1995). Seizure disorders. In L. Barker, J. Burton, & P. Zieve. Principles of ambulatory medicine (pp. 1178–1197, 4th ed.). Baltimore: Williams & Wilkins.

Kappas-Larson, P., & Lathrop, L. (1993). Early detection and intervention for hazardous ethanol use. Nurse Practitioner, 18(7), 50–55.

Karlowicz, K. A. (1995). Urologic nursing: Principles and practice. Philadelphia: W. B. Saunders.

Katz, J. (1996). The role of the sympathetic nervous system in phantom limb pain. Physical Medicine and Rehabilitation: State of the Art Reviews, 10(1), 153–175.

Katz, P. (2003). Peptic ulcer disease. In L. R. Baker, J. Burton, & P. Zieve. Principles of ambulatory medicine (6th ed.). Philadelphia: Lippincott Williams & Wilkins.

Kee, J. L. (1982). Fluids and electrolytes and clinical applications: A programmed approach (3rd ed.). New York: John Wiley & Sons.

Kelly, C., Dumenko, L., McGregor, S. E., & McHutcheon, M. E. (1992). A change in flushing protocols of central venous catheters. Oncology Nursing Forum, 19(4), 599–605.

Kelly, K. G. (1993). Advances in perioperative nutritional support. Medical Clinics of North America, 77(2), 465–475.

Kelsey, M. (1993). The antiplatelet effects of aspirin and related component drugs on the surgical patient. Journal of Post-Anesthesia Nursing, 8(2), 101–103.

Kemp, J. P., & Kemp, J. A. (2001). Management of asthma in children. 63(7), 1341–1348.

Kennedy, S., & Over, R. (1990). Psychophysiological assessment of male sexual arousal following spinal cord injury. Archives of Sexual Behavior, 19, 15–27.

Kersten, L. (1990). Changes in self concept during pulmonary rehabilitation: Parts 1 & 2. Heart & Lung, 19(5), 456–470.

Kessenich, C. (1996). Update on pharmacologic therapies for osteoporosis. Nurse Practitioner, 21(8), 19–20, 22–24.

Khoiny, E. E. (1996). Use of Depo-Provera in teens. Journal of Pediatric Health Care, 10(5), 195–201.

King, D., & Pippin, H. J. (1997). Community-acquired pneumonia in adults. American Family Physician, 56(2), 544–50.

King, I., & Tarsitano, B. (1982). The effect of structured and unstructured preoperative teaching: A replication. Nursing Research, 31(6), 324–329.

Klein, I., & Ojamaa, K. (1992). Cardiovascular manifestations of endocrine disease. Journal of Clinical Endocrinology and Metabolism, 75(2), 339–342.

Knight, L. et al. (1997). Caring for patients with third-generation implantable cardioverter defibrillators. Critical Care Nursing, 17(5), 46–63.

Kovach, T. (1990). Nip it in the bud: Controlling wound infection with preoperative shaving. Today's OR Nurse, 9, 23–26.

Kowdley, K. V. (1996). Update on therapy for hepatobiliary diseases. Nurse Practitioner: American Journal of Primary Healthcare, 21(7), 81–82, 84.

Kramer, M. C., & Reiter, R. C. (1997). Hysterectomy indications, alternatives and predictors. American Family Physician, 55(3), 827–834.

Krebs, L. U. (2000). Sexual and reproductive dysfunction. In S. L. Groenwald, M. H. Frogge, M. Goodman, & C. Yarbro (Eds.). Cancer nursing: Principles and practice (5th ed.). Boston: Jones and Bartlett.

Kruger, N. R. (1989). Case management: Is it a delivery system for my organization? Aspen's Advisor For Nurse Executives, 4(10), 4–6.

Krumberger, J. (1993). Acute pancreatitis. Critical Care Nursing Clinics of North America, 5(1), 185–202.

Kucharski, S. (1993). Fulminant hepatic failure. Critical Care Nursing Clinics of North America, 5(1), 141–151.

Kumar, U. M., & Pope, R. M. (1996). Balance therapeutic value against significant adverse effects: Corticosteroids. Journal of Musculoskeletal Medicine, 3(5), 21–24, 29.

Kupecz, D. (2000). Intermittent claudication treatment. The Nurse Practitioner, 25(5), 112–115.

LaForce, F. (1992). Antibacterial therapy for lower respiratory tract infections in adults: A review. Clinical Infectious Diseases, 14 (Suppl. 2), 5233–5237.

Lamm, B., Dungan, J., & Hiromoto, B. (1991). Long-term life-style management. Clinical Nurse Specialist, 5(4), 182–188.

Lancaster, L. E. (1991). Core curriculum for nephrology nursing, American Nephrology Nurses Association (2nd ed.). Pitman, NJ: Anthony J. Jannetti.

Lancaster, L. (1995). Core curriculum for nephrology nursing (3rd ed.). Pitman, NJ: Anthony J. Janetti.

Landoni, M. (2000). Group psychotherapy experiences for people with multiple sclerosis and psychological support for families. Journal of Neurovirology, May, 168–71.

Langenegger, T., & Michel, B. A. (1999). Drug treatment for rheumatoid arthritis. Clinical Orthopaedics and Relaxed Research, 366, 22–30.

Larkin, J. (1987). Factors influencing one's ability to adapt to chronic illness. Nursing Clinics of North America, 22 (3), 535–542.

Larsen, E., Lindbloom, L., & Davis, K. B. (1986). Development of the clinical nephrology practitioner: A focus on independent learning. Seattle: University of Washington Hospital.

Laughlin, R. M., & Clancy, G. J. (1982). Musculoskeletal assessment: Neurovascular examination of the injured extremity. Orthopedic Nursing, 1(1), 43–48.

Lawton, A. W. (1996). Sickle cell and the eye. The ABNF Journal, 7(3), 78–80.

Lazarus, R. S., & Folkman, S. (1980). Analysis of coping in a middle age community sample. Journal of Health Behavior, 21(9), 219–239.

Lazarus, R. S., & Folkman, S. (1984). Stress, appraisal and coping. New York: Springer-Verlag.

Lazarus, R. S., & Monat, A. (1977). Stress and coping: An anthology. New York: Columbia University Press.

Ledray, L. (1990). Counseling rape victims: The nursing challenge. Perspectives in Psychiatric Care, 36(2), 21–27.

Ledray, L. (1992). Home accommodation to self-determination: Nursing role in the development of health care policy: A nursing developed model for the treatment of rape victims . . . A nursing research demonstration project (American Academy of Nursing). American Nurses Association (ANA) Publications, 6-153, 68–76.

Ledray, L. (2001). The clinical care and documentation for victims of drug-facilitated sexual assault. Journal of Emergency Nursing, 27(3), 301–305.

Ledy, N. (1990). A structural model of stress, psychosocial resources and symptomatic experiences in chronic physical illness. Nursing Research, 39(4), 230–236.

Lee, B. Y., Karmakar, M. G., Herz, B. L., & Sturgill, R. A. (1995). Autonomic reflexia revisited. The Journal of Spinal Cord Medicine, 18(2), 75–87.

Lee, R., Graydon, J., & Ross, E. (1991). Effects of psychological well being, physical status and social support on oxygen dependent COPD patient's level of functioning. Research in Nursing and Health, 14(2), 323–328.

Leedom, J. M. et al. (1988). Pneumonia in compromised patients. Patient Care, 22(3), 153–165.

Leininger, S. (2002). The role of nutrition in wound healing. Critical Care Nursing Quarterly, 25(1), 13–21.

Lennie, T., Christman, S., & Jadack, R. (2001). Educational needs and altered eating habits following a total laryngectomy. Oncology Nursing Forum, 28(4), 667–674.

LeRoith, D., Taylor, S. I., & Olefsky, J. M. (1996). Diabetes mellitus: A fundamental and clinical text. Philadelphia: J. B. Lippincott.

Levine, D. (1997). Caring for the renal patient. Philadelphia: W. B. Saunders.

Lierman, L. M. (1988). Discovery of breast changes: Women's responses and nursing implications. Cancer Nursing, 11(6), 352–361.

List, M. A. (1996). Longitudinal assessment of quality of life in laryngeal cancer patients. Head and Neck, 18, 1–10.

Loewenhardt, P. M. (1989). Assuring successful home enteral feedings. Home Healthcare Nurse, 7(5), 16–20.

Logemann, J. (1994). Rehabilitation of the head and neck cancer patient. Seminars in Oncology, 21, 359–365.

Logston-Boggs, R., & Wooldridge-King, M. (Eds.). (1993). AACN procedure manual for critical care. Philadelphia: W. B. Saunders.

Long, L., & McAuley, J. (1996). Epilepsy: A review of seizure types, etiologies, diagnosis, treatment and nursing implications. Critical Care Nurse, 16(4), 83–91.

Lubkin, H. M. (1995). Chronic illness: Impact and interventions (3rd ed.). Boston: Jones and Bartlett.

Lucas, A. B. (1992). A critical review of venous access devices: The nursing perspective. In Current issues in cancer nursing practice. Philadelphia: J. B. Lippincott.

Luczum, M. E. (1984). Postanesthesia nursing: A comprehensive guide. Rockville, MD: Aspen Systems.

Lusis, S. A. (1997). Pathophysiology and management of idiopathic Parkinson's disease. Journal of Neuroscience Nursing, 29(1), 24–31.

Lydon, J. (1989). Assessment of renal function in the patient receiving chemotherapy. Cancer Nursing, 12(3), 133–143.

Maas, M. (1992). Impaired physical mobility. In M. Maas, K. Buckwalter, & M. Hardy (Eds.), Nursing diagnoses and interventions for the elderly. Redwood City, CA: Addison-Wesley Nursing.

MacFarlane, E. (1993). Sexual assault: Coping with crisis. Canadian Nurse, 6, 21–24.

MacIntyre, N. R. (1995). Mechanical ventilatory support. In T. Dantzimer & N. R. Macintyre (Eds.). Comprehensive respiratory care (pp. 439–455). Philadelphia: W. B. Saunders.

MacIntyre, N. R. (1995). Weaning from mechanical ventilatory support. In T. Dantzimer & N. R. Macintyre (Eds.). Comprehensive respiratory care (pp. 735–742). Philadelphia: W. B. Saunders.

Macklin, D. (1997). How to manage ICCS. American Journal of Nursing, 97(9), 26–35.

Maguire-Eisen, M. (1990). Diagnosis and treatment of adult acute leukemia. Seminars in Oncology Nursing, 6(1), 17–24.

Maher, A. B. (Ed.) (1998). Orthopedic nursing (2nd ed.). Philadelphia: W. B. Saunders.

Maher, L. (1998). Osteomyelitis: Diagnosis, staging, management. Patient Care, 32(2), 93–94, 99–109.

Mahon, S., et al. (1991). Managing the psychosocial consequences of cancer recurrence: Implications for nurses. Oncology Nursing Forum, 18(3), 577–583.

Mahoney, D. (2001). Nursing management of the patient with spinal cord injury. In J. Derstine & S. D. Hargrove (Eds.), Comprehensive rehabilitation nursing. Philadelphia: W. B. Saunders.

Maklebust, J. (1985). United Ostomy Association visits and adjustment following ostomy surgery. Journal of Enterostomal Therapy, 12(3), 84–89.

Maklebust, J. (1987). Pressure ulcers: Etiology and prevention. Nursing Clinics of North America, 22(2), 359–377.

Maklebust, J. (1990). Assisting with adjustment following ostomy surgery. Hospital Home Health, 7(7), 91–94.

Maklebust, J., & Magnan, M. (1992). Approaches to patient and family education for pressure ulcer management. Decubitus, 5(4), 18–28.

Maklebust, J. A., & Sieggreen, M. (1990). Pressure ulcers: Guideline for prevention and nursing management. West Dundee, IL: 5-N Publications.

Maklebust, J., & Sieggreen, M. (2001). Pressure ulcers: Guidelines for prevention and nursing management (3rd ed.). West Dundee, IL: SN Publications.

Malignant Hyperthermia Association of United States (MHS). (1992). Understanding malignant hypertension. Sherburne, NY.

Malinson, R. K. (1999). The lived experince of AIDS-related multiple losses by HIV-negative gay men. Journal of Association of Nurses in AIDS Care, 10(5), 22–31.

Maliski, S., Heilemann, M. S., & McCorkle, R. (2001). Mastery of postprostatectomy incontinence and impotence: His work, her work, our work. Oncology Nursing Forum, 28(6), 985–992.

Maloni, H. (2000). Pain in multiple sclerosis. Clinical Bulletin: National Multiple Sclerosis Society, New York, NY.

Malseed, R., Goldstein, F., & Balkon, N. (1995). Pharmacology: Drug therapy and nursing considerations. (4th ed.) Philadelphia: J. B. Lippincott.

Management and therapy of sickle cell disease. (1992). National Institutes of Health Publication No. 92-2117. Washington, DC: U.S. Department of Health and Human Services.

Managing the special problems of chronic lung disease. (1997). Patient Care, 31(7), 87–92, 95–98.

Mangan, C. M. (1992). Malignant pericardial effusions: Pathophysiology and clinical correlates. Oncology Nursing Forum, 19(8), 1215–1223.

Marchiondo, K., & Thompson, A. (1996). Pain management in sickle-cell disease.

Marrie, T. (1992). Pneumonia. Clinics in Geriatric Medicine, 8(4), 721–734.

Marsh, F. L. (1986). Refusal of treatment. Clinics in Geriatric Medicine, 2(3), 511–520.

Martens, K. H., & Mellor, S. D. (1997). A study of the relationship between home care services and hospital readmission of patients with congestive heart failure. Home Health Care Nurse, 15(2), 123–129.

Maryland Nurse Practice Act, July 1986, p. 4.

Masoorli, S., & Angeles, T. (1990, January). PICC lines: The latest home core challenge. RN, 53(1), 44–51.

Mauer, K., Abrahams, E., Arslanian, C., Schoenly, L., & Taggart, H. (2002). National practice patterns for the care of the patient with total joint replacement. Orthopedic Nursing, 21(3), 37–44.

Maves, M. (1992). Mutual goal setting. In G. Bulecheck & J. McCloskey (Eds.), Nursing interventions. Philadelphia: W. B. Saunders.

McCabe, S. M. (2001). Management of patients with neurologic dysfunction. In S. Smeltzer & B. Bare (Eds.), Brunner & Suddarth's textbook of medical surgical nursing (9th ed.). Philadelphia: Lippincott Williams & Wilkins.

McCaffery, M. & Beebe, A. (1989). Pain: Clinical manual for nursing practice. St. Louis: C.V. Mosby.

McCann, K., & Wadsworth, E. (1992). The role of informal carers in supporting gay men who have HIV related illness: What do they do and what are their needs? AIDS Care, 4(1), 25–34.

McCowan, C. B. (1998). Systemic lupus erythematosus. Journal of American Academy of Nurse Practitioners, 10(2), 225–231.

McCulloch, J. A. (1996). Focus issue on lumbar disc herniation: Macro and microdiscetomy spine. 21(245), 45S–56S.

McEwen, D. R. (1996). Management of alcoholic cirrhosis of the liver. AORN, 64(2), 209–225.

McGee, C. (1997). Secondary amenorrhea leading to osteoporosis: Incidence and prevention. Nurse Practitioner, 22(5), 38, 41–42, 44–45, 48, 51–52, 57–58, 63.

McIntyre, D. (1993). Cataract in adults: Management of functional impairment. Abstracts of Clinical Care Guidelines, 3, 1–6.

McKenry, L. M., & Salerno, E. (1995). Pharmacology in nursing (19th ed.). St. Louis: C. V. Mosby.

McLane, A., & McShane, R. (1992). Bowel management. In G. Bulechek & J. McCloskey (Eds.), Nursing interventions. Philadelphia: W. B. Saunders.

McMahon, K. (1995). Multiple organ failure: The final complication of critical illness. Critical Care Nurse, 15(6), 20–28.

Melroe, N., Stawarz, K., Simpsons, J., & Henry, W. (1997). HIV RNA quantification: Marker of HIV infection. Journal of the Association of Nurses in AIDS Care, 8, 31–38.

Mentzer, W., & Kan, Y. W. (2001). Prospect for research in hematologic disorders. Journal of the American Medical Association, 285(5), 640–642.

Metheny, N. (1993). Minimizing respiratory complications of nasoenteric tube feedings: State of the science. Heart and Lung, 22(3), 213–223.

Miaskowski, C., & Donovan, M. (1992). Implementation of the American Pain Society Quality Assurance standards for relief of acute pain and cancer pain in oncology nursing practice. Oncology Nursing Forum, 19(3), 411–415.

Michael, K. (2002). Fatigue and stroke. Rehabilitation Nursing, 27(3), 89–94.

Milde, F. K. (1988). Impaired physical mobility. Journal of Gerontological Nursing, 14(3), 20–40.

Milde, F. K., Hart, L. K., & Fearing, M. O. (1996). Sexuality and fertility concerns of dialysis patient. ANNA Journal, 23(3), 307–315.

Miller, A. C., et al. (1992). A distraction technique for control of burn pain. Journal of Burn Care and Rehabilitation, 13(5), 576–580.

Miller, C. A. (1999). Nursing care of older adults (3rd ed.). Philadelphia: J. B. Lippincott.

Miller, C. A. (2004). Nursing care of older adults (4th Ed.). Philadelphia: Lippincott Williams & Wilkins.

Miller, P., Wikoff, R., & Hiatt, A. (1992). Fishbein's model of reasoned action and compliance behavior of hypertensive patients. Nursing Research, 41(2), 104–109.

Mistovich, J. J., & Griffiths, B. (2001). Aortic dissection and aortic aneurysm: Pathophysiology, assessment and management. Emergency Medical Services, 9(1), 49–60.

Mitlak, B., & Nussbaum, S. (1993). Diagnosis and treatment of osteoporosis. Annual Reviews in Medicine, 44(1), 265–277.

Moe, K., & Grau, A. (2001). HIV prophylaxis within a treatment protocol for sexual assault victims: Rationale for the decision. Journal of Emergency Nursing, 27(5), 511–515.

Mohr, D. C., Goodkin, D. E., Likosky, W. et al. (1997). Treatment of depression improves adherence to interferon beta-1b therapy for multiple sclerosis. Archives of Neurology, 54, 531–533.

Mohr, W. K. (2003). Johnson's psychiatric mental health nursing (5th ed.). Philadelphia: Lippincott Williams & Wilkins.

Molzahn, A., Northcott H., Dossetor, J. (1997). Quality of life of individuals with end stage renal disease: Perceptions of patients: Nurses and physicians. ANNA Journal, 24(3), 325–333.

Mooney, T. (1975). Sexual options for paraplegics and quadriplegics. Boston: Little, Brown.

Moore, C., Heffernan, I., & Sheldon, S. (1992). Diagnosis and management of subclavian vein thrombosis. Journal of Infusional Chemotherapy, 2(3), 151–152.

Moore, J. (1988). Vaginal hysterectomy: Its success as an outpatient procedure. AORN Journal, 48(6), 1114–1120.

MS Exchange. (1997a). Intervening with hope. Partners in Medical Communications, 1(2), 3–4.

Mundy, A. (1999). Metabolic complications of urinary diversion. Lancet, 353(16), 1813–14.

Munin, M., Espejo-DeGuzman, Boninger, M., Fitzgerald, S., Penrod, L., & Singh, J. (2001). Predictive factors for successful early prosthetic ambulation annoy lower-limb amputees. Journal of Rehabilitation Research and Development, 38(4), 379–84.

Munkres, A., Aoerst, M. T., & Hughes, S. H. (1992). Appraisal of illness, symptom distress, self-care burden, and mood states in patients receiving chemotherapy for initial and recurrent cancer. Oncology Nursing Forum, 19(8), 1201–1209.

Muntzel M., & Drueke, T. (1992). A comprehensive review of the salt and blood pressure relationship. American Journal of Hypertension Supplement, 5, 15–25.

Murphy, D., Lu, M., Martin, D., Hoffman, D., & Marelich, W. (2002). Results of a pilot interventions trial to improve antiretroviral adherence among HIV-positive patients. Journal of the Association of Nurses in AIDS Care, 13(6), 57–69.

Murray, D. P. (1993). Impaired mobility: Guillain-Barré syndrome. Journal of Neuroscience Nursing, 25(2), 100–104.

National Association of Orthopedic Nurses. (1991). Core curriculum for orthopaedic nursing (2nd ed.). Pitman, NJ: Anthony J. Jannetti.

National Association of Orthopaedic Nurses. (2001). Core curriculum for orthopaedic nursing (4th Ed.). Pitman, NJ: Anthony J. Janetti.

National High Blood Pressure Education Program. (1997). The sixth report of the Joint National Committee on Prevention, Detection, Evaluation, and Treatment of High Blood Pressure. U.S. Department of Health and Human Services. National Heart, Lung & Blood Pressure Institute, National Institutes of Health (Pub. No. 98-4080). Washington, DC: DHHS.

National Institute of Neurological Disorders and Stroke. (2000). Prepared by Office of Communications and Public Liaison. National Institutes of Health, Bethesda, Maryland 20892-2540.

National Institutes of Health (NIH). (1994). Helicobacter pylori in peptic ulcer disease. Journal of the American Medical Association, 272, 65.

National Institutes of Health (NIH). (2000). Optimal calcium intake. U.S. Department of Health and Human Services, NIH Consensus Statement, 12(4), 1–31.

Nayduch, D. (2000). Emergency nursing. In S. Smeltzer, & B. Bare (2000). Brunner & Suddarth's textbook of medical—surgical nursing (9th ed.). Philadelphia: Lippincott Williams & Wilkins.

Newcombe, P. (2002). Pathophysiology of sickle cell disease crisis. Emergency Nurse, 9(9), 9–22.

Newell, F. (1992). Ophthalmology: Principles and concepts. St. Louis: C. V. Mosby.

Newman, D., & Smith, D. (1992). Pelvic muscle reeducation as a nursing treatment for incontinence. Urologic Nursing, 12(1), 9–15.

New options for deep vein thrombosis. (1998). Patient Care, 32(1), 91–100.

Nichols, R. I. (1991). Surgical wound infections. American Journal of Medicine, 91 (Suppl. 3B), 54–64.

Nighorn, S. (1988). Narcissistic deficits in drug abusers: A self-psychological approach. Journal of Psychosocial Nursing & Mental Health Services, 26(9), 22–26.

Nolde, T., Wong, S., & Wong, J. (1989). Teaching patients how to use a new hip: What elders said they needed to know and how nurses made sure they understood the information. Geriatric Nursing, 10(2), 69–70.

Norris, M. K. G. (1989). Acute tubular necrosis: Preventing complications. Dimensions in Critical Care Nursing, 8(1), 16–26.

North American Nursing Diagnosis Association (NANDA) nursing diagnosis definition (1990). Nursing Diagnosis, in press.

Northouse, L. L. (1989). The impact of breast cancer on patients and husbands. Cancer Nursing, 12(5), 276–284.

Northrop, C., & Kelly, M. (1987). Legal issues in nursing. St. Louis: C. V. Mosby.

Notowitz, L. B. (1993). Normal venous anatomy and physiology of the lower extremity. Journal of Vascular Nursing, 11(2), 39–42.

Nursing Practice Related to SCI & Disorders: A Core Curriculum. AASCIN. Editors Nelson, Zejdlik, & Love, 2002.

O'Berli, K., & Daries, B. (1992). Support and caring: Exploring the concepts. Oncology Nursing Forum, 19(5), 763–767.

O'Brien, L. A., Grisso, J. A., & Maislin, G. (1993). Hospitalized elders: Risk of confusion with hip fracture. Journal of Gerontological Nursing, 19(2), 25–33.

O'Donnell, L. (1996). An elusive weakness: Myasthenia gravis. Medsurg Nursing, 5(1), 44–49.

Ofman, U. S. (1993). Psychosocial and sexual implications of genitourinary cancer. Seminars in Oncology Nursing, 9, 286–292.

Oncology Nurses Society Clinical Practice Committee. (1992). Cancer chemotherapy guidelines: Recommendations for the management of vesicant extravasation, hypersensitivity and anaphylaxis. Princeton, NJ: Bristol-Meyers, Bristol Laboratories & Mead Johnson.

Pace, N. M., Long, J. B., Elerdin, S., et al. (1997). Clinical research: Performance model anchors successful nutrition support protocol. Nutrition in Clinical Practice, 12(6), 274–279.

Padberg, R. M. & Padberg, L. (1997). Patient education and support. In S. L. Groenwald, M. H. Frogge, M. Goodman, & C. H. Yarbro (Eds.). Cancer nursing: Principles and practice (4th ed.). Boston: Jones and Bartlett.

Pajeau, A. (2002). Identifying patients at high risk of ischemic stroke. Patient Care, 36(5), 36–51.

Palmer, J. (2000). Evaluation and Treatment of Swallowing Impairments. American Family Physician, 61(8): 2453–62.

Parker, J. (1998). Contemporary nephrology nursing. Pitman, NJ: Anthony J. Janetti, Inc.

Panke, J. T. (2002). Difficulties in managing pain at the end of life. American Journal of Nursing, 102(7).

Parkinson's Exercise Program. Parkinson's Disease and Movement Disorder Center, Graduate Hospital, 1800 Lombard St., Philadelphia, PA 19146.

Parobek, V. & Alaimo, I. (1996). Fluid and electrolyte management in the neurologically impaired patient. Journal of Neuroscience Nursing, 28(5), 322–328.

Pederson, B. (1992). Home care management of chronic obstructive pulmonary disease patient increases patient control and prevents rehospitalization. Home Healthcare Nurse, 10(2), 24–31.

Pellino, T., Polacek, L. A., Preston, M. A., Bell, N., & Evans, R. (1998). Complications of orthopaedic disorders and orthopedic surgery. In A. B. Maher, S. W. Salmond, & T. A. Pellino. Orthopedic nursing (2nd ed.). Philadelphia: W. B. Saunders.

Penrose, N. J. (1993). Guillain-Barré syndrome: A case study. Rehabilitation Nursing, 18(2), 88–90.

Peragallo-Dittko, (Ed.) & Godley, K. & Meyer, J. (Assoc. Eds.). (1993). A core curriculum for diabetes educators (2nd ed.). Chicago: American Association of Diabetes Educators.

Peretz, D. (1970). Reaction to loss. In A. C. Carr & D. Peretz (Eds.), Loss and grief: Psychological management in medicine. New York: Columbia University Press.

Perper, B., Mikals, C. (1996). Predischarge and postdischarge concerns of patients with an ostomy. Journal of Ostomy and Continence, (23)(2), 105–109.

Persons, C. B. (1987). Critical care procedures and protocols. Philadelphia: J. B. Lippincott.

Petajan, J. H., Gappmaier, E., White, A. T. et al. (1996). Impact of aerobic training on fitness and quality of life in multiple sclerosis. Annals of Neurology, 39, 432–447.

Phillips, T. J., & Dover, J. (1991). Leg ulcers. Journal of Academy of Dermatology, 25(6), 965–989.

Physicians Association for AIDS Care (PAAC). (1993). HIV Disease Nutrition Guidelines. PAAC.

Piasecki, P. A. (2001). Bone and soft tissue sarcoma. In S. Groenwald, M. Frogge, M. Goodman, & C. Yarbro (Eds.), Cancer nursing: Principles and practice. Boston: Jones and Bartlett.

Pieper, B., & Mikols, C. (1996). Predischarge and postdischarge concerns of persons with an ostomy. The Journal of WOCN, 23(2), 105–109.

Piepmeier, J. (1992). The outcome following traumatic spinal cord injury. Mount Kisco, NY: Futura Publishing.

Pierce, L. N. N. (1995). Mechanical ventilation and intensive respiratory care. Philadelphia: W. B. Saunders.

Pincus, J. H., & Barry, K. (1988). Protein redistribution that restores function in patients with dopa-resistant "off" periods. Neurology, 38, 481–483.

Poncar, P. J. (1994). Instilling hope in the oncology patient. Journal of Psychosocial Nursing, 32(1), 33–38.

Pons, V. G. (1991). Osteomyelitis: The case for aggressive diagnosis and treatment. Consultant, 31(10), 23–38.

Poor, G., Alkinson, E. J., & O'Fallon, W. (1995). Determinants of reduced survival following hip fractures in men. Clinical Orthopedics and Related Research, 319, 260–265.

Porte, D., & Sherwin S. (Eds.). (1997). Ellenberg & Rifkin's diabetes mellitus: Theory and practice (5th ed.). Stamford, CT: Appleton & Lange.

Porth, C. (2002). Pathophysiology: Concepts of altered health states (6th ed.). Philadelphia: Lippincott Williams & Wilkins.

Powell-Cope, G., & Brown, M. A. (1992). Going public as an AIDS family caregiver. Social Science Medicine, 34(5), 571–580.

Powers, M. (Ed.). (1996). Handbook of diabetes medical nutrition therapy (2nd ed.). Rockville, MD: Aspen Publishing.

Price, S., & Wilson, L. (1986). Pathophysiology: Clinical concepts of disease process. New York: McGraw-Hill.

Quality of Care Committee. (1989). Cataract in the otherwise healthy eye. San Francisco: American Academy of Ophthalmology.

Quality of Care Committee: Glaucoma Panel (1989). Primary open angle glaucoma. San Francisco: American Academy of Ophthalmology.

Queen, J. (2001). Transperitoneal laparoscopic radical prostatectomy. Seminars in Perioperative Nursing, 10(1), 24–28.

Quinn, C. (1994). The four A's of restraint reduction: Attention, assessment, anticipation, avoidance. Orthopedic Nursing, 13(2), 11–19.

Raad, I., Sherratz, R., Russell, B., & Reuman, P. (1990). Uncontrolled nosocomial rotavirus transmission during a community outbreak. American Journal of Infection Control, 18(1), 24–28.

Randall, H. T. (1984). Enteral nutrition: Tube feeding in acute and chronic illness. Journal of Parenteral Enteral Nutrition, 8(2), 113.

Ray, R. I. (2000). Complications of lower extremity amputations. Topics in Emergency Medicine, 22(3), 35–42.

Redman, B. K. (1988). The process of patient teaching in nursing. St. Louis: C. V. Mosby.

Redman, B., & Thomas, S. (1992). Patient teaching. In G. Bulechek & J. McCloskey (Eds.), Nursing interventions. Philadelphia: W. B. Saunders.

Redman, B., & Thomas, S. (1996). Patient teaching. In G. Bulechek & J. McCloskey (Eds.), Nursing interventions (2nd ed.). Philadelphia: W. B. Saunders.

Reeves, R. C. (1997). The role of nutrition in managing obesity, diabetes and heart disease. Journal of Women's Health, 6(6), 665–669.

Reich, H. (2001). Issues surrounding surgical menopause. The Journal of Reproductive Medicine, 46(2), 297–306.

Reilly, N. J. (1992). Urinary incontinence: New attitudes and treatment options. Innovations in Urology Nursing, 3(2), 1–15.

Renfroe, K. L. (1988). Effect of progressive relaxation on dyspnea and state of anxiety in patients with chronic obstructive pulmonary disease. Heart and Lung, 17(4), 408–413.

Report of the Expert Committee on the Diagnosis & Classification of Diabetes Mellitus. (1997). Diabetes Care, 20(7), 1183–1197.

Report of the U.S. Preventive Services Task Force. (2000). Guide to clinical prevention services (3rd ed.). Baltimore, MD: Williams & Wilkins.

Rhodes, V. A., Watson, P., & Johnson, M. H. (1988). Patterns of nausea and vomiting in antineoplastic postchemotherapy patients. Applied Nursing Research, 1(3), 143–144.

Riegel, B., & Vitello-Ciccio, J. (1996). Advanced heart failure. Journal of Cardiovascular Nursing, 10(2).

Riffle, K. L., et al. (1988). The relationship between perception of supportive behaviors of others and wives' ability to cope with initial myocardial infarctions in their husbands. Rehabilitation Nursing, 13(6), 310–315.

Righter, B. (1995). Uncertainty and the role of the credible authority during the ostomy experience. The Journal of WOCN, 22(2), 100–104.

Robbins, R., Serger, J., Kerhulas, S., & Fishbone, J. (1997). Iron management in ESRD and the role of the nephrology nurse. ANNA Journal, 24(2), 265–272.

Robinson, L. C. (1992). Atherosclerotic occlusive disease of the aorta. Journal of Vascular Nursing, 10(4), 17–23.

Rodts, M. F. (1998). Disorders of the spine. In A. B. Mahler, S. W. Salmond, and T. A. Pellino (Eds.), Orthopedic nursing (2nd ed.). Philadelphia: W. B. Saunders.

Rolstad, B., & Hoyman, K. (1992). Continent diversion and reservoirs. In B. Hampton & R. Bryant (Eds.). Ostomy and continent diversions: Nursing management. St. Louis: Mosby-Year Book.

Ropper, A. H. (1998). Neurological and neurosurgical intensive care (4th ed.). Philadelphia: J. B. Lippincott.

Rotello, L. C., Warren, J., Jastremski, M. S., & Milewski, A. (1992). A nurse-directed protocol using pulse axometry to wean mechanically ventilated patients from toxic oxygen concentrations. Chest, 102(6), 1833–1835.

Rubin, E., & Farber, J. L. (1995). Essential pathology (2nd ed.). Philadelphia: J.B. Lippincott.

Rubin, M. (1988). The physiology of bed rest. American Journal of Nursing, 88(1), 50–58.

Rucknagel, D. (1996). Incentive spirometry and sickle-cell disease—acute chest syndrome. RT: The Journal for Respiratory Care Practitioners, 9(6), 127–128, 130.

Rudolph, D. (1992). Limb loss in the elderly peripheral vascular disease patient. Journal of Vascular Nursing, 10(3), 8–13.

Ruehl, C., & Schremp, P. (1992). Nursing care of the cataract patient: Today's outpatient approach. Nursing Clinics of North America, 3, 727–744.

Salmond, S. (Ed.) (1996). Core curriculum for orthopedic nursing (3rd ed.). Pitman, NJ: National Association of Orthopedic Nurses.

Salmond, S. (1998). Infections of musculoskeletal system. In A. B. Maher, S. Salmond, & T. Pellino. Orthopedic nursing (2nd ed.). Philadelphia: W.B. Saunders.

Sanford, J., Sonde, M., & Gilbert, N. (1996). Guide to HIV/AIDS therapy (5th ed.). Vienna, VA: Antimicrobial Therapy.

Santilli, J. D. & Santilli, S. M. (1997). Diagnosis and treatment of abdominal, aortic aneurysms. American Family Physician, 56(4), 1081–1090.

Scheinberg, L. C., & Holland, N. J. (1987). Multiple sclerosis: A guide for patients and their families (2nd ed.). New York: Raven.

Scheld, W., & Mandell, G. (1991). Nosocomial pneumonia: Pathogenesis and recent advances in diagnoses and therapy. Review of Infectious Diseases, 13(Suppl. 9), 5743–5751.

Schoengrund, L., & Balzer, P. (1985). Renal problems in critical care. New York: John Wiley & Sons.

Schover, L. R. (1986). Sexual rehabilitation of the ostomy patient. In D. B. Smith & D. E. Johnson (Eds.). Ostomy care and the cancer patient. Orlando, FL: Grune & Stratton.

Schrag, A. (2001). What contributes to depression in Parkinson's disease? Psychological Medicine, 31(1), 65–73.

Schremp, P. (1995). Assessment of the eye and vision. In D. Ignatavicius, M. Workman, & M. Mishler (Eds.), Medical-surgical nursing: A nursing process approach (2nd ed.). Philadelphia: W. B. Saunders.

Schremp, P. (1995). Interventions for clients with eye and vision problems. In D. Ignatavicius, M. Workman, & M. Mishler (Eds.), Medical-surgical nursing: A nursing process approach (2nd ed.). Philadelphia: W. B. Saunders.

Schremp, P. (1999). Assessment of the eye and vision. In D. Ignatavicius, M. Workman, & M. Mishler (Eds.). Medical-surgical nursing: A nursing process approach (3rd ed.). Philadelphia: W. B. Saunders.

Schremp, P. (1999). Interventions for clients with eye and vision problems. In D. Ingnatavicius, M. Workman, & M. Mishler (Eds.). Medical-surgical nursing: A nursing process approach (3rd ed.). Philadelphia: W. B. Saunders.

Schumacher, H., Alvares, C., Blough, R., & Mazzella, F. (2002). Acute leukemia. Clinics in Laboratory Medicine, 22(1), 153–192.

Schuman, L. (1991). Care of the patient with major burns. In R. B. Trofino (Ed.), Nursing care of the burn injured patient. Philadelphia: F. A. Davis.

Schumann, L. (1995). Obstructive pulmonary disorders. In Copestead, L. E. C. Perspectives on pathophysiology. Philadelphia: W. B. Saunders.

Seeman, S. (2000). Interdisciplinary approach to a total knee replacement program. Nursing Clinics of North America, 35(2), 405–414.

Serger, J. M., & Weiss, R. J. (1996). Hematologic and erythropoietin responses to iron dextran in the hemodialysis environment. ANNA Journal, 23(3), 319–325.

Severson, A. L., Baldwin, L. R., & Dehoughery, T. G. (1997). International normalized ratio in anticoagulant therapy; understanding the issues. American Journal of Critical Care, 6(3), 88–94.

SGNA. (1993). Gastroenterology nursing: A core curriculum. St. Louis: Mosby-Year Book.

Shipes, E. (1987). Psychosocial issues: The person with an ostomy. Nursing Clinics of North America, 22(2), 291–302.

Shipton, S. (1996). Risk factors associated with multiple hospital readmissions. Home Care Provider, 1(2), 83–85.

Sieggreen, M. (1987). Healing of physical wounds. Nursing Clinics of North America, 22(2), 439–448.

Sieggreen, M. (1989). Nursing management of adults with venous and lymphatic disorders. In P. Beare & J. Myers (Eds.), Principles and practice of adult health nursing. St. Louis: C. V. Mosby.

Sigler, B. A., Edwards, A., Wilkerson, J. (1996). Nursing care. In E. N. Myers & J. Y. Sven (Eds.). Cancer of the head and neck (3rd ed.). Philadelphia: W. B. Saunders.

Simon, L. S. (1999). Arthritis: New agents herald more effective symptom management. Geriatrics, 54(6), 37–44.

Simmons, B. J. (1997). Management of intracranial hemodynamics in the adult: A research analysis of head positioning and recommendations for clinical practice and future research. Journal of Neuroscience Nursing, 29(1), 44–49.

Siris, E., & Schussheim, D. (1998). Osteoporosis: Assessing your patient's risk. Women's Health in Primary Care, 1(1), 99–106.

Sitton, E. (2000). Superior vena cava syndrome. In C. Yarbro, M. Frogge, M. Goodman, & S. Groenwald (Eds.), Cancer nursing: Principles & practice (5th ed.). Boston: Jones and Bartlett.

Skelton, N. K. (1992). Medical implications of obesity: Losing pounds and gaining years. Postgraduate Medicine, 92(1), 151–162.

Slye, D. A. (1991). Orthopedic complications. Nursing Clinics of North America, 26(1), 113–132.

Smeltzer, S. C. & Bare, B. G. (2000). Brunner & Suddarth's textbook of medical—surgical nursing (10th ed.). Philadelphia: Lippincott Williams & Wilkins.

Smeltzer, S. & Bare, B. (2004). Brunner & Suddarth's textbook of medical—surgical nursing (10th ed.). Philadelphia: Lippincott Williams & Wilkins.

Smith, D. B. (1992). Psychosocial adaptation. In B. Hampton & R. Bryant (Eds.). Ostomy and continent diversions: Nursing management. St. Louis, Mosby-Year Book.

Smith, L. J. (1992). Peritoneal dialysis in the critically ill patient. AACN Clinical Issues in Critical Care Nursing, 3(3), 558–569.

Smith, S. H. (1996). Principle exercise as an oncology nursing intervention to enhance quality of life. Oncology Nursing Forum, 23(4), 771–778.

Smith-DiJulio. (1994). People who depend on alcohol. In E. M. Varcarolis (Ed.), Foundations of psychiatric mental health nursing. Philadelphia: W. B. Saunders.

Smith-Di Julio, K. (2001). People who depend on alcohol. In E. M. Varcarolis (Ed.), Foundations of psychiatric mental health nursing (4th ed.). Philadelphia: W. B. Saunders.

Smith-DiJulio, K. (2001). Rape. In E. Varcarolis (Ed.), Foundations of psychiatric mental health nursing (4th ed.). Philadelphia: W. B. Saunders.

Snyder, P. (1998). Fractures. In A. B. Maher, S. Salmond, & T. Pellino. Orthopedic nursing (2nd Ed.) Philadelphia W. B. Saunders.

Society of Gastroenterology Nurses and Associates (SGNA) (1993). Gastroenterology nursing: A core curriculum. St. Louis: Mosby-Year Book.

Solomon, J., Yee, N., & Soulen, M. (2000). Aortic stent grafts: An overview of devices, indications and results. Applied Radiology Supplement, 7, 43–51.

Spector, S. L., & Nicklas, R. A. (1995). Practice parameters for the diagnosis and treatment of asthma. Journal of Allergy and Clinical Immunology, 96(5), 707–870.

Spencer, K. W. (1996). Significance of the breast to the individual and society. Plastic Surgical Nursing, 16(3), 131–132.

Spielberger, C., & Sarason, I. (Eds.). (1975). Stress and anxiety (Vol. 1). Washington, D.C.: Hemisphere.

Spollett, G. (1989). Irritable bowel syndrome: Diagnosis and treatment. Nurse Practitioner, 14(8), 32–44.

Sprangers, M. A. G., Taal, B. G., Aaronson, N. K., et al. (1995). Quality of life in colorectal cancer: Stoma vs. non-stoma patients. Disease of Colon and Rectum, 38, 361–69.

Stacey, T. (1989). Osteoporosis: Exercise therapy, pre- and postdiagnosis. Journal of Manipulative and Physiological Therapeutics, 12(3), 211–219.

Stein, J. H. (Ed.). (1990). Peritoneal dialysis new concepts and applications. Contemporary Issues in Nephrology, 22.

Stelzig, Y. (1999). Laryngeal manifestations in patients with Parkinson's disease. Laryngo-Rhino-Otogie, 78(10), 544–51.

Stetson, B., Schlundt, D. G., & Sbrocco, T., et al. (1992). The effects of aerobic exercise on psychological adjustment: A randomized study of sedentary obese women attempting weight loss. Women & Health, 19(4), 1–14.

Stevens, R. H. (1992). Patients who have undergone bone marrow transplantation: Their quest for meaning. Oncology Nursing Forum, 19(6), 899–905.

Stillwell, S. B. (1996). Mosby's critical care nursing reference. St. Louis: Mosby–Year Book.

Strandness, J. R., Eugene, D., & Arina Von, B. (1994). Vascular diseases, surgical and interventional therapy. Section XI. Acute and chronic venous disorders. New York: Churchill Livingstone, pp. 851–1044.

Strauss, A. (1984). Chronic illness and the quality of life. St. Louis: Mosby.

Stupczynski, J. S. (1984). Dealing with life-threatening complications of cancer. Consultant, 24(3), 207–223.

Styles, M. M. (1982). On nursing: Toward a new endowment. St. Louis: C. V. Mosby.

Sueppel, C., Kreder, K., & See, W. (2001). Improved continence outcomes with preoperative pelvic floor muscle strengthening exercises. Urologic Nursing, 21(3), 201–210.

Sullivan, I. (1989). Nursing interventions. Critical Care Nursing Clinics of North America, 1(1), 151–164.

Sullivan, J., et al. (1990). Ambulatory care for patients with acute leukemia: An alternative to frequent hospitalizations. Journal of Professional Nursing, 6(5), 300–309.

Sullivan, M. J., & Hawthorne, M. H. (1996). Nonpharmacologic interventions in the treatment of heart failure. Journal of Cardiovascular Nursing, 10(2), 47–57.

Summer, S., & Ebbert, D. W. (1992). Ambulatory surgical nursing: A nursing diagnosis approach. Philadelphia: J. B. Lippincott.

Taban, H. (1993). The nurse case manager in acute care settings. Journal of Nursing Administration, 23(10), 53–61.

Tanagho, E. A., & McAninch, J. W. (Eds.). (1995). Smith's general urology (14th ed.). Norwalk, CT: Appleton & Lange.

Tanner, D. C. (1989). Guidelines for treatment of chronic depression in the aphasic patient. Rehabilitation Nursing, 14(2), 77–80.

Task Force on Nutrition Support in AIDS. (1989). Guidelines for nutrition support in AIDS. Nutrition, 5(1), 39–46.

Tasman, W. (Ed). (2002). Duane's clinical ophthalmology. Philadelphia: Lippincott Williams & Wilkins.

Taylor, E. J., Baird, S., Malone, D., & McCorkle, R. (1993). Factors associated with anger in cancer patients and their caregivers. Cancer Practice, 1(2), 101–109.

Teasell, R. W., Malcolm, J., & Delaney, G. A. (1996). Sympathetic nervous dysfunction in high-level spinal cord injuries. Physical Medicine and Rehabilitation: State of the Art Reviews, 10(1), 37–55.

Thelan, L. A., Lough, M. L., Urden, L., & Stacy, K. M. (1998). Critical care nursing: Diagnoses and management (3rd ed.). St. Louis: Mosby–Year Book.

The Parkinson's Disease Association. (1994). Let's communicate. New York: American Parkinson's Disease Association.

The Parkinson's Disease Foundation. (1986). The Parkinson patient at home. New York: Parkinson's Disease Foundation.

Tilden, V., & Weinert, C. (1987). Social support and the chronically ill individual. Nursing Clinics of North America, 22(3), 613–620.

Tolley, F. & Henninger, D. (1991). Perceived stressors during the recovery period following enucleation. Insight, 3, 18–19.

Tortorice, P. U. (2000). Chemotherapy: Principles of therapy. In S. L. Groenwald, M. H. Frogge, M. Goodman, & C. H. Yarbro. Comprehensive cancer nursing review (5th ed.). Boston: Jones and Bartlett.

Tracey, C. (1992). Hygiene assistance. In G. Bulechek & J. McCloskey (Eds.), Nursing interventions. Philadelphia: W. B. Saunders.

Traver, G. A. (1988). Measures of symptoms and life quality to predict emergent use of institutional health care resources in chronic obstructive airways disease. Heart and Lung, 17(6), 689–697.

Tumbarello, C. (2000). Acute extremity compartmental syndrome. Journal of Trauma Nursing, 7(2), 30–36.

Twycross, R. (1988). The management of pain in cancer: A guide to drugs and dosages. Primary Care and Cancer, 12(5), 122–129.

United States Department of Health and Human Services. (1992). Management and therapy of sickle cell disease. U.S. Department of Health and Human Services, NIH Publication No. 92-2117. Washington, DC: U.S. Health Service.

United States Department of Health and Human Services. (2001). Guidelines for the use of antiretroviral agents in HIV-infected adults and adolescents.

USPHS/IDSA. (2001). Guidelines for the prevention of opportunistic infections in persons infected with human immunodeficiency virus.

Vail, B. A. (1997). Management of chronic viral hepatitis. American Family Physician, 55(8), 2749–2756.

Varella, L., & Utermohlen, U. (1993). Nutritional support for the patient with renal failure. Critical Care Nursing Clinics of North America, 5(1), 79–96.

Vaughn, D., Asbury, J., & Riordan-Eva, P. (1992). General ophthalmology (13th ed.). Los Altos, CA: Lange.

Vernon, G. (1989). Parkinson's disease. Journal of Neuroscience Nursing, 21(5), 273–281.

Viliani, T. (1999). Effects of physical training on straightening–up processes in patients with Parkinson's disease. Disability and Rehabilitation, 21(2), 68–73.

Visotsky, H. (1961). Coping behavior under extreme stress. Archives of General Psychiatry, 5, 27–32.

Walsh, B. (1992). Meeting the challenge of infection: A case study. Journal of Pediatric Oncology Nursing, 9(4), 146–158.

Walsh, B., Grunert, B., Telford, G., & Otterson, M. (1995). Multidisciplinary management of altered body image in the patient with an ostomy. Journal of Ostomy & Continence, 22(5), 227–235.

Walsh-D'Espiro, N. (1999). The new anticonvulsants: Dosing and adverse effects. Patient Care Archive, November 30, 1999.

Waltman, N. L., Bergstrom, N., Armstrong, N., Norvel, K., & Braden, B. (1991). Nutritional status, pressure sores and mortality in elderly patients with cancer. Oncology Nursing Forum, 18(5), 867–872.

Ward, G. E., Rennie, D. J., & Harper, W. (1998). Multidisciplinary assessment of outcome after hip fracture surgery. British Journal of Therapy and Rehabilitation, 5(1).

Waterbury, L. (2003). Anemia. In L. R. Barker, J. Burton, & P. Zieve (Eds.). Principles in ambulatory medicine (6th ed.). Philadelphia: Lippincott Williams & Wilkins.

Weaver, T., & Narsavage, G. (1992) Physiological and psychological variables related to functional status in chronic obstructive pulmonary disease. Nursing Research, 41(5), 286–291.

Webb, C., & Wilson-Barnet, J. (1983). Self-concept, social support, and hysterectomy. International Journal of Nursing Studies, 20(2), 97–107.

Webb, R. T., Lawson, A. L., & Neal, D. E. (1990). Clean intermittent self-catheterization in 172 adults. British Journal of Urology, 65(1), 20–23.

Weissman, C. (1996). Strategies for managing delirium in critically ill patients. Journal of Critical Illness, 11(5), 295–297, 301–302, 307.

Wickham, R. (2000). Hypercalcemia. In C. Yarbro, M. Frogge, M. Goodman, & S. Groewald (Eds.), Cancer nursing: Principles & practice (5th ed.). Boston: Jones and Bartlett.

Wiesel, P. (2000). Gut focused behavioral treatment (biofeedback) for constipation and fecal incontinence in multiple sclerosis. Journal of Neurology, Neurosurgery, and Psychiatry, 69(2):24003.

Wiggins, N. C. (1989). Education and support for the newly diagnosed cardiac family: A vital link in rehabilitation. Journal of Advanced Nursing, 14(1), 63–67.

Wijnands, G. (1992). Diagnosis and interventions in lower respiratory tract infections. The American Journal of Medicine, 92(Suppl. 4A), 91S–97S.

Williams, G. D. C. (1997). Preoperative assessment and health history interview. Nursing Clinics of North America, 32(2), 395–416.

Williams, M. A., Oberst, M. T., & Bjorklund, B. C. (1994). Early outcomes after hip fracture among women discharged home and to nursing homes. Research in Nursing and Health, 17(3), 175–183.

Williamson, D. F., Serdula, M. K., Anda, R. F., et al. (1992). Weight loss in adults: Goals, duration, and rate of weight loss. American Journal of Public Health, 82(9), 1251–1257.

Williamson, V. C. (1992). Amputation of the lower extremity: An overview. Orthopaedic Nursing, 11(2), 55–65.

Wujcik, D. (1996). Update on the diagnosis of and therapy for acute promyelocytic leukemia and chronic myelogenous leukemia. Oncology Nursing Forum, 23(3), 478–487.

Wujcik, D. (2000). Leukemia. In S. Groenwald, M. Frogge, M. Goodman, & C. Yarbro (Eds.). Cancer nursing: Principles and practice (5th ed.). Boston: Jones and Bartlett.

Woods, S. L., Froelicher, E. S., Sivaragin, S., & Matzer, C. (2000). Cardiac nursing (4th ed.). Philadelphia: Lippincott Williams & Wilkins.

Wysocki, T. (1997). Practical psychology for diabetes clinicians: How to deal with the key behavioral issues faced by patients and health care teams. Atlanta: American Diabetes Association.

Yates, P. C. (1993). Toward a reconceptualization of hope for patients with a diagnosis of cancer. Journal of Advanced Nursing, 18(4), 701–708.

Yetzer, E. A. (1996). Helping the patient through the experience of an amputation. Orthaepedic Nursing, 15(6), 45–49.

Yetzer, E., Kauffman, G., & Sopp, F. (1994). Development of a patient education program for new amputees. Rehabilitation Nursing, 19(6) 355–358.

Yetzer E., Winfree, M., & Scalione, C. (1989). An amputee support group. Rehabilitation Nursing, 14(3), 141, 142.

Zantl, J. A., Neuman, D. K., Colling, J., et al. (1996). Urinary incontinence in adults. Acute and chronic management, clinical practice guideline. No. 2 (1996 Update Agency for Health Care Policy and Research Publication No. 96-0682). Rockville, MD: AHCPR, Public Health Service, U.S. Department of Health and Human Services.

Zarifian, A. (1992). Sexual dysfunction in the male end stage renal disease patient. ANNA, 19(6), 527–532.

Zazworsky, D. J. (1997a). Exercise assessment for multiple sclerosis. Home Health Focus, 4(4), 30–31.

Zebrack, B. (2000). Quality of Life of long-term survivors of leukemia and lymphoma. Journal of Psychosocial Oncology. 18(4) 39–59.

LIST OF NIC INTERVENTIONS AND NOC OUTCOMES

Nursing Interventions Classification (NIC) Labels[1]

Abuse Protection Support
Abuse Protection Support: Child
Abuse Protection Support: Domestic Partner
Abuse Protection Support: Elder
Abuse Protection Support: Religious
Acid-Base Management
Acid-Base Management: Metabolic Acidosis
Acid-Base Management: Metabolic Alkalosis
Acid-Base Management: Respiratory Acidosis
Acid-Base Management: Respiratory Alkalosis
Acid-Base Monitoring
Active Listening
Activity Therapy
Acupressure
Admission Care
Airway Insertion and Stabilization
Airway Management
Airway Suctioning
Allergy Management
Amnioinfusion
Amputation Care
Analgesic Administration
Analgesic Administration: Intraspinal
Anaphylaxis Management
Anesthesia Administration
Anger Control Assistance
Animal-Assisted Therapy
Anticipatory Guidance
Anxiety Reduction
Area Restriction
Art Therapy
Artificial Airway Management
Aspiration Precautions
Assertiveness Training
Attachment Promotion
Autogenic Training
Autotransfusion

Bathing
Bed Rest Care
Bedside Laboratory Testing
Behavior Management
Behavior Management: Overactivity/Inattention

Behavior Management: Self-Harm
Behavior Management: Sexual
Behavior Modification
Behavior Modifications: Social Skills
Bibliotherapy
Biofeedback
Birthing
Bladder Irrigation
Bleeding Precautions
Bleeding Reduction
Bleeding Reduction: Antepartum Uterus
Bleeding Reduction: Gastrointestinal
Bleeding Reduction: Nasal
Bleeding Reduction: Postpartum Uterus
Bleeding Reduction: Wound
Blood Products Administration
Body Image Enhancement
Body Mechanics Promotion
Bottle Feeding
Bowel Incontinence Care
Bowel Incontinence Care: Encopresis
Bowel Irrigation
Bowel Management
Bowel Training
Breast Examination
Breastfeeding Assistance

Calming Technique
Cardiac Care
Cardiac Care: Acute
Cardiac Care: Rehabilitative
Cardiac Precautions
Caregiver Support
Case Management
Cast Care: Maintenance
Cast Care: Wet
Cerebral Edema Management
Cerebral Perfusion Promotion
Cesarean Section Care
Chemotherapy Management
Chest Physiotherapy
Childbirth Preparation
Circulatory Care: Arterial Insufficiency

---

[1]From McCloskey, J., & Bulechek, G. (Eds.). (2000). *Nursing interventions classification (NIC): Iowa intervention project* (3rd ed.). St. Louis, MO: Mosby. Reprinted with permission.

Circulatory Care: Mechanical Assist Device
Circulatory Care: Venous Insufficiency
Circulatory Precautions
Code Management
Cognitive Restructuring
Cognitive Stimulation
Communicable Disease Management
Communication Enhancement: Hearing Deficit
Communication Enhancement: Speech Deficit
Communication Enhancement: Visual Deficit
Community Disaster Preparedness
Community Health Development
Complex Relationship Building
Conflict Mediation
Conscious Sedation
Constipation/Impaction Management
Consultation
Contact Lens Care
Controlled Substance Checking
Coping Enhancement
Cost Containment
Cough Enhancement
Counseling
Crisis Intervention
Critical Path Development
Culture Brokerage
Cutaneous Stimulation

Decision-Making Support
Delegation
Delirium Management
Delusion Management
Dementia Management
Developmental Care
Developmental Enhancement: Adolescent
Developmental Enhancement: Child
Diarrhea Management
Diet Staging
Discharge Planning
Distraction
Documentation
Dressing
Dying Care
Dysreflexia Management
Dysrhythmia Management

Ear Care
Eating Disorders Management
Electrolyte Management
Electrolyte Management: Hypercalcemia
Electrolyte Management: Hyperkalemia
Electrolyte Management: Hypermagnesemia
Electrolyte Management: Hypernatremia
Electrolyte Management: Hyperphosphatemia
Electrolyte Management: Hypocalcemia
Electrolyte Management: Hypokalemia
Electrolyte Management: Hypomagnesemia
Electrolyte Management: Hyponatremia
Electrolyte Management: Hypophosphatemia

Electrolyte Monitoring
Electronic Fetal Monitoring: Antepartum
Electronic Fetal Monitoring: Intrapartum
Elopement Precautions
Embolus Care: Peripheral
Embolus Care: Pulmonary
Embolus Precautions
Emergency Care
Emergency Cart Checking
Emotional Support
Endotracheal Extubation
Energy Management
Enteral Tube Feeding
Environmental Management
Environmental Management:
    Attachment Process
Environmental Management: Comfort
Environmental Management: Community
Environmental Management:
    Home Preparation
Environmental Management: Safety
Environmental Management:
    Violence Prevention
Environmental Management: Worker Safety
Environmental Risk Protection
Examination Assistance
Exercise Promotion
Exercise Promotion: Strength Training
Exercise Promotion: Stretching
Exercise Therapy: Ambulation
Exercise Therapy: Balance
Exercise Therapy: Joint Mobility
Exercise Therapy: Muscle Control
Eye Care

Fall Prevention
Family Integrity Promotion
Family Integrity Promotion:
    Childbearing Family
Family Involvement Promotion
Family Mobilization
Family Planning: Contraception
Family Planning: Infertility
Family Planning: Unplanned Pregnancy
Family Process Maintenance
Family Support
Family Therapy
Feeding
Fertility Preservation
Fever Treatment
Financial Resource Assistance
Fire-Setting Precautions
First Aid
Fiscal Resource Management
Flatulence Reduction
Fluid Management
Fluid/Electrolyte Management
Fluid Monitoring
Fluid Resuscitation

Foot Care
Forgiveness Facilitation

Gastrointestinal Intubation
Genetic Counseling
Grief Work Facilitation
Grief Work Facilitation: Perinatal Death
Guilt Work Facilitation

Hair Care
Hallucination Management
Health Care Information Exchange
Health Education
Health Policy Monitoring
Health Screening
Health System Guidance
Heat Exposure Treatment
Heat/Cold Application
Hemodialysis Therapy
Hemodynamic Regulation
Hemofiltration Therapy
Hemorrhage Control
High-Risk Pregnancy Care
Home Maintenance Assistance
Hope Instillation
Humor
Hyperglycemia Management
Hypervolemia Management
Hypnosis
Hypoglycemia Management
Hypothermia Treatment
Hypovolemia Management

Immunization/Vaccination Management
Impulse Control Training
Incident Reporting
Incision Site Care
Infant Care
Infection Control
Infection Control: Intraoperative
Infection Protection
Insurance Authorization
Intracranial Pressure (ICP) Monitoring
Intrapartal Care
Intrapartal Care: High-Risk Delivery
Intravenous (IV) Insertion
Intravenous (IV) Therapy
Invasive Hemodynamic Monitoring

Kangaroo Care

Labor Induction
Labor Suppression
Laboratory Data Interpretation
Lactation Counseling
Lactation Suppression
Laser Precautions
Latex Precautions
Learning Facilitation

Learning Readiness Enhancement
Leech Therapy
Limit Setting

Malignant Hyperthermia Precautions
Mechanical Ventilation
Mechanical Ventilatory Weaning
Medication Administration
Medication Administration: Ear
Medication Administration: Enteral
Medication Administration: Epidural
Medication Administration: Eye
Medication Administration: Inhalation
Medication Administration: Interpleural
Medication Administration: Intradermal
Medication Administration: Intramuscular (IM)
Medication Administration: Intraosseous
Medication Administration: Intravenous (IV)
Medication Administration: Oral
Medication Administration: Rectal
Medication Administration: Skin
Medication Administration: Subcutaneous
Medication Administration: Vaginal
Medication Administration:
    Ventricular Reservoir
Medication Management
Medication Prescribing
Meditation Facilitation
Memory Training
Milieu Therapy
Mood Management
Multidisciplinary Care Conference
Music Therapy
Mutual Goal Setting

Nail Care
Nausea Management
Neurologic Monitoring
Newborn Care
Newborn Monitoring
Nonnutritive Sucking
Normalization Promotion
Nutrition Management
Nutrition Therapy
Nutritional Counseling
Nutritional Monitoring

Oral Health Maintenance
Oral Health Promotion
Oral Health Restoration
Order Transcription
Organ Procurement
Ostomy Care
Oxygen Therapy

Pain Management
Parent Education: Adolescent
Parent Education: Childrearing Family
Parent Education: Infant

Parenting Promotion
Pass Facilitation
Patient Contracting
Patient-Controlled Analgesia (PCA) Assistance
Patient Rights Protection
Peer Review
Pelvic Muscle Exercise
Perineal Care
Peripheral Sensation Management
Peripherally Inserted Central (PIC)
  Catheter Care
Peritoneal Dialysis Therapy
Pessary Management
Phlebotomy: Arterial Blood Sample
Phlebotomy: Blood Unit Acquisition
Phlebotomy: Venous Blood Sample
Phototherapy: Neonate
Physical Restraint
Physician Support
Pneumatic Tourniquet Precautions
Positioning
Positioning: Intraoperative
Positioning: Neurologic
Positioning: Wheelchair
Postanesthesia Care
Postmortem Care
Postpartal Care
Preceptor: Employee
Preceptor: Student
Preconception Counseling
Pregnancy Termination Care
Prenatal Care
Preoperative Coordination
Preparatory Sensory Information
Presence
Pressure Management
Pressure Ulcer Care
Pressure Ulcer Prevention
Product Evaluation
Program Development
Progressive Muscle Relaxation
Prompted Voiding
Prosthesis Care
Pruritus Management

Quality Monitoring

Radiation Therapy Management
Rape-Trauma Treatment
Reality Orientation
Recreation Therapy
Rectal Prolapse Management
Referral
Religious Addiction Prevention
Religious Ritual Enhancement
Reminiscence Therapy
Reproductive Technology Management
Research Data Collection
Resiliency Promotion

Respiratory Monitoring
Respite Care
Resuscitation
Resuscitation: Fetus
Resuscitation: Neonate
Risk Identification
Risk Identification: Childbearing Family
Risk Identification: Genetic
Role Enhancement

Seclusion
Security Enhancement
Seizure Management
Seizure Precautions
Self-Awareness Enhancement
Self-Care Assistance
Self-Care Assistance: Bathing/Hygiene
Self-Care Assistance: Dressing/Grooming
Self-Care Assistance: Feeding
Self-Care Assistance: Toileting
Self-Esteem Enhancement
Self-Modification Assistance
Self-Responsibility Facilitation
Sexual Counseling
Shift Report
Shock Management
Shock Management: Cardiac
Shock Management: Vasogenic
Shock Management: Volume
Shock Prevention
Sibling Support
Simple Guided Imagery
Simple Massage
Simple Relaxation Therapy
Skin Care: Topical Treatments
Skin Surveillance
Sleep Enhancement
Smoking Cessation Assistance
Socialization Enhancement
Specimen Management
Spiritual Growth Facilitation
Spiritual Support
Splinting
Sports-Injury Prevention: Youth
Staff Development
Staff Supervision
Subarachnoid Hemorrhage Precautions
Substance Use Prevention
Substance Use Treatment
Substance Use Treatment: Alcohol Withdrawal
Substance Use Treatment: Drug Withdrawal
Substance Use Treatment: Overdose
Suicide Prevention
Supply Management
Support Group
Support System Enhancement
Surgical Assistance
Surgical Precautions
Surgical Preparation

Surveillance
Surveillance: Community
Surveillance: Late Pregnancy
Surveillance: Remote Electronic
Surveillance: Safety
Sustenance Support
Suturing
Swallowing Therapy

Teaching: Disease Process
Teaching: Group
Teaching: Individual
Teaching: Infant Nutrition
Teaching: Infant Safety
Teaching: Preoperative
Teaching: Prescribed Activity/Exercise
Teaching: Prescribed Diet
Teaching: Prescribed Medication
Teaching: Procedure/Treatment
Teaching: Psychomotor Skill
Teaching: Safe Sex
Teaching: Sexuality
Teaching: Toddler Nutrition
Teaching: Toddler Safety
Technology Management
Telephone Consultation
Telephone Follow-Up
Temperature Regulation
Temperature Regulation: Intraoperative
Therapeutic Play
Therapeutic Touch
Therapy Group
Total Parenteral Nutrition (TPN) Administration
Touch
Traction/Immobilization Care
Transcutaneous Electrical Nerve
  Stimulation (TENS)

Transport
Triage: Disaster
Triage: Emergency Center
Triage: Telephone
Truth Telling
Tube Care
Tube Care: Chest
Tube Care: Gastrointestinal
Tube Care: Umbilical Line
Tube Care: Urinary
Tube Care: Ventriculostomy/Lumbar Drain

Ultrasonography: Limited Obstetric
Unilateral Neglect Management
Urinary Bladder Training
Urinary Catheterization
Urinary Catheterization: Intermittent
Urinary Elimination Management
Urinary Habit Training
Urinary Incontinence Care
Urinary Incontinence Care: Enuresis
Urinary Retention Care

Values Clarification
Vehicle Safety Promotion
Venous Access Devices (VAD) Maintenance
Ventilation Assistance
Visitation Facilitation
Vital Signs Monitoring
Vomiting Management

Weight Gain Assistance
Weight Management
Weight Reduction Assistance
Wound Care
Wound Care: Closed Drainage
Wound Irrigation

Nursing Outcomes Classifications (NOC) Approved for Clinical Testing[2]

Abuse Cessation
Abuse Protection
Abuse Recovery: Emotional
Abuse Recovery: Financial
Abuse Recovery: Physical
Abuse Recovery: Sexual
Abusive Behavior Self-Control
Acceptance: Health Status
Activity Tolerance
Adherence Behavior
Aggression Control
Ambulation: Walking

Ambulation: Wheelchair
Anxiety Control
Aspiration Control
Asthma Control

Balance
Blood Glucose Control
Blood Transfusion Reaction Control
Body Image
Body Positioning: Self-Initiated
Bone Healing
Bowel Continence

[2] From Johnson, M., Maas, M., et al. (Eds.). (2000). *Nursing outcomes classification* (2nd ed.). St. Louis, MO: Mosby. Reprinted with permission.

Bowel Elimination
Breastfeeding Establishment: Infant
Breastfeeding Establishment: Maternal
Breastfeeding: Maintenance
Breastfeeding: Weaning

Cardiac Pump Effectiveness
Caregiver Adaptation to Patient
  Institutionalization
Caregiver Emotional Health
Caregiver Home Care Readiness
Caregiver Lifestyle Disruption
Caregiver-Patient Relationship
Caregiver Performance: Direct Care
Caregiver Performance: Indirect Care
Caregiver Physical Health
Caregiver Stressors
Caregiver Well-Being
Caregiving Endurance Potential
Child Adaptation to Hospitalization
Child Development: 2 Months
Child Development: 4 Months
Child Development: 6 Months
Child Development: 12 Months
Child Development: 2 Years
Child Development: 3 Years
Child Development: 4 Years
Child Development: 5 Years
Child Development: Middle Childhood
  (6–11 Years)
Child Development: Adolescence (12–17 Years)
Circulation Status
Coagulation Status
Cognitive Ability
Cognitive Orientation
Comfort Level
Communication Ability
Communication: Expressive Ability
Communication: Receptive Ability
Community Competence
Community Health Status
Community Health: Immunity
Community Risk Control: Chronic Disease
Community Risk Control:
  Communicable Disease
Community Risk Control: Lead Exposure
Compliance Behavior
Concentration
Coping

Decision Making
Depression Control
Depression Level
Dialysis Access Integrity
Dignified Dying
Distorted Thought Control

Electrolyte & Acid-Base Balance
Endurance
Energy Conservation

Family Coping
Family Environment: Internal
Family Functioning
Family Health Status
Family Integrity
Family Normalization
Family Participation in Professional Care
Fear Control
Fetal Status: Antepartum
Fetal Status: Intrapartum
Fluid Balance

Grief Resolution
Growth

Health Beliefs
Health Beliefs: Perceived Ability to Perform
Health Beliefs: Perceived Control
Health Beliefs: Perceived Resources
Health Beliefs: Perceived Threat
Health Orientation
Health Promoting Behavior
Health Seeking Behavior
Hearing Compensation Behavior
Hope
Hydration

Identity
Immobility Consequences: Physiological
Immobility Consequences:
  Psycho-Cognitive
Immune Hypersensitivity Control
Immune Status
Immunization Behavior
Impulse Control
Infection Status
Information Processing

Joint Movement: Active
Joint Movement: Passive

Knowledge: Breastfeeding
Knowledge: Child Safety
Knowledge: Conception Prevention
Knowledge: Diabetes Management
Knowledge: Diet
Knowledge: Disease Process
Knowledge: Energy Conservation
Knowledge: Fertility Promotion
Knowledge: Health Behaviors
Knowledge: Health Promotion
Knowledge: Health Resources
Knowledge: Illness Care
Knowledge: Infant Care
Knowledge: Infection Control
Knowledge: Labor & Delivery
Knowledge: Maternal-Child Health
Knowledge: Medication
Knowledge: Personal Safety

Knowledge: Postpartum
Knowledge: Preconception
Knowledge: Pregnancy
Knowledge: Prescribed Activity
Knowledge: Sexual Functioning
Knowledge: Substance Use Control
Knowledge: Treatment Procedure(s)
Knowledge: Treatment Regimen

Leisure Participation
Loneliness

Maternal Status: Antepartum
Maternal Status: Intrapartum
Maternal Status: Postpartum
Medication Response
Memory
Mobility Level
Mood Equilibrium
Muscle Function

Neglect Recovery
Neurological Status
Neurological Status: Autonomic
Neurological Status: Central Motor Control
Neurological Status: Consciousness
Neurological Status: Cranial Sensory/
 Motor Function
Neurological Status: Spinal Sensory/
 Motor Function
Newborn Adaptation
Nutritional Status
Nutritional Status: Biochemical Measures
Nutritional Status: Body Mass
Nutritional Status: Energy
Nutritional Status: Food & Fluid Intake
Nutritional Status: Nutrient Intake

Oral Health

Pain Control
Pain: Disruptive Effects
Pain Level
Pain: Psychological Response
Parent–Infant Attachment
Parenting
Parenting: Social Safety
Participation: Health Care Decisions
Physical Aging Status
Physical Fitness
Physical Maturation: Female
Physical Maturation: Male
Play Participation
Prenatal Health Behavior
Preterm Infant Organization
Psychomotor Energy
Psychosocial Adjustment: Life Change

Quality of Life

Respiratory Status: Airway Patency
Respiratory Status: Gas Exchange
Respiratory Status: Ventilation
Rest
Risk Control
Risk Control: Alcohol Use
Risk Control: Cancer
Risk Control: Cardiovascular Health
Risk Control: Drug Use
Risk Control: Hearing Impairment
Risk Control: Sexually Transmitted
 Diseases (STDs)
Risk Control: Tobacco Use
Risk Control: Unintended Pregnancy
Risk Control: Visual Impairment
Risk Detection
Role Performance

Safety Behavior: Fall Prevention
Safety Behavior: Home Physical Environment
Safety Behavior: Personal
Safety Status: Falls Occurrence
Safety Status: Physical Injury
Self-Care: Activities of Daily Living (ADL)
Self-Care: Bathing
Self-Care: Dressing
Self-Care: Eating
Self-Care: Grooming
Self-Care: Hygiene
Self-Care: Instrumental Activities of Daily
 Living (IADL)
Self-Care: Non-Parenteral Medication
Self-Care: Oral Hygiene
Self-Care: Parenteral Medication
Self-Care: Toileting
Self-Direction of Care
Self-Esteem
Self-Mutilation Restraint
Sensory Function: Cutaneous
Sensory Function: Hearing
Sensory Function: Proprioception
Sensory Function: Taste & Smell
Sensory Function: Vision
Sexual Functioning
Sexual Identity: Acceptance
Skeletal Function
Sleep
Social Interaction Skills
Social Involvement
Social Support
Spiritual Well-Being
Substance Addiction Consequences
Suffering Level
Suicide Self-Restraint
Swallowing Status
Swallowing Status: Esophageal Phase
Swallowing Status: Oral Phase
Swallowing Status: Pharyngeal Phase
Symptom Control

CLINICAL SITUATIONS INDEX

NURSING DIAGNOSES INDEX

A

Activity intolerance
  related to claudication, in peripheral arterial disease, 128–129
  related to fatigue and inadequate oxygenation for activities, in chronic obstructive pulmonary disease, 151–154
  related to insufficient oxygenation for activities of daily living (ADLs) secondary to cardiac tissue ischemia, prolonged immobility, narcotics or medications, in myocardial infarction, 119–120
  related to pain and weakness secondary to anesthesia, tissue hypoxia, and insufficient fluids and nutrients, after surgery, 660–662

Activity intolerance, high risk for, related to deconditioning, with total parenteral nutrition, 1047–1048

Acute pain. *See* **Pain, acute**

Airway clearance, high risk for ineffective, related to relaxation of tongue and gag reflexes secondary to disruption in muscle innervation, in seizure disorders, 388–389

Airway clearance, ineffective
  related to excessive and tenacious secretions, in chronic obstructive pulmonary disease, 150–151
  related to increased mucus production, tenacious secretions, and bronchospasm, in asthma, 141–142
  related to increased secretions and diminished cough secondary to pain and fatigue, after thoracic surgery, 890–892

Anxiety
  related to actual or potential vision loss and perceived impact of chronic illness on life style, in glaucoma, 424–426
  related to anticipated surgery and unfamiliarity with preoperative and postoperative routines and postoperative sensations, before carotid endarterectomy, 721
  related to breathlessness and fear of suffocation, in chronic obstructive pulmonary disease, 154–155
  related to fear of embarrassment secondary to having a seizure in public, in seizure disorders, 389–390
  related to impending pacemaker insertion and prognosis, before permanent pacemaker insertion, 1002–1005
  related to impending surgery and insufficient knowledge of preoperative routines, intraoperative activities, and postoperative self-care activities, before thoracic surgery, 884–886
  related to impending surgery and perceived negative effects on life style, before cranial surgery, 775–777
  related to insufficient knowledge of postoperative routines, postoperative sensations, and crutch-walking techniques, before amputation, 687–688
  related to lack of knowledge of colostomy care and perceived negative effects on life style, before colostomy, 737–738
  related to lack of knowledge of ileostomy care and perceived negative effects on life style before ileostomy, 822–824
  related to lack of knowledge of impending surgical experience and implications of condition on life style, before laryngectomy, 851–853
  related to lack of knowledge of urostomy care and perceived negative effects on life style before urostomy, 908–909
  related to loss of control, memory losses, and fear of withdrawal, in alcohol withdrawal, 615–616
  related to perceived effects of injury on life style and unknown future, in spinal cord injury, 400–401
  related to prescribed chemotherapy, insufficient knowledge of chemotherapy, and self-care measures, 946–948
  related to prescribed radiation therapy and insufficient knowledge of treatment and self-care measures, with radiation therapy, 1035–1037
  related to sudden injury, treatment, uncertainty of outcome, and pain, in thermal injuries, 467–468
  related to unfamiliar environment, routines, diagnostic tests and treatments, and loss of control, in hospitalized adult client, 67–69
  related to unfamiliar hospital environment, uncertainty about outcomes, feelings of helplessness and hopelessness, and insufficient knowledge about cancer and treatment, at initial diagnosis of cancer, 560–562
  related to upcoming insertion of catheter/port and insufficient knowledge of procedure, with long-term venous access devices, 987–988
  related to upcoming surgery and insufficient knowledge of routine and postoperative activities, before radical prostatectomy, 874–875

Anxiety/Fear
  related to perceived mastectomy and prognosis, before breast surgery, 710–712
  related to surgical experience, loss of control, unpredictable outcome, and insufficient knowledge of preoperative routines, postoperative exercises and activities, and postoperative changes and sensations, before surgery, 642–646
  related to surgical experience, loss of control, unpredictable outcome, expected pain, and insufficient knowledge of preoperative routines, postoperative exercises and activities, and postoperative changes and sensations, before ambulatory surgery, 665–669

Anxiety/Fear (individual, family), related to unfamiliar situation, unpredictable nature of condition, fear of death, negative effects on life style, or possible sexual dysfunction, in myocardial infarction, 116–117

Aspiration, high risk for, related to position of tube and client, with enteral nutrition, 972–973

B

Body image, high risk for disturbed
  related to changes in appearance, with corticosteroid therapy, 962–963
  related to perceived negative effects of amputation and response of others to appearance, after amputation, 690–692

Bowel incontinence: areflexic, related to lack of voluntary sphincter control secondary to spinal cord injury involving sacral reflex arc (S2-S4), 415–418

Bowel incontinence: reflexic, related to lack of voluntary sphincter control secondary to spinal cord injury above eleventh thoracic vertebra (T11), 412–415

Breathing pattern, high risk for ineffective, related to immobility, pressure, pain, with peritoneal dialysis, 1023

COLLABORATIVE PROBLEMS INDEX

The prefix Potential Complication (PC) has been omitted for easier use of the index only.

A

Abscess
  bone, in osteomyelitis, 511
  in inflammatory bowel disease, 256–259
Acidosis
  metabolic
    in acute kidney failure, 282–287
    in chronic kidney disease, 291–299
    in thermal injuries, 458–467
Acute arterial thrombosis, in peripheral arterial disease, 127–128
Acute chest syndrome, in sickle cell disease, 434–438
Acute organic psychosis, in hypothyroidism, 217–220
Acute pulmonary edema, after thoracic surgery, 886–890
Acute renal failure, in pancreatitis, 235–239
Acute respiratory distress syndrome, in pancreatitis, 235–239
Acute respiratory failure, in Guillain-Barré syndrome, 334–336
Adult respiratory distress syndrome, in cerebrovascular accident, 315–319
Air embolism
  with hemodialysis, 978–981
  with total parenteral nutrition, 1041–1045
Alcohol hallucinosis, in alcohol withdrawal, 608–611
Anaphylactic reaction, with chemotherapy, 939–946
Anastomosis, disruption of, in arterial bypass grafting in lower extremity, 701–704
Anemia
  in chronic kidney disease, 291–299
  with hemodialysis, 978–981
  in inflammatory bowel disease, 256–259
  in sickle cell disease, 434–438
Aneurysm, ruptured, in abdominal aortic aneurysm resection, 681–682
Artery rupture, carotid, in neck dissection, 855–859
Arthritis, septic, in inflammatory joint disease, 492–494
Atelectasis
  in cerebrovascular accident, 315–319
  with mechanical ventilation, 994–996
Atherosclerotic heart disease, in hypothyroidism, 217–220
Autonomic hyperactivity, in alcohol withdrawal, 608–611
Autonomic nervous system failure, in Guillain-Barré syndrome, 334–336
Avascular necrosis
  of femoral head, after fractured hip and femur, 800–803
  in HIV/AIDS, 525–528

B

Bladder infection
  hemorrhagic, with chemotherapy, 939–946
  with radiation therapy, 1031–1035
Bladder perforation, with peritoneal dialysis, 1016–1021
Bladder trauma, after hysterectomy, 813–815
Bleeding. *See also* Hemorrhage
  after enucleation, 790–791
  gastrointestinal

  in cerebrovascular accident, 315–319
  in inflammatory bowel disease, 256–259
  with mechanical ventilation, 994–996
  in spinal cord injury, 395–400
  with radiation therapy, 1031–1035
  vaginal, after hysterectomy, 813–815
Bone abscess, in osteomyelitis, 511
Bone marrow depression
  with chemotherapy, 939–946
  in leukemia, 595–598
Bowel perforation, with peritoneal dialysis, 1016–1021
Bowel trauma, after hysterectomy, 813–815
Brain hemorrhage, hematoma, hygroma, after cranial surgery, 777–783

C

Cachexia, in end-stage cancer, 574–579
Calculi
  renal
    with chemotherapy, 939–946
    in inflammatory bowel disease, 256–259
    in neurogenic bladder, 364–365
  urinary
    after ileostomy, 824–826
    in urostomy, 909–911
Cardiac dysrhythmias
  in myocardial infarction, 113–116
  after pacemaker insertion (permanent), 1005–1008
  after thoracic surgery, 886–890
Cardiac output, decreased, with mechanical ventilation, 994–996
Cardiac tamponade
  in chronic kidney disease, 291–299
  in myocardial infarction, 113–116
Cardiogenic shock, in myocardial infarction, 113–116
Cardiotoxicity, with chemotherapy, 939–946
Cardiovascular dysfunction, in hospitalized adult client, 66–67
Cardiovascular insufficiency, after coronary artery bypass grafting, 760–765
Carotid artery rupture, in neck dissection, 855–859
Cellulitis, in thermal injuries, 458–467
Central nervous system edema, in neck dissection, 855–859
Central nervous system involvement, in leukemia, 595–598
Cerebellar dysfunction, after cranial surgery, 777–783
Cerebral dysfunction, after cranial surgery, 777–783
Cerebral edema, with radiation therapy, 1031–1035
Cerebral infarction, after carotid endarterectomy, 721–723
Cerebrospinal fistula, after laminectomy, 844–846
Cerebrospinal fluid leakage, after cranial surgery, 777–783
Chest syndrome, acute, in sickle cell disease, 434–438
Cholelithiasis, after ileostomy, 824–826
Cholinergic crisis, in myasthenia gravis, 357–360
Chronic leg edema, in deep venous thrombosis, 99–101
Circulatory problems, after carotid endarterectomy, 721–723
Clot formation
  with hemodialysis, 978–981
  after radical prostatectomy, 875–877

GENERAL INDEX

Page numbers in italics *indicate figures; those followed by* t *indicate tables; those followed by* b *indicate boxes*